HANDBOOK OF ANTICANCER PHARMACOKINETICS AND PHARMACODYNAMICS

CANCER DRUG DISCOVERY AND DEVELOPMENT

BEVERLY A. TEICHER, SERIES EDITOR

HANDBOOK OF ANTICANCER PHARMACOKINETICS AND PHARMACODYNAMICS

Edited by

WILLIAM D. FIGG, PharmD

Center for Cancer Research
National Cancer Institute, Bethesda, MD

and

HOWARD L. McLEOD, PharmD

Washington University School of Medicine, St. Louis, MO

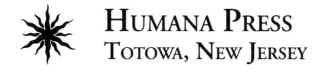

HUMANA PRESS
TOTOWA, NEW JERSEY

© 2004 Humana Press Inc.
999 Riverview Drive, Suite 208
Totowa, New Jersey 07512
www.humanapress.com

Cover design by Patricia F. Cleary.

This publication is printed on acid-free paper. ∞
ANSI Z39.48-1984 (American National Standards Institute)
Permanence of Paper for Printed Library Materials

For additional copies, pricing for bulk purchases, and/or information about other Humana titles, contact Humana at the above address or at any of the following numbers: Tel.:973-256-1699; Fax: 973-256-8341; Email: humanapr.com; or visit our Website: http://humanapress.com

Printed in the United States of America. 10 9 8 7 6 5 4 3 2 1
E-ISBN 1-59259-734-3
Library of Congress Cataloging-in-Publication Data

Handbook of anticancer pharmacokinetics and pharmacodynamics / edited by
William D. Figg, Howard L. McLeod.
    p. ; cm. -- (Cancer drug discovery and development)
  Includes bibliographical references and index.
  ISBN 1-58829-177-4 (alk. paper)
  1. Antineoplastic agents--Research--Handbooks, manuals, etc.
  [DNLM: 1. Antineoplastic Agents--pharmacology. 2. Antineoplastic
  Agents--pharmacokinetics. QV 269 H236 2004] I. Figg, William D. II.
  McLeod, Howard L. III. Series.
  RS431.A64H36 2004
  616.99'4061--dc21   2003013963

PREFACE

We embarked upon editing a text with the objective of having a single reference on clinical pharmacology to serve as a guide to drug development with a focus on cancer therapy. There are numerous textbooks that convey each of the components individually; however, we envisioned a text that went beyond individual topics and developed the *Handbook of Anticancer Pharmacokinetics and Pharmacodynamics.*

We have organized this handbook according to the following scheme (Figure 1), which outlines a logical flow of events from identification of a cancer-specific target to phase III clinical testing. This handbook includes two chapters that make it unique: "Identifying Agents to Test in Phase III Trials" by Roberts, Lynch, and Chabner and "Clinical Trials Designs for Approval of New Anticancer Agents: A Clinical Science" by Von Hoff. Together these chapters give a roadmap for moving an agent toward NDA submission. This handbook should be of interest to both the clinical pharmacologist and the pharmaceutical scientist.

Identify Potential Molecular Target

   Design Compound/Computational Analysis

     Synthesis

       Screen Agent Using In Vitro Models

        Understand Molecular Pharmacology

        SAR Analysis - Lead Optimization

       Preliminary Animal Toxicology

       In Vivo Experiments

        Formulation

        Preclinical Pharmacokinetics

        Formal Toxicology

         IND Submission for Clinical Evaluation

         Phase I Trial - Define MTD

          Characterize the Clinical Pharmacology

         Phase II Trial

          Translational Studies to Understand Pharmacology

         Phase III

         NDA Submission

Figure 1. Drug Development Plan

We would like to thank all of the authors for their thoughtful and thorough contributions. Our task of compiling this book was made easy by their high-quality efforts.

We would also like to thank our post-doctoral fellows and graduate students who have stimulated us to continue to learn over the years. Furthermore, we appreciate the tolerance of our careers from our families and their continued support (Jennifer Figg and William Figg, II and Donya, Katie, and Max McLeod). Lastly, we continue to be conscious of our patients who keep us focused on the goal of finding treatments and cures for all types of cancer.

William D. Figg, PharmD
Howard L. McLeod, PharmD

CONTENTS

CONTRIBUTORS

H. RICHARD ALEXANDER, MD • *Surgery Branch, Center for Cancer Research, National Cancer Institute, Bethesda, MD*

YUICHI ANDO, MD, PhD • *Department of Clinical Oncology, Saitama Medical School, Saitama, Japan*

PHILIP M. ARLEN, MD • *Tumor Immunology and Biology, Center for Cancer Research, National Cancer Institute, Bethesda, MD*

SHARYN D. BAKER, PharmD • *Sidney Kimmel Comprehensive Cancer Center at Johns Hopkins University, Baltimore, MD*

UDAI BANERJI, PhD • *Cancer Research UK Centre for Cancer Therapeutics, Institute of Cancer Research, Sutton, Surrey, UK*

SUSAN E. BATES, MD • *Cancer Therapeutics Branch, Center for Cancer Research, National Cancer Institute, Bethesda, MD*

KENNETH S. BAUER, PharmD, PhD • *University of Maryland School of Pharmacy, Greenebaum Cancer Center, Baltimore, MD*

ANDREW P. BEELEN, MD, BS Pharm • *Section of Clinical Pharmacology, Dartmouth Hitchcock Medical Center, and Dartmouth Medical School, Lebanon, NH*

JONAS BERGH, MD, PhD • *Department of Oncology, Radiumhemmet, Karolinska Institute and Hospital, Stockholm, Sweden*

SUSAN M. BLANEY, MD • *Texas Children's Cancer Center, Baylor College of Medicine, Houston, TX*

ALAN V. BODDY, PhD • *Northern Institute for Cancer Research, University of Newcastle, Newcastle upon Tyne, UK*

ANGELIKA M. BURGER, PhD • *Tumor Biology Center at the University of Freiburg, Freiburg, Germany*

KEVIN CAMPHAUSEN, MD • *Radiation Oncology Branch, Center for Cancer Research, National Cancer Institute, Bethesda, MD*

JAMES CASSIDY, MB, ChB, MSc, MD, FRCP • *Department of Oncology, Cancer Research UK, Beatson Laboratories, Glasgow, UK*

BRUCE A. CHABNER, MD • *Division of Hematology/Oncology, Massachusetts General Hospital and Harvard Medical School, Boston, MA*

STEVE Y. CHO, MD • *Neuro-Oncology Branch, National Cancer Institute, National Institutes of Neurological Disorders and Stroke, NIH, Bethesda, MD*

SALLY A. COULTHARD, PhD • *Northern Institute for Cancer Research, University of Newcastle, Newcastle upon Tyne, UK*

HANS EHRSSON, PhD • *Karolinska Hospital, Stockholm, Sweden, and Department of Oncology-Pathology, Karolinska Institutet, Stockholm, Sweden*

STAFFAN EKSBORG, PhD • *Karolinska Hospital, Stockholm, Sweden, and Department of Woman and Child Health, Karolinska Institutet, Stockholm, Sweden*

ENE I ETTE, PharmD, PhD, FCP, FCCP • *Vertex Pharmaceutical Corporation, Cambridge, MA*

HEINZ-HERBERT FIEBIG, MD • *Tumor Biology Center at the University of Freiburg, Freiburg, Germany*

HOWARD A. FINE, MD • *Neuro-Oncology Branch, National Cancer Institute, National Institutes of Neurological Disorders and Stroke, NIH, Bethesda, MD*

TITO FOJO, MD • *Cancer Therapeutics Branch, Center for Cancer Research, National Cancer Institute, Bethesda, MD*

JAN-ERIK FRÖDIN, MD, PhD • *Departments of Oncology and Haematology, Cancer Centre Karolinska, Karolinska Hospital, Stockholm, Sweden*

JACQUES GALIPEAU, MD • *Department of Experimental Medicine, Lady Davis Institute for Medical Research, McGill University, Montreal, PQ, Canada*

VICTOR GHETIE, PhD • *The Cancer Immunobiology Center, University of Texas Southwestern Medical Center at Dallas, Dallas, TX*

JAMES GULLEY MD, PhD • *Tumor Immunology and Biology, Center for Cancer Research, National Cancer Institute, Bethesda, MD*

HOWARD GURNEY, MB, BS, FRACP • *Medical Oncology and Palliative Care, Westmead Hospital, Westmead, Australia*

MELINDA HOLLINGSHEAD, DVM, PhD • *Developmental Therapeutics Program, National Cancer Institute, Frederick, MD*

LISA C. IACONO, PharmD • *Department of Pharmaceutical Sciences, St. Jude Children's Research Hospital, Memphis, TN*

SYMA IQBAL, MD • *Norris Comprehensive Cancer Center, Keck School of Medicine, University of Southern California, Los Angeles, CA*

IAN JUDSON, PhD • *Cancer Research UK Centre for Cancer Therapeutics, Institute of Cancer Research, Sutton, Surrey, UK*

H. THOMAS KARNES, PhD • *Department of Pharmaceutics, Virginia Commonwealth University School of Pharmacy, Richmond, VA*

MAIHGAN A. KAVANAGH, MD • *Surgery Branch, Center for Cancer Research, National Cancer Institute, Bethesda, MD*

JILL M. KOLESAR, PharmD • *School of Pharmacy, University of Wisconsin—Madison, Madison, WI*

HEINZ-JOSEF LENZ, MD, FACP • *Norris Comprehensive Cancer Center, Keck School of Medicine, University of Southern California, Los Angeles, CA*

LIONEL D. LEWIS MB, BCh, MD, FRCP (LONDON) • *Section of Clinical Pharmacology, Dartmouth Hitchcock Medical Center, and Dartmouth Medical School, Lebanon, NH*

STEVEN K. LIBUTTI, MD • *Surgery Branch, Center for Cancer Research, National Cancer Institute, Bethesda, MD*

WALTER J. LOOS, PhD • *Laboratory of Translational and Molecular Pharmacology, Department of Medical Oncology, Erasmus MC—Daniel den Hoed Cancer Center, Rotterdam, The Netherlands*

THOMAS J. LYNCH JR., MD • *Division of Hematology/Oncology, Massachusetts General Hospital and Harvard Medical School, Boston, MA*

JOHN L. MARSHALL, MD • *Lombardi Cancer Center, Georgetown University Medical Center, Washington, DC*

HÅKAN MELLSTEDT, MD, PhD • *Departments of Oncology and Haematology, Cancer Centre Karolinska, Karolinska Hospital, Stockholm, Sweden*

CYNTHIA MÉNARD, MD • *Radiation Oncology Branch, Center for Cancer Research, National Cancer Institute, Bethesda, MD*

LAURETTA ODOGWU, MD • *Lombardi Cancer Center, Georgetown University Medical Center, Washington, DC*

ANDERS ÖSTERBORG, MD, PhD • *Departments of Oncology and Hematology, Cancer Centre Karolinska, Karolinska Hospital, Stockholm, Sweden*

WILLIAM P. PETROS, PharmD, FCCP • *West Virginia University School of Pharmacy, Mary Babb Randolph Cancer Center, Morgantown, WV*

JAMES F. PINGPANK, MD • *Surgery Branch, Center for Cancer Research, National Cancer Institute, Bethesda, MD*

ATIQUR RAHMAN, PhD • *Center for Drug Evaluation and Research, Food and Drug Administration, Rockville, MD*

LAURENT P. RIVORY, PhD • *Medical Oncology, Sydney Cancer Centre and Department of Pharmacology, University of Sydney, NSW, Australia*

THOMAS G. ROBERTS JR., MD • *Division of Hematology/Oncology, Massachusetts General Hospital and Harvard Medical School, Boston, MA*

MICHELLE A. RUDEK, PharmD, PhD • *Sidney Kimmel Comprehensive Cancer Center at Johns Hopkins University, Baltimore, MD*

EDWARD A. SAUSVILLE, MD • *Developmental Therapeutics Program, National Cancer Institute, Rockville, MD*

DAVID S. SCHRUMP, MD • *Thoracic Oncology Section, Surgery Branch, Center for Cancer Research, National Cancer Institute, Bethesda, MD*

PATRICIA W. SLATTUM, PharmD, PhD • *Department of Pharmacy, Virginia Commonwealth University, Richmond, VA*

ALEX SPARREBOOM, PhD • *Clinical Pharmacology Research Core, Center for Cancer Research, National Cancer Institute, Bethesda, MD*

H. TRENT SPENCER, PhD • *Division of Hematology/Oncology and BMT, Department of Pediatrics, Emory University School of Medicine, Atlanta, GA*

CLINTON F. STEWART, PharmD • *Department of Pharmaceutical Sciences, St. Jude Children's Research Hospital, Memphis, TN*

JAN STOEHLMACHER, MD • *Norris Comprehensive Cancer Center, Keck School of Medicine, University of Southern California, Los Angeles, CA*

JEFF STONE, MD • *Texas Children's Cancer Center, Baylor College of Medicine, Houston, TX*

P. KELLIE TURNER, PharmD • *Department of Pharmaceutical Sciences, St. Jude Children's Research Hospital, Memphis, TN*

JAMES A. UCHIZONO, PharmD, PhD • *Department of Pharmaceutics and Medicinal Chemistry, University of the Pacific, Stockton, CA*

JÜRGEN VENITZ, MD, PhD • *Department of Pharmaceutics, Virginia Commonwealth University, Richmond, VA*

ELLEN S. VITETTA, PhD • *Cancer Immunobiology Center and the Department of Microbiology, University of Texas Southwestern Medical Center at Dallas, Dallas, TX*

DANIEL D. VON HOFF, MD • *Departments of Medicine, Pathology and Molecular and Cellular Biology, Arizona Health Sciences Center, Arizona Cancer Center, University of Arizona, Tucson, AZ*

E. SALLY WARD, PhD • *The Cancer Immunobiology Center and the Center for Immunology, University of Texas Southwestern Medical Center at Dallas, Dallas, TX*

PAUL J. WILLIAMS, PharmD, MS, FCCP • *Trials by Design LLC, Stockton, CA*

PAUL WORKMAN, PhD • *Cancer Research UK Centre for Cancer Therapeutics, Institute of Cancer Research, Sutton, Surrey, UK*

SUOPING ZHAI, MD, PhD • *Clinical Pharmacology Research Core, Center for Cancer Research, National Cancer Institute, Bethesda, MD*

WILLIAM C. ZAMBONI, PharmD • *Program of Molecular Therapeutics and Drug Development, University of Pittsburgh Cancer Institute, Hillman Cancer Research Center Pittsburgh, and Department of Pharmaceutical Sciences, School of Pharmacy and Department of Medicine, School of Medicine, University of Pittsburgh, Pittsburgh, PA*

VALUE-ADDED eBOOK/PDA ON CD-ROM

This book is accompanied by a value-added CD-ROM that contains an eBook version of the volume you have just purchased. This eBook can be viewed on your computer, and you can synchronize it to your PDA for viewing on your handheld device. The eBook enables you to view this volume on only one computer and PDA. Once the eBook is installed on your computer, you cannot download, install, or e-mail it to another computer; it resides solely with the computer to which it is installed. The license provided is for only one computer. The eBook can only be read using Adobe® Reader® 6.0 software, which is available free from Adobe Systems Incorporated at www.Adobe.com. You may also view the eBook on your PDA using the Adobe® PDA Reader® software that is also available free from Adobe.com. You must follow a simple procedure when you install the eBook/PDA that will require you to connect to the Humana Press website in order to receive your license. Please read and follow the instructions below:

1.   Download and install Adobe® Reader® 6.0 software

You can obtain a free copy of the Adobe® Reader® 6.0 software at www.adobe.com.

*Note: If you already have the Adobe® Reader® 6.0 software installed, you do not need to reinstall it.

2.   Launch Adobe® Reader® 6.0 software

3.   Install eBook: Insert your eBook CD into your CD-ROM drive

PC: **Click on the "Start" button, then click on "Run"**

At the prompt, type "d:\ebookinstall.pdf" and click "OK"

*Note: If your CD-ROM drive letter is something other than d: change the above command accordingly.

MAC: Double click on the "eBook CD" that you will see mounted on your desktop.

Double click "ebookinstall.pdf"

4.   Adobe® Reader® 6.0 software will open and you will receive the message

"This document is protected by Adobe DRM" Click "OK"

*Note: If you have not already activated the Adobe® Reader® 6.0 software, you will be prompted to do so. Simply follow the directions to activate and continue installation.

Your web browser will open and you will be taken to the Humana Press eBook registration page. Follow the instructions on that page to complete installation. You will need the serial number located on the sticker sealing the envelope containing the CD-ROM.

If you require assistance during the installation, or you would like more information regarding your eBook and PDA installation, please refer to the eBookManual.pdf located on your cd. If you need further assistance, contact Humana Press eBook Support by e-mail at ebooksupport@humanapr.com or by phone at 973-256-1699.

*Adobe and Reader are either registered trademarks or trademarks of Adobe Systems Incorporated in the United States and/or other countries.

1

Molecular Targets

Udai Banerji, PhD, Ian Judson, PhD and Paul Workman, PhD

1. INTRODUCTION

Cancer continues to be one of the major causes of mortality throughout the world. There will be an estimated 15 million new cases and 10 million new deaths in 2020, even if the current trends remain unchanged *(1)*. Since the use of mustine to treat a patient with acute lymphoblastic leukemia in 1943 *(2)*, 92 anticancer drugs have been approved by the U.S. Food and Drug Administration (FDA). A recent World Health Organization (WHO) consultation considered only 17 drugs and two anti-emetics as high priority and 12 more to have some advantage in particular clinical settings *(3)*. Although the development of new anticancer drugs has improved survival in a few diseases such as childhood leukemia and testicular cancer, there is an urgent need to continue to develop new and improved agents, as well as to optimize the use of conventional drugs.

Cancer cells differ from normal cells by the following hallmark traits *(4)*: (1) their ability to proliferate due to self-sufficiency in growth signals; (2) insensitivity to growth inhibitory signals; (3) evasion of apoptosis and senescence; (4) limitless replicative potential; (5) sustained angiogenesis; and (6) potential to invade tissue and metastasize. Although each of these traits may be targeted for drug development, two additional areas are important: chemoprevention and modulation of resistance (Fig. 1).

Traditionally, anticancer drug development has focused on DNA as a target, based on the fact that a high turnover of nucleic acids in cancer cells will provide a therapeutic margin. More recent efforts in drug development focus on a better understanding of the molecular basis of cancer and the use this information to identify and validate new targets for rational drug development programs *(5)*.

Handbook of Anticancer Pharmacokinetics and Pharmacodynamics
Edited by: W. D. Figg and H. L. McLeod © Humana Press Inc., Totowa, NJ

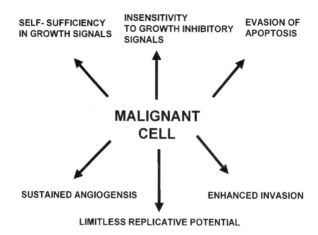

Fig. 1. Characteristic hallmark traits of a malignant cell that are targeted for anticancer drug development. For more details see text and *ref.* 4.

Some of the ways targets are identified and validated include:

- Evidence of pathological deregulation, that is, mutation or over- or underexpression in disease.
- Evidence of adverse clinical outcome correlating with the particular target locus.
- Creation of a malignant phenotype by mutation or increasing or decreasing expression of proposed target.
- Reversal of a malignant process by correcting the genetic abnormality, for example, knockout, RNA interference, transfection, and so forth.

The emergence of high-throughput mutation screening *(6)* and gene expression analysis *(7)* will add to the already large number of targets that are a focus for new anticancer drug development. Once a target has been validated, it can be channeled into the drug discovery process that includes screening, lead identification, lead optimization, preclinical toxicology, and clinical trials *(8)*. Better understanding of the biology and molecular pathology of cancer coupled to improvements in innovative technology is crucial to every step of the drug development process. High-throughput screening, combinatorial chemistry, and the input of structural biology play important roles in lead identification and optimization.

The pharmacokinetic, efficacy and toxicology profiles were previously the most important criteria as to whether a compound would be a viable candidate for clinical development. With identification and validation of new molecular targets, rational drug design now provides anticancer drugs with potential for a greatly improved therapeutic index. Furthermore, pharmacokinetic–pharmacodynamic relationships are playing an increasingly important role in decisions on the rational development and use of new anticancer drugs.

Cancer chemotherapy has reached a fascinating stage, in which new molecular therapeutics such as Gleevec, Herceptin, and Iressa are being introduced alongside, tested and tried traditional cancer drugs such as the hormonal and cytotoxic agents. It is hoped that agents targeted to the molecular pathology of cancer may eventually replace the more traditional drugs. A future in which patients will be prescribed personalized mechanism-based anticancer drugs targeted to their individual molecular and genomic profiles can be envisaged. However, for the next several years it is likely that both novel designer molecular therapeutics and traditional agents will be used side by side and indeed in combination.

Rational development of both new and old drugs requires a thorough understanding of their pharmacokinetics and pharmacodynamics. To develop meaningful pharmacokinetic–pharmacodynamic relationships it is also essential to have a detailed knowledge of the mechanism of action of the drugs concerned and an understanding of the molecular targets on which they act. A detailed analysis of every molecular target, novel and traditional, is not practical because of space constraints. Instead, the objective is to give an overview of the breadth of approaches that are involved in routine treatment and particularly in developmental cancer therapeutics. Selected examples and a detailed listing of literature references are included.

For the purpose of this chapter, targets have been categorized as either established or novel types. Established targets include those against which most currently licensed anticancer drugs were developed and include DNA, microtubules, and nuclear hormone receptors. Novel targets include those against which more recent efforts of drug development have concentrated. They include the products of oncogenes and the genes responsible for the multistep transformation of normal cells into cancer cells, including receptors and receptor tyrosine kinases. The section on novel targets emphasizes the relationships of the novel targets described to the biological traits of cancer as described earlier in this section.

2. ESTABLISHED MOLECULAR TARGETS

2.1. DNA

DNA is one the most successfully exploited targets for anticancer drug development. The use of mustine to treat leukemia in 1943 (2), predated the discovery of the double helical structure of DNA by Watson and Crick in 1953. However, some of the early attempts at rational drug design led to highly effective drugs such as 5-flurouracil (5-FU). With further understanding of the structure and function of DNA and molecules that regulate it, there may be new targets within and around DNA that can be further exploited for anticancer drug development (Fig. 2).

2.1.1. BASE PAIRS

The bases of DNA are heterocyclic rings; adenine and guanine are purines whereas cytosine and thymine are pyrimidines. Adenine binds to thymine and guanine binds to cytosine, via noncovalent interactions involving two and three hydrogen bonds, respectively. Alkylating agents have an active moiety that in the case of nitrogen mustards includes the ethylene immonium ion where the terminal carbon of the mustard chlorethyl group binds to the DNA. The most frequent site of alkylation of DNA by these molecules is the N7 position of the guanine (9). Platinum compounds react with the N7 position of guanine to form a variety of monofunctional and bifunctional DNA adducts. Although covalent adduct formation is the mechanism of cytotoxicity of all antitumor alkylating agents, these drugs exhibit widely different potencies, toxicities, and disease selectivities. These can be attributed to the effects of the nonalkylating structural elements in the agents giving rise to differences in pharmacokinetics, biodistribution, and toxicity to normal tissue.

2.1.2. PURINE AND PYRIMIDINE INCORPORATION

Native purine and pyrimidine nucleotides are natural targets for rational drug design. Pyrimidines such as cytosine are incorporated into DNA as deoxycytidine tri-phosphate (dCTP) and competitive inhibition of this incorporation by Ara-C triphosphate (Ara-CTP) causes deregulation and inhibition of a wide range of enzymes including DNA polymerase (10) and ribonucleotide reductase (11). Enzymes important to de novo purine synthesis such as phosphoribosyl pyrophosphate amidotransferase are inhibited by monophosphate deriva-

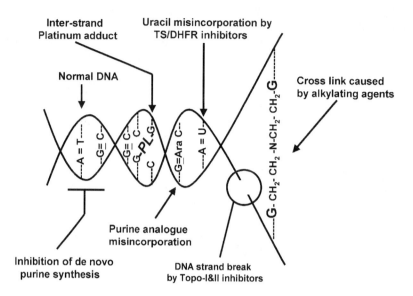

Fig. 2. DNA as a target for anticancer agents.

tives of 6-mercaptopurine (6-MP) and 6-thioguanine (6-TG). Misincorporation of ribonucleotide and deoxyribonucleotide metabolites of thiopurines can cause DNA strand breaks *(12)*. Of the pyrimidine analogues used successfully in the clinic cytosine arabinoside *(13)* and gemcitabine *(14)* are good examples, whereas 6-MP *(15)* and 6-TG *(16)* are purine analogs used routinely.

2.1.3. DIHYDROFOLATE REDUCTASE AND THYMIDYLATE SYNTHASE

Thymidylate synthase (TS) is essential for the production of dTTP and inhibition of TS leads to depletion of dTTP as well as increased levels of dUMP, which when phosphorylated leads to the misincorporation of dUTP into DNA causing DNA damage by uracil DNA glycosylase *(17)*. Dihydrofolate reductase (DHFR) is important in maintaining the reduced folate pool, which in turn is essential for the conversion of dUMP to dUTP by TS. Reduced folate pools are important for *de novo* purine biosynthesis *(18)* (Fig. 3).

Both TS and DHFR are important targets and offer a degree of therapeutic selectivity. Both TS and DHFR are important for ongoing DNA replication and repair; thus, malignant cells can be more susceptible due to their rapid multiplication. Unfortunately, cancer cells can be selected to overexpress TS *(19)* and DHFR *(20)* as a mechanism to develop resistance to TS inhibitors such as 5-FU and methotrexate, respectively. Also of importance is the fact that folate receptors are known to be overexpressed in malignancies such as mesothelioma *(21)*. Clinically, drugs that have been developed to exploit DHFR and TS include methotrexate *(22)*, 5-FU *(23)*, and raltitrexed *(24)*.

2.1.4. TOPOISOMERASE I AND II

Eukaryotic DNA has a complex structure and is frequently supercoiled, knotted, or interlinked. Topoisomerase I and II are enzymes that modify the topological state of DNA by first cleaving the phosphodiester backbone of the DNA so as to allow the passage of another single- or double-stranded DNA, following which the topoisomerase reseals the strand, thus relieving DNA torsional strain. Opening up of DNA by relaxing the tertiary

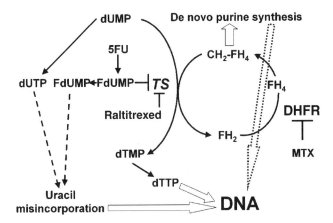

Fig. 3. Mechanism of action of inhibitors of dihydrofolate reductase and thymidylate synthase.

structure is essential for processes such as transcription, replication, and repair of DNA. There are two topoisomerases that are current targets for anticancer drugs. Topoisomerase I causes single-stranded DNA breaks and is not ATP dependent, whereas topoisomerase II causes double-stranded DNA breaks and is ATP and Mg^{2+} dependent (25). Both topoisomerase I (26) and II (27) have been found to be overexpressed in cancer, confirming their importance as valid targets. Successfully used topoisomerase I inhibitors include topotecan and irinotecan (28) whereas etoposide (29) and doxorubicin (30) are examples of topoisomerase II inhibitors that are used in the clinic.

2.2. Microtubules

Microtubules are components of the mitotic spindles that are essential for mitosis. They are in dynamic equilibrium with the pool of soluble tubulin dimers present in the cell. There is a constant incorporation of free dimers into the polymerized structures together with the release of the dimers into the soluble tubulin pool (31). Although tubulin and microtubules are present in normal as well as tumor tissue, their fundamental involvement in cell division makes them important targets for anticancer drug development.

Vinca alkaloids bind to distinct high-affinity binding sites on tubulin, causing alteration of microtubular dynamics at the ends of the mitotic spindle (32). Clinically used drugs known to interact with tubulin include the vinca alkaloids vincristine, vinblastine, and venorelbine, whereas interesting preclinical candidates include dolastatin and cryptophycins, which compete with vinca alkaloids at their tubulin binding site (33).

Taxanes bind mainly to polymerized tubulin. They decrease the lag time and shift the dynamic equilibrium between tubulin dimers and microtubules toward polymerization, thus stabilizing the microtubules (34). Clinically important drugs known to act as microtubule stabilizers include paclitaxel and docitaxel (35), whereas the macrolide epothilones A and B (36) are in various stages of clinical development. Interesting preclinical candidates include the sponge derivative discodermolide (33).

2.3. Nuclear Hormone Receptors

Hormones are known to influence a wide variety of malignancies. Most have intracellular receptors, which once stimulated, activate intranuclear transcription factors. The hormone receptors estrogen, androgen, glucocorticoid, and retinoic acid are discussed in this section.

2.3.1. ESTROGEN RECEPTORS

Intranuclear estrogen receptors have transactivation domains (AF-1 and AF-2) that when activated lead to transcription *(37)*. Apart from binding to specific DNA binding sites, they are involved in considerable crosstalk with the insulin-like growth factors *(38)* and the oncogenic transcription factors c-*fos* and c-*jun (39)*. Modulating estrogen receptors by selective estrogen receptor modulators (SERMs) is now the standard treatment for metastatic breast cancer and for reducing the incidence of contralateral breast cancer. Drugs in clinical use and research include the triphenyethylates tamoxifen and toremifene, the benzothiophene derivatives raloxifene, and the steroidal antiestrogen faslodex *(40)*.

2.3.2. ANDROGEN RECEPTORS

Androgen receptor (ARs) bind both testosterone and dehydrotestosterone before activating transcription *(41)*. Although overexpression of androgen receptors is not seen in all prostate carcinomas, these cancers are known to rely uniquely on androgenic stimulation for growth and evasion of apoptosis *(42)*. Mutations of AR hormone binding domain or amplification of the AR gene along with alteration of coactivators of AR lead to increased sensitivity of AR to very low levels of androgens and constitutive activation of the AR signaling pathway has been shown to confer hormone refractory status *(43)*. Various ways to prevent AR activation are currently in use including reduction of testosterone (medical or surgical castration) and blocking the binding of testosterone to AR by agents such as flutamide and bicalutamide *(44)*.

2.3.3. GLUCOCORTICOID RECEPTORS

As members of the steroid hormone superfamily, intracellular glucocorticoid receptors (GRs) have both a hormone binding site and a DNA binding domain. Stimulation of GR leads to the activation and transcription of GR-dependent genes known to inhibit growth in malignant cells in acute lymphoblastic leukaemia (ALL), whereas mutations in GR have been shown to confer resistance to dexamethasone *(45)*. Dexamethasone is part of standard chemotherapy regimens in ALL and multiple myeloma.

2.3.4. RETINOIC ACID RECEPTORS

Retinoic acid receptors are also members of the nuclear steroid receptor superfamily. In acute promyelocytic leukemia (APL) a t(15;17) translocation fuses a nuclear receptor, that is, retinoic acid receptor (RAR)-α, to a nuclear matrix protein PML (promyelocytic leukemia protein). The oncogenic PML–RAR product impairs nuclear receptor–induced differentiation and leads to a leukemic phenotype. Retinoic acid and arsenic trioxide cause degradation of PML–RAR and induce remissions in APL *(46)*.

3. NOVEL MOLECULAR TARGETS

This section discusses molecular targets in relation to the key hallmarks of cancer highlighted earlier: (1) ability to proliferate due to self-sufficiency in growth signals; (2) insensitivity to growth inhibitory signals; (3) evasion of apoptosis and senescence; (4) limitless replicative potential; (5) sustained angiogenesis; and (6) potential to invade tissue and metastasize (Fig. 1) *(4)*.

3.1. Self-Sufficiency in Growth Signals

Self-sufficiency in growth signals is an extremely important hallmark of the cancer cell. It is possible to target a number of processes that contribute to the self-sufficiency of growth signals in the cancer cell. The broad areas illustrated in this section include signal transduction pathways, control of chromatin regulation, and protein folding and degradation.

3.1.1. SIGNAL TRANSDUCTION

3.1.1.1. Receptors

Receptors involved in signal transduction are important targets for cancer (Table 1). They may be overexpressed, mutated, or lie upstream of other signal transduction defects. Inhibiting receptors that are overexpressed or mutated has been successful in the cases of epidermal growth factor receptor (EGFR, also known as Erb-B1) *(47)*, Erb-B2 *(48)*, platelet-derived growth factor receptor (PDGFR) *(49)*, and vascular endothelial growth factor receptor (VEGFR) *(50,51)*. Stimulating receptors that modulate signal transduction, as in the case of interleukin-2 (IL-2) *(52)* and interferon *(53)*, have also proved successful anticancer strategies. Some of the successful ways that these targets have been exploited include monoclonal antibodies, small molecule inhibitors, and antisense technology. Trastuzumab (Herceptin) is a monoclonal antibody already licensed for treatment of Erb-B2-positive breast cancer *(54)*, while the quinazolines gefitinib (Iressa) *(55)* and erlotinib (Tarceva) *(56)* targeting the EGFR receptor are in advanced stages of clinical development. Gefitinib is now approved for the treatment of non-small cell lung cancer. An example of the stimulation of receptors that influence signal transduction is interferon-α which is licensed for renal cell carcinoma *(57)*, malignant melanoma *(58)* and chronic myelogenous leukemia (CML) *(53)*.

3.1.1.2. Cytoplasmic Signalling Proteins

Src. Src is a cytosolic nonreceptor tyrosine kinase that is activated by PDGFR *(59)* and focal adhesion kinase (FAK) *(60)* and is upstream of Sam68, which is important in regulating mitosis *(61)*. Src kinase activity has been shown to be elevated in colon *(62)* and breast cancers *(63)* while mutations in Src have been identified in colon cancer *(64)*. This has led to interest in developing Src inhibitors *(65,66)*.

Bcr–Abl. The (9:22) translocation can result in the formation of the fusion protein Bcr–Abl, which functions as a constitutively active tyrosine kinase and crosstalks with Ras, phosphatidylinositol 3-kinase (PI3 kinase), and Crkl *(67)*. Bcr-Abl is present in the myelogenic progenitors of 95% of CML patients *(68)* and transgenic mice with Bcr–Abl promoter under the control of a tetracycline-repressible promoter develop reversible leukemia in the presence or absence of tetracycline *(69)*. Imatinib (Gleevec) is a potent inhibitor of Bcr–Abl and trials have shown hematological responses of 95%, 53%, and 29% in chronic, accelerated, and blast phases, of CML respectively, which has led to the drug being licensed for this indication *(67,70)*.

Ras–Raf–Mek–Erk Pathway. Members of the Ras superfamily of proteins that are implicated in cancer include H-Ras, N-Ras, and K-Ras. Ras mutations are found in a variety of tumor types *(70)* and have also been shown to be a marker for poor prognosis *(71,72)*. Ras undergoes prenylation, a lipid posttranscriptional modification required for proper localization to the inner surface of the plasma membrane. Some members of the Ras family require farnesylation and others also undergo geranylgeranylation along with Rho, Rac, and cdc42, which are important to malignant transformation mediated by Ras. The enzymes that mediate farnesylation and geranylgeranylation are farnesyl transferase (FT) and geranygeranyl transferase (GGT), respectively *(73)*. While H-Ras prenylation is inhibited by FT inhibitors, K-Ras is more difficult to inhibit and may require both FT and GGT inhibitors to block malignant transformation *(74)*. Examples of FT inhibitors that have already reached the clinic include R115777, L778,123, SCH66336, and BMS214662 *(73)*. There is increasing evidence that FT inhibitors may not in fact act solely or even partly via Ras. Research to identify the downstream targets continues, with one candidate being the Rho B apoptotic control protein.

Table 1
Receptors and Receptor Tyrosine Kinases Targeted in Cancer

Receptors/receptor tyrosine kinases targeted for inhibition

Receptor	Malignancy	Inhibitor
EGFR (Erb-1)	Breast, lung head and neck, colorectal, ovary	Gefitinib (Iressa)
Erb-B2	Breast	Trastuzumab (Hereptin)
PDGFR	Breast, ovary	Imatinib (Gleevec)
c-KIT	Sarcoma	Imatinib, SU6668
VEGF (FLt1)	Breast, ovarian, lung	SU6668
FGFR	Breast	SU6668

Receptors targeted for stimulation

Receptor	Disease
Interferon	Renal cell carcinoma, CML, multiple myeloma
Interleukin-2	Renal cell carcinoma

The Raf family of serine threonine kinases are important players in signal transduction pathways involved in malignancies. They are activated by Ras proteins *(75)* or by protein kinase C (PKC) *(76)* in a Ras-independent manner. Also, Bcl-2 targets Raf-1 to mitochondria *(77)*. Importantly, mutations in the genes encoding BRAF have recently been identified in a high proportion of melanoma and in a lower proportion of colorectal and other cancers *(78)*. Several drugs are in the advanced stages of preclinical development including a small molecule kinase inhibitor, BAY-43-9006, and an antisense oligonucleotide *(79,80)*.

MEK is phosphorylated by Raf, and once activated, phosphorylates the MAP kinases ERK-1 and ERK-2. Although MEK has not been identified as an oncogene product, no other substrates apart from ERK have been identified, thus making it an important focal point for signal transduction mitogenic pathways, activated by proven oncogenes. Drug development programs are actively pursuing MEK inhibitors, and CI-1040 (formally PD184352) has shown promising xenograft activity and is now undergoing clinical trials *(81)*. Once activated, a fraction of cytosolic ERK-1 and -2 translocates into the nucleus and affects gene regulation *(82)*. There are theoretical concerns that null mutations of the p38 MAP kinase family have led to embryonic lethal phenotypes *(83)* and that ERK inhibitors may be toxic; however, until specific ERK inhibitors are developed, these questions will not be resolved *(81)*.

PI3 Kinase. PI3 kinase is a lipid kinase activated by Ras *(84)* and a number of receptor tyrosine kinases including PDGFR *(85)* and EGFR *(86)*. Downstream of PI3 kinase, PKB/Akt (activated via PDK1) and m-TOR are important kinases that are critical for cell proliferation *(87)*. The tumor suppressor gene *PTEN* (phosphate and tensin homolog deleted from chromosome 10) dephosphorylates and inactivates phosphatidylinositol 3,4,5-triphosphate (PIP-3) which is the lipid product formed by the activation of PI3 kinase *(88)*. Amplification of genes encoding PI3 kinases is seen in ovarian *(89)* and cervical cancer *(90)*, and the fact that PI3 kinase lies downstream of receptor tyrosine kinases that are overexpressed or mutated in cancer and is upstream of known oncoproteins such as PKB/Akt make it an attractive target for anticancer drug development *(91)*. In further support of PI3 kinase as an exciting drug target is that mutation and loss of *PTEN* is the second most common tumor suppressor gene abnormality in human cancers *(92)*. The PI3 kinase inhibitors wortmannin and LY294002 do not have favorable pharmacokinetic profiles but are prototypes for further drug development *(93)*.

m-TOR. m-TOR is a protein kinase that phosphorylates the initiation factor 4E binding protein (4E-BP1); this in turn binds eIF-4E, which is important for the translation of cyclin D1 mRNA. This crucial link to the cell cycle control pathway and the fact that it is downstream of the PI3 kinase pathway (described above) make m-TOR an interesting target for drug development *(94)*. Rapamycin binds to the immunophilin FKBP12 that inactivates m-TOR; and athough this agent has poor pharmacokinetic properties, rapamycin analogs such as CCI-779 are in early stages of clinical development *(95)*.

STAT. Signal transducers and activators of transcription (STAT) are cytoplasmic transcription factors that are activated by growth factor receptors (interferons) and cytoplasmic tryosine kinases such as JAK and Src *(96)*. In addition to the evidence that STAT3 is required for the activation of v-Src transformation *(97)*, new evidence that a constitutionally active STAT3 mutation alone is sufficient to induce malignant transformation makes STAT3 an interesting anticancer drug target *(98)*. STAT3 activation is seen in a variety of cancers including breast *(99)*, head, and neck cancers *(100)*. Different approaches to try and modulate STAT activity based on STAT dimerization, translocation, and DNA binding are being targeted *(96)*. The various points for pharmacological intervention downstream of membrane receptors are shown in Fig. 4.

3.1.1.3. Transcription Factors

AP-1 Family. The biological role of the activator protein-1 family (AP-1), consisting of Fos, Jun, and ATF, in cancer is still emerging *(101)*. Over expression of c-Fos has been shown to induce cartilaginous tumors *(102)* and absence of c-Fos is associated with reduced expression of matrix metalloproteinases, thus affecting angiogenesis and invasion *(103)*. c-Jun is known to transform mammalian cells but requires coexpression of other oncogenes such as Ras and Src *(104)* and is also known to cooperate with c-Fos in the formation of cartilaginous tumors *(102)*. Better understanding of these transcription factors will help develop specific inhibitors. However, inhibition of protein–protein and protein–DNA interactions in which these proteins participate is technically demanding.

c-Myc. c-Myc is a prototype for oncogene activation by chromosomal translocation *(105)*. It is involved in several prooncogenic events such as protein synthesis *(106)*, cell cycle progression by inactivation of cell cycle inhibitor p27 *(107)*, and activation of cyclin E and E2F *(108)*. Myc targets genes that regulate apoptosis such as p53 *(109)* and affects cell adhesion by down regulation of LFA-1 *(110)*. Finally c-Myc has been associated with a number of malignancies including Burkitt's lymphoma, multiple myeloma and T-cell ALL *(105)*, making it an attractive target for anticancer drug development.

NF-κB. NF-κB is an antiapoptotic transcription factor that is normally inhibited by IκB *(111)*. Amplification or overexpression of the *NFκB* gene has been seen in a variety of malignancies such as Hodgkin's disease *(112)* and colon *(113)* and non-small-cell cancer *(114)*, whereas inactivation of IκB has been demonstrated in Hodgkin's lymphoma *(115)* Various inhibitors of *NFκB* such as triptolide *(116)* and BAY11-7082 *(117)* are prototypes for further developments.

3.1.2. Control of Chromatin Regulation

3.1.2.1. Methylation

Methylation of cytosine residues in adjacent cytosine and guanine nucleotides in DNA (Cpg) is achived by DNA methyltransferase (DNMT) *(118)*. Conseqences of CpG methyla-

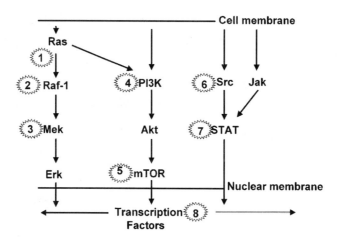

Fig. 4. Signal transduction pathways and non-receptor sites targeted for anticancer drug development: (1) Ras prenylation; (2) Raf-1; (3) Mek; (4) P13 Kinase; (5) m-TOR; (6) Src; (7) STAT; (8) Transcription factors.

tion include silencing of a variety of tumor suppressor genes including *Rb, p16, p14, BRCA1*, and *MLH1 (119,120)*. There is evidence that, although tumors may exhibit global hypomethylation, there are large areas of CpG island hypermethylation in tumors *(121,122)*. Various possibilities for the use of DNMT inhibitors exist; they could be used as single agents with the aim to reactivate methylation-silenced genes such as *Rb* and *p16*, or in combination with conventional cytotoxics, where reactivation of the genes encoding the mismatch repair protein MLH1 affects the sensitivity of cancer cells to carboplatin and epirubicin *(119)*. Examples of DNMT inhibitors that are in the clinic or those in various stages of development include 5-aza-2-demethoxycytidine *(123)* and *S*-adenosyl homocystine (SAH) *(124)*.

3.1.2.2. Acetylation

Acetylation of histones and the control of gene transcription were linked several decades ago, but it was only after the discovery of the histone acetylase and deacetylase enzymes that this phenomenon has been pursued as an approach to the development of anticancer agents. Nucleosomes containing hypoacetylated histones bind tightly to the phosphate backbone of DNA, inhibiting transcription because transcription factors and RNA polymerase do not have access to the DNA. Acetylation neutralizes the charge on the histones, generating a more open DNA configuration, hence providing the transcription apparatus access to the DNA *(125)*.

Histone Acetylases (HAT). Four major groups of HATs have been identified and some of them are shown to have relevance to cancer *(125)*. AIB1 (SRC1 homolog) overexpression has been demonstrated in breast cancers and has been reported to deregulate steroid receptor genes *(126)*. p300/CBP translocation has been observed in AML *(127)*, whereas point mutations are seen in colorectal and gastric carcinomas *(128)*. A combination of microdeletions, translocations, and point mutations of *p300* is seen Rubinson–Tyabi syndrome, in which patients have a propensity to develop cancer *(129)*. Thus, the rationale for targeting HAT for anticancer drug development lies in the fact that if mutated they can cause loss of tumor suppression and in certain situations, when overexpressed they may lead to an oncogenic phenotype.

Histone Deacetylases (HDACs). Four different classes of HDACs have been identified *(130)*. Studies in yeast in which specific HDACs were deleted indicate that Rpd3, Sir2, and Hda1 have distinct functions in cell cycle progression, amino acid synthesis, and carbohydrate transport *(131)*. HDACs also have nonhistone targets and can regulate the deacetylation of p53 and E2F *(128)*. The binding of HDAC with the PML–RAR translocation product leads to inhibition of differentiation, which is known to be one of the driving forces in certain subtypes of AML. The treatment of such patients with retinoic acid results in the displacement of HDACs and allows ligand-dependent coactivators such as SRC-1 to bind and activate transcription, which leads to reactivation of the differentiation process *(132)*.

Early inhibitors of HDAC include trichostatin A (TSA) and trapoxin (TPX), while a novel hybrid compound of TSA and TPA called cyclic hydroxamic acid containing peptide 1 (CHAP1) along with FK228 and MS-275 are at various stages of clinical development *(133)*. Another agent, suberoylanilide hydroxamic acid (SAHA), is currently undergoing clinical trial *(130)*.

3.1.3. PROTEIN FOLDING AND DEGRADATION

3.1.3.1. Proteasome

Rapid and irreversible proteasomal protein degradation is the key to the activation or repression of many cellular processes. The primary component of the protein degradation pathway in the cell is the 26S proteasome *(134)* which, degrades proteins that have been marked for degradation by a process of additon of polyubiquitin chains. The proteins are denatured to short (3- to 22-residue) polypeptides while the ubiquitin chain is recycled *(135,136)*. Proteins with tumor suppressor functions such as p27 *(137)* (inhibits CDK 2, 4, and 6), and IκB *(138)* (inhibits NF-κB) are degraded by the ubiquitin proteasome pathway, and proteasomal inhibition has been shown to cause growth inhibition both in vitro and in vivo. The boronic acid derivative shows promising activity in multiple myeloma, chronic lymphocytic leukemia and in combination with doxetaxel for prostate cancer *(135,139)*. It has now been approved for the treatment of multiple myeloma.

3.1.3.2. Molecular Chaperone Complex—Heat Shock Protein 90

Heat-shock protein 90 (HSP90) and its endoplasmic reticulum homolog GRP78 are important molecular chaperones involved in posttranslational folding of client proteins. Client proteins such as Erb-B2, Bcr-Abl, Src, c-Raf-1, Akt/PKB, and CDK4/6 are either oncoproteins or are integral elements of signal transduction pathways that are deregulated in cancer *(140)*. The ability to affect the signal transduction pathway at multiple levels makes HSP90 an attractive target, and the benzoquinone ansamycin geldanamycin *(141)* and radicicol *(142)* are important lead compounds. The geldanamycin analogue 17AAG has shown promising preclinical activity and is in early clinical trials *(143)*.

3.2. Insensitivity to Antigrowth Signals

3.2.1. G_1–S CHECKPOINT

The G_1–S checkpoint controls the orderly progression of cells from the G_1 phase to the S phase where DNA duplication occurs. The key events include the phosphorylation of the retinoblastoma (Rb) protein leading to its inability to inhibit the transcription factor E2F. The phosphorylation of Rb is regulated by cyclins D and E and cyclin dependent kinases (CDK) 4, 6, and 2 *(144)* (Fig. 5). The G_1–S checkpoint is deregulated in cancer in many ways. Point mutations and loss of RB have been reported in different cancers *(145,146)*. Cyclin D acts to funnel a number of signal transduction pathways such as Ras-Mek or PI3 kinase *(147)* pathway. More important, low levels of natural inhibitors of the WAF-KIP family (p21/p27) and the *INK* gene family (p15/p16) have been found in breast, colon, and head and neck tumors *(148)*. The importance of low levels of inhibitors has been validated further by knockout models that have shown increased incidences of cancer *(149)*. At present a number of drugs targeting the CDKs such as flavopiridol and CYC202 (R-rosovitine) are in early clinical trials and a large number of potential leads such as indirubin and nitropaullones have shown promise *(150,151)*. A number of other CDK inibitors with various levels of selectivity of individual CDKs (e.g., CDK2 or CDK4) are now in preclinical and clinical development.

3.2.2. G_2–M Checkpoint

DNA damage causes cells to either arrest at G_1–S or G_2–M checkpoints. In cases where the G_1–S checkpoint is deregulated (Rb mutation, mutant *P53*, or inappropriately low CDKIs of the CIP/KIP or ARF families), cells progress to the G_2–M checkpoint where they accumulate as a result of the inhibition of cyclin B and Cdc2 by Wee1 and Chk1. The accumulation of cells at G_2–M is advantageous to the damaged cell as it gives it time to repair DNA before committing itself to mitosis, and abrogation of the G_2–M checkpoint can cause premature mitosis and subsequent apoptosis *(151)*. The staurosporine analog UCN01 causes abrogation of the G_2–M checkpoint by inhibiting Wee1 kinase *(152)* and potentiates cytotoxicity of DNA damaging agents such as cisplatin *(153)* and mitomycin C *(154)*.

3.2.3. *p53* Tumor Suppressor Gene

p53 is a tumor suppressor gene that acts as a powerful transcription factor that binds to as many as 300 different promoter elements in the genome, broadly altering patterns of specific gene expression. The *p53* mutation is the most common genetic mutation in cancer, with more than 1700 different mutations being reported *(155)*, the most common sites being exons 5 and 8 *(156)*. p53 is activated by a variety of cellular stresses including UV light, ionizing radiation, and DNA damage by cytotoxic agents. p53 is inactivated by a variety of factors including its binding to Mdm2 that promotes its conjugation with ubiquitin, thus leading to proteasomal degradation. Mdm2 is, in turn, stimulated by the *INK4/ARF* locus. *p53* exerts its antigrowth activity in two broad areas, cell cycle inhibition and induction of apoptosis. The inhibtion of the cell cycle by p53 is predominantly by induction of p21(Waf1/Cip1), which in turn inhibits the CDK4/6. p53 has proapoptotic functions by virtue of its ability, among other effects, to stimulate cytochrome *c* release by Bax and to induce genes that produce reactive oxygen molecules.

p53 can be deregulated in cancer in multiple ways; it can be defective as a result of mutations, and alternately this can induce loss of upstream activators or loss of downstream effector genes. Approaches to exploit p53 as a target for cancer therapeutics can target two genetic backgrounds present in cancers: first a situtation in which *p53* is mutant and second, the case where it is wild type.

When the *p53* gene is mutant, it is possible to try and deliver the normal gene into the tumor by an adenoviral or other vectors. This approach has reached Phase III trials *(157–159)*. Another strategy in a *p53* mutant setting includes therapy with adenovirus with a *E1B* deletion. Adenovirus induces *p53* through the action of the *E1A* gene product, while the *E2B* gene product inhibits this, thus allowing the virus to replicate in cells expressing the *E1B* gene product. A virus with a *E1B* gene deletion, however, will allow selective replication of the adenovirus in cells with an inactive p53 pathway *(160)* and this approach has now reached Phase I trials *(161)*. Reactivation of the function of mutant p53 is an attractive option and numerous attempts to find small molecules *(162)* and peptides *(163)* are underway.

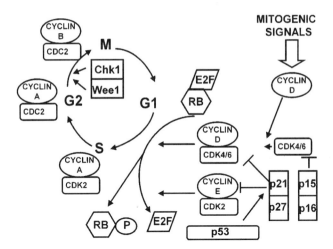

Fig. 5. Targets for cell cycle modulation.

In a setting when the p53 status is wild type, strategies include blocking the interaction between p53 and MDM2, an oncogene that inhibits *p53*. Screens for small molecules that block the interactions between p53 and MDM2 are underway *(164)*. Mdm2 can be inactivated by an antisense approach *(165)* or by novel peptides *(166)*. Both p53 and Mdm2 are regulated by nuclear export processes and a small molecule of CRM-1 nuclear exportin, leptomycin B is a potent activator of p53 response *(167)*.

3.3. Evasion of Apoptosis and Senescence

Apoptosis or programmed cell death is characterized by morphological changes (shrinkage, condensation of nuclei, and loss of microvilli) *(168)*, and the biochemical hallmark of cleavage of chromosomal DNA into nucleosomal units by caspases *(169)* and reactive oxygen molecules *(170)*. Apoptosis is governed by proapoptotic events, which include: (1) death receptor signaling, (2) release of cytochrome *c* from the mitochondria triggered by Bax, (3) *p53* activation, which stimulates *Bax* and genes whose product generate reactive oxygen species. Antiapoptotic factors include: (1) antiapoptotic protein Bcl-2, (2) cellular inhibitor of apoptosis 2 (c-IAP), and (3) NF-κB (*see* section on transcription factors). Deregulation of any of these key factors can lead to inhibition of apoptosis and an inappropriate survival advantage to the affected cell *(171)* (Fig. 6).

3.3.1. DEATH RECEPTORS

Loss of the proapoptotic function of Fas due to mutations in Fas receptors has been seen in plasmacytomas *(172)* and non-Hodgkin's lymphoma *(173)* and can confer a survival advantage to affected cells. TRAIL (TNF-related apoptosis inducing ligand) has been used target death receptors in malignant cells in xenograft models *(174)*.

3.3.2. PROAPOPTOIC INTRACELLULAR APOPTOSIS INHIBITORS

p53 has proapoptotic functions by virtue of its ability , among other effects, to stimulate cytochrome *c* release by Bax and induce genes that produce reactive oxygen molecules. The importance of p53 as a target is covered on the section on insensitivity to growth signals.

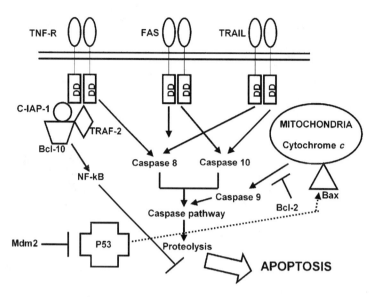

Fig. 6. Targets for apoptosis modulation.

3.3.3. APOPTISIS INHIBITOR PROTEINS

Bcl-2 is an antiapoptotic protein *(175)* that is overexpressed in a variety of malignancies *(176,177)*. Attempts to inhibit Bcl-2 by adenoviral vectors carrying a dominant negative gene or by an antisense approach are in varying stages of clinical development *(178,179)*. Various signal transduction pathways, particularly the PI3 kinase pathway, are known to be involved in survival cell signaling. Inhibitors of PI3 kinase (*see* above) have potential to induce apoptosis and to potentiate the effects of cytotoxics. Elucidation of the genes and pathways involved in in the regulation of apoptosis is expected to generate a range of novel targets for drug development.

3.4. Limitless Replicative Potential—Telomerase

Telomeres are specialized DNA–protein structures that cap the ends of linear chromosomes, preventing their ends from degrading and subsequent end-to-end fusion with other chromosomes *(180)*. Telomerase and importantly its catalytic subunit hTERT are crucial to maintaining these telomere caps *(181)*. It is possible to immortalize normal cell lines with the introduction of hTERT *(182)*. The fact that significantly elevated telomerase activity is found in various tumors (acute myeloblastic leukemia, breast, prostate, lung) while activity in normal tissue is generally negligible *(180)* helps support the concept of telomerase as a valid target. On the other hand, expression of telomerase in normal stem cells has caused concern. Telomerase has been targeted by transcriptase inhibitors such as AZT-TP *(183)*, other small molecule inhibitors that bind to the G-quadriplex structure of telomeric DNA *(180)*, and an antisense approach *(184)*.

3.5. Sustained Angiogenesis

Angiogenesis is the formation of new blood vessels from the existing vascular bed and is essential for tumor growth, invasion, and metastasis *(185)*. Angiogenesis occurs as a multi-step process with initial events involving tumor hypoxia leading to release of proangiogenic factors followed by hyperpermeability and matrix formation before immature vessels are formed to supply the tumor. On completion of vessel formation several antiangiogenic factors are released (Fig. 7).

A number of factors highlight the importance of angiogensis as a target for anticancer treatment. First, increased abnormal intratumoral vascularization is demonstrable in multiple cancers and was associated with a poor prognosis in breast, prostate, ovarian, and head and neck cancers (186). Second, increased levels of proangiogenic factors were found in breast (187), gastric (188), and ovarian cancers (189). Finally inhibition of such factors influencing angiogenesis by small molecules (190), antisense (191) and knockout models (192) have resulted in delayed tumor growth and metastasis in preclinical models.

3.5.1. ACTIVATORS OF ANGIOGENESIS

Drugs inhibiting VEGF receptor tyrosine kinases, including SU5416 (193), SU6668 (194), and interferon-α (195), have shown preclinical and clinical activity. FGF activity has been modulated by heparin-like compounds such as RG-13577 (196), whereas PDGF signaling is inhibited by drugs such as Gleevec (197). TNP470 is a potent angiogenesis inhibitor that acts on the cell cycle regulator MetAP-2 (198). The transcription factor HIF-1 is the key regulator of angiogenesis induction by hypoxia (186). Activation of HIF-1 results in the increased expression of VEGF and other proangiogenic gene products. The targeting of HIF-1 α is of major interest for anticancer drug development.

3.5.2. ENDOTHELIAL CELLS

Drugs targeting existing endothelial cells are classified as antivascular rather than antiangiogenic but have been included here for the sake of convenience. Vascular targeting drugs such as Combretastatin A destabilize vasculature by targeting the tubulin in endothelial cells, resulting in the rapid destruction of blood vessels (199). The mechanism of endothelial cell selectivity remains unclear, but may involve pharmacokinetic and access issues.

3.5.3. MATRIX FORMATION

Matrix metalloproteinase inhibitors are discussed in the section on metastasis, see below. The alpha (v) integrin inhibitor EMD-121974 shows promising activity (200).

3.5.4. MISCELLANEOUS AGENTS

Thalidomide inhibits a variety of proangiogenic factors (201), whereas interleukin-12 up-regulates interferon-γ receptors (202). Conventional cytotoxic agents such as paclitaxel also negatively influence angiogenesis (203).

3.5.5. NATURALLY OCCURRING ANTIANGIOGENIC AGENTS

Low levels of the antiangiogenic protein thrombospondin are reported to correlate with an aggressive malignant phenotype (204) and preclinical models confirm thrombospondin inhibits angiogensis (205). Endostatin is being evaluated in clinical trials (206). Angiostatic steroids such as squalamine derived from shark liver have a mechanism of action that is thought to involve the inhibition of the NH_3, Na–H exchange pump (207).

3.6. Potential to Invade and Metastasise

The major cause of death from cancer is often not the primary tumor but metastasis to a distant site. The search for the mechanisms that regulate metastasis has led investigators to study features in both the primary tumor cells (seed) and the microenvironment (soil) to which they metastasized. The relative importance of each of the above factors is still debated, but there is a consensus that targeting the factors that are prometastatic will eventually lead to improved cancer care in the adjuvant setting (208). Targeting the metastatic potential of

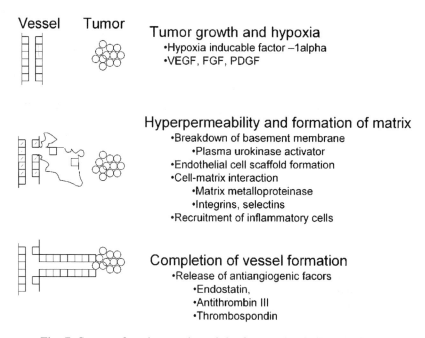

Vessel   Tumor

Tumor growth and hypoxia
•Hypoxia inducable factor –1alpha
•VEGF, FGF, PDGF

Hyperpermeability and formation of matrix
•Breakdown of basement membrane
•Plasma urokinase activator
•Endothelial cell scaffold formation
•Cell-matrix interaction
•Matrix metalloproteinase
•Integrins, selectins
•Recruitment of inflammatory cells

Completion of vessel formation
•Release of antiangiogenic facors
•Endostatin,
•Antithrombin III
•Thrombospondin

Fig. 7. Stages of angiogenesis and the factors that influence them.

cancer includes inhibiting tumor cell invasion or reduction of the potential of the cancers to aggregate or seed in distant organs.

3.6.1. TUMOR CELL INVASION

The ability of cancer cells to invade the extracellular stroma involves matrix metallo-proteinases *(209)*, cysteine proteases *(210)*, and plasminogen activators *(211)* . These are involved in the degradation of basement membrane and invasion of the extracellular matrix. Elevated levels of matrix metalloproteinase *(209)*, and urokinase plasminogen activator *(212)* have been shown to correlate to the metastatic potential of cancers. Inhibitors of MMPs that have been developed clinically include Marimastat *(213)* and BMS 275291 *(214)*. During the extensive evaluation of these agents they have proved disappointing. This may have been due in part to their testing against relatively advanced tumors, whereas it might be imagined that they would be more effective in an adjuvant setting.

3.6.2. TUMOUR CELL ADHESION

The transportation of the malignant cell through the extracellular matrix, vascular spread, subsequent aggregation, and seeding are influenced by extracellular components that influ-ence cell adhesion. Overexpression of factors such as integrins *(215)*, proteoglycans *(216)*, lecithins *(217)* and hepatocyte growth factor/scatter factor *(218)* correlate with increased potential to metastasise. Protein kinase C (PKC) isoforms affect metastasis differentially; although overexpression of PKC-ε *(219)* correlates with increased metastasis, PKC-δ inhibits metastasis *(220)*. Prostacyclins are known to inhibit metastasis by inhibition of tumor cell adhesion to endothelial cells *(221)*. Integrin activation is inhibited by the compound EMD121974 *(200)*, where the glycosidase inhibitor swainsonine has reached Phase I trials *(222)*. Bryostatin inhibits the TPA-induced down-regulation of PKC-δ thus maintaining contact inhibition and preventing metastasis *(220)*. The prostacylin analog cicaprost has shown promising antimetastaic activity in preclinical models *(221,223)*.

4. CHEMOPREVENTION

Given the challenges associated with inhibition of the multiple oncogenic abnormalities involved in the late stages of cancer, the concept of chemoprevention is an attractive one. Chemoprevention can be either primary, secondary, or tertiary. Primary prevention is aimed at healthy individuals, while secondary prevention is directed at patients with a preclinical or early stage disease. Tertiary prevention is aimed at patients who have undergone initial treatment and aims to prevent recurrence *(224)*. Whereas targets for tertiary prevention have been covered under previous sections, primary and secondary prevention are discussed below.

4.1. Retinoic Acid Receptors

As described earlier, retinoic acid receptors belong to the nuclear receptor superfamily. They have been shown to influence the malignant potential of mammalian cells and are exploited in two principal ways in anticancer treatment: first to treat acute promyelocytic leukemia (see Subheading 2.3.4.) *(46)* and second in secondary prevention of a variety of cancers. Epidemiological data suggest that geographical areas where vitamin A deficiency was endemic had an increased incidence of aerodigestive cancers *(225)*. Coupled with the fact that underexpression of retinoic acid receptor β has been demonstrated in bronchial biopsies of chronic smokers *(226)* have prompted research into retinoic acid receptors for cancer prevention. Retinoids used in chemoprevention in vitro include receptor-independent apoptotic retinoids such as 4-HPR (4-hydroxyphenyl retinamide) *(227)*, receptor-active apoptotic retinoids such as 9-c-RA (9-*cis*-retinoic acid), and receptor-active growth inhibitory retinoids such as the benzoate, Nhet17 *(228)*.

4.2. Cycloxygenase-2 (COX-2)

COX-2 expression has been linked to hepatocellular *(229)* and ovarian *(230)* carcinomas. The fact that population-based studies showed a 40–50% decrease in the relative risk of colorectal cancer in persons who were prolonged users of nonsteroidal antiiflammatory drugs (NSAIDs) *(231)* makes COX-2 an interesting target for cancer chemoprevention. The selective COX-2 inhibitor celecoxib has been shown to reduce both the size and number of adenomas in patients with adenomatous polyposis coli who are susceptible to colorectal cancer *(232)*.

4.3. Curcumin

The diferuloylmethane curcumin, a component of the food flavor turmeric, has been shown to be chemopreventive by inducing apoptosis *(233)* and has been tested in a wide variety of premalignant lesions *(234)*.

As we gain greater understanding of the molecular basis of early stage cancers and preneoplasias, there will be increasing potential to define mechanism based molecular targets for rational chemoprevention.

5. DRUG RESISTANCE

A large number of mechanisms have been associated with the development of drug resistance. A detailed discussion is outside the scope of this chapter. The transmembrane efflux pump known as P-glycoprotein (Pgp) causes ATP-dependent efflux of a variety of drugs including anthracylines, vinca alkaloids, taxanes, and steroid hormones. The fact that Pgp expression has been negatively correlated with chemosensitivity and survival in various malignancies *(235)* and that transfection of the *MDR1* gene encoding Pgp causes initially sensitive cell lines to acquire resistance *(236)* makes Pgp a valid target for anticancer drug development. Attempts have been made to overcome multidrug resistance by inhibiting Pgp by calcium channel blockers such as verapamil *(237)* and cyclosporin analog PSC 833 *(238)*. One of the major factors that contribute to the drug resistance is likely to be genetic instability. This likely provides a driving force for the generation of resistance, especially in the presence of selection pressure of drug treatment. Understanding the molecular basis of genetic instability should provide a way forward for preventing the development of resistance. The use of signal tranduction modulators in conjunction with cytotoxic agents has potential to overcome drug resistance.

6. CONCLUDING REMARKS

The development and use of new cancer therapeutics continues to progress at an exciting pace, accelerated both by the discovery of new molecular targets that have arisen from molecular oncology and genomics, and also by the implementation of new discovery technologies *(239)*. The rational development and application of new and established cancer therapeutics requires a thorough understanding and consideration of the mechanisms of action and molecular target involved, coupled to a firm linkage to the principles of pharmacokinetics and pharmacodynamics *(240)*. This chapter has provided an overview of many of the molecular targets that are modulated by cancer drugs, from the relatively nonspecific effect on DNA to highly selective agents that are designed to attack particular loci responsible for malignant progression. It is challenging to cover such a broad field, but it is hoped that this review has sufficiently illustrated the principles and exciting potential of molecularly targeted anticancer drugs.

REFERENCES

1. Parkin MD. Global cancer statistics in the year 2000. Lancet Oncol 2001; 2:533–543.
2. Karnofsky DA. Summary of the results obtained with nitrogen mustard in the treatment of neoplastic disease. Ann NY Acad Sci 1958; 68:899.
3. Sikora K, Advani S, Koroltchouk V, et al. Essential drugs for cancer therapy: a world health organization consultation. Ann Oncol 1999; 10:385–390.
4. Hanahan D, Weinberg RA. The hallmarks of cancer. Cell 2000; 100:57–70.
5. Workman P. Scoring a bull's-eye against cancer genome targets. Curr Opin Pharmacol 2001; 1: 342–352.
6. Futreal PA, Kasprzyk A, Birney E, et al. Cancer and genomics. Nature 2001; 409:850–852.
7. Clarke PA. Pole R, Wooster R, et al. Gene expression microarray analysis in cancer biology, pharmacology, and drug development: progress and potential. Biochem Pharmacol 2001; 62:1311–1336.
8. Workman P, Garrett MD. Discovering novel chemotherapeutic drug targets for the third millennium. Eur J Cancer 1999; 35:2010–2030.
9. Hartley AJ, Gibson WN, Kohn KW, Mattes BW. DNA sequence selectivity by three antitumour chlorethylating agents. Cancer Res 1986; 46:1943.
10. Townsend AJ, Cheng YC. Sequence specific effects of ara-5-aza-CTP and ara-CTP on DNA synthesis by purified human DNA polymerises in vitro: visualization of chain elongation on a defined template. Mol Pharmacol 1987; 32:320.
11. Baker CH, Banzon J, Bollinger JM et al. 2'-Deoxy-2'-methylenecytidine and 2'-deoxy 2',2'-defluorocytidine 5' diphosphates: potent mechanism based inhibitors of ribonucleotide reductase. J Med Chem 1991; 34:1879.
12. Christie NT, Drake S, Meyn RE, et al. 6-Thiopurine induced DNA damage as a determinant of cytotoxicity in cultured Chinese hamster ovary cells. Cancer Res 1984; 44:3665.
13. Rai KR, Holland JF, Glidiwell OJ, et al. Treatment of acute myelocytic leukaemia: a study by cancer and leukaemia group B. Blood 1981; 58:1203.
14. Kaye SB. Gemcitabine: current status of phase I and II trials. J Clin Oncol 1994; 12:1527.
15. Schmiegelow K, Bretton-Myer U. 6-Mercaptopurine dosage and pharmacokinetics influence the degree of bone marrow toxicity following high dose methotrexate in children with acute lymphoblastic leukaemia. Leukaemia 2001; 15:74–79.

16. Casseileth PA, Lych E, Hines JD, et al. Varying intensity of postremission therapy of acute myeloid leukaemia. Blood 1992; 79:1924.

17. Webley SD, Welsh SJ, Jackman AL, Aherne GW. The ability to accumulate deoxyuridine triphosphate and cellular response to thymidylate synthetase inhibition. Br J Cancer 2001; 85:446–452.

18. Chabner BA, Myers CE, Coleman CN, Johns DG. The clinical pharmacology of antineoplastic agents (first of two parts). N Eng J Med 1975; 292:1107–1113.

19. Lacopetta B, Grieu F, Joseph D, Elsaleh H. A polymorphism in the enhancer region of the thymidylate synthetase promoter influences survival in colon cancer patients treated with 5-flurouracil. Br J Cancer 2001; 85:827–830.

20. Matherly LH, Taub JW, Ravindranath Y, et al. Elivated dihydrofolate reductase and impaired methotrexate transport as elements I methotrexate resistance in childhood acute lymphoblastic leukaemia. Blood 1995; 85:500–509.

21. Bueno R, Appasani K, Mercer H, Lester S, Sugarbaker D. The alpha folate receptor is higly activated in malignant pleural mesothelioma. J Thorac Cardiovasc Surg 2001; 121:225–233.

22. Otten J, Philippe N, Suciu S, et al. The children leukaemia group. 30 years of research and achievements. Eur J Cancer 2002; 38(S4):44–49.

23. Mayer R. Oral versus intravenous fluropyrimidines for advanced colorectal cancer: by either route, its all the same. J Clin Oncol 2001; 19:4093–4096.

24. Caponigro F, Avallone A, Budillon A, Comella P, Comella G. Raltitrexed/5-flurouracil based combination chemotherapy regimens in anticancer therapy. Anticancer Drugs 2001; 12:489–497.

25. Kellner U, Rudolph P, Parwaresch R. Human DNA-topoisomerases—diagnostic and therapeutic implications in cancer. Onkologie 2000; 23:424–430.

26. Lynch BJ, Bronstien IB, Holden JA. Elevations of DNA topoisomerase I in invasive c.arcinoma of the breast. Breast J 2001; 7:176–180

27. Nakopoulou L, Zervas A, Lazaris AC, et al. Predictive value of topoisomerase II alpha immumostaining in urothelial bladder cancer. J Clin Pathol 2001; 54:309–313.

28. Garcin-Carbonero R, Supko J. Current perspectives on the clinical experience, pharmacology and continued development of the camptothecins. Clin Cancer Res 2002; 8:641–661.

29. Hainsworth JD. Extended-schedule oral etoposide in selected neoplasms and overview of administration and scheduling issues. Drugs 1999; 58(S3):51–56.

30. Holmes FA, Rowinsky EK. Pharmacokinetic profiles of doxorubicin in combination with taxanes. Semin Oncol 2001; 28(S12):8–14.

31. Weisenberg RC, Deery WJ, Dickinson PJ. Tubulin nucleotide interactions during the polymerization and depolymerization of microtubules. Biochemistry 1976; 21:4248–4254.

32. Himes RH. Interactions of the catharanthus (vinca) alkaloids with tubulins and microtubules. Pharmacol Ther 1991; 51:257–267.

33. Dumontet C, Sikic BI. Mechanism of action of and resistance to antitubular agents: microtubule dynamics, drug transport and cell death. J Clin Oncol 1999; 17:1061–1070.

34. Dye RB, Fink SP, Williams RC. Taxol induced flexibility of microtubules and its reversal by MAP-2 and tau. J Biol Chem 1993; 268:6847–6850.

35. du Bois A. Treatment of advanced ovarian cancer. Eur J Cancer 2001; 37(S9):1–7.

36. Bollag DM, McQueney PA, Zhu J, et al. Epothilones, a new class of microtubule stabilizing agents with a taxol like mechanism of action. Cancer Res 1995; 55:2325–333.

37. Kumar V, Green S, Staub A, Chambon P. Localization of the estradiol binding and putative DNA binding domains of the human oestrogen receptor. EMBO J 1986; 5:2231–2236.

38. Lee AV, Jackson JG, Gooch JL, et al. Enhancement of insulin-like growth factor signaling in human breast cancer: estrogen regulation of insulin receptor substrate-1 expression in vitro and in vivo. Mol Endocrinol 1999; 13:787–796.

39. Webb P, Lopez GN, Uht RM, Kushner PJ. Tamoxifen activation of the estrogen receptor AP-1 pathway: potential origin for the cell specific estrogen like effects of antiestrogens. Mol Endocrinol 1995; 9:443–456.

40. Osborne CK, Zhao H, Fuqua SAW. Selective estrogen receptor modulators: structure, function and clinical use. J Clin Oncol 2000; 18:3172–3186.

41. Maclean HE, Warne GL, Zajac JD. Localization of functional domains in the androgen receptor. J Steroid Biochem Mol Biol 1997; 62:233–242.

42. Denmeade SR, Lin XS, Isaacs JT. Role of programmed (apoptotic) cell death during the progression and therapy of prostate cancer. Prostate 1996; 28:251–265.

43. Grossmann ME, Huang H, Tindall D. Androgen receptor signalling in androgen refractory prostate cancer. J Natl Cancer Inst 2001; 93:1687–1697.
44. Taplin ME, Ho S. Clinical review 134: the endocrinology of prostate cancer. J Clin Endocrinol Metab 2001; 86:3467–3477.
45. Hillmann AG, Ramda J, Multanen K, Norman MR, Harmon JM. Glucocorticoid receptor gene mutations in leukemic cells acquired in vitro and in vivo. Cancer Res 200; 60:2056–2062.
46. Zhu J, Gianni M, Kofp E, Honore N, et al . Retinoic acid induces proteasome dependent degradation of retinoic acid receptor alpha (RAR alpha) and oncogenic RAR alpha fusion proteins. Proc Natl Acad Sci USA 1999; 96:14,807–14,812.
47. Anabell J, Rojo F, Averbuch S, et al. Pharmacodynamic studies of epidermal growth factor receptor inhibitor ZD1839 in skin from cancer patients: histopathological and molecular consequences of receptor inhibition. J Clin Oncol 2002; 20:110–124.
48. Slamon D, Pegram M. Rationale for trastuzumab (Herceptin) in adjuvant breast cancer trials. Semin Oncol 2001; 28(S3):9–13.
49. Heinrich MC, Griffith DJ, Druker BJ, et al. Inhibition of c-kit receptor tyrosine kinase activity by STI 571, a selective tyrosine kinase inhibitor. Blood 2000; 96:925–932.
50. Hoekman K. SU6668 a multitargeted angiogenesis inhibitor. Cancer J 2001; 7:(S3)134–138.
51. Ellis LM, Takahashi Y, Liu W, Shaheen M. Vascular endothelial growth factor in human colon cancer: biology and therapeutic implications. Oncologist 2000; 5:(S1):11–15.
52. Buzio C, Andrulli S, Santi R, et al. Long term immunotherapy with low dose interleukin 2 and interferon alpha in the treatment of patients with advanced renal cell carcinoma. Cancer 2001; 92: 2286–2296.
53. Mahon FX, Delbrel P, Cony-Makhoul P, et al. Follow up of complete cytogenetic remission in patients with chronic myelogenous leukaemia after cessation of interferon alpha. J Clin Oncol 2002; 20:214–220.
54. Baselga J, Albanell J, Molina MA, et al. Mechanism of action of trastuzumab and scientific update. Semin Oncol 2001; 28(S16):4–11.
55. Goss GD, et al. Final results of the dose escalation study phase of a phase I pharmacokinetics, pharmacodynamics and biological activity study of ZD1839; NCIC CTG IND122. Proc Am Soc Clin Oncol 2001; 20:85a.
56. Finkler N, et al. Phase 2 evaluation of OSI-774, a potent oral antagonist of the EGFR-TK in patients with advanced ovarian cancer. Proc Am Soc Clin Oncol 2001; 20:208a.
57. Glaspy JA. Therapeutic options in the management of renal cell carcinoma. Semin Oncol 2002; 29(S7): 41–46.
58. Lens MB, Dawes M. Interferon alpha therapy for malignant melanoma: a systematic review of randomised controlled trials. J Clin Oncol 2002; 20:1818–1825.
59. Kypta RM, Goldberg Y, Ulug ET, Courtneidge SA. Association between the PDGF receptor and members of the src family of tyrosine kinases. Cell 1990; 10:481–492.
60. Cobb BS, Schaller MD, Leu TH, Parsons JT. Stable association of pp60Fyn with the focal adhesion-associated protein tryrosine kinase pp125FAK. Mol Cell Biol 1994; 14:147–155.
61. Taylor SJ, Anafi M, Pawson T, Shalloway D. Functional interaction between c-Src and its mitotic target, Sam 68. J Biol Chem 1995; 28:10,120–10,124.
62. Bolen JB, Veillette A, Schwartz AM, DeSeau V, Rosen N. Activation of pp60c-src protein kinase activity in human colon carcinoma cell lines. Proc Natl Acad Sci USA 1987; 84:2251–2255.
63. Egan C, Pang A, Durda D, Cheng HC, Wang JH, Fujita DJ. Activation of Src in human breast cancer cell lines: elevated levels of phosphotyrosine phosphatase activity that preferentially recognizes the Src carboxy terminal negative regulatory tyrosine kinase 530. Oncogene 1999; 18:1227–1237.
64. Irby RB, Mao W, Coppola D, et al. Activating SRC mutation in a subset of advanced human colon cancers. Nat Genet 1999; 21:187–190.
65. Sawyer T, Boyce B, Dalgarno D, Iuliucci J. Src inhibitors: genomics to therapeutics. Expert Opin Invest Drug 2001; 10 :1327–1344.
66. Vu CB. Recent advances in the design and synthesis of SH2 inhibitors of Src, Grb2 and ZAP-70. Curr Med Chem 2000; 7:1081–1100.
67. Mauro MJ, O'Dwyer M, Heinrich MC, Druker BJ. STI571: a paradigm of new agents for cancer therapeutics. J Clin Oncol 2002; 20:325–334.
68. Deininger MWN, Goldman JM, Melo JV. The molecular biology of chronic myeloid leukaemia. Blood 2000; 96:3343–3356.

69. Huettner CS, Zhang P, Van Etten RA, Tenen DG. Reversibility of acute B-cell leukaemia induced by BCR-ABL1. Nat Genet 2000; 24:57–60.
70. Adjei AA. Blocking oncogenic Ras signalling for cancer therapy. J Natl Cancer Inst 2001; 93:1062–1074.
71. Keohavong P, DeMichele MA, Melacrinos AC, et al. Detection of K-ras mutations in lung carcinomas: relationship to prognosis. Clin Cancer Res 1996; 2:411–418.
72. Nelson HH, Christiani DC, Mark EJ, et al. Implications and prognostic value of K-ras mutation for early stage lung cancer in women. J Natl Cancer Inst 1999; 91:2032–2038.
73. Sebti SM, Hamilton AD. Farnesyltransferase and gernylgernyltransferase I inhibitors and cancer therapy: lesions from mechanism and bench-to-bedside translational studies. Oncogene 2000; 19: 6584–6593.
74. Lerner E, Zhang TT, Knowles, Quan Y, Hamiltion AD, Sebti S. Inhibiton of the prenylation of K-Ras, but not H- or N-Ras, is highly resistant to CAAX peptidomimetics and requires both farnesyltrasferase and gernygernyltransferase I inhibitor in human tumour cell lines. Oncogene 1997; 15:1283–1288.
75. Weber CK, Slupsky JR, Herrmann C, et al. Mitogenic signalling of Ras is regulated by differential interaction with Raf isoenzymes. Oncogene 2000; 19:169–176.
76. Kolch W. Meaningful relationships: the regulation of the Ras/Raf/MEK/ERK pathway by protein interactions. Biochem J 2000; 351:289–305.
77. Wang HG, Rapp UR, Reed JC. Bcl-2 targets the protein kinase Raf-1 to mitochondria. Cell 1996; 87: 629–638.
78. Davis H, Bignell GR, Cox C, et al. Mutations in the *BRAF* gene in human cancer. Nature 2002; 417:949–954.
79. Lyons JF, Wilhelm S, Hibner B, Bollag G. Discovery of a novel Raf kinase inhibitor. Endocrinol Relat Cancer 2001; 8:219–225.
80. Rudin C, Holmlund J, Fleming GF, et al. Phase I trial of ISIS 5132, an antisense oligonucleotide inhibitor of c-raf-1, administred by 24 hrs weekly infusion to patients with advanced cancer. Clin Cancer Res 2001; 7:1214–1220.
81. Sebolt-Leopold J. Development of anticancer drugs targeting the MAP kinase pathway. Oncogene 2000; 19:6549–6599.
82. Lenormand P, Brondello JM, Brunet A, Pouyssegur J. Growth factor induced p42/p44 MAPK nuclear translocation and retention requires both MAPK activation and neosynthesis of nuclear anchoring proteins. J Cell Biol 1998; 142:625–633.
83. Allen M, Svensson L, Roach M, et al. Deficiency of the stress kinase p38 alpha results in embryonic lethality: characterization of the kinase dependence of stress responses of enzyme-deficient embryonic stem cells. J Exp Med 2000; 191:859–869.
84. Ramirez de Molina A, Penalva V, Lucas L, Lacal JC. Regulation of choline kinase activity by Ras proteins involves Ral-GDS and PI3K. Oncogene 2002; 21:937–946.
85. Stephens L, Anderson KE, Hawkins P. Src family kinase mediate receptor stimulated phosphoinositide-3 kinase dependent tyrosine phosphorylation of dual adaptor for phosphotyrosine and 3-phospho-inositides in endothelial and B cell lines. J Biol Chem 2001; 276:42,767–42,773.
86. Rodrigues G, Falasca M, Zhang Z, et al. A novel positive feedback loop mediated by the docking protein Gab 1 and phosphatidylinositol 3-kinase in epidermal growth factor receptor signalling. Mol Cell Biol 2000; 20:1448–1459.
87. Scheid MP, Woodgett JR. PKB/AKT: functional insights from genetic models. Nat Rev Mol Cell Biol 2001; 2:760–768.
88. Cristofano AD, Pandolfi PP. The multiple roles of PTEN in tumour suppression. Cell 2000; 100:387–390.
89. Shayesteh L, Lu Y, Kuo WL, et al. PI3CA is implicated as an oncogene in ovarian cancer. Nat Genet 1999; 21:99–102.
90. Ma YY, Wei SJ, Lin YC, et al. PILCA as an oncogene in cervical cancer. Oncogene 2000; 19:2739–2744.
91. Stein R, Waterfield MD. PI3-kinase inhibition: a target for drug development. Mol Med Today 2000; 6:347–357.
92. Ali IU, Schriml LM, Dean M. Mutational spectra of PTEN/MMAC1 gene: a tumour suppressor with lipid phosphatase activity. J Natl Cancer Inst 1999; 91:1922–1932.
93. Hu L, Zaloudek C, Mills GB, Gray J, Jafe RB. In vivo and in vitro ovarian carcinoma growth inhibition by a phosphatidylinoitol 3-kinase inhibitor (LY294002). Clin Cancer Res 2000; 6:880–886.
94. Hidalgo M, Rowinsky E. The rapmycin-sensitive signal transduction pathway as a target for cancer therapy. Oncogene 2000; 19:6680–6686.

95. Garber K. Rapamycin's resurrection: a new way to target the cancer cell cycle. J Natl Cancer Inst 2001; 93:1517–1519.
96. Turkson J, Jove R. STAT proteins: novel molecular targets for cancer chemotherapy. Oncogene 2000; 19:6613–6626.
97. Bromberg JF, Horvath CM, Besser D, et al. Stat3 activation is required for cellular trasformation by v-src. Mol Cell Biol 1998; 18:2553–2558.
98. Bromberg JF, Wrzeszczynska MH, Devgan G, et al. Stat 3 as an oncogene. Cell 1999; 98:239–303.
99. Garcia R, Yu CL, Hudnall A, Catlett R. Constitutive activation of Stat3 in fibroblasts transformed by diverse oncoproteins and in breast carcinoma cells. Cell Growth Different 1997; 8:1267–1276.
100. Grandis JR, Drenning SD, Zeng Q, et al. Constitutive activation of Stat 3 signalling abrogates apoptosis in squamous cell carcinogenesis in vivo. Proc Natl Acad Sci USA 2000; 97:4227–4232.
101. Jochum W, Passegue E, Wagner EF. AP-1 in mouse development and tumourigenesis. Oncogene 2001; 20:2041–2412.
102. Wang ZQ, Grigoriadis AE, Mohle-Steinlein U, Wagneer EF. A novel target cell for c-fos-induced oncogenesis: development of chondrogenic tumours in embryonic stem cell chimeras. EMBO J 1991; 10:2437–2450.
103. Saez E, Rutberg SE, Mueller E, et al. c-fos is required for malignant progression of skin tumours. Cell 1995; 8:721–723.
104. Schutte J, Minna JD, Birrer MJ. Deregulated expression of human c-jun transforms primary rat embryo cells in cooperation with an activated c-Ha-ras gene and transforms rat-1a cells as a single gene. Proc Natl Acad Sci USA 1989; 86:2257–2261.
105. Boxer LM, Dang CV. Translocation involving c-myc and c-myc function. Oncogene 2001; 20: 5595–5610.
106. Schmidt EV. The role of c-myc in cellular growth control. Oncogene 1999; 18:2988–2996.
107. Bouchard C, Thieke K, Maier A, et al. Direct induction of cyclin D2 by Myc contributes to cell cycle progression and sequestration of p27. EMBO J 1999; 18:5321–5333.
108. Beier R, Burgin A, Kiermaier A, et al. Induction of cyclin E-cdk-2 activity , E2F dependent transcription and cell growth by Myc are generally separable events. EMBO J 2000; 19:5813–5823.
109. Reisman D, Selkind NB, Roy B. c-myc trans activates the p53 promoter through a required downstream CACGTG motif. Cell Growth Different 1993; 4:57–65.
110. Inghirami G, Grignani F, Sternas L. Down regulation of LFA-1 adhesion receptors by C-myc oncogene in human B lymphoblastoid cells. Science 1990; 250:682–686.
111. Rayet B, Gelinas C. Aberrant rel/nfkb genes and activity in human cancer. Oncogene 1999; 18: 6938–6947.
112. Krappmann D, Emmerich F, Kordes U, Scharschmidt E, Dorken B, Scheidereit C. Molecular mechanisms of constitutive NF-κB/Rel activation in Reed Sternberg cells . Oncogene 1999; 18:943–953.
113. Lind DS, Hochwald SN, Malaty J, et al. Nuclear factor-kappa B is upregulated in colorectal cancer. Surgery 2001; 130:363–369.
114. Mukhopadhyay T, Roth JA, Maxwell SA. Altered expression of the p50 subunit of the NF-kappa B transcription factor complex in non-small-cell lung carcinoma. Oncogene 1995; 11:999–1003.
115. Cabannes E, Khan G, Aillet F, Ruth J, et al. Mutations in IKBa gene in Hodgkin's disease suggest a tumour suppressor role of IkB alpha. Oncogene 1999; 18:3063–3070.
116. Liu H, Liu ZH, Chen ZH, et al. Triptolide: a potent inhibitor of NF-kappa B in T- lymphocytes. Acta Pharmacol Sin 2000; 21:782–786.
117. Weldon CB, Burow ME, Rolfe KW, et al. NF-kappa B-mediated chemoresistance in breast cancer cells. Surgery 2001; 130:143–150.
118. Razin A, Riggs AD. DNA methylation and gene function. Science 1980; 210:604–610.
119. Brown R, Strathdee. Epigenomics and epigenetic therapy of cancer. Trends Mol Med 2002;8:S43–S48.
120. Ohtani-Fujiata N, Fujita T, Aoike A, Osifchin NE, Robbins PD, Sakai T. CpG methylation inactivates the promoter activity of the human retinoblastoma tumour suppressor gene. Oncogene 1993; 8:1063–1067.
121. Yan PS, Perry MR, Laux DE, et al. CPG island arrays: an application towards deciphering epigenetic signatures of breast cancer. Clin Cancer Res 2000; 6:1432–1438.
122. Costello JF, Fruhwald MC, Smiragalia DJ, et al. Aberrant CpG island methylation has nonrandom and tumour type specific patterns. Nat Genet 2000; 25:132–138.
123. Jones PA. Altering gene expression with 5-azacytadine. Cell 1985; 40:485–486.

124. Sibani S, Melnyk S, Pogribny I, et al. Studies of methionine cycle intermediates (SAM, SAH) DNA methylation and the impact of folate deficiency on tumour numbers in Min-mice. Carcinogenesis 2002; 23:61–65.
125. Kouzarides T. Histone acetylases and deactylases in cell proliferation. Curr Opin Geneti Dev 1999; 9:40–48.
126. Anzic SL, Kononen J, Walker L, et al. AIB1, a steroid receptor coactivator amplified in breast cancer. Science 1997; 277:965–968.
127. Borrow J, Stanton VP, Anderson JM, et al. The translocations t(8;16)(p11;p13) of acute myeloid leukaemia fuse a putative acetyltransferase to the CREB-binding protein. Nat Genet 1996; 14:33–41.
128. Muraoka M, Konishi M, Kikuchi-Yanoshita R, et al. p300. p300 gene alterations in colorectal and gastric carcinomas. Oncogene 1996; 12:1565–1569.
129. Giles RH, Peters DJM, Breuning MH. Conjunction dysfunction: CBP/p300 in human disease. Trends Genet 1998; 14:178–183.
130. Marks P, Rifkind RA, Richon VM, et al. Histone deacetylases and cancer: causes and therapies. Nat Rev Cancer 2001; 1:194–202.
131. Bernstein BE, Tong JK, Schreiber SL. Genome wide studies of histone deacetylase in yeast. Proc Natl Acad Sci USA 2000; 97:13708–13713.
132. Lyn RJ, Nagy L, Inoue S, Shao W, Miller WH, Evans RM. Role of the histone deacetylase complex in acute promyelocytic leukaemia. Nature 1998; 391:811–814.
133. Minoru Y, Furumai, Makoto N, Komatsu Y, Nishino N, Horinouchi S. Histone deacetylase as a new target for cancer chemotherapy. Cancer Chemother Pharmacol 2001; 48(S1):20–26.
134. Rock KL, Gramm C, Rothstein L, et al. Inhibitors of proteasome inhibition of most cell proteins and the generation of peptides presented on MHC class I molecules. Cell 1994; 79:761–771.
135. Adams J. Proteasome inhibiton: a novel approach to cance therapy. Trends Mol Med 2002; 8(S):49–54.
136. Goldberg AL, Stein R, Adams J. New insights into proteasome function: from archaebacteria to drug dvelopment. Chem Biol 1995; 2:503–508.
137. An B, Goldfarb RH, Siman R, Dou QP. Novel dipeptidyl proteasome inhibitors overcome Bcl-2 protective function and selectively accumulate the cyclin dependant kinase inhibitor p27 and induces apoptosis in transformed, but not normal human fibroblasts. Cell Death Diff 1998; 5:1062–1075.
138. Palombella VJ, Rando OJ, Goldberg AL. The ubiquitin–proteasome pathway is required for processing the NF-kappa B1 precursor protein and the activation of the NF-kappa B. Cell 1994; 78:773–785.
139. Adams J, Palombella VJ, Sausville EA et al. Proteasome inhibitors: a novel class of potent and effective antitumour agents. Cancer Res 1999; 59:2615–2622.
140. Maloney A, Workman P. HSP90 as a new therapeutic target for cancer therapy: the story unfolds. Expert Opin Biol Ther 2002; 2:3–24.
141. Neckers L, Shculte TW, Mimnaugh E. Geldanamycin as a potential anti-cancer agent: its molecular target and biochemical activity. Invest New Drugs 1999; 17:361–373.
142. Soga S, Sharma SV, Shiotsu Y, et al. Sterioispecific antitumour activity of radicicol oxime derivatives. Cancer Chemother Pharmacol 2001; 48:435–445.
143. Banerji U, O'Donnel A, Scurr M, et al. Phase I trial of the heat shock protein 90 (HSP90) inhibitor 17-allylamino-17 demethoxy-geldanamycin (17AAG). Pharmacokinetic profile and pharmacodynamic endpoints. Proc Am Soc Clin Oncol 2001; 20:326.
144. Sherr CJ. The Pezcoller lecture: cancer cell cycles revisited. Cancer Res 2000; 60:3689–3695.
145. Sarbia M, Tekin U, Zeriouh M, et al. Expression of the RB protein, allelic imbalance of RB gene amplification of the CDK4 gene in metaplasias, dysplasias and carcinomas in Barrett's oesophagus. Anticancer Res 2001; 21:387–392.
146. Gras E, Pons C, Machin P. Loss of hetrozygosity at the RB-1 locus and pRB immunostaining in epithelial ovarian tumours: a molecular immunohistochemical and clinicopathological study. Int J Gynecol Pathol 2001; 20:335–340.
147. Gille H, Downwards J. Multiple Ras effector pathways contribute to the G1 cell cycle progression. J Biol Chem 1999; 274:22,033–22,040.
148. Tsihlias J, Kapusta L, Slingerland J. The altered significance of altered cyclin-dependent kinase inhibitors in human cancer. Annu Rev Med 1999; 50:401–423.
149. Labuhn M, Jones G, Speel EJ, et al. Quantitative real time PCR does not show selective targeting of P14 (ARF) but concomitant inactivation of both P16 (INK4A) and P14 (ARF) in 105 pituitary gliomas. Oncogene 2001; 20:1103—1109.

150. Senderowicz AM. Small molecule modulators of cyclin-dependent kinases for cancer therapy. Oncogene 2000; 19:6600–6606.
151. Senderowicz AM, Sausville E. Preclinical and clinical development of cyclin-dependent kinase modulators. J Natl Cancer Inst 2000; 92:376–387.
152. Yu L, Orlandi L, Wang P, et al. UCN-01 abrogates G2 arrest through a Cds2 dependent pathway that is associated with the inactivation of the Wee1HU kinase and activation of the Cdc25c phosphatase. J Biol Chem 1998; 273:33,455–33,464.
153. Bunch PT, Eastman A. Enhancement of cisplatin induced cytotoxicity by 7-hydroxystaurosporine (UCN-01), a new G2 checkpoint inhibitor. Clin Canc Res 1996; 2:791–797
154. Akinaga S, Normura K, Gomi K, et al. Enhancement of antitumour activity of mitomycin C in vitro and in vivo by UCN-01, a selective inhibitor of protein kinase C. Cancer Chemother Pharmacol 1993; 32:183–189.
155. Hollstein M, Shomer B, Greenblatt M, et al. Somatic point mutations in the p53 gene of human tumours and cell lines: updated compilation. Nucleic Acids Res 1996; 24:141–146.
156. Lain DP, Lain S. Therapeutic exploitation of the p53 pathway. Trends Mol Med 2002; 8(S):38–42.
157. Schuler M, Herrmann R, Jacques LP, et al. Adenovirus mediated wildtype P53 gene transfer in patients receiving chemotherapy for advanced non-small-cell lung cancer: results of a multicenter phase II study. J Clin Oncol 2001; 19:1750–1758.
158. Nemunaitis J, Swisher SG, Timmons T, et al. Adenovirus mediated p53 gene transfer in sequence with cisplatin to tumours of patients with non-small-cell lung cancer. J Clinical Oncol 2000; 18:609–622.
159. Dummer R, Bergh J, Karlsson Y, et al. Biological activity and safety of adenoviral vector expressed wild type p53 after intratumoral injection in melanoma and breast cancer in patients with p53 overexpressing tumours. Cancer Gene Ther 2000; 7:1069–1076.
160. Bischoff JR, Kirn DH, Williams A, et al. An adenovirus mutant that selectively replicates in p-53 deficient human tumour cells. Science 1996; 274:373–376.
161. Vasey PA, Shulman LN, Campos S, et al. Phase I trial of intraperitoneal injection of the E1B-55 kd-gene-deleted adenovirus ONYX-015 (dl1520) given on days 1 through 5 every 3 weeks in patients with recurrent/ refractory epithelial ovarian cancer. J Clin Oncol 2002; 20:1562–1569.
162. Foster BA, Coffey HA, Morin MJ, et al. Pharmacological rescue of mutant p53 conformation and function. Science 1999; 286:2507–2510.
163. Friedler A, Hansson LO, Veprintsev DM, et al. A peptide that binds and stabilizes p53 core domain. Chaperone strategy for rescue of oncogenic mutants. Proc Natl Acad Sci USA 2002:99:937–942.
164. Zhang R, Wang H. MDM2 oncogene as a novel target for human cancer therapy. Curr Pharmaceut Design 2000; 6:393–416.
165. Wang H, Nan L, Yu D, et al. Antisense anti-MDM2 oligonucleotides as a novel therapeutic approach to human breast cancer. In vitro and in vivo activities and mechanisms. Clin Cancer Res 2001; 7:3613–3624.
166. Bottger V, Bottger A, Howard SF, et al. Identification of novel mdm2 binding peptides by phage display. Oncogene 1996; 13:2141–2147.
167. Lain S, Xirodimas D, Lane DP. Accumulating active p53 in the nucleus by inhibition of nuclear export: a novel strategy to promote the p53 tumour suppressor function. Exp Cell Res 1999;253:315–324.
168. Manjo G, Joris I. Apoptosis, oncosis and necrosis. Am J Pathol 1995; 146:3–15.
169. Enarl M, Sakahira H, Yokoyama H, et al. A caspase activated DNase that degrades DNA during apoptosis and its inhibitor ICAD. Nature 1998; 391:43–50.
170. Polyak K, Xia Y, Zweier JL, et al. A model for p53 induced apoptosis. Nature 1997; 389:300–305.
171. Mullauer L, Gruber P, Sebinger D, et al. Mutations in apoptosis genes: a pathogenetic factor for human disease. Mutat Res 2001; 488:211–231.
172. Landowski TH, Qu N, Buyuksal I, et al. Mutations in the Fas antigen in patients with multiple myeloma. Blood 1997; 90:4266–4270.
173. Gronbaek K, Straten PT, Ralfkiaer E, et al. Somatic fas mutations in non Hodgkin's lymphoma: associated with extranodal disease and autoimmunity. Blood 1998; 92:3018–3042.
174. Walczak H, Miller RE, Ariail K, et al. Tumoricidal acitivity of tumour necrosis factor related apoptosis inducing ligand in vivo. Nat Med 1999; 5:157–163
175. Adams JM, Cory S. The Bcl-2 protein family: arbiters of cell survival. Science 1998; 281:1322–1326.
176. Rantanen S, Monni O, Joensuu H, et al. Causes and consequences of BCL2 overexpression in diffuse large B cell lymphoma. Leuk Lymphoma 2001; 42:1089–1098.
177. Uchida T, Minei S, Gao JP, et al. Clinical significance of p53, MDM2 and bcl-2 expression in transitional cell carcinoma of the bladder. Oncol Rep 2002; 9:253–259.

178. Ayash LJ, Clarke M, Adams P, et al. Clinical protocol. Purging of autologous stem cell sources with bcl-x adenovirus for women undergoing high dose chemotherapy for stage IV breast carcinoma. Hum Gene Ther 2001; 12:2023–2025.

179. Tolcher AW. Preliminary phase I results of G3139 (bcl-2 antisense oligonucleotide) therapy in combination with docetaxel in hormone refractory prostate cancer. Semin Oncol 2001; 28(S4):67–70.

180. Bearss DJ, Hurley LH, Von Hoff DD. Telomere maintenance mechanisms as a target for drug development. Oncogene 2000; 19:6632–6641.

181. Mayerson M. Role of telomerase in normal and cancer cells. J Clin Onc 2000; 18:2626–2634.

182. Hahn W, Counter Cm, Lundberg AS, et al. Creation of tumour cells with defined genetic elements. Nature 1999; 400:464–468.

183. Strahl C, Blackburn E. Effects of reverse transcriptase inhibitors on telomere length and telomerase activity in two immortalized human cell lines. Mol Cell Biol 1996; 16:53–65.

184. Glukhov AI, Zimnik OV, Gordeev SA, et al. Inhibition of telomerase activity of melanoma cell in vitro by antisense oligonucliotieds. Biochem Biophys Res Commun 1998; 248:368–371.

185. Folkman J. What is the evidence that tumours are angiogenesis dependent? J Natl Cancer Inst 1990; 82:4–6.

186. Fox SB, Giampietro G, Harris A. Angiogenesis: pathological, prognostic and growth factor pathways and their link to trial design and anticancer drugs. Lancet Oncol 2001; 2:278–289.

187. Kanzaki A, Takebayashi Y, Bando H, et al. Expression of uridine and thymidine phosphorylase genes in human breast carcinoma. Int J Cancer 2002; 97:631–635.

188. Ikeguchi M, Cai J, Fukuda K, et al. Correlation between spontaneous apoptosis and expression of angiogenic factors in advanced gastric adenocarcinoma. J Exp Clin Cancer 2001; 20:257–263.

189. Fujimoto J, Sakaguchi H, Akoi I, et al. Clinical implications of expression of vascular endothelial growth factor in metastatic lesions of ovarian cancers. Br J Cancer 2001; 85:313–316.

190. Raymond M, Shaheen M, William W, et al. Tyrosine kinase inhibition of multiple angiogenic growth factor receptors improves survival in mice bearing colon cancer liver metastasis by inhibition of endothelial cell survival mechanisms. Cancer Res 2001; 61:1464–1468.

191. Gu ZP, Wang YJ, Li JG, et al. VEGF165 antisense RNA suppresses oncogenic properties of human esophageal squamous cell carcinoma. World J Gastroenterol 2002; 8:44–48.

192. Koolwijk P, Peters E, Van der Vecht B, et al. Involvement of VEGFR-2 (kdr/flk-1) but not VEGFR-1 (flt-1) in VEGF-A and VEGF-C induced tube formation by human microvascular endothelial cells in fibrin matrices in vitro. Angiogenesis 2001; 4:53–60.

193. Rosen LS. Angiogenesis inhibition in solid tumours. Cancer J 2001; 7(S3):120–128.

194. Hoekman K. SU6668 a multitargeted angiogenesis inhibitor. Cancer J 2001; 7(S3):134–138.

195. Di Raimondo F, Palumbo GA, Molica S, et al. Angiogenesis in chronic myeloproliferative diseases. Acta Haematol 2001; 106:177–183.

196. Miao HQ, Ornitz DM, Aingorn E, et al. Modulation of fibroblast growth factor-2 receptor binding, dimerization, signalling and angiogenic activity by a synthetic heparin mimicking polyanionic compound. J Clin Invest 1997; 99:1565–1575.

197. George D. Platelet derived growth factor receptors: a therapeutic target in solid tumours. Semin Oncol 2001; 28(5):27–33.

198. Kruger EA, Figg WD. TNP-470: an angiogenesis inhibitor in clinical development for cancer. Expert Opin Investig Drugs 2000; 9:1383–1396.

199. Malcontenti-Wilson C, Muralidharan V, Skinner S, et al. Combretastatin A4 prodrug study of effect on the growth and the microvascular of colorectal liver metastasis in a murine model. Clin Cancer Res 2001; 7:1052–1060.

200. MacDonald TJ, Taga T, Shimada H, et al. Preferential susceptibility of brain tumours to the antiangiogenic effects of an alpha (v) integrin antagonist. Neurosurgery 2001; 48:151–157.

201. Gupta D, Treon SP, Shima Y. Adherence of multiple myeloma cells to bone marrow stromal cells upregulates vascular endothelial growth factor secretion: therapeutic applications. Leukemia 201; 15: 1950–1961.

202. Voest EE, Kenyon BM, O'Reilly MS, et al. Inhibition of angiogenesis in vivo by interleukin 12. J Natl Cancer Inst 1995; 87:581–586.

203. Lau DH, Xue L, Young LJ. Paclitaxel (taxol): an inhibitor of angiogenesis in a highly vascularized transgenic breast cancer. Cancer Biother Radiopharmaceut 1999; 14:31–36.

204. Tokunaga T, Nakamura M, Oshika Y. Thrombospondin 2 expression is correlated with inhibition of angiogenesis and metastasis of colon cancer. Br J Cancer 1999; 79:354–359.

205. Tolsma SS, Volpert OV, Good DJ, et al. Peptides derived from two separate domains of the matrix protein thrombospondin-1 have antiangiogenic activity. J Cell Biol 1993; 122:497–511.
206. Mundhenke C, Thomas JP, Wilding G, et al. Tissue examination to monitor antiangiogenic therapy: a phase I clinical trial with endostatin. Clin Cancer Res 2001; 7:3366–3374.
207. Bhargava P, Marshall JL, Dahut W, et al. A phase I and pharmacokinetic study of squalamine, a novel antiangiogenic agent in patients with advanced cancer. Clin Cancer Res 2001; 7:3912–3919.
208. Fidler IJ. Critical determinants of cancer metastasis: rationale for therapy. Cancer Chemother Pharmacol 1999; 43(S):3–10.
209. Kawata R, Shimada T, Maruyama S, et al. Enhanced production of matrix metalloproteinase-2 in human head and neck carcinoma is correlated with lymph node metastasis. Acta Otolaryngol 2002; 122:101–106.
210. Krepela E. Cysteine proteinases in tumour cell growth and apoptosis. Neoplasma 2001; 48:332–349.
211. Brownstein C, Falcone DJ, Jacovina A, et al. A mediator of cell surface specific plasmin generation. Ann NY Acad Sci 2001; 947:143–155.
212. Ahmed N, Pansino F, Baker M, et al. Association between alphabeta6 integrin expression, elevated p42/44 kDa MAPK, and plasminogen-dependent matrix degeneration in ovarian cancer. J Cell Biochem 2002; 84:675–686.
213. Groves MD, Puduvalli VK, Hess KR, et al. Phase II trial of temozolomide plus the matrix metalloproteinase inhibitor marimastat in recurrent and progressive glioblastoma multiforme. J Clin Oncol 2002; 20:1383–1388.
214. Naglich JG, Jure-Kunkel M, Gupta E, et al. Inhibition of angiogenesis and metastasis in two murine models by matrix metalloproteinase inhibitor BMS- 275291. Cancer Res 2001; 61:8480–8485.
215. Ziober BL, Lin CS, Kramer RH. Laminin binding integrins in tumour progression and metastasis. Semin Cancer Biol 1996; 7:119–128
216. Benchimol S, Fuks A, Jothy S, et al. Carcinoembryonic antigen, a human tumour marker as an intercellular adhesion molecule. Cell 1989; 57:327–334
217. Raz A, Lotan R. Endogenous galactoside binding lectins: a new class of functional tumour cell surface molecules related to metastasis. Cancer Metastas Rev 1987; 6:433–452.
218. Maulik G, Shrikhande A, Kijima T, et al. Role of hepatocyte growth factor receptor c-met in oncogenesis and potential for therapeutic inhibition. Cytokine Growth Factor Rev 2002; 13:41–59.
219. Jansen AP, Verwiebe EG, Dreckschmidt NE, et al. Protein kinase C epsilon transgenic mice. A unique model for metastatic squamous cell carcinoma. Cancer Res 2001; 61:808–812.
220. Heit I, Wieser RI, Herget T, et al. Involvement of protein kinase C delta in contact dependent inhibition of growth in human and murine fibroblasts. Oncogene 2001; 20:5143–5154.
221. Schneider MR, Tang DG, Schirner M, et al. Prostacyclin and its analogues: antimetastatic effects and mechanism of action. Cancer Metastas Rev 1994; 13:349–364.
222. Goss PE, Baptiste J, Fernandes B, et al. A phase I study of swainsonine in patients with advanced malignancies. Cancer Res 1994; 54:1450–1457.
223. Schneider MR, Schirner M, Lichtner RB, et al. Antimetastatic action of the prostacylin analogue cicaprost in experimental mammary tumours. Breast Cancer Res Treat 1996; 38:133–141.
224. De Flora S, Izzotti A, D'Agostini F, et al. Multiple points of intervention in the prevention of cancer and other mutation related diseases. Mutation Res 2001; 480–481:9–22.
225. Lippman SM, Lee JS, Lotan R, et al. Chemoprevention of upper aerodigestive tract in cancers: a report of the third upper aerodigestive cancer task force worksop. Head Neck 1990; 12:5–20.
226. Xu XC, Lee JS, Lee JJ, et al. Nuclear retinoid acid receptor beta in bronchial epithelium of smokers before and during chemoprevention. J Natl Cancer Inst 1999; 91:1317–1321.
227. Sharp RM, Bello-DeOcampp D, Salmaan TA. N-(4-Hydroxyphenyl)retinamide (4-HPR) decreases neoplastic properties of human prostate cells: an agent for prevention. Mutat Res 2001; 496:163–170.
228. Guruswamy S, Lightfoot S, Gold MA, et al. Effects of retinoids on cancerous phenotype and apoptosis in organotypic cultures of ovarian carcinoma. J Natl Cancer Inst 2001; 93:516–525.
229. Bae HS, Jung ES, Park YM, et al. Expression of cycloxygenase-2 (COX-2) in hepatocellular carcinoma and growth inhibition of hepatoma cell lines by a COX-2 inhibitor NS-398. Clin Cancer Res 2001; 17:1410–1418.
230. Rodriguez-Burford C, Barnes MN, Oelschlager DK, et al. Effects of nonsteroidal antiinflammatory agents (NSAIDs) on ovarian carcinoma cell lines: preclinical evaluation of NSAIDs as chemopreventive agents. Clin Canc Res 2002; 8:202–209.

231. Thun MJ, Namboodri MM, Heath CW, et al. Aspirin use and reduced risk of fatal colon cancer. N Engl J Med 1991; 325:1593–1596.
232. Abiy-Issa HM, Alshafie GA, Seibert K, et al. Dose response effects of the COX-2 inhibitor, celecoxib on the chemoprevention of mammary carcinogenesis. Anticancer Res 2001; 21:3425–3432.
233. Anto RJ, Mukhopadhyay A, Denning K, et al. Curcumin (diferuloylmethane) induces apoptosis through the activation of caspase-8, BID cleavage and cytochrome c release: its suppression by ectopic expression of Bcl-2 and Bcl-xl. Carcinogenesis 2002; 23:143–150.
234. Cheng AL, Hsu CH, Hsu JK, et al. Phase I clinical trial of curcumin, a chemopreventative agent in patients with high risk or pre-malignant lesions. Anticancer Res 2001; 21:2895–2900.
235. Lehne G. P-glycoprotein as a drug target in the treatment of multidrug resistant cancer. Curr Drug Targets 2000; 1:85–99.
236. Gros P, Ben Neriah YB, Croop JM, et al. Isolation and expression of a complementary DNA that confers multidrug resistance. Nature 1986; 323:728–731.
237. Shah A, Gaveriya H, Motohashi N, et al. 3,5-Diacetyl-1,4-dihydropyridines: synthesis and MDR reversal in tumour cells. Anticancer Res 2000; 20:373–377.
238. Bates S, Kang M, Meadows B, et al. A phase I study of infusional vinblastine in combination with the P-glycoprotein antagonist PSC 833 (valspodar). Cancer 2001; 92:1577–1590.
239. Workman P. The opportunities and challenges of personalized genome-based molecular therapies for cancer: Targets, technologies, and molecular chaperones. Cancer Chemother Pharmacol 2003: 52(Suppl 1): S45–S56.
240. Workman P. How much gets there and what does it do?: The need for better pharmacokinetic and pharmacodynamic endpoints in contemporary drug discovery and development. Curr Pharmaceut Des 2003;9: 891–902.

2   Preclinical Screening for New Anticancer Agents

Angelika M. Burger, PhD
and Heinz-Herbert Fiebig, MD

Contents

1. INTRODUCTION

Cancer chemotherapy is a rather young discipline. It has been pursued with scientific vigor and multinational collaborations only since the mid-20th century. Although 92 approved anticancer drugs are available today for the treatment of more than 200 different tumor entities, effective therapies for most of these tumors are lacking *(1)*. Out of the 92 registered drugs, 17 are considered by oncologists to be more broadly applicable and 12 additional agents are perceived as having certain advantages in some clinical settings *(2)*. They are mostly cytotoxic in nature and act by a very limited number of molecular mechanisms. Thus, the need for novel drugs to treat malignant disease requiring systemic therapy is still pressing. Public institutions, the pharmaceutical industry, and, more recently, small business and biotech companies create hundreds of thousands of compounds with potential anticancer activity. Only a certain number of drugs and concepts, however, can be evaluated clinically because of cost and ethical considerations. A preselection, called the screening process, is therefore required. The aim of screening efforts is to identify products that will produce antitumor effects matching the activity criteria used to define which compounds can progress to the next stage in the preclinical development program. Anticancer drug screening can be performed using various types of in vitro and in vivo tumor models. The ideal screening system, however, should combine speed, simplicity, and low costs with optimal predictability of pharmacodynamic activity.

Handbook of Anticancer Pharmacokinetics and Pharmacodynamics
Edited by: W. D. Figg and H. L. McLeod © Humana Press Inc., Totowa, NJ

2. HISTORY OF ANTICANCER DRUG SCREENS

Initial screening and drug development programs were small in scale and directed toward the evaluation of antitumor activity of small numbers and specific types of potential drugs *(3)*. Stimulated by the approaches of Ehrlich and Warburg, studies were conducted on the effects on tumor growth of dyes or respiratory poisons, respectively *(4,5)*. In the 1930s several researchers engaged in systematic studies of certain classes of compounds such as Boyland in the United Kingdom, who tested aldehydes in spontaneous tumors in mice, and Lettre in Germany, who studied colchicine derivatives and other mitotic poisons in tissue culture and ascites tumors *(6)*. In the United States, Shear, first at Harvard and then at the National Cancer Institute (NCI), inaugurated a screening program for testing and isolation of bacterial polysaccharides employing mice bearing sarcoma 37 as test systems for necrosis and hemorrhage. The program was quickly extended to plant extracts and synthetic compounds. In the early 1950s the program had evaluated more than 300 chemicals and several hundreds of plant extracts. Two of these materials were tested clinically *(7)*.

Larger-scale screens emerged around 1955, stimulated by the discovery that chemical agents, such as nitrogen mustard and folic acid antagonists, were capable of producing remissions of malignant lymphomas *(8,9)*. As a result, the program of Shear at the NCI was extended to incorporate the evaluation of synthetic agents and natural products for antitumor activity. Further institutions that engaged in screening programs were Sloan-Kettering in New York, the Chester Beatty Research Institute in London, and the Southern Research Institute in Alabama *(3)*. In addition, screening, evaluation, and development programs were instituted at chemical and pharmaceutical companies, research institutions, medical schools, and universities in various countries in the world.

As a result of these efforts, several agents were found with clinical activity, particularly against leukemias and lymphomas. Currently they provide the battery of available drugs for systemic treatment of cancer and encompass alkylating agents (cyclophosphamide, bis(chloroethyl)nitrosourea [BCNU], 1-(2-chloroethyl)-3-cyclohexyl-1-nitrosourea [CCNU], antimetabolites (methotrexate, 5-fluorouracil [5-FU], 6-mercaptopurine), antibiotics (mitomycin C, adriamycin), and hormones (androgens, estrogens, corticoids) *(3)*.

3. THE NCI SCREEN

The NCI Developmental Therapeutics Program (DTP) anticancer drug screen has undergone several changes since its inception in 1955 *(10)*. It has become the foremost public screening effort worldwide in the area of cancer drug discovery, not the least because the experimental screening models used were always adopted to novel emerging knowledge and technologies. The early philosophy from which the NCI endeavor proceeded was that the elucidation of empirically defined antitumor activity in a model would translate into activity in human cancers. The choice of specific screening models was guided by sensitivity to already identified clinically active agents, and in the early period was exclusively focused on in vivo testing procedures *(11)*. Initially, three transplantable murine tumors were employed, namely, the sarcoma 180, the carcinoma 755, and the leukemia L1210. The latter was found to be the most predictive rodent model among the available panel and was retained in 1975, when the NCI screening process was changed in that the P388 murine leukemia model was utilized as a prescreen and followed by a panel of tumors now also including human xenografts (breast MX-1, lung LX-1, colon CX-1) *(12)*. The human xenografts were utilized with the intent to achieve a better prediction for clinical response against solid human malignancies as compared to hematological malignancies.

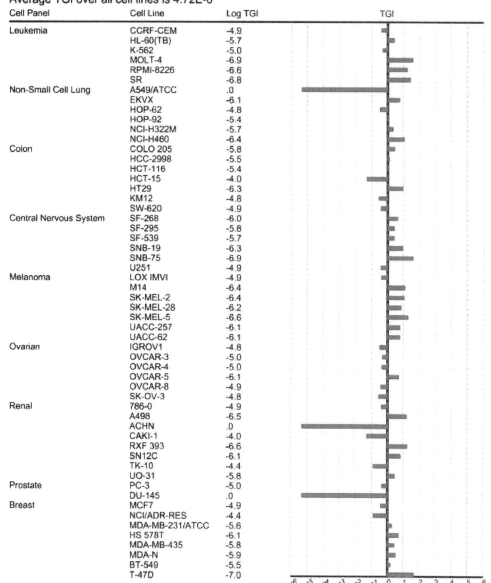

TGI Mean Graph for Compound 123127
Average TGI over all cell lines is 4.72E-6

Cell Panel	Cell Line	Log TGI
Leukemia	CCRF-CEM	-4.9
	HL-60(TB)	-5.7
	K-562	-5.0
	MOLT-4	-6.9
	RPMI-8226	-6.6
	SR	-6.8
Non-Small Cell Lung	A549/ATCC	.0
	EKVX	-6.1
	HOP-62	-4.8
	HOP-92	-5.4
	NCI-H322M	-5.7
	NCI-H460	-6.4
Colon	COLO 205	-5.8
	HCC-2998	-5.5
	HCT-116	-5.4
	HCT-15	-4.0
	HT29	-6.3
	KM12	-4.8
	SW-620	-4.9
Central Nervous System	SF-268	-6.0
	SF-295	-5.8
	SF-539	-5.7
	SNB-19	-6.3
	SNB-75	-6.9
	U251	-4.9
Melanoma	LOX IMVI	-4.9
	M14	-6.4
	SK-MEL-2	-6.4
	SK-MEL-28	-6.2
	SK-MEL-5	-6.6
	UACC-257	-6.1
	UACC-62	-6.1
Ovarian	IGROV1	-4.8
	OVCAR-3	-5.0
	OVCAR-4	-5.0
	OVCAR-5	-6.1
	OVCAR-8	-4.9
	SK-OV-3	-4.8
Renal	786-0	-4.9
	A498	-6.5
	ACHN	.0
	CAKI-1	-4.0
	RXF 393	-6.6
	SN12C	-6.1
	TK-10	-4.4
	UO-31	-5.8
Prostate	PC-3	-5.0
	DU-145	.0
Breast	MCF7	-4.9
	NCI/ADR-RES	-4.4
	MDA-MB-231/ATCC	-5.6
	HS 578T	-6.1
	MDA-MB-435	-5.8
	MDA-N	-5.9
	BT-549	-5.5
	T-47D	-7.0

Fig. 1. Example of NCI 60-cell-line screening data. Shown is the sensitivity profile of adriamycin in 9 different tumor histologies on the basis of the total growth inhibition (TGI). Bars to the *left* indicate more resistant and *bars* to the right, more sensitive cell lines.

For the same reason, starting in 1985, the human tumor cell line panel comprised of 60 different cell types, including mainly solid malignancies, was introduced and replaced the P388 in vivo leukemia prescreen in the 1990s (Fig. 1; see also http://dtp.nci.nih.gov./branches/ btb/). This project has been designed to screen up to 20,000 compounds per year for potential anticancer activity. Selection criteria for preclinical drug candidates are cytotoxic potency and differential activity against particular tumor types and/or a few specific cell lines (13).

The screen is unique in that the complexity of a 60-cell-line dose response produced by a given compound results in a biological response pattern that can be utilized in pattern recognition algorithms *(14)*. Using these algorithms, it is possible to assign a putative mechanism of action to a test compound, or to determine that the response pattern is unique and not similar to that of any of the standard prototype compounds included in the NCI database. Such agents are then tested against the sensitive cell line grown as subcutaneous xenografts in nude mice in vivo *(15)*. Because of the vast number of molecules emerging from the in vitro screen for nude mouse testing, in 1995 the preclinical development cascade was amended to include the hollow fiber (HF) assay *(16)*. The HF assay is a short-term in vivo assay combined with in vitro culture methods. It has been proven as a rapid and efficient means of selecting compounds with the potential for in vivo activity in conventional xenografts *(10,16)*.

In parallel with the implementation of the HF "in vivo filter system," a three-cell-line prescreen preceding the 60-cell-line screen was established in early 1995 as it became obvious that many agents were completely inactive under the conditions of the assay. This prescreen (MCF-7 breast, H460 lung, and SF268 brain cancer lines) would test for the presence of toxicity at a drug concentration of $10^{-4}\,M$ and could eliminate a large proportion of the inactive agents, but preserve "active" agents for multidose 60-cell-line testing. Computer modeling indicated that approx 50% of drugs could be eliminated without a significant decrease in ability to identify active agents, and should be able to increase the throughput and efficiency of the main cancer screen with limited loss of information (http://dtp.nci.nih.gov./branches/btb/).

Thus, the current NCI preclinical anticancer drug screening process is summarized in Fig. 2. Although the NCI drug development scheme is still empirical as it is based on selection of in vitro and in vivo antiproliferative activity, a number of new agents that were adopted for clinical use have been identified based on their unique patterns of activity in the in vitro screen such as spicamycin (NSC 650425), a glycoprotein synthesis inhibitor; the protein kinase C inhibitor UCN-01; or depsipeptide (NSC 630176), a histone deacetylase (HDAC) inhibitory agent *(17)*.

Recent insights into the molecular basis of human cancer and high-throughput profiling of the genome and proteome of the NCI 60-cell-line panel initiated a transition to rational molecular targeted discovery and development of anticancer agents in vitro and also in vivo *(18,19)*.

4. STRENGTHS AND PITFALLS OF CELL-BASED SCREENS VS CELL-FREE HTS ON ISOLATED TARGETS

Large-scale screening using animal systems as practiced in the past (the P388 model; see above) is highly unethical and, particularly in Europe, strictly regulated. In the majority of cases, either cellular or target-based high-throughput assays will precede in vivo evaluation of potential anticancer drugs.

High-throughput screening (HTS) plays an essential role in contemporary drug discovery processes. Miniaturization, robot-aided automatization, and data management by novel information technologies have provided the means of testing large compound libraries comprising several hundreds of thousands of molecules either from collections or combinatorial chemistry approaches that emerged recently *(2)*. Estimates of HTS screening capacity range from 100,000 to 1 million compounds per week. Whereas cell-based assay formats can be performed in 96- to 384-well plates, high-density formats such as 1536-well plates with an assay volume of only 10 µL are suitable only for a cell-free isolated target-based screening setup *(20)*.

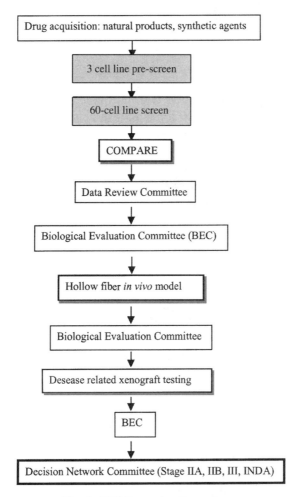

Fig. 2. NCI Screening Procedure.

4.1. Cell-Based Screening Assays

4.1.1. CONVENTIONAL CELLULAR SCREENS

Cellular screens in cancer research employ mainly permanent human tumor cell lines; their immortal nature and hence manageable, reproducible growth behavior make them suitable test systems. Of critical importance, however, is the detection method, the choice of which depends on the cell number used and thus the desired sensitivity. Various procedures to determine cell growth are employed in screening laboratories. The earliest broadly used growth inhibition assays were developed by Mosmann and the NCI screening staff, namely, the methylthiazoldiphenyl tetrazolium (MTT) assay. The yellow MTT dye is reduced by mitochondria into a purple formazan, which can be read with ultraviolet/visible light scanners *(21,22)*. Its limitations are the use of large quantities of a hazardous solvent, dimethyl sulfoxide, which is required to dissolve the resulting formazan crystals and the varying number of mitochondria in cells.

Currently employed in the NCI 60-cell-line screen is the sulforhodamine B (SRB) assay; SRB is a dye that stains protein *(23)*.

Most industrial-scale cellular screens prefer the use of fluorescence or luminescence detection systems. The latter include, for example, the propidium iodide (PI) assay staining for DNA content *(24)* or use of a luciferase reporter *(25,26)*. They appear to offer the most advantages, such as high sensitivity and easy handling.

The use of one-dimensional or monolayer cultures to measure cell growth is the most convenient and frequently applied method. Owing to tumor heterogeneity and three-dimensional in vivo growth, however, currently employed monolayer assays of human tumor (epithelial) cells are oversimplistic and have some disadvantages for the in vitro evaluation of certain anticancer agents:

1. Short-term culture conditions (2–6 d) may select for cytotoxic drugs.
2. Tumor cell growth can continue despite the fact that clonogenic cells are reduced, missing certain classes of cytostatic agents (e.g., inducers of cellular senescence).
3. Extracellular matrix and blood vessel targets (angiogenesis) are absent.
4. Gradients of oxygen tension, extracellular pH, nutrients, catabolites, and cell proliferation rate are a function of distance in solid tumors from blood vessels and are also not possible to mimic by monolayers *(27)*.
5. Drug penetration barriers occur only in multilayered solid tumors.

Drugs that are encompassed by this list include signal transduction inhibitors, antibodies, bioreductive drugs, anti-angiogenic peptides, small molecules, or antitelomerases. These classes of drugs therefore might best be examined in either specially designed cell systems and tailored screens or biochemical assays.

4.1.2. TAILORED CELLULAR SCREENS

Examples of successful in vitro models of a tumor environment using multicellular spheroids or postconfluent multicell layers for screening of bioreductive agents have been reported by Phillips et al. *(27,28)*. The latter showed that agents requiring bioactivation by the microenvironment such as mitomycin C or EO9 were differentially chemosensitive in plateau-phase multilayered cells as compared to exponentially growing monolayers. The novel structures RSU 1069 and SR4233 were found by this procedure *(27,28)*.

Over the past couple of years, the enzyme telomerase has been causally linked to immortalization and cancer and thus has arisen as a promising anticancer target *(29,30)*. Telomerase acts at the end of chromosomes termed telomeres by synthesizing telomeric repeat sequences. Telomeres are important noncoding sequences that protect chromosomes from end-to-end fusions and maintain chromosomal stability. In each round of cell division telomeric sequences (approx 30–100 bp) are lost owing to the end replication problem. As a result, cells expressing telomerase have an unlimited proliferation capacity, for example, cancer or renewal stem cells, while telomerase-negative cells will undergo replicative senescence when their telomeres become critically short *(30)*. Specific telomerase inhibition has been shown to require a certain number of population doublings or in vitro passages of tumor cells, a so-called lag time, to induce cessation of cell growth *(29,31)*. Such agents would be missed in, for example, the NCI screen based on a 48-h drug incubation period and most other conventional cellular screens.

Nonetheless, Nassani's and colleagues' approach to the identification of telomerase inhibitory agents employed parts of the NCI screening procedure, namely, the COMPARE algorithm *(14)*, which is an bioinformatic analysis of sensitivity patterns generated in preliminary random screens *(32)*. Nassani had carefully characterized a panel of tumor cell lines for telomerase and its components and used a "seed" compound with telomerase inhibitory activity, but low cytotoxic potency, berberine ($IC_{50} \sim 35 \ \mu M$), for search of better analogs.

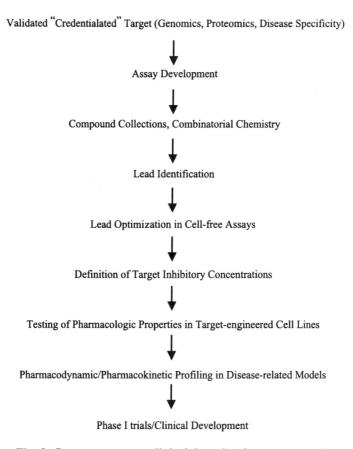

Validated "Credentialated" Target (Genomics, Proteomics, Disease Specificity)

↓

Assay Development

↓

Compound Collections, Combinatorial Chemistry

↓

Lead Identification

↓

Lead Optimization in Cell-free Assays

↓

Definition of Target Inhibitory Concentrations

↓

Testing of Pharmacologic Properties in Target-engineered Cell Lines

↓

Pharmacodynamic/Pharmacokinetic Profiling in Disease-related Models

↓

Phase I trials/Clinical Development

Fig. 3. Contemporary preclinical drug development cascade.

FJ5002 was found as a genuine and effective antitelomerase agent ($IC_{50} \sim 2$ μM) and is currently in preclinical development *(33)*.

A third example for tailored screens is the NCI angiogenesis screen, which was established after recommendations that NCI should facilitate research into mechanisms of tumor angiogenesis and the development of drugs that target the essential tumor vasculature (http://dtp.nci.nih.gov./aa-resources/aa_index.html). This program is unique inasmuch as it not only offers the screening of potential antiangiogenic drugs, but also distributes validated endothelial cells and the required reagents, controls (TNP470 [IC_{50} = 0.5–1.5 n*M*]), and reproducible angiogenesis bioassay procedures. A 72-h proliferation at passage 1–6 of primary endothelial cells is guaranteed to retain TNP470 sensitivity and endothelial markers in terms of proliferation, growth inhibition, cord formation, and migration. Because the screen has been inaugurated only recently, the discovery of new agents has not been reported so far.

4.2. Biochemical Screening Assays

Biochemical assays are compared to cellular assays "target-driven" and provide the means for evaluating high numbers of compounds *(2)*. These screens are primarily employed in the pharmaceutical industry and institutions that harbor large compound libraries for systematic search of novel agents. Figure 3 summarizes the procedure for such an approach.

An important advantage of biochemical screens is that they can be fully automated; thus, most steps can be performed by robot or computer systems such as dispensing of targets, addition of drugs and detection reagents, as well as compound library storage and management. Key requirements for target-oriented screening are:

1. The molecular target must be validated, shown to be causally linked to disease initiation or progression.
2. The target required for in vitro assays must be made available in large quantities, for example, by recombinant DNA techniques.
3. Defined, pure compound libraries comprising hundred of thousands of structures derived from combinatorial approaches or collections of natural substances should be available.
4. Simple, cost-effective, highly reproducible assay and detection systems, which can be performed in microplate formats *(34)*.

Suitable platforms have been proven to be enzyme linked immunoadsorbent assays (ELISA) and other enzyme-based colorimetric methods. Further technologies that are frequently used are: (1) radiometric assays dependent on scintillation proximity counting by employing scintillant-coated beads in microtiter plates; (2) time-resolved fluorescence based on highly fluorescing rare-earth metal–ligand chelates (europium, samarium, terbium); (3) fluorescence polarization; and (4) luminescence detection including chemiluminescence or electrochemiluminescence *(2)*.

Prominent targets for which these strategies have been employed and led to drugs that have progressed to advanced clinical development or even FDA approval are the protein kinases. For example, Gleevec™ (STI571) was found in an effort to develop bcr-abl kinase inhibitors. Bcr-abl is a chromosomal translocation product causing chronic myeloid leukemia, Gleevec has proven to be able to produce complete hematological and cytogenetic responses in this disease in patients *(35)*. Only careful testing of STI571 and its analogs in in vitro kinase assays and structural optimization of pharmacologic properties led to its success. If the agent would have been evaluated in a conventional cellular screen, it would have failed common activity criteria. In the NCI 60-cell-line screen, for example, only one cell line, namely K562, possesses the bcr-abl abnormality; in addition, STI571 antiproliferative activity as a means of IC_{50} concentration is rather low. Mow et al. found even in the K562 cell line values for colony formation in the order of 12 μM and IC_{90}s of target and growth inhibition of approx 20 μM *(36,37)*.

4.3. Combination of Target and Cell Screens

Both cell- and target-based screening procedures have clear advantages and disadvantages, while cell-based approaches will miss agents with certain defined modes of action such as, for example, specific telomerase inhibitors owing to lack of cytotoxic potency in short-term assays. They might, on the other hand, identify compounds as active with previously unknown targets and hence allow for identification of novel mechanisms of action as well as the elucidation of their interplay in certain pathways. An example of this from the NCI 60-cell-line screen is the spicamycin analog KRN5500. The compound was found potently active in the 48-h SRB assay over 68 cell lines, however, showing differential cytotoxicity in that six cell lines were exquisitely sensitive (IC_{50} = 5 nM), and 17 were resistant (IC_{50} > 10 μM), the pattern of activity in the screen was unique, indicating a novel mechanism of action *(14,38)*. Careful studies in the molecular mechanism of KRN5500 using sensitive and resistant cell lines revealed that the agent might target the enzymatic machinery or organelles important for proper glycoprotein processing, representing novel targets in cancer treatment. Thus, KRN5500-resistant cells had elevated levels of enzymes associated with the endoplasmic reticulum (ER), namely, glucose-6-phosphatase and

GalNAc transferase, while KRN5500-sensitive cells in contrast had high levels of ceramidase, an enzyme that is localized in the ER and Golgi apparatus and has been linked to carcinogenesis *(38–41)*.

Another advantage of compounds identified in cellular screens are their proven cell-permeable properties, which might be missing in cell-free systems. In addition, ligand interactions might be more appropriate in the biological environment.

Considering these facts, a combination of rational biochemical and "more" empirical cellular screening systems would therefore be the most optimal methodology in new cancer drug discovery.

We have recently applied this combination successfully in the identification of the novel CDK inhibitory agent E224 (5-methyl indirubin) *(42,43)*. Figure 4 shows the discovery process followed in our laboratories. E224 emerged from a discovery program that aimed to exploit active ingredients of Chinese traditional anticancer medicines for rational drug design. The *Indigo naturalis* constituent indirubin had previously been shown to possess activity against leukemia cells; hence, 20 analogs were synthesized and tested for in vitro antiproliferative activity using permanent cell lines in the propidium iodide assay *(24)* as well as xenografts in the clonogenic assay *(44)*. Whereas the compounds were inactive in the cell line screen ($IC_{50} > 30 \mu M$, Fig. 5), they showed some activity ranging from approx 10 to 50 μM in the clonogenic assay (data not shown). Had they been evaluated based only on monolayer cell line screening, these agents might have been discarded because of lack of potency. E224 and related compounds were further "rescued" by molecular mechanism based investigations into their effects on the cell cycle that revealed that they were able to block cell proliferation in the late G_1 and G_2/M phases. The latter effects gave an indication that cyclin-dependent kinases (CDKs) might be the target of indirubin analogs *(34,42)*. Indeed crystal structures of CDK2 with indigoids had shown atomic interactions with the kinase's ATP-binding pocket. Moreover, in a panel of more than 25 kinases, indirubin derivatives specifically inhibited the activity of CDK1 over CDK2, and CDK5 over CDK4 *(42)*. Because the IC_{50}s of kinase inhibition were similar to those of agents currently in clinical trials such as flavopiridol and roscovitine, the five most potent novel CDK inhibitors were selected for in vivo testing against the large-cell lung cancer xenograft LXFL 529, which was a very responsive line in the clonogenic assay. E224 showed marked in vivo activity against LXFL 529 lung cancer xenografts at doses of 100 mg/kg given once daily for 5 d for 3 wk intraperitoneally (Fig. 6). At a dose that was well tolerated, E224 was able to produce tumor remissions ($T/C = 9\%$). Thus, it seems that E224 has the pharmacodynamic and pharmacokinetic properties required for further preclinical development and that target-oriented combined with empirical assays (Fig. 4) are powerful screening methods.

5. USING MODEL ORGANISMS FOR SCREENING

Nonmammalian organisms as systems for anticancer drug screening arose in the late 1990s as a potential alternative to human models in the light of advances in genomic research. A group at the Fred Hutchinson Cancer Research Center in Seattle headed by Steven Friend proposed to use yeast (*Saccharomyces cerevisiae*), the nematode *Caenorhabditis elegans*, or the fruit fly *Drosophila melanogaster*, because they share similar signaling and growth regulatory pathways with humans *(45)*. The advantage, particularly of yeast, is that the complete genome comprises only 6250 defined genes, and, most importantly, many genes that are altered in human tumors have homologs in this model organism. For example, the *p53* tumor suppressor gene has its structural homolog in *RAD9*, the mismatch repair genes *MSH2* and *MSH1* in *MSH2^Sc^* and *MLH1^Sc^* or the *cyclins D* and *E* in *cyclin D^Dm^* and *cyclin E^Dm^*, respectively *(45)*. These models are therefore

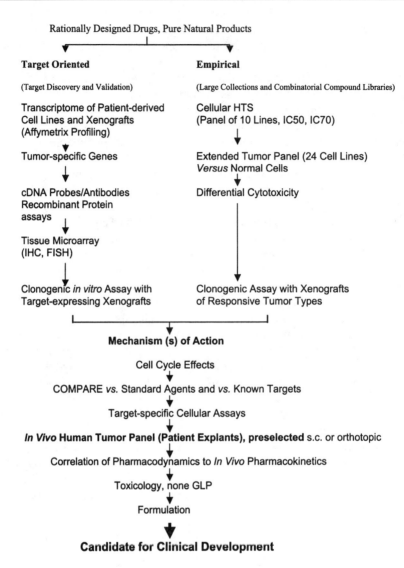

Fig. 4. The Freiburg approach to anticancer drug screening.

thought to provide a valuable resource to achieve a greater understanding about human cancer and hopefully give insights into new approaches for therapy. Friend and co-workers have chosen to employ DNA damage response elements/pathways to delineate mechanisms of actions of known, very effective anticancer agents (e.g., cisplatin in germ cell tumors) and to find novel targets for therapy by defining molecular changes underlying genetic instability of cancers, which they believe are mainly defects in DNA repair pathways, cell cycle checkpoints, and cell cycle transition. The group has determined the effects of cancer mutations on sensitivity or resistance to various chemotherapeutic agents in a panel of isogenic yeast strains, each defective in a particular DNA repair or cell cycle checkpoint function. Widely different toxicity profiles were observed for 23 standard

```
IN-VITRO ACTIVITY OF E224Q IN HUMAN TUMOR XENOGRAFTS (Monolayer Assay)                        13.04.99  09:46:11
```

TUMOR/ PASSAGE NO.	EXP. NO.	CTRL FLUOR. UNITS	Distribution of IC70 related to Mean log.scaled axis				IC50 ug/ml	IC70 ug/ml	IC90 ug/ml
			*0.01	*0.1	Mean ????????	*10	*100		

```
BCL
T24       ZF049AT  1474    >                   |                  .   >30.000    >30.000    >30.000
CCL
HT29      ZF052AT  7727    >                   |                  .   >30.000    >30.000    >30.000
SW620     ZG051AT  3275    >                   |                  .   >30.000    >30.000    >30.000
CXF
94L       ZG122AT  2350    >                   |                  .   >30.000    >30.000    >30.000
GXF
251L      ZG060AT  3434    >                   |                  .   >30.000    >30.000    >30.000
LCLS
DMS114    ZF110AT  1897    >                   |                  .   >30.000    >30.000    >30.000
DMS273    ZG048AT  ****    >                   |                  .   >30.000    >30.000    >30.000
LXFA
526L      ZG110AT  2047    >                   |                  .   >30.000    >30.000    >30.000
629L      ZG111AT  2580    >                   |                  .    46.377    >30.000    >30.000
LXFE
66NL      ZF111AT  2405    >                   |                  .   >30.000    >30.000    >30.000
A549      ZG049AT  6323    >                   |                  .   >30.000    >30.000    >30.000
LXFL
1072L     ZF048AT   570    >                   |                  .   >30.000    >30.000    >30.000
529L      ZF051AT  5287    >                   |                  .   >30.000    >30.000    >30.000
MACL
MCF7      ZF060AT  6064    >                   |                  .   >30.000    >30.000    >30.000
MDAMB46   ZF191AT   610    >                   |                  .   >30.000    >30.000    >30.000
MAXF
401NL     ZG115NT  2157    .                   |                  .
MEXF
462NL     ZF119AT  3166    >                   |                  .   >30.000    >30.000    >30.000
514L      ZG064AT  4119    >                   |                  .   >30.000    >30.000    >30.000
OVCL
OVCAR3    ZF115NT  3589    .                   |                  .
OVXF
899L      ZF192AT  1088    >                   |                  .   >30.000    >30.000    >30.000
PRCL
DU145     ZG109AT  3647    >                   |                  .   >30.000    >30.000    >30.000
PC3M      ZF109AT  4322    >                   |                  .   >30.000    >30.000    >30.000
RXF
486L      ZF122AT  3064    >                   |                  .   >30.000    >30.000    >30.000
944L      ZG119AT  4600    >                   |                  .   >30.000    >30.000    >30.000
UXF
1138L     ZF064AT  4670    >                   |                  .   >30.000    >30.000    >30.000

Mean               n=0         ????????                               46.377    ????????   ????????
```

Fig. 5. Sensitivity profile of E224 over 25 human tumor cell lines comprising the Freiburg panel. The mean IC_{50} and IC_{70} (inhibitory concentrations 50% and 70%) of E224 was >30 μM and thus the agent was considered inactive according to our selection criteria.

anticancer agents and X-ray treatment, indicating that the type of DNA repair and cell cycle checkpoint mutations in individual tumors could strongly influence the outcome of a particular chemotherapeutic regimen (46,47). While cisplatin was specifically toxic to yeast strains defective for the Rad6/Rad18-controlled pathway of damage tolerance during the S phase, sensitivity to the ribonucleotide reductase inhibitor hydroxyurea was seen in the intra-S-phase checkpoint-deficient mec1 and mec2 strains. Hence, some of the commonly used anticancer agents showed significant specificity in their killing in yeast, and this provides strong evidence that new molecular diagnostics could improve the utility of the standard therapies (46).

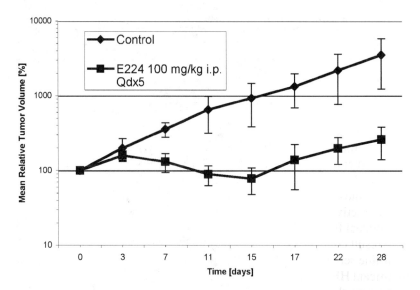

Fig. 6. Activity of E225 against the s.c. growing large cell lung carcinoma xenograft LXFL 529 in nude mice. The drug was given intraperitoneally five times a week for 3 wk. In this schedule E224 was very well tolerated and produced a tumor growth inhibition compared to control of 91% accompanied by partial regressions between d 11 and 15.

However, screening and predicting activity of anticancer agents in yeast is limited by some differences in biology of yeast and mammalian cells such as tubulin. Spindle poisons are not toxic to *S. cerevisiae* and are therefore not active against yeast tubulin. Hormones, growth factors, and prodrugs requiring metabolic activation also cannot be modeled in yeast *(45,46)*.

6. PREDICTIVITY OF SCREENING DATA

One of the key criteria for the strength/power of screening programs is their predictiveness of clinical response. Unfortunately, these analyses are very time consuming, as the process of preclinical and clinical development requires several years, so that outcomes of screens employing novel strategies are not yet foreseeable.

6.1. NCI Analysis of Activity in Preclinical Models and Early Clinical Trials

6.1.1. XENOGRAFTS

The review of NCI in vitro and in vivo screening efforts based on the 60 human cell line panel and xenograft testing in the 1990s has recently been published. The methods of the NCI procedures were mainly empirical during this time period and disease rather than target based *(10,47)*. Data were available on 39 agents with both xenograft data and Phase II trial results. The analysts found that histology of a particular preclinical model showing in vivo activity did not correlate with activity in the same human cancer histology. However, drugs with in vivo activity in a third of the tested xenograft models did correlate with ultimate activity in some Phase II trials. This and the fact that none of the currently registered anticancer drugs was devoid of activity in preclinical tumor models, but showed activity in the clinic, led to the conclusion that activity in in vivo models of compounds demonstrating in vitro activity remains desirable *(10,48)*.

The hollow fiber assay has proven a valuable interface for selecting development candidates from large pools of compounds with in vitro antiproliferative activity for expensive and time-consuming subcutaneous xenograft testing (Fig. 2).

6.1.2. HOLLOW-FIBER ASSAY

The HF assay was developed by Hollingshead et al. (16) at the NCI and is composed of 2-cm tubes filled with tumor cell lines. These fibers are implanted into mice at two sites (intraperitoneal and subcutaneous). The fibers are removed after 4–6 d in the animal and processed in vitro for quantification of tumor cell growth. By determining net cell kill, one can examine whether drugs administered via different routes are bioavailable and can reach the tumor sites (47).

Of 564 compounds tested in the HF model and that were also tested in in vivo xenografts, 20% showing HF activity also responded in xenograft models. This response was most likely if the intraperitoneal fiber activity was found in more than six intraperitoneal fibers. While a positive HF result could correctly predict in vivo xenograft response in one-fourth of the cases, 60-cell-line screening activity was able to predict correctly HF response in the order of 50%. Significant HF activity in more than six intraperitoneal fibers was likely if the mean IC_{50} for in vitro growth inhibition of a compound was below $10^{-7.5}$ M. These analyses showed that the HF assay is a very valuable, rapid model system with predictive value.

6.2. Predictive Value of the Colony-Forming Assay

Another combined in vitro/in vivo testing procedure is the soft agar colony-forming assay, also termed tumor clonogenic assay (TCA). The TCA can either be used for sensitivity screening of patient tumor material in vitro predicting direct clinical response, or with fresh xenograft tissue for selecting the most appropriate in vivo model (49–51). However, its high throughput application is limited by lack of reproducibility (unique sample material) and the elaborative assay procedure.

A correlation between in vitro human tumor sensitivities and clinical responses of the same patients was first established by Salmon and co-workers. Their results demonstrated a highly significant correlation of in vitro tumor resistance to specific drugs with failure of the patient to respond to the same drugs clinically. Although the prediction for resistance was very high, that for sensitivity was less precise. Although in vitro tumor sensitivity was noted in every case where the patient responded, there was a significant fraction of false-positive tests resulting in clinical therapy failure (49). Similar results were found in our laboratories when the response of xenograft tissue derived from patient tumors was compared to that of the patient. The TCA predicted correctly for tumor response in 62% and for resistance in 92% of the examined cases (50,51). The latter is mirrored by the even better response prediction of the Freiburg nude mouse xenografts if used in vivo.

6.3. Relationship Between Clinical Response and Patient Explants in Nude Mice

6.3.1. THE FREIBURG EXPERIENCE

Unlike the NCI in vivo screen, the Freiburg xenograft panel is derived directly from patient explants and not established from permanent human tumor cell line material. By comparing drug efficacy in patients and their tumors grown in nude mice, a total of 21 patients reached a remission. The same result was observed in 19 tumors growing as xenografts. 59 patients did not respond to treatment and the same result was found in 57 cases in the nude mouse system. Overall, xenografts gave a correct prediction for resistance in 97% (57/59) and for tumor responsiveness in 90% (19/21) (52).

Although most analyses of predictivity and usefulness of in vitro and in vivo screening procedures indicate clearly a high value of anticancer drug screens, particularly if validated by employing agents that have made it to the clinic, it remains uncertain how the new molecular targeted agents with no prior defined clinical activity will translate into patient benefit.

It also seems further to be certain that pure in vitro screening methodology will not be sufficient to delineate potential clinical activity, particularly because pharmacokinetics have a major impact on pharmacodynamic activity. Data derived from in vivo model systems deem necessary to ensure that drug concentrations inhibiting the target and in vitro cell growth to 100% or at least 50% can be reached.

7. CONCLUSIONS AND PERSPECTIVES

Preclinical screening is necessary to prioritize compounds for further development. In the era of target-oriented molecular cancer therapeutics, screening procedures are tailored toward the desired mechanism of tumor inhibition. They require, however, careful design and validation. In the past, empirical screens designed to find highly potent cytotoxic agents produced an arsenal of clinically used drugs with low selectivity and efficacy in solid tumors. Although antiproliferative activity is generally a desirable effect, it might bias toward finding compounds poisoning DNA and the cytoskeleton in the commonly used short-term cultures rather than drugs with novel mechanisms. However, empirical screening approaches combined with novel knowledge emerging from genome and proteome research as well as bioinformation technologies might be the most efficient way forward. The work reported recently by Scherf et al. from the NCI on a gene expression database for the molecular pharmacology of cancer is pointing in this very promising direction (19). The NCI group used cDNA microarray technology to assess the transcriptome of the 60 human cancer cell line panel. Clustering of the cell lines on the basis of their responses to drugs yielded unique gene patterns indicating mechanisms of sensitivity and resistance. For example, a negative correlation could be found between expression of the enzyme asparagine synthetase (ASNS) and L-asparaginase sensitivity in the panel lines. Certain leukemias lack ASNS and depend on exogenous L-asparagine for growth. By treating these cells with L-asparaginase, L-asparagine is depleted and they will cease growth, which was well demonstrated by employing genomics (19). If the bioinformatic and chemoinformatic analyses of the currently assembled RNA, DNA, and protein profiles of human cancer cells lead to credential/valid results such as the described ASNS sensitivity pattern, major advances will be made in new drug discovery with respect to speed of preclinical development and prediction of therapeutic usefulness.

ACKNOWLEDGMENTS

This work was supported by grants from the German Ministry for Education and Research (BMBF) and the US National Cancer Institute, Developmental Therapeutics Program as well as from the European Commission with a grant to A. M. B. (QLG1-CT-1999-01341).

REFERENCES

1. Sikora K, Advani S, Koroltchouk V, et al. Essential drugs for cancer therapy: a World Health Organization consultation. Ann Oncol 1999; 10:385–390.
2. Aherne W, Garret M, McDonald T, Workman P. Mechanism-based high-throughput screening for novel anticancer drug discovery. In: Baguley BC, Kerr DJ (eds). Anticancer Drug Development. London, UK; San Diego, CA: Academic Press, 2002, pp. 249–267.

3. Goldin A, Woolley PV, Tew KD, Schein PS. Sources of agents and their selection for antitumor activity screening. In: Hilgard P, Hellman K (eds). Anticancer Drug Development, Barcelona, Spain: Prous, 1983, pp. 9–45.

4. Simpson BT, Marsh MC. Chemotherapeutic experiments with coaltar dyes on spontaneous mouse tumors. J Cancer Res 1926; 10:50–60.

5. Mendel B. Action of ferricyanide on tumor cells. Am J Cancer 1937; 30:549–552.

6. Boyland E. Experiments on the chemotherapy of cancer. I. The effects of certain antibacterial substances and related compounds. Biochem J 1938; 32:1207–1213.

7. Shear MJ, Hartwell JL, Peters VB, et al. Some aspects of a joint institutional research program on chemotherapy of cancer: current laboratory and clinical experiments with bacterial polysaccharide and with synthetic organic compounds. In: Moulton FR (ed). Approaches to Tumor Chemotherapy. Washington DC: American Association for the Advancement Science, 1947, pp. 236–284.

8. Gilman A, Philips FS. The biological actions and therapeutic applications of the B-chloroethyl amines and sulfides. Science 1946; 103:409–415.

9. Faber S, Diamond LK, Mercer RD, et al. Temporary remissions in acute leukemia in children produced by folic acid antagonists, 4-aminopteroyl-glutamic acid (aminopterin). N Engl J Med 1948; 238:787–793.

10. Johnson JI, Decker S, Zaharevitz D, et al. Relationships between drug activity in the NCI preclinical in vitro and in vivo models and early clinical trials. Br J Cancer 2001; 84:1424–1431.

11. Zubrod CG, Schepartz S, Leiter J, et al. The chemotherapy program of the National Cancer Institute: history, analysis and plans. Cancer Chemother Rep 1966; 50:349–540.

12. Venditti JM. Preclinical drug development: rationale and methods. Semin Oncol 1981; 8:349–361.

13. Monks A, Scudiero D, Shoemaker R, et al. Feasibility of a high-flux anticancer drug screen using a diverse panel of cultured human tumor cell lines. J Natl Cancer Inst 1991; 83:757–766.

14. Paull KD, Shoemaker RH, Hodes L, et al. Display and analysis of patterns of differential activity of drugs against human tumor cell lines: development of mean graph and COMPARE algorithm. J Natl Cancer Inst 1989; 81:1088–1092.

15. Dykes DJ, Abbott BJ, Mayo JG, et al. Development of human tumor xenograft models for in vivo evaluation of new antitumor drugs. In: Fiebig HH, Berger DP (eds). Contributions to Oncology, Vol. 42: Immunedeficient Mice in Oncology. Basel: Karger, 1992, pp. 1–22.

16. Hollingshead M, Plowman J, Alley MC, Mayo J, Sausville E. The hollow fibre assay. In: Fiebig HH, Burger AM (eds). Contributions to Oncology, Vol. 54: Relevance of Tumor Models for Anticancer Drug Development. Basel: Karger, 1999, pp. 109–120.

17. Plowman J, Camalier R, Alley M, Sausville E, Schepartz S. US-NCI testing procedures. In: Fiebig HH, Burger AM (eds). Contributions to Oncology, Vol. 54: Relevance of Tumor Models for Anticancer Drug Development. Basel: Karger, 1999, pp. 121–135.

18. Sausville EA, Feigal E. Evolving approaches to cancer drug discovery and development at the National Cancer Institute, USA. Ann Oncol 1999; 10:1287–1291.

19. Scherf U, Ross DT, Waltham M, et al. A gene expression database for the molecular pharmacology of cancer. Nat Genet 2000; 24:236–244.

20. Beveridge M, Park YW, Hermes J, Marenghi A, Brophy G, Santos A. Detection of p56ick kinase activity using scintillation proximity assay in 384-well format and imaging proximity assay in 384- and 1536-well format. J Biomol Screen 2000; 5:205–211.

21. Mosmann T. Rapid colorimetric assay for cellular growth and survival: application to proliferation and cytotoxicity assays. J Immunol Methods 1983; 65:55–63.

22. Alley MC, Scudiero DA, Monks A, et al. Feasibility of drug screening with panels of human tumor cell lines using a microculture tetrazolium assay. Cancer Res 1988; 48:589–601.

23. Skehan P, Storeng R, Scudiero D, et al. New colorimetric assay for anticancer-drug screening. J Natl Cancer Inst 1990; 82:1107–1112.

24. Dengler W, Schulte J, Berger DP, Mertelsmann R, Fiebig HH. Development of a propidium iodide fluorescence assay for proliferation and cytotoxicity assays. Anticancer Drugs 1995; 6:522–532.

25. Crouch SPM, Kozlowski R, Slater KJ, Fletcher J. The use of ATP bioluminescence as a measure of cell proliferation and cytotoxicity. J Immunol Methods 1993; 160:81–88.

26. Andreotti PE, Cree IA, Kurbacher CM, et al. Chemosensitivity testing of human tumors using a microplate adenosine triphosphate luminescence assay: clinical correlation for cisplatin resistance of ovarian carcinoma. Cancer Res 1995; 55:5276–5282.

27. Phillips RM. In vitro models of solid-tumour biology and drug delivery: implications for and applications to target-oriented screening for novel anticancer drugs. In: Fiebig HH, Burger AM (eds). Con-

tributions to Oncology, Vol. 54: Relevance of Tumor Models for Anticancer Drug Development. Basel: Karger, 1999, pp. 67–80.

28. Phillips RM, Clayton MRK. Plateau phase cultures: an experimental model for identifying drugs which are bioactivated within the microenvironment of solid tumours. Br J Cancer 1997; 75:196–201.

29. Kelland RL. Telomerase: biology and phase I trials. Lancet Oncol 2001; 2:95–102.

30. Holt SE, Shay JW, Wright WE. Refining the telomere-telomerase hypothesis of aging and cancer. Nat Biotechnol 1996; 14:1734–1741.

31. Damm K, Hemmann U, Garin-Chesa P, et al. A highly selective telomerase inhibitor limiting human cancer cell proliferation. EMBO J 2001; 20:6958–6968.

32. Nassani I, Yamori T, Tsuruo T. Screening with COMPARE analysis for telomerase inhibitors. In: Double JA, Thompson MJ (eds). Methods in Molecular Biology, Vol. 191: Telomeres and Telomerase. Totowa, NJ: Humana Press, 2002, pp. 197–207.

33. Nassani I, Seimiya H, Yamori T, Tsuruo T. FJ5002: a potent telomerase inhibitor identified by exploiting the disease-oriented screening program with COMPARE analysis. Cancer Res 1999; 59:4004–4011.

34. Schächtele C, Trotzke F, Mundt M, Finkenzeller G, Marme D. Robot screening: a new dimension in target-oriented drug discovery. In: Fiebig HH, Burger AM (eds). Contributions to Oncology, Vol. 54: Relevance of Tumor Models for Anticancer Drug Development. Basel: Karger, 1999, pp. 249–260.

35. Goldman JM. Tyrosine-kinase inhibition in treatment of chronic myeloid leukaemia. Lancet 2000; 355:1031–1032.

36. Mow BM, Chandra J, Svingen PA, et al. Effects of the Bcr/abl kinase inhibitors STI571 and adaphostin (NSC 680410) on chronic myelogenous leukemia cells in vitro. Blood 2002; 99:664–671.

37. Krystal GW, Honsawek S, Litz J, Buchdunger E. The selective tyrosine kinase inhibitor STI571 inhibits small cell lung cancer growth. Clin Cancer Res 2000; 6:3319–3326.

38. Burger AM, Kaur G, Hollingshead M, et al. Antiproliferative activity in vitro and in vivo of the spicamycin analogue KRN5500 with altered glycoprotein expression in vitro. Clin Cancer Res 1997; 3:455–463.

39. Kamishohara M, Kenney S, Domergue R, Vistica DT, Sausville EA. Selective accumulation of the endoplasmic reticulum–Golgi intermediate compartment induced by the antitumor drug KRN5500. Exp Cell Res 2000; 256:468–479.

40. Kenny S, Kamishohara M, Boswell J, Sausville EA, Vistica D. KRN5500: an antileukemic analog of ceramide. Proc Am Assoc Cancer Res 2002; 43:409.

41. Seelan RS, Qian C, Yokomizo A, Bostwick DG, Smith DI, Liu W. Human acid ceramidase is overexpressed but not mutated in prostate cancer. Genes Chromosomes Cancer 2000; 29:137–146.

42. Hoessel R, Leclerc S, Endicott JA, et al. Indirubin, the active constituent of a Chinese antileukaemia medicine, inhibits cyclin-dependent kinases. Nat Cell Biol 1999; 1:60–67.

43. Marko D, Schatzle S, Friedel A, et al. Inhibition of cyclin-dependent kinase 1 (CDK1) by indirubin derivatives in human tumour cells. Br J Cancer 2001; 84:283–289.

44. Fiebig HH, Schmid JR, Bieser W, Henss H, Löhr GW. Colony assay with human tumor xenografts, murine tumors and human bone marrow. Potential for anticancer drug development. Eur J Cancer Clin Oncol 1987; 23:937–948.

45. Hartwell LH, Szankasi P, Roberts CJ, Murray AW, Friend S. Integrating genetic approaches into the discovery of anticancer drugs. Science 1997; 278:1064–1068.

46. Simon JA, Szankasi P, Nguyen DK, et al. Differential toxicities of anticancer agents among DNA repair and checkpoint mutants of Saccharomyces cerevisiae. Cancer Res 2000; 60:328–333.

47. Gura, T. Systems for identifying new drugs are often faulty. Science 1997; 278:1041–1042.

48. DeVita JV. Principles of chemotherapy. In: DeVita VT, Hellmann S, Rosenberg SA (eds). Cancer Principles & Practice of Oncology, 3rd Edit. Philadelphia, PA: Lippincott, 1989, pp. 277–300.

49. Salmon, SE, Hamburger AW, Soehnlen B, Durie BGM, Alberts DS, Moon TE. Quantitation of differential sensitivity of human-tumor stem cells to anticancer drugs. N Engl J Med 1978; 298:1321–1327.

50. Scholz CC, Berger DP, Winterhalter BR, Henss H, Fiebig HH. Correlation of drug response in patients and in the clonogenic assay using solid human tumor xenografts. Eur J Cancer 1990; 26:901–905.

51. Burger AM, Fiebig HH. Screening using animal systems. In: Baguley BC, Kerr DJ (eds). Anticancer Drug Development. San Diego, CA: Academic Press, 2001, pp. 285–297.

52. Fiebig HH, Dengler WA, Roth T. Human tumor xenografts: predictivity, characterization and discovery of new anticancer agents. In: Fiebig HH, Burger AM (eds). Contributions to Oncology, Vol 54: Relevance of Tumor Models for Anticancer Drug Development. Basel: Karger, 1999, pp. 29–50.

3

Mouse Models in Cancer Drug Discovery and Development

Edward A. Sausville, MD
and Melinda Hollingshead, DVM, PhD

CONTENTS

1. INTRODUCTION

The basis for proceeding with development of an anticancer agent has historically resulted in part from the capacity of the agent to inhibit tumor cell proliferation either in tissue culture (in vitro) or in animals (in vivo), without specific reference to a molecular or cellular target of action. Indeed, the potentially useful effects of the vast majority of agents currently approved for use as safe and effective as oncologic therapeutics in humans were initially detected by their favorable performance in mouse models of human cancer. This chapter provides an overview of the types of mouse models used in cancer drug discovery and development, their strengths and limitations, how to interpret them, and caveats in the consideration of results from commonly used murine model studies. The algorithm currently in use at the National Cancer Institute (NCI) in the United States is presented. This chapter is meant to be a practical, working summary of practice rather than a comprehensive review of the topic. For the latter, the reader is encouraged to seek more encyclopedic treatments (*1–3*, among others).

2. GOALS OF PRECLINICAL MOUSE MODEL STUDIES

The scientific goal to which the use of mouse models extends is the detection and refinement of lead structures to develop a clinical candidate. Murine efficacy models are

Handbook of Anticancer Pharmacokinetics and Pharmacodynamics
Edited by: W. D. Figg and H. L. McLeod © Humana Press Inc., Totowa, NJ

usually used in conjunction with chemical and pharmacology studies to develop a series of analogs and to compare handling of development candidates by the physiologic milieu of a living host. These developmental iterations require that useful animal models be geared to accommodate reasonable throughput to assess several, perhaps dozens, of lead structures. The ultimately successful clinical agent will have an impact on the survival of the patient cohort treated with the new agent compared to "standard" approaches. Therefore, mouse models must be useful in predicting either response (measured by tumor shrinkage) or protracted cytostatic effect.

A key point to be emphasized is that no single mouse model is appropriate for use throughout a drug's development. The information obtained from each model depends on the question asked, and drugs actually require different types of models at different times in their development cycle. "Pharmacology" models may be used to qualify a compound for more detailed studies, whereas "efficacy" models define the potential for a biologic effect. The latter may be specifically driven by a particular presumptive molecular target (e.g., activated oncogene or deleted tumor suppressor gene) or may be target nonselected. "Biological" models constructed to reflect the operation of a single target or defined multiple targets may be useful in confirming that the drug target or downstream events dependent on the target(s) are affected by the drug.

One option to accommodate the need for high to medium throughput is to use rodent tumors grown in syngeneic or allogeneic rodent hosts. This includes "classic" models such as Lewis lung carcinoma and L1210 or P388 leukemia. These have the advantage of immunocompetence of the host, and they often allow assessment of metastasis and tissue invasion into homologous stroma. Immunocompromised models such as athymic "nude" mouse models or mice with severe combined immunodeficiency (SCID) have the advantage that human cells may actually be studied. These tumors may be implanted in the animal in an "artificial" site to facilitate measurement of drug effect (e.g., subcutaneously), or in an "orthotopic" location to mimic the site of tumor origin. Orthotopic implants may offer a physiology more like the disease state being modeled, and they certainly provide different pharmacodynamic profiles from subcutaneous implants.

In contrast, "biology" models are geared for close correspondence to the human disease, and therefore the throughput of compounds must necessarily be of lesser concern when developing and implementing these models. Typically, such models have long latency and incomplete incidence or penetrance of the cancer phenotype. Examples include *bona fide* spontaneous tumor occurrences usually seen in senescent or virally infected (e.g., mouse mammary tumor virus) animals, as well as carcinogen-induced models. "Metastasis" models are optimized by removal of a primary transplanted tumor followed by an incubation period to allow microscopic lesions to grow to detectable levels. These have similarities to the outcomes obtained following surgical resection of a primary human tumor. Engineered animals are created by "transgenic" or "knockout" technologies that manipulate embryos in vitro and reintroduce the marked embryonic cells in a way that leads to animals chimeric for the gene desired. Through serial crosses, lineages of animals with or without a gene of interest can be generated and genetically stabilized.

3. ISSUES IN ANY MOUSE MODEL

The potential usefulness of any murine model is critically dependent on the "take rate" or fraction of animals in which the tumor grows following implantation. The tumor "take rate" determines the number of mice required for each experiment and thus governs the practicality and cost of an experiment. A key requirement in conducting an efficacy experiment is the need to properly randomize treatments equitably across the incidence or "take rates" intrinsic to the model. Without a clear explanation as to the randomization scheme used, interlaboratory reproducibility of the model or its results can be hampered. Whether a tumor is propagated by serial animal passage or by inoculation of cultured cells, it is critical to data interpretation that similar inoculum sizes be compared. This should drive selection of a randomization method that distributes variations in the tumor "take rate" and inoculum (e.g., viability, cell aggregation) across treatment groups to avoid inadvertent accumulation of these effects in a single treatment group.

When selecting a treatment schema, the route of drug administration and its relevance to the clinic can convey greater or lesser confidence in the utility and validity of the model. For example, intraperitoneal treatment of tumors propagated in the abdominal cavity, and intratumoral treatments in general, are less useful evidence supporting a compound for development than activity observed across physiological barriers, for example, intravenous or intraperitoneal treatment of subcutaneously growing tumor. The desire to mimic clinically relevant treatment schemes is one area in which murine models fall short. Because of the physical limitations of mice, it is extremely difficult to mimic the continuous or frequent intravenous administration schedules possible in the human patient.

The importance of proper vehicle selection cannot be overstated. The vehicle affects the solubility, absorbability, and toxicity of a compound in ways that can impair detection of activity. Where possible, the selected vehicle should be practical in humans. For example, in the United States, dimethyl sulfoxide or high concentrations of ethanol, dimethyl formamide, or dimethyl acetamide are not readily translated to clinical use despite their facile use for mouse studies. The use of "suspensions" of incompletely dissolved compounds is to be discouraged.

How and when to evaluate efficacy in the selected tumor model is an additional key variable. The time at which treatment is initiated can profoundly affect the degree of activity detected. Generally, the treatment starting time is selected based on what is known about the compound mechanism of action and its pharmacological profile. Treatment can be initiated before tumors are detected, or it can be delayed until the tumors "stage." In "staged" models the tumors are allowed to achieve a preselected size before treatment is initiated. "Early treatment" models (in which treatment starts within a few days after tumor implantation and before the animal has evidence of disease) are less demanding than "staged" models. Early treatment schedules can truly be used only for robustly growing tumors with predictable growth kinetics and a 90–100% "take rate." "Early-stage" models, in contrast to "early-treatment" models, are defined as those in which treatment commences when the tumor stages (described below) to between 63 and 200 mg wet weight. In "advanced-stage" models treatment initiates when the tumors stage at 200 mg or more. The later, or more advanced, the stage of tumor to be treated, the larger the number of animals that must be entumored, as heterogeneity in growth rates will frequently limit the number of animals that reach the desired "staging" size at the same time. In addition to the measurement of response rates described below, advanced-stage models allow scoring of the number and type of regressions ("partial" or "complete") and duration of survival, and more faithfully mimic the clinically important endpoints.

During conduct of efficacy models, it is important to determine whether treatment-related toxicities are occurring. In addition to the obvious significance of lethality, indications of treatment toxicity can be deduced from body weight loss. Generally, weight loss in excess of 20% of the starting body weight, in the absence of an analogous effect in the tumor-bearing, vehicle-treated groups, is evidence of drug toxicity.

The schedule of administration may be empirical, based on the tumor growth rate, or it may be designed around the pharmacology of the compound or its known capacity to affect the desired target. The need to explore a variety of schedules is one reason why efficacy models are frequently geared to high throughput, as optimization of a schedule often requires different schedules to be systematically examined. Empirical schedules utilize frequent administration for rapidly doubling tumors, to weekly schedules for tumors with doubling times of 6–10 d. Ideally, in the future the empirical approach will be tied to knowledge of the concentrations and exposure times of drug required to achieve an effect on the tumor's biological target(s) of interest.

Selection of the tumor model for efficacy evaluations is another factor to consider in the development of a clinical candidate. Models can be selected empirically using various factors (e.g., cost, availability, familiarity). However, many drug development programs select the tumor models based on in vitro data demonstrating the capacity of the test agent to modulate cell proliferation, molecular target expression, or other desired endpoints. While this is a viable method for tumor selection, it is not without complications. For example, human tumor cell lines propagated in the subcutaneous compartment of immunocompromised animals have enormous variations in growth rate (from a doubling time of approx 1–3 d, e.g., LOX IMVI and SK-MEL-28 to >12 d for the M19-MEL melanomas; ref. 1) and highly variable take rates (10–100%). These factors significantly limit the feasibility of developing murine tumor models from many of the well-characterized tumor cell lines currently available.

4. GENERAL PROCEDURES FOR MOUSE MODEL STUDIES

To evaluate a compound in animal models, a starting treatment dose must be selected. This is most commonly based on the maximum tolerated dose (MTD) of the compound. Thus, an initial study commences with determination of the MTD of the agent. Typically, one mouse each of the same strain to be used in the efficacy model is treated with 50% deescalating doses from 400 mg/kg. Animals are held for up to 14 d, quantifying morbidity (weight loss) and mortality. Dose levels are sought that define an LD_{10}, or lethal dose for 10% of the animals treated. This dose is used as a basis for calculating an initial dosing scheme. Although larger numbers of animals and additional dose levels provide more robust data, they also consume large amounts of the test material, which often is available in limited supply particularly early in its development.

A convenient way of displaying data from mouse model experiments in which reliable tumor measurements can be obtained (e.g., subcutaneous implant sites) is to calculate an approximate tumor weight. For this approximation, the tumor is measured in two dimensions and the mass is calculated using the formula for the volume of a prolate ellipsoid and assuming unit specific gravity:

$$\text{Tumor weight} = \text{Tumor volume} = \frac{\text{Length (mm)} \times [\text{Width (mm)}]^2}{2} \qquad (1)$$

On a particular treatment schedule, evidence of drug effect is described by the following parameters:

$$\% \ T/C = \frac{\Delta \text{ Tumor weight (median) of treated group}}{\Delta \text{ Tumor weight (median) of control group}} \times 100 \qquad (2)$$

or, for $\Delta T < 0$,

$$\% \ T/C = \frac{\Delta \text{ Tumor weight (median) of treated group}}{\text{Initial tumor weight}} \times 100 \qquad (3)$$

$$\text{Growth delay} = (T - C)/C \times 100 \qquad (4)$$

where T and C are the median times to reach a predetermined weight or number of tumor doublings in the treated and control groups, respectively.

$$\text{Net log cell kill} = \frac{\left[(T - C) - \text{treatment duration}\right] \times 0.31}{\text{Tumor doubling time}} \qquad (5)$$

where T and C are as given for growth delay.

Not all tumor models can be defined by direct measurement of tumor volume during the in-life experimental phase. More often than not, the orthotopic models do not afford the opportunity to observe tumor growth without sacrificing the host. Many of these can be monitored by recording the time required to produce a lethal tumor burden. These "challenge" survival models include intraperitoneally propagated tumors as well as many other orthotopic implant sites, for example, intracerebrally administered glioma models or intravenously administered lymphomas. For these, the "increased lifespan" (ILS), or increased time to some easily definable endpoint such as hind limb paralysis in the case of the lymphoma models, is defined by

$$\% \text{ ILS} = \left[(T - C)/C\right] \times 100 \qquad (6)$$

where T and C are the median times to reach the defined endpoint for the treated group and vehicle-treated control group, respectively.

The degree of activity to support further development of a compound is to a certain extent a matter of interpretation. A fairly stringent position (e.g., see ref. 2) is that suitable candidates for further development should possess at least two $\log_{10}$ cell kill, implying obvious significant regressions of measurable tumors. A distinct position that is less stringently demanding would utilize a T/C <40% at some point in the compound's treatment course as evidence of an antineoplastic action, particularly if occurring in a model that is resistant to the known antineoplastic agents. The number of treated animals influences the strength of the conclusion. A T/C <40% as a minimal criterion of activity is based on models with control groups of at least 20 mice in the vehicle-treated group, and with at least three treatment groups of six mice in each dose level, and where evidence of drug toxicity occurs only in the top dose group, with activity in the absence of drug toxicity occurring at least one dose level below the dose level demonstrating toxicity. A valid experiment likewise will ideally not have evidence of "no takes" or spontaneous regressions in the control groups.

5. STANDARD NCI APPROACHES

The standard NCI xenograft protocol initially expands cells from in vitro culture by implanting 10^7 cells/mouse subcutaneously on the lateral body wall just caudal to the front limb near the axillary region. These implants are monitored for growth and are passed to recipient mice when they reach about 400 mg. This is achieved by collecting the donor tumor, mincing it into 30- to 40-mg fragments, and transferring these fragments into recipient mice. With each serial passage the doubling time between 200 and 400 mg is determined, and the tumor is used for a treatment experiment when the doubling time appears stable.

Additional issues to consider in the design and interpretation of xenograft experiments include tumor dependency on hormonal supplementation, for example, estradiol for MCF-7 breast tumor xenografts; the need for special matrices, for example, Matrigel®, to support optimal tumor growth, the superiority of SCID mice to athymic mice for hematological tumors, and for some of the genetically manipulated models the need for antibiotic-driven modulation of specific gene products. The presence of a vehicle-treated control group is absolutely necessary for proper data interpretation. Often, an untreated control group can aid in data interpretation, particularly if there are vehicle-related effects. An adequate number of mice must be used so as to be confident of differences in the treatment groups. The number used depends on the degree of significance desired and the number of spontaneously regressing tumors. Although more extensive statistical treatment has been given to the issues (4) in general, as noted above, for tumors with 100% take rates, and a minimal response threshold set at % T/C of ≤40, one needs 16–20 vehicle control mice and 6–10 for each dose group. To maintain the statistical validity of the data, one must randomize animals to treatment groups to avoid experimental bias. The method of randomization will depend on the tumor treatment protocol being used. For staged tumor models, randomization should produce groups with comparable tumor burdens at the start of each experiment. For early treatment subcutaneous models, intraperitoneal tumors, and other orthotopic models, randomization should produce groups that are not biased by potential variability in tumor inoculation. Ideally, the operator should be also blinded to the treatment and control injections, but this is not always feasible.

Early-treatment (treatment is begun before tumor is measurable) or early-stage (tumor is 63–200 mg) models are suitable for use only with tumors with take rates of 90% or greater and spontaneous regression rate of 10% or less. Advantages of this type of model are the ability to assess the effect of chronic dosing, the ability to initiate treatment before the tumor has vascularized, and the potential to use essentially all mice inoculated. A major disadvantage is the questionable relevance to the advanced tumors encountered in humans. Conversely, these models may be highly relevant for assessing adjuvant treatment potential.

Advanced-stage tumor models (> 200 mg tumor size) have the contrasting advantage of the ability to score parameters relevant to the clinic such as partial and complete regressions and tumor-free survivors and the ability to score the effect of drug on some aspects of tumor stroma formation. The disadvantages include a relatively long duration for each experiment (6–12 wk in some models), the need for larger numbers of mice to be entumored to allow randomization for comparable groups of tumor sizes, and the possibility that an active compound will be missed in these more strenuous models if the dose, route, schedule, and formulation have not been optimized.

6. CORRELATION OF ACTIVITY IN MOUSE MODELS WITH CLINICAL ACTIVITY

Mouse model testing is ultimately of value only if the process identifies compounds with the potential for subsequently demonstrating activity in the clinic. Early studies (5) employed mouse leukemia models grown intraperitoneally to detect activity of agents subsequently found to be active in human leukemia. To increase the likelihood of detecting compounds with activity in solid tumors, from 1975 to 1985 the NCI screened compounds in a series of murine syngeneic and human xenograft models. A recent review of compounds entered into clinical trials on the basis of activity in these models, or of standard agents studied in these models as controls, has been reported (6). There was, in general, little correlation between the activity of a compound in a particular tumor histology in the mouse and activity in the homologous tumor type in humans. However, of agents demonstrating activity in > 33% of the mouse models tested, approx 50% went on to demonstrate activity in at least two disease types in humans. In contrast, no compounds had activity in at least two diseases among the understandably small number of compounds that were advanced to clinical testing despite activity in < 33% of the models tested. Other monographs (1,7) have demonstrated that subcutaneous xenografts from human solid tumors in general tend to be resistant to most of the currently used "standard" agents, at least when assessed in terms of the induction of partial or complete responses. Thus, mouse models actually reliably predict resistance and seem to indicate compounds with the potential for clinical utility. Moreover, advanced-stage mouse models are easily related to response criteria that can be turned into clinically useful endpoints. A clear problem with the empirical use of tumor response in only some fraction of human xenograft mouse models remains the practical implications for a drug development plan based not on the clear ability of a drug to alter a defined physiologic process, but on drug behavior in arbitrarily available or experimentally tractable models. How to translate evidence of activity in preclinical models to maximal efficiency in clinical development remains problematic. A related issue to current interest in developing nontoxic, potentially "cytostatic" therapies is that mice are suitable for assessing cytostatic effects in a variety of tumor models; however, translating these results into clinically relevant, easily adoptable cytostatic endpoints in humans is less clear.

7. CAUTIONS IN THE USE OF MOUSE MODELS

Implicit in the data described above is the concern that mouse xenograft models are, at best, generally but not specifically, predictive of drug activity in the human. Caveats in the interpretation of mouse model efficacy data can be assigned to reasons in one of four major categories. First, murine pharmacology and metabolism of compounds can differ significantly from humans. For example, camptothecins are highly active in several murine xenograft models (8). However, the drugs as a class are active only in the lactone form, and mouse plasma can stabilize the lactone (9). In contrast, human plasma actually favors production of the hydrolyzed form, so one should expect mouse models to overstate the potential of camptothecins in humans. Second, intrinsic differences between the susceptibility of mouse and human target normal organs to the toxic effects of an agent may skew the assessment of therapeutic index. An example of this is the bone marrow sensitivity of different species to bizelesin, a DNA minor groove-binding agent. It causes inhibition of murine bone marrow proliferation at concentrations in the nanomolar range. In contrast, human marrow is inhibited at concentrations in the picomolar range. Thus, the compound was predicted to have a much larger therapeutic index than was ultimately observed in the human (10). Third, the target affected by the drug may have an intrinsically different activity in murine vs human tumor and normal cells. This issue is exemplified by brefeldin, a cyclic lactone, which causes inhibition of secretory processes in human cells at concentrations of approx 0.1 μM, whereas the same process in murine cells is affected at concentrations of approx 1 μM (11). Thus, human tumors growing in mice have an intrinsically very favorable therapeutic index (12). Finally, an issue that arises most commonly during evaluations of biologically based reagents such as immunotoxins or growth factors is the absence of a murine homolog of the human target. Alternatively, the target may exist but have a radically different affinity for the agent. The most egregious example of this problem occurred in the evaluation of an anti-Le[y]-directed doxorubicin conjugate, which produced dramatic cures of human tumors in mice (13). However, mice do not possess the Le[y] antigen so they did not predict for the noteworthy gastrointestinal toxicity that occurred when the construct was introduced into human use (14).

Strategies to leverage the risks associated with using mouse models to prioritize compounds for development build on efforts to avoid these types of problems. An initial guiding principle is that the activity of a candidate compound in mouse models should be understood very clearly in relation to its plasma concentration versus time profile. Thus, even if the target of drug action is unknown or ambiguous, relatively small human Phase I trials can indicate whether analogous levels are achievable in humans, and thus avoid committing to full-scale development until human pharmacology is considered. Second, in the current age of targeted therapy, linking activity in a mouse model to the achievement of target modulation when administered by the favored clinical route is an important advantage. For example, STI-571 (Gleevec®) was qualified for use in humans not only on the basis of its capacity to modulate differentially p210$^{bcr-abl}$ tyrosine phosphorylation in vitro but also on the capacity of oral and parenteral dose forms to accomplish this in subcutaneous xenografts of target-bearing cells *(15)*. Third, where a target for toxicity is known, building an assessment of the plasma area under the curve for toxic as well as efficacious concentrations, across a range of species, may place the degree of activity observed in the mouse in context of the likely human therapeutic index. Although this is most readily achieved for bone marrow cultures, efforts to define suitable endpoints for cardiac, hepatic, and other large organ toxicities are underway. The most informed use of mouse models therefore considers not only the degree of compound activity *per se* but also the pharmacodynamic features of activity and toxicity.

A final caution relates to the type and nature of activity seen. Again as emphasized by Corbett et al. *(2)*, any drug that performs well only in syngeneic models should be considered as possibly having an immune basis for its action, or contributing to its efficacy. In allogeneic or xenografted models, "excessive" activity with cures across multiple dose levels should raise the possibility of greatly different intrinsic susceptibilities to the agent on the part of the host organism as compared to the tumor cells, and furthermore raises the possibility of differential metabolism of the agent by the tumor compartment.

8. SPECIALIZED, ENGINEERED MODELS

Recent technological advances have allowed the derivation of mouse strains containing genes important in the pathogenesis of cancer to be either introduced (transgenic) or deleted (knockout) from inbred strains of mice *(16)*. These models have clearly been of enormous utility in enhancing our understanding of the biological basis of cancer development. Mating strains with defined lesions in complementary pathways has allowed assessment of the interaction between multiple targets. Initial enthusiasm for the use of these models in the drug discovery and development process has given way to uncertainty as to how best to use these resources.

The first issue relates to how representative or validated the engineered mouse models might be with respect to human disease. Although in many cases the engineered mouse models have several features that recall the human disease, in no case has the correspondence been exact. A second concern is where in the development process these models should be used. There is, depending on the model and the strain, a degree of variability in the latency and penetrance of the phenotype. Because of this, many animals must be maintained to have sequential cohorts of animals uniformly reach the tumor size or stage that allows comparisons among different treatments. Indeed, some efforts to use engineered animal models have identified three phases for treatment approaches in the natural course of their evolution. These include "prevention," "early intervention," and "late intervention" phases of the same model within mice of the same genetic background (e.g., ref. *17*). Several study agents have documented differences in efficacy in each of the different phases of these models, resulting in a lack of certainty in how to translate the results obtained in the models to particular analogous stages in the natural history of human tumors. Furthermore, this circumstance is not amenable to the evaluation of more than a few compounds or combinations at once even in the largest industrial or academic laboratories. Thus, engineered animal models of the transgenic or knockout variety may be ill suited to evaluations of multiple analogs and schedules, as is often required for the earlier stages of development. In addition, compounds at an early point in their development are often poorly defined in terms of optimal dose, route, and schedule as well as formulation. This causes a real concern as to how comparable the different treatment groups in an engineered model actually are in the absence of correlative pharmacology studies. For many drugs that target pathogenic mechanisms, treatments of extended duration are likely necessary. This requires large amounts of compound, protracted treatment schedules, frequent mouse handling, and significant time commitments, further complicating the issues of tumor latency, penetrance, and disease "phase" at which treatment is initiated.

If a genetically engineered model is used later in a compound's development, after pharmaceutical optimization, concerns as to the validity of negative results and their capacity to convey certainty that a compound should be "dropped" exist considering the investment to that point. A classic example of where a transgenic mouse model overpredicted efficacy is the response of mice engineered to overexpress the Ha-*ras* oncogene to farnesyltransferase inhibitors (FTIs). Very good activity was reported for these agents *(18)*. Unfortunately, the clinical experience with these agents produced more modest evidence of the drug's effect *(19)*. Although one might argue this outcome could have been predicted as most human tumors do not express Ha-*ras*, and that the FTIs do not *per se* actually target an essential feature unique to *ras* action in carcinogenesis, it might be argued that the FTIs as a class should not have been expected to be "*ras*" specific. Nonetheless, this result clearly indicates the care that must be taken to address the comparability and context of the model for comparison to the human disease. Finally, concerns about the issues surrounding engineered mice created in academia and covered by patents (e.g., ref. *20*) have diminished corporate enthusiasm and engendered academic frustration surrounding their use in defining agents for eventual clinical use.

9. A NEW ALGORITHM FOR ANIMAL MODEL USE

The ideal animal model for early cancer drug development would allow rapid turnaround of information, possess a capacity for evaluating large numbers of compounds, and be amenable to statistical analysis. It would predict, in a useful way, the probability of activity in more stringent mouse models, and ultimately correlate with clinical activity. It should be able to allow facile assessment of mechanistic information pertinent to the drug. No one model possesses all these features. Recently, in an effort to address a perceived lack of efficiency resulting in a bottleneck to throughput on the part of the classical human xenograft models, the *hollow-fiber assay* was developed by Hollingshead *(21)*.

In the routine conduct of this assay, cells initially growing in cell culture are loaded into polyvinylidine fluoride fibers that are permeable to compounds with $M_r < 500,000$ Da. The fibers can be placed in murine peritoneal, subcutaneous, and other compartments. Following exposure to drug, either administered in the same compartment or given in a way that requires action at a pharmacological distance, the viable cell mass is estimated in fibers removed from the animal and evidence of an antiproliferative effect is adduced. The phosphorylation state of targets or gene expression changes after treatment can be measured with various techniques (e.g., protein blots, polymerase chain reaction). By measuring alterations of these targets in cells harvested from fibers following in vivo treatments, evidence of an effect on the purported drug target can begin to be assessed.

Compounds with evidence of antiproliferative effects in hollow fibers could then either be advanced directly to studies of pharmacology associated with this outcome, or be scheduled for xenograft studies. A recent study of the correlation between activity in NCI's preclinical models and activity in the clinic *(6)* concluded there was a strong correlation between the number of hollow fibers of a given histologic cell type with evidence of an antiproliferative effect and the subsequent demonstration of xenograft activity in the same tumor type. An additional important observation was the relationship between the concentration of drug causing antiproliferative effects in cell culture and evidence of activity in the hollow-fiber activity: in vitro activity at concentrations only > 1 μM was associated with a low likelihood of activity in cells growing in vivo in the hollow fibers.

The availability of this model suggests a discovery and development strategy in which the hollow-fiber model is used to quantitate the effect of drug on a molecular target of drug action and to assess the pharmacologic parameters associated with that activity. Dosing regimens are optimized to achieve the necessary drug levels in a sustained way. This is followed by assessing activity in a xenograft model selected for its expression of the target of interest. Ideally, a pair of engineered cell lines isogenic but for the target of interest is also assessed. Studies of compound activity should capture effects on the target as well as on tumor cell proliferation. Confirmatory studies in transgenic animals might be contemplated to confirm that the observed activity of the compound is actually target relatable.

10. CONCLUSIONS

Despite the recognized pitfalls and shortcomings associated with the use of mouse models of the type described here for the discovery and refinement of cancer treatments, essentially no successful cancer therapeutic has advanced to the clinic without robust, well-defined, or easily reproduced activity in an animal model, usually syngeneic murine tumors or immunodeficient mice bearing human tumor xenografts. Although the use of treatments with defined molecular targets that can be assessed in real time may improve the predictive power of models expressing those targets, the gold standard for securing drug licensure will remain the safety and efficacy of the drug in human clinical trials. It is hoped that the linking of efforts to define the pharmacology of active regimens in mice to the effects of these agents on a molecular target responsible in part for the tumor's growth and the drug's action will provide a very firm basis to make decisions concerning the logic of pursuing a given compound for further development.

REFERENCES

1. Plowman J, Dykes D, Hollingshead M, Simpson-Herren L, Alley M. Human tumor xenografts in NCI drug development. In: Teicher BA (ed). Anticancer Drug Development Guide: Preclinical Screening, Clinical Trials, and Approval. Totowa, NJ: Humana Press, 1997, pp. 101–126.
2. Corbett T, Valeriote F, LoRusso P, et al. In vivo methods for screening and preclinical testing: use of rodent solid tumors for drug discovery. In: Teicher BA (ed). Anticancer Drug Development Guide: Preclinical Screening, Clinical Trials, and Approval. Totowa, NJ: Humana Press, 1997, pp. 75–100.
3. Fiebig HH, Dengler WA, Roth T. Human tumor xenografts; predictivity, characterization, and discovery of new anti-cancer agents. In: Fiebig HH, Burger AM (eds). Contributions to Oncology, Vol. 54: Relevance of Tumor Models for Anticancer Drug Development. Basel: Karger, 1999, pp. 29–50.
4. Schabel FM Jr, Griswold DP Jr, Laster WR Jr, Corbett TH, Lloyd HH. Quantitative evaluation of anticancer agent activity in experimental animals. Pharmaceut Ther A 1977; 1:411–435.
5. Waud WR. Murine L1210 and P388 leukemias. In: Teicher BA (ed). Anticancer Drug Development Guide: Preclinical Screening, Clinical Trials, and Approval. Totowa, NJ: Humana Press, 1997, pp. 59–74.
6. Johnson JI, Decker S, Zaharevitz D, et al. Relationships between drug activity in NCI preclinical in vitro and in vivo models and early clinical trials. Br J Cancer 2001; 84:1424–1431.
7. Dykes DJ, Abbott BJ, Mayo JG, et al. Development of human tumor xenograft models for in vivo evaluation of new antitumor drugs. In: Fiebig HH, Berger DP (eds). Contributions to Oncology, Vol. 42: Immunodeficient Mice in Oncology. Basel: Karger, 1992, pp. 1–22.
8. Thompson J, Stewart CF, Houghton PJ. Animal models for studying the action of topoisomerase targeted drugs. Biochim Biophys Acta 1998; 1400:301–319.
9. Mi Z, Burke TG. Marked interspecies variations concerning the interactions of camptothecin with serum albumins: a frequency domain fluorescence study. Biochemistry 1994; 33:12,540–12,545.

10. Volpe DA, Tomaszewski JE, Parchment RE, et al. Myelotoxic effects of the bifunctional alkylating agent bizelesin on human, canine, and murine progenitor cells. Cancer Chemother Pharmacol 1996; 39:143–149.

11. Ishii S, Nagasawa M, Kariya Y, Yamamoto H. Selective cytotoxic activity of brefeldin A against human tumor cell lines. J Antibiot (Tokyo) 1989; 42:1877–1878.

12. Sausville EA, Duncan KLK, Senderowicz A, et al. Antiproliferative effect in vitro and antitumor activity in vivo of brefeldin A. Cancer J Sci Am 1996; 2:52.

13. Trail PA, Willner D, Lasch SJ, et al. Cure of xenografted human carcinomas by BR96-doxorubicin immunoconjugates. Science 1994; 263:1076.

14. Saleh MN, Sugarman S, Murray J, et al. Phase I trial of the anti-Lewis Y drug immunoconjugate BR96-doxorubicin in patients with lewis y-expressing epithelia tumors. J Clin Oncol 2000; 18:2282–2292.

15. LeCoutre P, Mologni L, Cleris L, et al. In vivo eradication of human BCR/ABL-positive leukemia cells with an ABL kinase inhibitor. J Natl Cancer Inst 1999; 91:163–168.

16. Van Dyke T, Jacks T. Cancer modeling in the modern era: progress and challenges. Cell 2002; 108:135–144.

17. Bergers G, Javaherian K, Lo KM, Folkman J, Hanahan D. Effects of angiogenesis inhibitors on multistage carcinogenesis in mice. Science 1999; 284:808–812.

18. Kohl NE, Omer CA, Conner MW, et al. Inhibition of farnesyltransferase induces regression of mammary and salivary carcinomas in ras transgenic mice. Nat Med 1995; 1:792–797.

19. Britten CD, Rowinsky EK, Soignet S, et al. A Phase I and pharmacological study of the farnesyl protein transferase inhibitor L-778,123 in patients with solid malignancies. Clin Cancer Res 2001; 7:3894–3903.

20. Marshall E. Intellectual property. Dupont ups ante on use of Harvard's OncoMouse. Science 2002; 296:1212.

21. Hollingshead M, Plowman J, Alley M, Mayo J, Sausville E. The hollow fiber assay. In: Fiebig HH, Burger AM (eds). Contributions to Oncology, Vol. 54: Relevance of Tumor Models for Anticancer Drug Development. Basel: Karger, 1999, pp. 109–120.

4 Defining the Starting Dose

Should It Be Based on mg/kg, mg/m², or Fixed?

Howard Gurney, MB, BS, FRACP

CONTENTS

1. INTRODUCTION

There are three issues that set the scene for defining the starting dose of new anticancer drugs:

1. There is a revolution in the understanding and identification of drug elimination mechanisms at the molecular level.
2. Some of the new targeted therapies will have a larger therapeutic window than traditional cytotoxic agents.
3. The traditional monopoly held by body surface area for dose calculation of cytotoxic agents is inaccurate for many drugs and is probably dangerous.

Cytotoxic drug disposition is minimally affected by body size. At best body size accounts for < 30% of the interindividual variation in drug effect. Most of the variation is the result of genetic and phenotypic differences in elimination and absorption processes. Drug elimination is largely determined by mechanisms that are unrelated to body size, and other methods that account for these variations are needed for dose calculation. Even with new drugs that may have a large safety margin, reduction in interpatient variability in drug effect is critical to minimizing underdosing.

Handbook of Anticancer Pharmacokinetics and Pharmacodynamics
Edited by: W. D. Figg and H. L. McLeod © Humana Press Inc., Totowa, NJ

2. WHAT IS BSA AND WHY DO WE USE IT?

In 1916, when Delafield and Eugene DuBois developed a formula to approximate body surface area (BSA) using height and weight, they would not have realized the implications that this would later have on the millions of cancer patients treated with cytotoxic chemotherapy *(1)*. They developed the nomogram to normalize measurement of basal metabolic rate between individuals, but in the late 1950s it was suggested after minimal investigation that BSA should be used to normalize for cytotoxic drug elimination. This practice continues almost half a century later.

BSA is the two-dimensional surface area of an individual's skin. Skin surface area was previously directly measured by the use of molds or paper cutouts applied to the skin surface. If we still used that method today to calculate BSA, the obvious question would be clear to everyone. How is it that an estimation of the skin surface area has become the conventional tool for predicting an individual's ability to eliminate cytotoxic drugs? Instead, the practice became mystified by the use of formulas, slide rules, and calculators, so oncologists were led to believe that they could determine an "accurate" dose of chemotherapy to a few decimal places.

BSA correlates with basal metabolic rate, and BSA nomograms were originally devised for this purpose *(1)*. BSA is also known to be proportional to blood volume *(2)*. It has been claimed that BSA is also proportional to glomerular filtration rate (GFR) *(3)*, but a more recent assessment has questioned this relationship *(4)*. Liver function decreases with advancing age in parallel to the loss of liver volume *(5)*. However, interpatient variation in hepatic function remains large even in healthy subjects *(6)*. Liver volume as determined by helical computed tomography (CT) scanning has been shown to correlate with BSA ($r^2 = 0.54$) and total body weight ($r^2 = 0.61$) in 21 patients with a history of cancer but without liver metastases *(7)*.

One of the first uses of BSA in drug dose calculation was in 1950, when Crawford et al. *(8)* showed that plasma drug levels for sulfadiazine (an acetylated and renally excreted antibiotic) and acetylsalicylic acid (a renally excreted analgesic) linearly correlated with dose when patients were divided into four groups according to surface area. BSA has also been used to extrapolate toxic doses in experimental animals to allow an estimation of a safe starting dose for Phase I studies of cytotoxic agents in humans *(9,10)*. In 1958, an attempt was made to define a more accurate method of dose calculation for cytotoxic drugs in children *(11)*. Pinkel examined the literature and found that the "conventional" dose of five cytotoxic drugs (mercaptopurine, methotrexate, mechlorethamine, triethylenethiophosphoramide, and actinomycin) for pediatric and adult humans and for experimental animals were similar if corrected for "representative" BSAs for humans and animals. Pharmacokinetic analyses were not performed and actual patients were not included in the study, so a comparison of other variables such as antitumor effect or toxicity could not be undertaken. Three of the drugs are renally excreted (mercaptopurine, methotrexate, and actinomycin) and the apparent relationship may have been the result of the known correlation of BSA and renal function. Pinkel recommended that the potential use of BSA for dose calculation should be investigated further but this was not undertaken until the last decade. In the meantime, the use of BSA for dose calculation in oncology became dogma, without further investigation into the relationship between dose and BSA or other parameters of body size.

3. DOES BODY SIZE CORRELATE WITH DRUG DISPOSITION?

3.1. Lean Body Mass, Ideal Body Weight, and Obesity

Lean body mass (LBM) consists of body cell mass, extracellular fluid, and nonfat connective tissue and is essentially fat-free mass *(7)*. LBM is commonly measured by dual-energy X-ray absorptiometry, which distinguishes fat, fat-free mass, and bone.

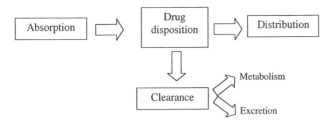

Fig. 1. Determinants of drug disposition.

It has been suggested that LBM correlates with systemic drug clearance but so far this has not yet been substantiated *(12)*. Nawaratne et al. showed that LBM correlates with liver volume and antipyrine clearance, a nonspecific quantitative test of hepatic drug oxidation *(7)*. However, in this study there was no correlation between liver volume and antipyrine clearance, indicating that other unknown factors account for the relationship. Further studies are required to determine the importance of LBM in dose calculation of hepatically eliminated drugs.

Ideal body weight (IBW) is the weight that insurance companies consider appropriate for height and is determined by a formula. The use of IBW for dose calculation (sometimes as a function for BSA) attempts to account for excess adipose tissue. Body constitution in the obese is characterized by a higher percentage of fat and a lower percentage of lean tissue and water. The effect of obesity on some cytotoxic drugs has been examined. In obese patients methotrexate clearance is increased, busulfan and ifosfamide clearances are unchanged, and doxorubicin and cyclophosphamide clearances are reduced *(13–17)*. Hepatic oxidative metabolism is unaffected by obesity as measured by antipyrine clearance or the erythromycin breath test *(18,19)*. It would be expected that the volume of distribution be affected in obese patients especially for drugs that are lipid soluble. However, this expected relationship is variable with some lipid-soluble drugs increasing the volume of distribution (e.g., benzodaizepines, verapamil) whereas others have no effect (e.g., cyclosporin, propranolol) *(20)*. Given these data there is little to suggest the routine use of IBW for dose calculation either alone or to calculate BSA. However, obesity and cachexia should be considered extreme variations from the norm and the effect of these body states on drug disposition should be examined in separate studies (see below).

3.2. Volume of Distribution and Clearance

Drug disposition or blood concentration is determined by absorption, distribution, and clearance (Fig. 1). Absorption and clearance are largely determined by the activities of metabolizing enzymes and transmembrane pumps in the gut, kidney, and liver. For some drugs, hepatic and renal blood flow are also important. Drug distribution is dictated by the degree of plasma protein binding and whether the drug freely distributes into extravascular tissue. For instance, drugs that are highly plasma protein bound such as warfarin, tolbutamide, and ibuprofen have a low volume of distribution (approx 0.1 L/kg) that roughly equates to blood volume *(21)*. Because blood volume and the amount of total body water are related to body size, volume of distribution may relate to body size in some circumstances *(2)*. Aminoglycosides, phenobarbitone, ibuprofen, carboplatin, vinorelbine, irinotecan, and tacrolimus are some drugs for which measures of body size have correlated with the apparent volume of distribution *(22–28)*.

However, it must be remembered that volume of distribution (V_d) is not a physiological measurement but a pharmacokinetic ratio. It is the theoretical volume into which a drug is distributed and is described by the formula: V_d = dose/concentration.

Table 1
Pharmacokinetic Correlation
With Toxicity and Tumor Response[a]

Toxicity	Tumor response
AUC, CL, or steady-state concentration	
Etoposide	Teniposide
Carboplatin	Methotrexate
Vincristine	Etoposide
Vinorelbine	5-Fluorouracil
5-Fluorouracil	Docetaxel *(70)*
Docetaxel *(70)*	
Doxorubicin	
Irinotecan and SN-38	
Topotecan	
Trimetrexate	
N-Methyl formamide	
Hexamethylene bisacetamide	
Menogaril	
Plasma concentration	
Cisplatin	Doxorubicin
6-Mercaptopurine	
Paclitaxel *(34)*	
Methotrexate	

[a] See ref. *37* for complete reference list unless otherwise indicated.

Therefore, the volume of distribution for an intravenous dose is determined by peak blood concentration. The possible relationship between body size and volume of distribution may be important in circumstances where peak plasma concentration determines toxicity or drug efficacy. Intuitively, one would expect a relationship between peak plasma concentration and toxicity for cytotoxic agents. However, limited information is available. No correlation was found between toxicity and peak concentration of irinotecan SN-38, or epirubicin *(29,30)*. A correlation has been shown for oral etoposide *(31)*. However, for this drug and also for paclitaxel, the time above a critical plasma concentration, rather than peak concentration, appears to be more important *(32–34)*. Where a relationship has been shown between a pharmacokinetic parameter and drug efficacy or toxicity for anticancer treatment, it is usually the area-under-the time–concentration curve (AUC) or steady-state plasma concentration rather than V_d or peak plasma concentration that correlates (Table 1).

The AUC is determined by dose and clearance and defined by the formula: AUC = clearance/dose. As mentioned above, metabolism and elimination by the kidneys and liver determine drug clearance. Very few of these processes would be expected to be determined by body size. A few drugs such as aminoglycosides are almost solely eliminated by glomerular filtration. It has been suggested that the GFR correlates with body size *(3)*, and doses of gentamicin and tobramycin are now determined by adjusting for body weight. However, even for carboplatin, a cytotoxic drug that is mostly eliminated by glomerular filtration, a dose calculated using GFR is more accurate than one using BSA *(19)*.

Table 2
Correlation of Body Size With Drug Clearance

Drug	Correlation/comments	References
Docetaxel	Interpatient variability of CL correlates with BSA.	71
Paclitaxel	BSA explains 53% of interpatient variability in CL.	62
Temozolamide	BSA reduced interpatient variability of CL from 20% to 13% on d 1 and 16% to 10% on d 5.	72, 73
Oral busulfan	CL correlates with BSA ($r^2 = 0.28$) and weight ($r^2 = 0.3$).	14
Vinorelbine	CL correlates with BSA ($r^2 = 0.27$).	74

Table 3
No Correlation for Body Size With Clearance or AUC

Class	Drug	References
Topoisomerase inhibitors	Etoposide	75
	Irinotecan	61, 76
	Topotecan	77
Antibiotics	Epirubicin	63, 78
	Piroxantrone	37
Spindle poisons	Vinorelbine	64
	Paclitaxel	35
Antimetabolites	5-Fluorouracil	37
	Methotrexate	37
	Trimetrexate	37
	Dichloromethotrexate	37
Alkylating agents	Ifosfamide	37
	Busulfan	37
	Cisplatin	60, 79
	Carboplatin	43
Miscellaneous	N-Methyl formamide	37
	Hexamethylene bisacetamide	37
	Menogaril	37
	Brequinar	37

3.3. BSA Does Not Affect Clearance of Most Cytotoxic Agents

Over the last decade, the relationship between BSA and drug disposition of cytotoxic drugs has been revisited (35–38). Table 2 is a list of drugs that have been reported to show a correlation between drug clearance and BSA. Even for some of these drugs the correlation coefficients are low, indicating that BSA accounts for < 30% of the variability in clearance between individuals. For most cytotoxic drugs, no correlation can be seen with BSA and drug clearance when this relationship has been examined (Table 3). The most compelling evidence against the use of BSA for dose calculation is the fact that a large interpatient variability in drug effect remains despite "normalization"' of dose by BSA. Drug clearance varies widely for any given drug even when dose is calculated as a function of BSA.

Most of these studies have been in adults where the variation in body size is minimal. In adult populations the extremes of BSA vary from approx 1.4 to 2.2 m^2—only a 1.5-fold range. Furthermore, the majority of individuals fall into a range of BSA much lower than this. Even for drugs for which the use of BSA may reduce variability, in practice there is minimal contribution in reduction in variability from the use of body size for a person measuring 1.7 m^2 compared to 1.8 m^2. The real issue is whether an individual of 40 kg should get the same dose as one weighing 120 kg. Studies have not been performed to examine the contribution of BSA in drug disposition for the situations of extremes of body size, although obese patients have been shown to have reduced clearance of some drugs such as doxorubicin and cyclophosphamide (16,17). However, assuming a maximum contribution of BSA to drug disposition of 30%, it is only in the situations of extreme BSA that this parameter may become a significant factor in dose calculation.

The issue of substantial variation in body size is amplified in pediatric oncology, where body weight ranges from a few kilograms to adult size. In these situations of extreme differences, body size must come into play. This is more akin to the interspecies scaling of chemotherapy dose, such as in estimating the dose for humans based on toxicology studies in rodents. BSA has proved useful in this situation of interspecies scaling of dose (9,10). It would therefore be reasonable to use BSA to scale an approximate starting dose of a drug for clinical trials in children based on adult data. However, even here it is unreasonable to use BSA as the sole determinant of dose for individual infants. The same inaccuracies of using BSA alone would hold when differentiating doses between children within a small range of body size.

It has been pointed out previously that the higher dose per meter squared for a drug that is often adopted in pediatric patients as compared to the same drug in adults is not necessarily attributable to better tolerance in children (37). This practice may also have come about to compensate for the inaccuracies of using BSA for dose calculation. An 11-yr-old with normal drug elimination mechanisms should probably get the same dose as a larger adult with similar drug elimination capabilities. We see that this is the case by default. An 11-yr-old with a BSA of 1.2 m^2 will get a 420-mg dose of paclitaxel based on the pediatric recommendation of 350 mg/m^2. A 1.7-m^2 adult will receive the same dose (425 mg) based on the recommended dose for adults of 250 mg/m^2.

4. THE SIGNIFICANCE OF GETTING THE WRONG DOSE

A common argument in support of the continued use of BSA for dose calculation of chemotherapy is that the degree of inaccuracy is not clinically significant. The obvious consequence of incorrect dose calculation is overdose and excessive toxicity, a situation most oncologists have learned to accept. A more common but less appreciated consequence is underdosing and reduced drug effect.

Individuals vary in their capability to eliminate xenobiotics by 4- to 10-fold (37). For drugs with a wide therapeutic window such as antibiotics, this problem is not crucial because the recommended dose can be pitched toward the high end of the dose range without fear of significant dose-related toxicity. On the other hand, cytotoxic chemotherapy has a narrow therapeutic window. The dose that causes unacceptable or even fatal toxicity is not much higher than the optimal dose needed for the anticancer effect. For this reason, the main endpoint of dose-finding studies has traditionally been prevention of unacceptable toxicity. Couple this with the wide interpatient variability in drug disposition and conservatism becomes intrinsic to the dose-recommendation process for anticancer drugs. The mean dose is pitched toward the low range to minimize the number of patients with severe toxicity, and, consequently, many cancer patients are inadvertently underdosed (Fig. 2) (39).

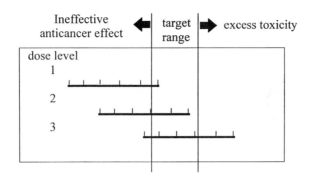

Fig. 2. Scheme of a Phase I study for a drug with linear pharmacokinetics. The *horizontal lines* represent the variations in systemic exposure at various dose levels. At dose level 3, patients with lower drug elimination capability develop dose-limiting toxicity and subsequently that dose level is defined as the maximum tolerated dose. Dose level 2 is recommended for Phase II studies because it causes tolerable toxicity in all patients. However, because of the variation in drug handling, a proportion of patients will be relatively underdosed, as they are more capable of eliminating the drug. This means the wide distribution of systemic exposure is skewed toward the ineffective range when dose is calculated using BSA.

A few studies have shown a significantly worse antitumor effect for those patients who failed to develop myelosuppression after treatment compared to those who did among patients receiving adjuvant treatment for breast cancer or chemotherapy for advanced testicular cancer. If lack of myelosuppression is accepted as an indication of underdosing, the frequency of this event can then be estimated to be between 30% and 75% for common chemotherapeutic regimens. It has been estimated that this inadvertent underdosing may lead to a relative reduction in cure rate for breast cancer and testis cancer by as much as 10–20% *(39)*.

Pharmacokinetic evidence for inadvertent underdosing can be found in a study by Gamelin et al. *(40)*. This group had defined the optimum 5-fluorouracil (5-FU) plasma concentration with a regimen using 5-FU in a dose of 1300 mg/m^2 infused over 8 h every week. For a group of 81 patients treated with a dose calculated using BSA, 80% of patients were found to have an ineffective 5-FU plasma concentration after the first dose.

Furuta et al. have shown that even for noncytotoxic drugs, underdosing can be a problem *(41)*. They showed in Japanese patients that a difference in efficacy of amoxicillin and omeprozole treatment for gastritis caused by *Helicobacter pylori* infection depended on the presence of a single nucleotide polymorphism (SNP) in the *CYP 2C19* gene. Those who did not have a SNP were poor metabolizers and had a 100% cure rate. Patients who were homozygous had extensive metabolism of omperazole and had a < 30% cure rate. Those who were heterozygous had an intermediate (60%) cure rate of *Helicobacter*-induced gastritis.

5. WHAT CAUSES INTERINDIVIDUAL VARIATIONS IN DRUG EFFECTS?

The variation in cytotoxic drug clearance between individuals is mostly due to differing activity of drug elimination processes because of genetic and environmental factors *(37)*. It is therefore prudent to summarize the current knowledge regarding the drug elimination processes.

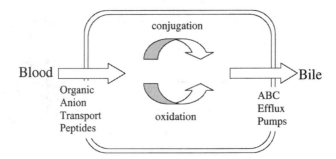

Fig. 3. Xenobiotic hepatic elimination.

Most cytotoxic drugs are eliminated by the liver. A minority of drugs have renal elimination as the major route. Most of these are excreted by efflux pumps in the proximal tubules utilizing the organic anion (OAT) and cation transporters (OCT) as well as multidrug resistance pump 1 (MDR1) *(42)*. In these cases, the hepatic biliary pumps are also usually involved to some extent. The occasional cytotoxic drug is predominantly eliminated by glomerular filtration. The best know example is carboplatin, in which at least 75% of unmetabolized drug is eliminated by glomerular filtration. In this uncommon situation Calvert and colleagues were able to relate the AUC to GFR allowing dose calculation by a simple formula: dose = target AUC × (GFR + 25) *(43)*. Almost all other cytotoxic drugs have complex elimination, and it is unlikely that other simple formulas can be developed for these drugs.

Hepatic elimination is summarized in Fig. 3. Many drugs enter the hepatocyte by way of the OAT polypeptides *(44)*. These xenobiotics are then handled by a combination of metabolism and biliary pump excretion. Phase 1 metabolism consists of oxidation usually to an inactive but sometimes active metabolites. The major drug oxidizing enzymes are the cytochrome P450s. These transmembrane proteins are bound to the inner mitochondrial membrane and bind multiple substrates, allowing the exchange of an oxygen radical from the P450s iron molecule to the substrate.

Phase 2 metabolism involves inactivation of the molecule by conjugation with glucuronide, sulfate, or glutathione. These are usually then excreted by the kidney or into the bile by an ATP binding cassette (ABC) pump, multidrug resistance protein 2 (MRP2), also known as canalicular multipurpose organic anion transporter (c-MOAT). Many cytotoxic drugs are also pumped directly into the bile without metabolism by another ABC pump, the MDR1. The importance of MDR1 in hepatic drug elimination has been underestimated. Almost 50% of drugs such as doxorubicin, paclitaxel, vinca alkaloids, and etoposide are excreted directly into the bile unchanged *(45,46)*. MDR1 therefore may play an important role in interindividual variation in drug elimination along with variations in metabolism.

All of these processes are now known to be transcriptionally regulated by orphan nuclear receptors such as pregnane and xenobiotic receptor (PXR) and constitutive androstane receptor (CAR) *(47)*. These promiscuous receptors bind multiple disparate ligands such as dexamethasone and rifampicin in the cytosol and then translocate to the nucleus. Here multiple drug elimination genes are upregulated including MDR1, MRP2, and many CYP enzymes *(47,48)*. By upregulation of OATP they also enhance entry of more substrate into the cell, providing a positive feedback loop for drug elimination (Fig. 4) *(49)*.

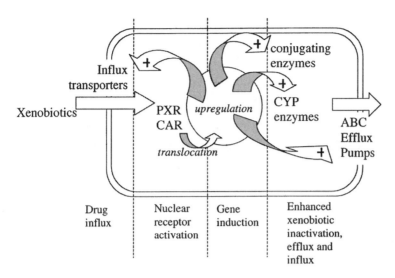

Fig. 4. Regulation of hepatic drug elimination.

6. VARIATIONS IN ELIMINATION PROCESSES

Cytochrome P450 (CYP) 3A, the major oxidizing enzymes for many cytotoxic drugs, varies by as much as 50-fold in vitro although the reasons for this are not clear *(50)*. Fifteen percent of caucasians and 50% of blacks and Asians have an allele that codes for a functional CYP3A5 protein. In this situation, CYP3A5 contributes 50% of CYP3A activity, and it has been proposed that this may be the cause of the variation in CYP3A activity between individuals *(51)*. Most of the polymorphisms described for CYP3A4 do not significantly alter activity of this enzyme. CYP3A4 is highly conserved across species, and given its importance in detoxification it is not surprising that few (if any) polymorphisms that render CYP3A4 inactive have been propagated. Competitive inhibition of CYP3A activity occurs between substrates, and this is a common cause for drug interactions because of reduced elimination.

Less is known about the variation in other critical hepatic elimination processes such as active biliary excretion by MDR1, MRP2, and the other members of the ABC family of efflux pumps, although some polymorphisms have been identified *(52)*. It may be that polymorphisms of the orphan nuclear receptors (PXR, CAR) are important in determining interindividual variations in drug elimination. A number of SNPs have been identified for PXR, but the significance of these needs to be determined *(53)*.

Dihydropyrimidine dehydrogenase (DPD), the enzyme that catabolizes 5-FU, varies by eightfold in activity *(54)*. Approximately 15% of individuals have markedly reduced DPD activity owing to an SNP of the DPD gene and are subject to unexpected life-threatening toxicity after a standard 5-FU dose *(55)*. UDP-glucuronosyltransferase, a major conjugation enzyme, is also subject to a number of polymorphisms that affect function. Patients with Dubin–Johnson syndrome who have a deficiency in glutathione *S*-transferase activity due to various SNPs have increased toxicity from irinotecan and its active metabolite SN-38, as the latter compound is inactivated by this enzyme *(56)*.

7. IS DOSE CALCULATION IMPORTANT
FOR TARGETED THERAPIES?

Variation in drug elimination is important even for the new targeted therapies. These compounds have a larger therapeutic window than traditional cytotoxic agents, so overdosage is not such a problem. However, Iressa, a tyrosine kinase inhibitor for epithelial growth factor receptor, does have dose-related toxic effects including diarrhea and skin rash that cause some patients to stop therapy. Iressa has a 3- to 10-fold interpatient variation in drug exposure. The drug is metabolized by CYP3A4. There is minimal renal elimination and it is unkown at this stage whether MDR1 is involved in elimination *(57)*.

Rituximab, a monoclonal antibody to CD20, is active against B-cell lymphoma. Low blood rituximab concentration relates to poor response, and a large interpatient variation has been demonstrated *(58)*. The mechanism of drug elimination is not clear. Dose is determined as a function of BSA, although no relationship has been demonstrated between the clearance of this antibody and BSA.

Imatinib, a tyrosine kinase inhibitor active against chronic myelogenous leukemia (CML) and gastrointestinal stroma tumors, is metabolized by CYP3A4 and also CYP2D6 and CYP2C9. Twenty-five percent is unmetabolized, and so biliary MDR1 may be important. Body weight has minimal effect on clearance. Drug discontinuation attributable to toxicity is rare but there is a four- to sixfold variation in drug exposure between individuals. There is a dose–efficacy relationship for CML, and so underdosing because of inaccurate dose calculation may be a problem with this drug *(59)*.

It can be seen that accurate dose calculation is important even for the novel anticancer therapies, not only to reduce toxicity but also to prevent underdosage and reduced efficacy.

8. CAN WE USE FIXED DOSES?

Because body size is not useful for the majority of anticancer drugs is it reasonable to use a fixed dose for all patients *(60,61)*? The advantages of using fixed doses of cytotoxic drugs are many, including financial and safety issues. For example, what is the additional cost of prescribing 305 mg of paclitaxel instead of 300 mg? Can 215 mg of DTIC (instead of 200 or 220 mg), 85 mg of docetaxel (instead of 80 or 90 mg), or 63 mg of methotrexate be compounded accurately? The decimal point can easily be missed by an inexperienced technician when 2.2 mg of vincristine is prescribcd.

At least three studies have examined the safety of this approach. Smorenburg et al. randomized patients to fixed-dose paclitaxel or a conventional dose calculation arm and found that BSA accounted for approx 50% of the interpatient variability in clearance. They hypothesized that this was related to the cremophor vehicle, the distribution of which is related to blood volume *(62)*. In this case the BSA dose was more accurate than a fixed dose of paclitaxel.

The main disadvantage of using a fixed dose is that it is no more accurate than a BSA-derived dose. A large interpatient variation in drug exposure will remain, with all the implications of overdosing and underdosing discussed above. Our group has examined the use of epirubicin (150 mg continuous infusion) and vinorelbine (60 mg every 21 d) in separate studies and found that this approach was safe for both drugs. However, interpatient variability in clearance was still eightfold and fourfold, respectively, for each drug, which is similar to the variability if BSA was used for dose calculation *(63,64)*.

It is unlikely therefore that using a single fixed dose of anticancer drugs for all patients is the answer. For that matter, this is not the case for noncytotoxic drugs either. As one example, it has been shown that there is a wide variation in effective dose for omeprozole because of differences in drug metabolism capability. The recommended dose of this drug is 20 mg for all patients. However, when variations in drug elimination are taken into account, a more accurate dose recommendation is 20 mg, 60 mg, 80 mg, or 120 mg depending on CYP2C19 status *(41)*. A similar fixed dose–range system for dose calculation could be applied for anticancer drugs.

9. TOXICITY-ADJUSTED DOSES

One popular method of dose individualization is to adjust subsequent doses of chemotherapy based on the level of myelosuppression, eventually avoiding overdosing and underdosing—so called "toxicity-adjusting dosing" *(37)*. A Swedish group has adopted this approach in the adjuvant treatment of breast cancer *(65)*. Using the 5-FU, epirubicin, and cyclophosphamide (FEC) regimen, dose adjustments were made on each cycle to ensure a target level of myelosuppression. After a number of dose adjustments this method of individualizing the dose gave a threefold interpatient range of cyclophosphamide dose (450–1800 mg/m^2) and a fourfold range for epirubicin (38–120 mg/m^2). This is more in keeping with the known interpatient variation in drug clearance for these drugs. However, it would be better to achieve an individualized dose variation from the first dose rather than the third, fourth, or fifth dose. To achieve this, the dose calculation method must take into account the activity of the elimination processes for the drug(s) in question *before* the first treatment is given.

10. A COMPROMISE

Consideration should be given to using a range of "fixed doses" for a particular drug that could be used as the starting dose and for dose adjustments. However, the original question remains. How should we determine the starting dose for anticancer drugs? The answer must be in defining ways to predict drug handling in each individual. We do this currently when carboplatin is dosed using GFR. However, as previously stated, the use of simple formulas for other drugs will not be possible because of complex elimination mechanisms. Complex formulas using obscure parameters also should not be favored. Dose calculation must be kept relatively simple to allow the busy clinician to adopt any new system. The best system will determine drug handling capability for an individual and be useful across a range drugs. This should be possible because coupling of CYP3A4/5 metabolism and MDR1 biliary excretion accounts for a large proportion of xenobiotic elimination.

Studies are underway to define the drug-handling genotype and phenotype *before* drug administration so an individualized dose can be given on the first cycle *(64,66–69)*. Assessment of both hepatic metabolism and active biliary excretion is essential, as these are the important elimination processes for the majority of cytotoxic drugs. Such in vivo tests of drug handling would have the advantage of being applicable to a range of cytotoxic and noncytotoxic drugs cleared by similar mechanisms. Measurement of the activity of linchpin nuclear receptors such as PXR and CAR may allow determination of drug elimination across an even wider palette of elimination routes. Efforts should be made to determine the activities of these receptors by genotype or phenotype in humans.

One scenario is that the majority of patients who have "normal" drug elimination receive a standard fixed dose of drug according to the regimen. Pretreatment in vivo tests of genotype or phenotype will identify the estimated 20–30% of patients who fall into the extremes of drug elimination capability. If body size is found to be important in determining variability in drug exposure, then this can also be accounted for. These patients will receive significantly lower or higher fixed doses. In other words, starting doses will be a range of fixed doses according to low, normal, or high drug elimination or disposition type. Fine-tuning of doses will be based on the presence or absence of toxicity or some other parameter that measures biological effect.

11. DOSE CALCULATION SCHEMA IN NEW DRUG DEVELOPMENT

Special Reference to Body Size

1. Treat body size as an identified parameter that may potentially influence the drug effect as already occurs for renal function, hepatic function, genetic polymorphism, and so forth. Exclude patients with extremes of body size from initial Phase 1 studies, as one would for patients with abnormal renal or hepatic function.
2. Because body size is unlikely to be critical in determining variability for most drugs, it is not necessary to be too stringent regarding the limits for inclusion in adult studies. A recommended range of BSA is < 1.5 or > 2.2. Body weight may be used as an alternative (e.g., <40 kg and >120 kg) or a body mass index (e.g., 18–32).
3. Use fixed doses for various levels in a Phase 1 study.
4. Undertake Phase 1 studies based on appropriate endpoint that may not be toxicity (see Chapter 5). Pharmacokinetic and pharmacodynamic studies should be undertaken as usual to describe the pharmacological behavior of the agent as well as pharmacokinetic endpoints. At this time determine whether body size, along with other parameters, affects drug disposition.
5. If body size is related to drug disposition, other factors for drug elimination (known and unknown) are likely to be equally or more important in determining drug disposition. Try not to incorporate body size measures in complex algorithms for dose calculation but rather offer a range of fixed doses for various body size (and drug elimination) categories.
6. If there is no obvious effect of body size, again examine any correlations with body size and drug disposition in population pharmacokinetic/pharmacodynamic studies in Phase II, and if necessary, Phase III studies.
7. Do not develop dose calculation methods that require formulas resulting in a myriad of doses for a particular drug. Aim for the majority of patients to receive a fixed dose. Use tests (as yet not developed) that define the "outliers" in drug elimination capability and use alternative fixed doses in these patients.
8. After a dose calculation system is determined for a new drug, this should be tested in a subsequent Phase II study to ensure that interindividual variability in drug effect has been significantly reduced by this system.
9. Be mindful that any dose calculation system cannot account for all variables and will be inaccurate to a degree. Biological surrogates should be employed such as neutropenia, other toxicity, or blood drug levels to adjust dose up or down after initial dose calculation. An example of development of a method for dose calculation of a theoretical new drug is summarized in Table 4.

In summary, body size should be only one of a number of key parameters that are considered when determining chemotherapy dose for a new drug. For some drugs the affect of body size on drug disposition will be insignificant. For others, body size may contribute up to 30% of interpatient variability. Body size may theoretically affect peak plasma concentrations for drugs with a low volume of distribution and care should be exercised when examining these drugs in Phase 1 studies.

Table 4
Development of a Dose Grid for Drug Z

---

1. In a Phase 1 study using a different fixed dose levels for drug Z, the effects of various parameters such as body size, drug elimination measures, protein binding, and so forth on drug disposition were examined. It was found that;

   a. Drug exposure varied by four- to sixfold between individuals.

   b. BSA contributes 30% of variation in drug disposition and effect.

   c. Drug elimination contributes 70% of variation in drug disposition and effect.

2. It was also confirmed that drug Z is metabolized by CYP3A4 and eliminated by MDR1 and MRP2 biliary pumps. Simple tests exist to measure these processes in individuals (genotype and/or phenotype).

3. A dose grid is developed using a range of fixed doses and to take into account the two most important determinants of drug exposure. Four categories were selected for drug elimination and three for body size to reflect their relative contribution to drug disposition. Values are expressed in or as percent of the base dose.

   Drug Elimination Capability

Body size	Very poor	Poor	Efficient	Ultraefficient
Small	30	50	80	100
Medium	50	80	100	120
Large	80	100	120	150

   Note there are six fixed doses and the range of dose is fivefold which approximated the known variation in drug exposure for drug X.

4. This dose grid is tested in a Phase II study. It is found that variability in drug exposure falls from four- to sixfold to 1.5-fold. This is considered clinically significant and the dose grid is accepted for use for drug Z as a single agent.

It should not be assumed that body size affects drug disposition of a new drug. This parameter should be examined in Phase 1 studies along with other parameters after a fixed dose is given. For this reason, individuals with extremes of body size should be excluded from initial Phase 1 studies. Drug disposition in individuals with extremes of body size should be examined in separate studies if appropriate, as occurs with other factors such as renal and hepatic function. Special attention should be applied to factors that are probably more important in determining variability such as measures of drug elimination phenotype and genotype. These should not be confined to drug metabolism alone but also include transmembrane influx and efflux pumps and key regulatory nuclear receptors.

REFERENCES

1. Du Bois D, Du Bois EF. A formula to estimate the approximate surface area if height and weight be known. Arch Intern Med 1916; 17:863–871.
2. Baker RJ, Kozoli DD, Meyer KA. The use of surface area for establishing normal blood volume. Surg Gynecol Obstet 1957; 104:183–189.

3. Smith HW. The Kidney: Structure and Function in Health and Disease. New York, NY: Oxford University Press, 1951.

4. Dooley MJ, Poole SG. Poor correlation between body surface area and glomerular filtration rate. Cancer Chemother Pharmacol 2000; 46:523–526.

5. Schnegg M, Lauterburg BH. Quantitative liver function in the elderly assessed by galactose elimination capacity, aminopyrine demethylation and caffeine clearance. J Hepatol 1986; 3:164–171.

6. Lauterburg BH, Preisig R. Quantitation of liver function. In: McIntyre N, Benhamou J, Bircher J, Rizzetto M, Rodes J (eds). Oxford Textbook of Clinical Hepatology. Oxford, UK: Oxford University Press, 1991, pp. 309–314.

7. Nawaratne S, Brien JE, Seeman E, et al. Relationships among liver and kidney volumes, lean body mass and drug clearance. Br J Clin Pharmacol 1998; 46:447–452.

8. Crawford JD, Terry ME, Rourke GM. Simplification of drug dosage calculation by application of the surface area principle. Pediatrics 1950; 5:783–790.

9. Freireich EJ, Gehan EA, Rall DP, Schmidt LH, Skipper HE. Quantitative comparison of toxicity of anticancer agents in mouse, rat, hamster, dog, monkey, and man. Cancer Chemother Rep 1966; 50:219–231.

10. Goldsmith MA, Slavik M, Carter SK. Quantitative prediction of drug toxicity in humans from toxicology in small and large animals. Cancer Res 1975; 35:1354–1364.

11. Pinkel D. The use of body surface area as a criterion of drug dosage in cancer chemotherapy. Cancer Res 1958; 18:853–856.

12. Morgan DJ, Bray KM. Lean body mass as a predictor of drug dosage. Implications for drug therapy. Clin Pharmacokinet 1994; 26:292–307.

13. Fleming RA, Eldridge RM, Johnson CE, Stewart CF. Disposition of high-dose methotrexate in an obese cancer patient. Cancer 1991; 68:1247–1250.

14. Gibbs JP, Gooley T, Corneau B, et al. The impact of obesity and disease on busulfan oral clearance in adults. Blood 1999; 93:4436–4440.

15. Lind MJ, Margison JM, Cerny T, Thatcher N, Wilkinson PM. Prolongation of ifosfamide elimination half-life in obese patients due to altered drug distribution. Cancer Chemother Pharmacol 1989; 25:139–142.

16. Rodvold KA, Rushing DA, Tewksbury DA. Doxorubicin clearance in the obese. J Clin Oncol 1988; 6:1321–1327.

17. Powis G, Reece P, Ahmann DL, Ingle JN. Effect of body weight on the pharmacokinetics of cyclophosphamide in breast cancer patients. Cancer Chemother Pharmacol 1987; 2:219–222.

18. Caraco Y, Zylber-Katz E, Berry EM, Levy M. Antipyrine disposition in obesity: evidence for negligible effect of obesity on hepatic oxidative metabolism. Eur J Clin Pharmacol 1995; 47:525–530.

19. Hunt CM, Westerkam WR, Stave GM. Effect of age and gender on the activity of human hepatic CYP3A. Biochem Pharmacol 1992; 44:275–283.

20. Cheymol G. Clinical pharmacokinetics of drugs in obesity. An update. Clin Pharmacokinet 1993; 25:103–114.

21. Roland M, Tozer T. Clinical Pharmacokinetics. Concepts and Applications, 3rd Edit. Baltimore, MD: Williams & Wilkins, 1994.

22. Xuan D, Lu JF, Nicolau DP, Nightingale CH. Population pharmacokinetics of tobramycin in hospitalized patients receiving once-daily dosing regimen. Int J Antimicrob Agents 2000; 15:185–191.

23. Touw DJ, Graafland O, Cranendonk A, Vermeulen RJ, van Weissenbruch MM. Clinical pharmacokinetics of phenobarbital in neonates. Eur J Pharmaceut Sci 2000; 12:111–116.

24. Murry DJ, Oermann CM, Ou CN, Rognerud C, Seilheimer DK, Sockrider MM. Pharmacokinetics of ibuprofen in patients with cystic fibrosis. Pharmacotherapy 1999; 19:340–345.

25. Madden T, Sunderland M, Santana VM, Rodman JH. The pharmacokinetics of high-dose carboplatin in pediatric patients with cancer. Clin Pharmacol Ther 1992; 51:701–707.

26. Nguyen L, Tranchand B, Puozzo C, Variol P. Population pharmacokinetics model and limited sampling strategy for intravenous vinorelbine derived from phase I clinical trials. Br J Clin Pharmacol 2002; 53:459–468.

27. Miya T, Goya T, Fujii H, et al. Factors affecting the pharmacokinetics of CPT-11: the body mass index, age and sex are independent predictors of pharmacokinetic parameters of CPT-11. Invest New Drugs 2001; 19:61–67.

28. Sam WJ, Aw M, Quak SH, et al. Population pharmacokinetics of tacrolimus in Asian paediatric liver transplant patients. Br J Clin Pharmacol 2000; 50:531–541.

29. Rothenberg ML, Kuhn JG, Schaaf LJ, et al. Phase I dose-finding and pharmacokinetic trial of irinotecan (CPT-11) administered every two weeks. Ann Oncol 2001; 12:1631–1641.

30. Tjuljandin SA, Doig RG, Sobol MM, et al. Pharmacokinetics and toxicity of two schedules of high dose epirubicin. Cancer Res 1990; 50:5095–5101.
31. van der Gaast A, Vlastuin M, Kok TC, Splinter TA. What is the optimal dose and duration of treatment with etoposide? II. Comparative pharmacokinetic study of three schedules: 1×100 mg, 2×50 mg, and 4×25 mg of oral etoposide daily for 21 days. Semin Oncol 1992; 19(6 Suppl 14):8–12.
32. Millward MJ, Newell DR, Yuen K, et al. Pharmacokinetics and pharmacodynamics of prolonged oral etoposide in women with metastatic breast cancer. Cancer Chemother Pharmacol 1995; 37:161–167.
33. Gianni L, Kearns CM, Giani A, et al. Nonlinear pharmacokinetics and metabolism of paclitaxel and its pharmacokinetic/pharmacodynamic relationships in humans. J Clin Oncol 1995; 13:180–190.
34. Huizing MT, Vermorken JB, Rosing H, et al. Pharmacokinetics of paclitaxel and three major metabolites in patients with advanced breast carcinoma refractory to anthracycline therapy treated with a 3-hour paclitaxel infusion: a European Cancer Centre (ECC) trial. Ann Oncol 1995; 6:699–704,
35. Grochow LB, Baraldi C, Noe D. Is dose normalization to weight or body surface area useful in adults? J Natl Cancer Inst 1990; 82:323–325.
36. Reilly JJ, Workman P. Normalisation of anti-cancer drug dosage using body weight and surface area: is it worthwhile? A review of theoretical and practical considerations. Cancer Chemother Pharmacol 1993; 32:411–418.
37. Gurney H. Dose calculation of anticancer drugs: a review of the current practice and introduction of an alternative. J Clin Oncol 1996; 14:2590–2611.
38. Ratain MJ. Body-surface area as a basis for dosing of anticancer agents: science, myth, or habit? J Clin Oncol 1998; 16:2297–2298.
39. Gurney H. How to calculate the dose of chemotherapy. Br J Cancer 2002; 86:1297–1302.
40. Gamelin E, Boisdron-Celle M, Guerin-Meyer V, et al. Correlation between uracil and dihydrouracil plasma ratio, fluorouracil (5-FU) pharmacokinetic parameters, and tolerance in patients with advanced colorectal cancer: a potential interest for predicting 5-FU toxicity and determining optimal 5-FU dosage. J Clin Oncol 1999; 17:1105–1110.
41. Furuta T, Ohashi K, Kamata T, et al. Effect of genetic differences in omeprazole metabolism on cure rates for *Helicobacter pylori* infection and peptic ulcer. Ann Intern Med 1998; 129:1027–1030.
42. Motohashi H, Sakurai Y, Saito H, et al. Gene expression levels and immunolocalization of organic ion transporters in the human kidney. J Am Soc Nephrol 2002; 13:866–874.
43. Calvert AH, Newell DR, Gumbrell LA, et al. Carboplatin dosage: prospective evaluation of a simple formula based on renal function. J Clin Oncol 1989; 7:1748–1756.
44. Kullak-Ublick GA, Ismair MG, Stieger B, et al. Organic anion-transporting polypeptide B (OATP-B) and its functional comparison with three other OATPs of human liver. Gastroenterology 2001; 120: 525–533.
45. van Asperen J, van Tellingen O, Beijnen JH. The role of mdr1, a P-glycoprotein in the biliary and intestinal secretion of doxorubicin and vinblastine in mice. Drug Metab Dispos 2000; 28:264–267.
46. Yamaguchi K, Yasuzawa T, Sakai T, Kobayashi S. Identification of novel metabolites of vinorelbine in rat. Xenobiotica 1998; 28:281–291.
47. Liddle C, Goodwin B. Regulation of hepatic drug metabolism: role of the nuclear receptors PXR and CAR. Semin Liver Dis 2002; 22:115–122.
48. Kast HR, Goodwin B, Tarr PT, et al. Regulation of multidrug resistance-associated protein 2 (ABCC2) by the nuclear receptors pregnane X receptor, farnesoid X-activated receptor, and constitutive androstane receptor. J Biol Chem 2002; 277:2908–2915.
49. Guo GL, Staudinger J, Ogura K, Klaassen CD. Nucleotide induction of rat organic anion transporting polypeptide 2 by pregnenolone-16alpha-carbonitrile is via interaction with pregnane X receptor. Mol Pharmacol 2002; 61:832–839.
50. Wrighton SA, VandenBranden M, Ring BJ. The human drug metabolizing cytochromes P450. J Pharmacokinet Biopharm 1996; 24:461–473.
51. Kuehl P, Zhang J, Lin Y, et al. Sequence diversity in CYP3A promoters and characterization of the genetic basis of polymorphic CYP3A5 expression. Nat Genet 2001; 4:383–391.
52. Tanabe M, Ieiri I, Nagata N, et al. Expression of P-glycoprotein in human placenta: relation to genetic polymorphism of the multidrug resistance (MDR)-1 gene. J Pharmacol Exp Ther 2001; 297:1137–1143.
53. Zhang J, Kuehl P, Green ED, et al. The human pregnane X receptor: genomic structure and identification and functional characterization of natural allelic variants. Pharmacogenetics 2001; 7:555–572.
54. Etienne MC, Lagrange JL, Dassonville O, Fleming R, Thyss A. Population study of dihydropyrimidine dehydrogenase in cancer patients. J Clin Oncol 1994; 12:2248–2253.

55. Maring JG, van Kuilenburg AB, Haasjes J, et al. Reduced 5-FU clearance in a patient with low DPD activity due to heterozygosity for a mutant allele of the DPYD gene. Br J Cancer 2002; 86: 1028–1033.
56. Iyer L, Das S, Janisch L, et al. UGT1A1*28 polymorphism as a determinant of irinotecan disposition and toxicity. Pharmacogenomics J 2002; 2:43–47.
57. Iressa investigators brochure on file, Astra Zeneca.
58. Berinstein NL, Grillo-Lopez AJ, White CA, et al. Association of serum Rituximab (IDEC-C2B8) concentration and anti-tumor response in the treatment of recurrent low-grade or follicular non-Hodgkin's lymphoma. Ann Oncol 1998; 9:995–1001.
59. Imatinib investigators' brochure on file, Novartis.
60. de Jongh FE, Verweij J, Loos WJ, et al. Body-surface area-based dosing does not increase accuracy of predicting cisplatin exposure. J Clin Oncol 2001; 19: 3733–3739.
61. Mathijssen RHJ, Verweij J, Maja JA, et al. Impact of body-size measures on irinotecan clearance: alternative dosing recommendations. J Clin Oncol 2002; 20:81–87.
62. Smorenburg CH, Sparreboom A, Botenbal M, Stoter G, Nooter K, Verweij J. Randomized-crossover evaluation of body-surface area-based dosing versus flat-fixed dosing of paclitaxel. J Clin Oncol 2003; 21:197–202.
63. Gurney HP, Ackland S, Gebski V, Farrell G. Factors affecting epirubicin pharmacokinetics and toxicity: evidence against using body-surface area for dose calculation. J Clin Oncol 1998; 16: 2299–3004.
64. Gurney H, Ackland S, Liddle C, et al. Determining the drug elimination phenotype: hepatic sestamibi scan and midazolam clearance as in vivo tests for drug metabolism and biliary elimination. Proc Am Soc Clin Oncol 2001; 20: abstract 305.
65. Bergh J, Wiklund T, Erikstein B, et al. Tailored fluorouracil, epirubicin, and cyclophosphamide compared with marrow-supported high-dose chemotherapy as adjuvant treatment for high-risk breast cancer: a randomised trial. Scandinavian Breast Group 9401 study. Lancet 2000; 356:1384–1391.
66. Schott AF, Taylor LB, Baker L. Individualized chemotherapy dosing based on metabolic phenotype. Proc Am Soc Clin Oncol 2001; 20:abstr 306.
67. Rivory LP, Slaviero K, Seale JP, et al. Optimizing the erythromycin breath test for use in cancer patients. Clin Cancer Res 2000; 6:3480–3485.
68. Innocenti F, Iyer L, Ratain MJ. Pharmacogenetics: a tool for individualizing antineoplastic therapy. Clin Pharmacokinet 2000; 39:315–325.
69. Stoehlmacher J, Park DJ, Zhang W, et al. Association between glutathione S-transferase P1, T1, and M1 genetic polymorphism and survival of patients with metastatic colorectal cancer. J Natl Cancer Inst 2002; 94:936–942.
70. Bruno R, Hille D, Riva A, et al. Population pharmacokinetics/pharmacodynamics of docetaxel in Phase II studies in patients with cancer. J Clin Oncol 1998; 16:187–196.
71. Bruno R, Vivler N, Vergniol JC, De Phillips SL, Montay G, Sheiner LB. A population pharmacokinetic model for docetaxel (Taxotere): model building and validation. J Pharmacokinet Biopharmacol 1996; 24:153–172.
72. Jen JF, Cutler DL, Pai SM, Batra VK, Affrime MB, Zambas DN, Heft S, Hajian G. Population pharmacokinetics of temozolomide in cancer patients. Pharm Res 2000; 17:1284–1289.
73. Hammond LA, Eckardt JR, Baker SD, et al. Phase I and pharmacokinetic study of temozolomide on a daily-for-5-days schedule in patients with advanced solid malignancies. J Clin Oncol 1999; 17: 2604–2613.
74. Nguyen L, Tranchand B, Puozzo C, Variol P. Population pharmacokinetics model and limited sampling strategy for intravenous vinorelbine derived from phase I clinical trials. Br J Clin Pharmacol 2002; 53:459–468.
75. Nguyen L, Chatelut E, Chevreau C, et al. Population pharmacokinetics of total and unbound etoposide. Cancer Chemother Pharmacol 1998; 41:125–132
76. Miya T, Goya T, Fujii H, et al. Factors affecting the pharmacokinetics of CPT-11: the body mass index, age and sex are independent predictors of pharmacokinetic parameters of CPT-11. Invest New Drugs 2001; 19:61–67.
77. Loos WJ, Gelderblom H, Sparreboom A, Verweij J, de Jonge MJ. Inter- and intrapatient variability in oral topotecan pharmacokinetics: implications for body-surface area dosage regimens. Clin Cancer Res 2000; 6:2685–2689.

78. Dobbs NA, Twelves CJ. What is the effect of adjusting epirubicin doses for body surface area? Br J Cancer 1998; 78:662–666.
79. Miya T, Goya T, Yanagida O, Nogami H, Koshiishi Y, Sasaki Y. The influence of relative body weight on toxicity of combination chemotherapy with cisplatin and etoposide. Cancer Chemother Pharmacol 1998; 42:386–390.

5 Phase I Trials in Oncology

Design and Endpoints

James Cassidy, MB, ChB, MSc, MD, FRPC

CONTENTS

INTRODUCTION
SELECTION OF PATIENTS
STARTING DOSE SELECTION
SCHEDULE SELECTION
DOSE ESCALATION
ENDPOINTS
SURROGATE ENDPOINTS
LIMITATIONS
CONCLUSIONS

1. INTRODUCTION

Development of drugs to treat cancer is different from that for other diseases for a number of important reasons. Some of these are self evident, but all have a profound influence on drug development in this therapeutic area.

Cancer is perceived by patients as an immediate life-threatening event. In many cases this perception is correct and therefore there is a sense of urgency to initiate therapy and an understandable reluctance to take part in trials that involve a placebo of any sort. It is thus rare to conduct the "gold standard" double-blinded randomized controlled trial that is common in other disease entities.

The majority of cancer drugs that have come through the drug development process are traditional cytotoxics that target DNA or the mechanics of cell division. As such they usually have antiproliferative side effects such as myelosuppression, mucositis, hair loss, and teratogenic effects. It is therefore impossible to employ normal volunteer studies, which again are a mainstay of noncancer clinical pharmacology. Thus, we are almost always trying to develop drugs in patients with cancer. It is clear that few (if any) patients will volunteer for an experimental therapy when standard care is available. The problem is then compounded by the need to use end-stage patients for our Phase I studies in cancer.

Often comparatively little is known about many of the fundamental issues of mechanism of action, schedule dependency, toxicity, pharmacodynamics, and pharmacokinetics when a new anticancer drug is first administered to humans. So we are forced to develop safety-

Handbook of Anticancer Pharmacokinetics and Pharmacodynamics
Edited by: W. D. Figg and H. L. McLeod © Humana Press Inc., Totowa, NJ

conscious clinical plans, but also ones that will allow the therapeutic goals to be achieved as quickly and efficiently as possible. It is clear that these competing tensions result in a decision-making process that is far from ideal.

The paradigms that have been used for drug development in oncology have been designed to cope with traditional cytotoxic drugs, and these will not likely be applicable to drugs that are cytostatic or act on a particular aspect of the malignant phenotype such as angiogenesis, invasion, or metastatic capacity.

The normal volunteer study used in traditional pharmacology has more than one endpoint. It is usual to measure the expected effect in volunteers (e.g., blood pressure in response to an antihypertensive drug). It is also usual that toxicity will not be observed and thus placebo controls are commonly used to exclude nonspecific effects such as nausea or headache. In cancer the commonly applied endpoint for a Phase I study is the observation of a dose-limiting side effect (DLT), which is then used to define a maximal tolerated dose (MTD). We monitor tumor response but realistically do not expect to see any such response in most cases. Cancer Phase I studies therefore should be more appropriately thought of as toxicological investigations in humans. The traditional aim of a Phase I study is to define a safe dose and schedule to be taken into Phases II and III with the aim of determining activity in these later trials. It is self-evident that declaring an inappropriate dose after Phase I will have serious consequences—usually lack of activity if MTD is set too low, or conversely, too much toxicity if MTD is set too high.

This chapter outlines the usual methodology for "cytotoxic" drugs and highlights the important limitations of this approach. In many instances we have not yet found ideal ways of developing some classes of agents, and continued methodological developments are required to improve efficiency in this area of therapeutics (1,2).

2. SELECTION OF PATIENTS

As has been demonstrated, we usually cannot employ normal volunteers for Phase I studies in cancer. Mainly because of potential toxicity, we are limited to working with cancer patients who have either failed standard therapy or for whom no standard therapy exists. It is self evident that such patients tend to have widespread metastases, limited life expectancy, and numerous manifestations of the underlying cancer. These can be nonspecific such as malaise, nausea, anorexia, lethargy, or cachexia. Alternatively, they can be organ-specific, such as neuropathy, renal dysfunction, diarrhea, or hepatic dysfunction.

This has important ramifications for drug testing in this group. It can be difficult to tease out drug-related effects from the clinical manifestations of the disease; intercurrent comedication is the rule, with all of the potential for drug interactions, and the handling of the drug may be altered by organ dysfunction.

To attempt to limit such problems we select patients within very careful entry criteria. They usually should have at least a 3-mo life expectancy to allow time to observe any side effects. They should have critical organ function (liver, renal) that is normal or near normal. This will help limit variable pharmacokinetics between patients and allow for some comparison to be made between animal pharmacokinetics (done with normal organ function) and the human experience (3). Unfortunately, this leads to a high degree of patient selection, as most people with advanced intractable cancer will have deranged organ function.

3. STARTING DOSE SELECTION

At the start of the first Phase I trial of an anticancer drug, we will have some (limited) data on dosing in animal model systems. Usually this will have been derived from toxicity (lethality) experiments and will have been performed across a limited dose range *(4)*. In the case of standard cytotoxics with marrow toxicity, there is fairly good correlation with human toxicology (reviewed in ref. *1*). The convention with such drugs is to employ as a starting dose 1/10th of the lethal dose in 10% of animals (LD_{10})—in the most sensitive animal species— and this has been shown to be generally safe if somewhat conservative *(5)*.

It is quite unlikely that such a correlation will exist for agents with alternative mechanisms of action. More subjective side effects such as malaise, nausea, headache, and myalgia cannot be observed in animals, yet it is these that are emerging in many instances as the dose-limiting effects for drugs aimed at "new targets." The real dilemma is to select a starting dose that will be safe but not so low as to then make the trial last very long and give the early-dose patients no chance of responding to therapy.

4. SCHEDULE SELECTION

Preclinical knowledge of schedule dependency with a new agent is usually sketchy at best. At most one will have some idea of an appropriate route of administration and a concept of whether the drug needs to be given often or as a single dose with time allowed for normal tissue recovery. The dilemma is then how often to give the new drug in early-phase studies? Considerations of mechanism of action, expected toxicities, and convenience will all have an influence here. Often sponsors and investigators try to avoid this issue by setting up studies with a variety of schedules; this does not usually solve the dilemma, but simply delays the decision-making process until the Phase II plans are made.

5. DOSE ESCALATION

The same dilemma applies in the case of dose escalation schema. If the most efficient Phase I is that which reaches the MTD as quickly as possible, the temptation is to be aggressive with dose escalation *(6)*. In the absence of toxicity at the previous dose, how much of an increase should be made for the next dose level? A variety of fairly arbitrary methods are utilized to try to overcome this dilemma. Traditionally dose escalation has been performed using a "modified" Fibonacci scheme; if level 1 is the starting dose X1, level 2 is X1 + 100%, level 3 is X2 plus 67%, level 4 is X3 plus 50%, and level 5 and above are Xn + 30–35%. This method was introduced in the early 1970s with nitrosourea and epipodophyllotoxin. It has a few inherent problems. The "modified" part is usually a preset number of drug dose doublings that will be allowed before the more conservative part is commenced. This is too often decided in an arbitrary fashion but can have a profound effect on the trial. Too many doublings might lead to excessive toxicity, and too few leads to a trial that lasts longer than it should and exposes too many patients to subtherapeutic drug doses. A widely practiced method to avoid this pitfall is to maintain drug dose doubling until the first drug-related adverse events are observed and then to employ the Fibonacci element. This also has limitations, because of the amount of non-drug-related problems that such patients encounter it is sometimes difficult to define accurately the relationship to the study drug. The tendency is to err on the side of caution, enter the Fibonacci phase, and then find that these "toxicities" are absent in subsequent dose cohorts. How many patients should be treated at each dose level? This is usually arbitrarily set at three patients per dose cohort in the absence of toxicity that would mandate expansion of the cohort. However, many investigators have switched to single-patient cohorts at least for the very early low doses to limit exposure of patients to doses that are too low to have a realistic expectation of efficacy. It is worth noting that although this aim may be achieved, the use of single-patient cohorts will not necessarily result in more rapid escalation through the doses.

Dose escalation usually tales place with each new cohort. Intrapatient dose escalation is less common, but at times the same patient has been re-entered at a later (higher-dose) cohort. The argument against it is that, if cumulative toxicities occur, it will be more complex to attribute them correctly if intrapatient escalation is performed. However, if an adequate washout period is allowed, it may be reasonable to allow patients to have a higher dose with more expectation of therapeutic benefit.

This method is considered by many to be over-conservative (6) and, as a result, alternatives have been sought based on pharmacokinetics (7) and, more recently, Bayesian approaches (8,9). As yet none have reached as widespread acceptance as the "modified" Fibonacci. One particularly intriguing possibility is to allow patients to select their own doses using a linear analog scale that ranges from "low dose–low toxicity with less chance of a response" up to "high dose–toxicity likely with more chance of a response."

6. ENDPOINTS

The accepted dogma in oncology is, the higher the dose, the better the antitumor effect. This can be verified for some cytotoxic drugs up to a threshold value beyond which toxicity becomes limiting or even lethal. Conversely, we do not often have an identifiable lower dose threshold for activity with a cytotoxic agent. In fact, most drugs we use have an apparently very narrow therapeutic index. The usual endpoint for a cytotoxic Phase I study thus is the occurrence of grade 3–4 reversible toxicity in the majority of patients treated at that dose level. Objective measures of blood parameters can be simply applied to predefine acceptable levels of toxicity. Subjective toxicity causes much more of a problem. A lethargy that one person might consider intolerable may be of little significance to a more stoical individual.

Even the apparently simple objective measures such as blood count parameters are under question now. The discovery and widespread use of hematological growth factors to support blood counts means that we could define MTD with and without such support (or even a cocktail of such "support" molecules). This has some merit in that we commonly define MTD in terms of nausea and vomiting *despite* maximal antiemetic support. Conceptually similar though these situations are, it is not yet widely accepted to perform initial Phase I trials of drug plus growth factor.

It is also possible to influence such endpoints by patient selection. Prior exposure to cytotoxics or extensive radiotherapy with fields encompassing marrow primes patients to experience myelosuppression. It is necessary to take account of this, usually by including a cohort of "good risk" patients at the end of the trial to ensure that the MTD has not been set too low.

7. SURROGATE ENDPOINTS

The schema outlined above has been shown over the years of development of "cytotoxics" to be fairly efficient. Individual drugs or clinical circumstances require that the basic plan be altered slightly to take such factors into account. A good example is the situation when acute toxicity is not dose limiting but a cumulative effect such as neuropathy is expected to be the DLT.

The world of oncology has now moved into a new and exciting era when the explosion in molecular knowledge about the cellular phenotype that defines cancer is being translated into drugs designed to inhibit some aspects of this phenotype. Examples are drugs that inhibit invasion (matrix metalloproteinase inhibitors [MMPIs]) (10), that inhibit angiogenesis (11), and that interfere with growth regulatory signals within cells, such as Ras farnesylation inhibitors.

The clinical testing of these agents is complicated by the expectation that they will have a novel spectrum of toxicity and lack the usual "cytotoxic" effects such as marrow damage. In addition, it is unreasonable to expect such agents to cause tumor volume shrinkage in the context of bulky disease. So we have lost both of our familiar markers of activity and toxicity. This has led to the development of so-called "surrogate" markers. The ideal such marker would be able to define rapidly and efficiently that the target had been affected in the appropriate tissue in the manner and extent that one would predict. In the case of MMPI, one could assay the activity of the target enzymes in the target tissues (i.e., tumor and normal tissue to define selectivity). Because it is uncommon to be able to get serial tumor biopsies, the ideal surrogate tissue is likely to be the peripheral blood. The complexities in developing such surrogate markers immediately become apparent. However, when compared with the time and expense of developing a drug that fails to reach the clinic, the expenditure to develop worthwhile clinically applicable and validated surrogate endpoints can be viewed as good value.

An alternative (overlapping) strategy is to apply the more modern imaging modalities to measure more directly the functional effect of the drug rather than just volume change in the tumor mass. The simplest example is the measure of blood flow in the tumor under the influence of drugs that purport to alter this, for example, combretastin. More information is also available from positron emission tomography (PET) and magnetic resonance imaging (MRI), but these methodologies are still in development and will require prospective validation before drug development "stop–go" decisions would be possible.

A further approach taken by many investigators in this field is to combine the new cytostatic agent with a known cytotoxic, thereby allowing our original paradigm to be used *(12)*.

8. LIMITATIONS

The generic design of Phase I outlined in this chapter has several limitations that are particularly relevant when considering the evaluation of non-DNA-targeted drugs.

1. The MTD may be far in excess of the dose required to optimize efficacy. One example might be the inhibition of a target enzyme that is complete and durable at dose X. So dose 2X has no additional benefit and, even worse, causes an additional toxicity that may be unrelated to specific target inhibition.

2. Chronic dosing is almost impossible to achieve in the standard Phase I population because of disease progression and cancer-related adverse events that prevent further dosing. In addition, because MTD is usually defined by acute events, the long-term dosing required in Phase II or III may be found to be impossible. A good example is the case of MMPIs, which as a group tend to be limited both by daily dose and duration of therapy that is tolerable.

3. Patients in Phase I are selected for good organ function. The reasons for this are outlined above and are based mainly on safety considerations. However, because those same considerations apply in Phases II and III, we end up with a population that is *not* representative of the average patient with advanced cancer. This has two important long-term consequences:

    a. Response rates in Phase II (and even some Phase III) trials are higher than one might expect in a less select group of patients. This is often the basis for press reports of "wonder drugs" that can immeasurably damage the psychological well-being of cancer patients.

    b. The response rates from Phase II are used to set the parameters for statistical considerations in the ensuing Phase III trials—which then turn out to be insufficiently powered to reveal the smaller (but still clinically significant) advantage that one might realistically expect.

4. The small numbers of patients enrolled in Phase I trials are not sufficient to define fully the toxicity pattern of a drug. For this reason, not only should response rates be viewed with some suspicion, but also reports of little or no toxicity should be treated with caution.

9. CONCLUSIONS

Fairly sound methodology has been developed over the last 30 yr for the development of cytotoxic agents. However, many elements in the overall plan are reliant on empirical decision making. This may not have been so crucial when developing drugs with "standard" antiproliferative effects. It is very likely that this same plan will not apply to cytostatic-type agents. Further scientific protocols for the clinical development of such agents are urgently needed. It seems highly likely that time and energy spent developing surrogate markers of activity will pay dividends in the long run.

REFERENCES

1. Arbuck SG. Workshop on Phase 1 design. Ann Oncol 1996; 7:567–573.
2. Korn EL, Arbuck SG, Pluda JM, et al. Clinical trial designs for cytoststic agents: Are new approaches needed? J Clin Oncol 2001; 19:265–272.
3. Newell DR. Phase 1 clinical studies with cytotoxic drugs: pharmacokinetic and pharmacodynamic considerations. Br J Cancer 1990; 61:189–191.
4. Burtles SS, Newell DR, Henrar REC, Connors TA. Revisions of general guidelines for the preclinical toxicology of new cytotoxic anticancer agents in Europe. Eur J Cancer 1995; 31:408–410.
5. Newell DR, Burtles SS, Fox BW, Jodrell DI, Connors TA. Evaluation of rodent only toxicology for early clinical trials with novel cancer therapeutics. Br J Cancer 1999; 81:760–768.
6. Penta JS, Rosner LR, Trump DL. Choice of starting dose and escalation for phase 1 studies of antitumor agents. Cancer Chemother Pharmacol 1992; 31:247–250.
7. Evans WE, Rodman JH, Relling MV, et al. Concept of maximum tolerated systemic exposure and its application to Phase I–II studies of anticancer drugs. Med Pediatr Oncol 1991; 19:153–159.
8. O'Quigley J, Shen LZ. Continual reassessment methodology: a likelihood approach. Biometrics 1996; 52:673–684.
9. O'Quigley J, Pepe M, Fisher L. Continual reassessment method: a practical design for Phase 1 clinical trials in cancer. Biometrics 1990; 46(1):33–48.
10. Denis LJ, Verweij J. Matrix metalloproteinase inhibitors: present achievements and future prospects. Invest New Drugs 1997; 15:175–185.
11. Kerbel RS. Clinical trials of antiangiogenic drugs: opportunities, problems and assessment of initial results. J Clin Oncol 2001; 19:45s–51s.
12. Baselga J, Averbuch SD. ZD1839 (Iressa) as an anticancer agent. Drugs 2000; 60:33–40.

6 Analytical Methods

*Development, Validation,
and Clinical Applicability*

Hans Ehrsson, *PhD*, Staffan Eksborg, *PhD*, and Jonas Bergh, *MD*, *PhD*

CONTENTS

1. INTRODUCTION

The anticancer drugs constitute an extremely heterogeneous group of chemical entities. Inorganic compounds (cisplatin, arsenic trioxide) and low-molecular-weight (hydroxyurea) as well as high-molecular-weight organic compounds (bleomycin) are represented. Thus, almost every drug will require evaluation of optimal conditions for sample handling and analytical procedures. The situation is complicated further by the fact that the given drug can be inactive *per se* and requires biotransformation to be pharmacologically active. For example, cyclophosphamide has to be enzymatically converted to 4-hydroxycyclophosphamide in the liver and temozolamide must be degraded in vivo to the linear triazine MTIC, which exerts the antitumor activity. There are also examples where both the parent compound and the formed metabolites contribute to the cytotoxic activity, for example, chlorambucil and its main metabolite phenylacetic acid mustard. It is therefore essential to establish which substance(s) should be quantified when performing pharmacokinetic/pharmacodynamic studies and that sufficient sensitivity and selectivity are obtained by the analytical procedure used.

In this chapter we focus on some important areas that in our opinion have not previously been sufficiently penetrated. The examples discussed will mostly come from our own

Handbook of Anticancer Pharmacokinetics and Pharmacodynamics
Edited by: W. D. Figg and H. L. McLeod © Humana Press Inc., Totowa, NJ

research concerning alkylating agents, platinum-containing drugs, and antraquinone glycosides.

Those interested in an overview of analytical techniques for anticancer drugs are referred
to a recent review *(1)*.

2. CHEMICAL STABILITY IN BIOLOGICAL MATERIAL

2.1. Alkylating Agents and Cisplatin

The stability of most anticancer drugs, for example, cisplatin, oxaliplatin, and busulfan,
is mostly lower in biological material as compared to pure aqueous solutions. Cisplatin, for
example, is stable in an acidic aqueous solution containing 0.1 M sodium chloride whereas
the degradation half-life in human plasma is only about 0.9 h (37°C) *(2)*. The low stability
in plasma is attributable to the fact that the compound has a high propensity to react with
thiol-containing endogenous compounds, for example, albumin, glutathione, and cysteine.
The stability of cisplatin in whole blood is higher than in plasma, the half-life being approx
1.43 h, most probably because cisplatin is in a chemical environment with lower nucleophilic
character when partitioned to the red blood cells.

The low stability of cisplatin places stringent requirements on the handling of the blood
samples. The blood is collected in prechilled tubes, stored on ice, and ultrafiltrated centrip-
etally (20 min, 4°C) within 1 h using a 10,000 mol wt cutoff filter. Centripetal ultrafiltration
allows the free fraction of cisplatin in whole blood to be determined. Less than 5% of
cisplatin will be decomposed following this handling procedure *(2)*.

Anticancer drugs containing the nitrogen mustard group (chlorambucil, melphalan) have
for a long time been used in anticancer therapy. Recently, small peptides containing the
alkylating group have been suggested to mediate a more selective delivery to cancer cells
(3). The compounds are chemically unstable but, in contrast to the platinum-containing
drugs, show an increased stability in plasma. Thus, chlorambucil has a degradation half life
of 0.45 h in buffer (pH 7.4, 37°C) but is considerably more stable in the presence of albumin
($t_{1/2}$ = 15.8 h in 45 mg/mL of albumin). Chlorambucil is extensively bound to albumin, and
when bound it is about 100 times more stable than in the free form *(4)*. Formation of the
cyclic aziridinium ion is the rate-determining step in the hydrolysis of aromatic nitrogen
mustards. The rate of formation is drastically affected by the dielectric constant of the
solvent, and it can be concluded that chlorambucil when bound to albumin is in a chemical
environment with solvating properties quite different from those in pure aqueous solution.

2.2. Anthraquinone Glycosides

The antraquinone glycosides are extensively metabolized to their corresponding 13-
hydroxyderivatives by aldo–ketoreductase. This enzyme is present in most human tissues,
which has to be taken into account in the bioanalysis. The formation rate of the reduced
metabolites is increased with increasing lipophilic character of the drug. Incubation studies
in whole blood reveal fast formation of large amounts of daunorubicinol and idarubicinol
from the two most lipophilic anthraquinone glycosides commercially available *(5,6)*. The
conversion could be diminished by immediate cooling of the blood samples on ice or by
treatment of the samples by an ultrasonic cell disruptor. None of the anthraquinone glycosides are metabolized in cell-free plasma.

3. STABILITY DURING STORAGE

It is of utmost importance that the stability of the compound during storage conditions is
thoroughly investigated. For example, both cisplatin and oxaliplatin have a degradation half-

life of approx only 2 d in plasma at –20°C, which means that 10% of the compounds have decomposed already after 8 h during this storage condition. In ultrafiltrate both substances are stable for at least 1 mo at –80°C.

The concentration of doxorubicin in spiked-frozen (–20°C) plasma samples decreased during storage. Most likely the decrease was not the result of chemical degradation of the drug but caused by changes in the plasma matrix. The amount of precipitates in the thawed samples increased with increasing storage time and also by repeated freezing and thawing of plasma samples. Probably the anthraquinone glycosides are adsorbed on the precipitate, resulting in a decrease of the extraction yield during the analytical procedure *(5)*.

4. SELECTIVITY

Selectivity is a measure of the extent to which an analytical procedure can determine a particular compound without interference from matrix components, metabolites, or degradation products. Irrelevant conclusions have been drawn concerning the pharmacokinetics and the fate of the platinum-containing drugs in in vitro cell systems because of the use of analytical methods with insufficient selectivity. The pharmacokinetics of oxaliplatin has almost exclusively been based on the determination of the platinum content in plasma or ultrafiltrate using flameless atomic absorption spectroscopy (FAAS) or inductively coupled plasma mass spectrometry (ICPMS). The reported terminal half-lives in humans show large variations, the shortest 31–47 h, being obtained by FAAS and the longest, 189–273 h, by the more sensitive ICPMS *(7)*. Using highly selective liquid chromatography in combination with postcolumn derivatization with *N,N*-diethyldithiocarbamate in a microwave field, the kinetics was studied in patients with colorectal carcinoma. A median terminal half-life of 14 min was found *(8)*. Oxaliplatin rapidly reacts with endogenous low-molecular-weight species such as cysteine and methionine and high-molecular-weight compounds such as albumin, globulin, and hemoglobin. The long terminal half-lives reported (> 200 h) by measuring ultrafiltrate platinum most probably reflect the turnover rates of endogenous high-molecular-weight species representing inactive platinum conjugates.

The extensive studies of chromatographic properties of the anthraquinone glycosides using reversed phase systems showed that the chromatographic selectivity increased with decreasing concentration of organic modifier in the mobile phase. The choice of organic modifier is also of importance in pharmacokinetic studies of anthraquinone glycosides. Acetonitrile is superior to alcohols and acetone because of a higher chromatographic selectivity in separation of intact drugs and their corresponding active 13-hydroxy metabolites *(9)*. Thus, a number of pharmacokinetic studies have been conducted using reversed phase liquid chromatography with this organic modifier in the mobile phase, for example, a study of the influence of the infusion time on the pharmacokinetics of doxorubicin and a comparative pharmacokinetic study of doxorubicin after intravenous and intrahepatic administration *(10,11)*.

5. LIMIT OF QUANTIFICATION (LOQ)

LOQ is the lowest concentration of an analyte that can be measured with an acceptable level of precision and accuracy. The LOQ should be measured using the anticancer drug in the biological matrix and is usually the lowest point of the calibration curve. This value must of course be determined experimentally and never by extrapolation. An acceptable precision at LOQ is in general considered to be 10–20% coefficient of variation. It is essential that the analytical technique has sufficient sensitivity to establish accurately the terminal elimination half-life of the drug.

Photometric detection at 600 nm gives a high detection selectivity and sensitivity for quantification of the anthraquinone glycosides. Fluorometric detectors can preferably be used, as recent technical improvements have increased their sensitivity considerably.

Cisplatin has a low molar absorptivity but can be determined photometrically at 344 nm after postcolumn derivatization with N,N-diethyldithiocarbamate (12), giving a derivative with a molar absorptivity of 20,000 M^{-1} cm^{-1}. Busulfan, initially used in the treatment of chronic myelogenous leukemia, has today an important place in combination with bone marrow transplantation. A gas chromatographic method was developed for the analysis of busulfan in patients (13). The method comprises derivatization with iodide, extraction, and sample concentration in one single step. Replacing the methane sulfonate groups by iodide gives a derivative that can be determined with high sensitivity using electron capture detection as well as mass spectrometry.

6. CALIBRATION CURVES

Calibration curves are usually constructed by making up a series of the biological material, for example, blood or plasma, containing known amounts of the analyte and taking each sample separately through the analytical procedure. The analytical instrument generates a signal, which is plotted on the y-axis of a calibration graph with the standard concentrations on the x-axis. A straight line (or sometimes a curve) is drawn through the calibration points. Calculated regression coefficients are then used for the determination of sample concentrations.

The use of improper techniques for the determination of the regression coefficients might, however, introduce large systematic errors. Unless a proper test of accuracy is performed, these errors are difficult to detect.

Calibration curves are generally evaluated by ordinary linear (unweighted) regression. This technique might, however, be less accurate in the lower part of the calibration curves when a wide range of concentrations is to be determined, because of the regression equation to a great extent is determined by values in the high concentration range. In such cases, calibration curves sometimes are generated for different concentration ranges, that is, different regression equations are used. The choice of the various concentration ranges with corresponding regression equations is mostly arbitrary. The use of nonparametric statistical methods has become increasingly important for the evaluation of experimental data because these methods are valid even when the underlying distribution is not normal. Moreover, nonparametric regression procedures are less sensitive to outliers than least-squares regression.

Nonparametric linear regression (14,15) is almost as efficient as the least-squares method when the errors are normally distributed but much more efficient when the errors are not normally distributed, especially when n is small (16). The precision of the regression parameters is expressed by nonparametric confidence intervals (17). Nonparametric linear regression can easily be implemented with modern computers, for example, by the use of basic programming (18) or spreadsheet programs. Least median of squares regression is an alternative robust regression technique, minimizing the median squared residual (19). The median squared residual is not changed by outlying observations, and hence robust estimates of regression parameters are obtained. Extended least-squares regression, a general statistical estimation method, is a powerful tool for analysis of individual pharmacokinetic data, used to avoid the weighting problem in the data analysis (20).

Visual inspection of the corresponding calibration curves often gives the impression that almost identical sample concentrations are obtained irrespective of which of the previous principles for evaluation of calibrations curves has been used for quantification (21).

The ratio plot is an indispensable tool also for the validation of calibration curves. Calculated values of C_{est}/C_{actual} (C_{est} is the sample concentration in the standard solution determined from the regression coefficients and C_{actual} is the known concentration in the standard solution) have demonstrated that nonparametric, least median of squares regressions and extended least-squares regression are more suited for calculation of regression coefficients of calibration curves than ordinary linear regression in cases with large concentration intervals. Weighted least-squares regression might possibly increase the accuracy of estimated concentrations in the low concentration range, but the proper choice of weights is not obvious (20).

The high selectivity of the chromatographic system enables construction of calibration curves with two different anthraquinone glycosides as internal standards at different concentrations to cover the wide concentration ranges of doxorubicin and doxorubicinol expected in plasma samples from cancer patients. For pharmacokinetic studies two calibration curves were prepared for doxorubicin, one with a plasma concentration range of 2–200 ng/mL, using daunorubicin (30 ng/mL) as internal standard (IS) and one with a plasma concentration range of 200–1400 ng/mL, using idarubicin (400 ng/mL) as IS. A standard curve for doxorubicinol, 2–45 ng/mL, was prepared with daunorubicin (30 ng/mL) as IS. Daunorubicin and idarubicin were added as internal standards for all plasma samples from patients receiving doxorubicin giving concentrations of 30 ng/mL and 400 ng/mL, respectively.

7. CLINICAL APPLICABILITY

7.1. Cisplatin

It has generally been assumed that cisplatin is present as intact drug in plasma as a result of a high chloride concentration and is converted to the monohydrated complex (MHC) intracellularly because of the lower chloride concentration. MHC is supposed to exert the cytotoxic effect by binding to DNA. The use of liquid chromatography in combination with postcolumn derivatization with N,N-diethyldithiocarbamate made it possible for the first time to study the pharmacokinetics of both cisplatin and MHC in whole blood in patients (22). This study suggested that the kinetics of MHC was formation-rate-limited. The presence of MHC in blood is due to the fact that the pK_a for MHC is 6.56 (23) and at physiological pH it will be present mainly in its less reactive monohydroxo form. Preparative isolation of MHC on porous graphitic carbon using an alkaline mobile phase (24) also made it possible to evaluate its cytotoxicity in an in vitro system (25) and to study its nephrotoxic and ototoxic activity in an animal model (26). Previous studies on the toxicity of MHC have used hydrolysis mixtures of cisplatin in water that contained both the parent compound, MHC, the dihydrated complex, and possibly di- and trimeric platinum containing compounds.

Ototoxicity is one dose-limiting and unpredictable side effect of cisplatin treatment that together with nephro- and neurotoxicity has attracted a large amount of interest. Administration of sulfur-containing chemoprotectors, for example, D-methionine, has shown promising results regarding protection in animal models (27,28). We have recently shown that administration of D-methionine results in lower blood concentrations of cisplatin in an animal model, most probably as a result of a chemical interaction between cisplatin and the protector (29). It is essential to use selective techniques when performing these types of studies because analytical techniques measuring only total platinum concentration (e.g., by atomic absorption spectroscopy) will codetermine the drug and its reaction products with the protector.

7.2. Anthraquinone Glycosides

Doxorubicin, an anthraquinone glycoside, is currently one of the clinically most important antineoplastic drugs. In early clinical studies epirubicin appears to be one of the most promising new anthracycline derivatives, which is suggested to have a considerably higher therapeutic index than doxorubicin *(30)*.

Weenen et al. *(31)* stated that accurate comparison of the pharmacokinetics of doxorubicin and epirubicin must await evaluation of a large number of patients because of the considerable interindividual variability. However, by simultaneous administration or the two drugs combined with the use of a highly selective analytical technique, it has been possible to overcome intra- and interindividual variation and to compare their pharmacokinetics. Thus, by this method even minor differences in pharmacokinetics can be evaluated.

The plasma pharmacokinetics of doxorubicin and epirubicin have been studied after simultaneous intravenous bolus injection of equal amounts of the two drugs in patients with ovarian carcinoma and after simultaneous intrahepatic administration in patients with nonresectable and symptomatic liver cancer *(32,33)*.

The plasma concentration of epirubicin as well as of doxorubicin after intravenous and intrahepatic administration followed a three-compartment open model. The plasma concentration of doxorubicin was in all cases higher than that of epirubicin. On average the area under the plasma concentration time curve (AUC) and the maximum plasma concentration (C_{max}) were 2.1 and 1.7 times larger for doxorubicin than for epirubicin, respectively. Epirubicin was eliminated faster than doxorubicin, the terminal half-life time being, on average, 1.5 times longer for doxorubicin.

The reduced toxicity of epirubicin in comparison with doxorubicin after intravenous administration has been suggested to be the consequence of the pharmacokinetic behavior of epirubicin, characterized by constantly lower plasma levels as compared to doxorubicin, that is, a reduction in AUC and C_{max}. The importance of the differences in the pharmacokinetics of doxorubicin and epirubicin in relation to therapeutic efficacy is unclear.

The plasma concentrations of the 13-hydroxy metabolites did not exceed 20 ng/mL. Their AUC values averaged 23% of those of the intact drugs. The clinical importance of the 13-hydroxy metabolites, that is, influence on the therapeutic efficiency and side effects, is not fully understood. Extensive formation of these metabolites has been associated with a high therapeutic response. In model systems doxorubicinol in general has cytotoxic properties similar to those of doxorubicin.

Factors influencing the pharmacokinetics of doxorubicin and epirubicin administered simultaneously in equal doses as a 24-h constant rate infusion have been investigated in children (0.73–15.3 yr) with acute lymphocytic leukemia (ALL) *(34)*. In this pharmacokinetic study our previously published simplified sampling procedure comprising only one blood sample taken prior to the end of the infusion, that is, at pseudo-steady state, was used *(35)*.

The plasma pharmacokinetics of neither doxorubicin nor epirubicin correlated with the age of the pediatric patients. It was not possible to demonstrate a statistical difference of the dose-normalized maximum concentrations between males and females. The interpatient variations of the dose-normalized maximum concentrations of both drugs were, however, larger among females than among males.

The doxorubicin/epirubicin C_{max} ratio was 1.39. The pharmacokinetic differences in children are less pronounced than in adults. Hence, the reduction of systemic side effects obtained by substituting doxorubicin with epirubicin might be less pronounced in children than in adults. However, the pharmacokinetic differences of the two drugs in children are still of such a magnitude that substituting doxorubicin with epirubicin most likely will be of clinical importance.

A comparison of C_{max} values in the pediatric patients and in a previous study of adult breast cancer patients *(36)* shows that dosing based on body surface area results in similar plasma concentrations of epirubicin in children and adults, under the assumption that identical infusion rates are used. In contrast, dosing based on body weight results in lower plasma concentrations of epirubicin in children than in adults. The interpatient variation of the dose-normalized C_{max} values of epirubicin were higher in children with ALL than in breast cancer patients, underlining the difficulties in a proper dosing of anthraquinone glycosides to children. The rather marked interpatient variation in clearance has previously been demonstrated when epirubicin was used in the 5-FU, epirubicin, and cyclophosphamide (FEC) combination *(37)*.

8. CAPILLARY AND VENOUS BLOOD SAMPLING

The plasma pharmacokinetics for doxorubicin (area under plasma concentration time curve and maximum plasma concentration) show more than a 10-fold interindividual variability despite dosing based on body surface area *(10)*. An individualized doxorubicin dose, based on determined plasma concentrations, would therefore most likely result in an improvement of treatment *(38,39)*. The drug concentration in one single venous plasma sample drawn at the end of a constant infusion (2 h or longer) gives highly accurate estimates of the systemic exposure of the anthraquinone glycosides doxorubicin and epirubicin *(35)* and may substitute a complete pharmacokinetic evaluation requiring at least 12 blood samples collected over a 24-h period. The clinical applicability of this method has been established *(36)*. Plasma levels of anthraquinone glycosides have so far been measured using blood samples obtained by puncturing of a peripheral vein. With increased sensitivity of analytical techniques, for example, by using modern fluorometric detectors it is now possible to quantify anthraquinone glycosides in capillary samples, collected by a finger lancet puncture.

Potential concentration differences of doxorubicin in plasma from capillary and venous blood samples were evaluated in 16 patients (7 females and 9 males; median age: 37 yr, range: 1–77 yr) *(40)*. The quantitative analysis of doxorubicin was carried out by reversed phase liquid chromatography with fluorometric detection. The very high correlation between concentrations of doxorubicin in capillary and venous plasma samples ($r = 0.98$; $p < 0.0001$) might falsely give the impression that capillary and venous sampling sites can be used interchangeably. In contrast, the ratio plots *(41)* clearly demonstrate minor but significantly higher capillary plasma concentrations, the median capillary/venous plasma concentration ratio being 1.13 (95% confidence interval [CI]: 1.06–1.20). The wide plasma concentration range of doxorubicin, because of inclusion of samples from patients treated with large variations in dose and infusion times, did not affect the relative concentrations of doxorubicin in capillary and venous samples. Multiple regression with stepwise variable selection revealed that gender was the only variable tested affecting the capillary/venous plasma concentration ratio, the concentration ratio being significantly higher in males (median: 1.18) than in females (median: 1.01). Gender differences in plasma protein binding, body composition, or blood flow might influence the amount of doxorubicin diffusing into the tissue, thereby affecting the capillary/venous concentration ratio. The observed concentration differences of doxorubicin in plasma from capillary and venous samples are, however, of minor importance only.

The practical advantage of collecting capillary blood instead of venous blood is evident, but is most pronounced in pediatric patients, who often find venous blood sampling very traumatic. In addition, deterioration of the veins caused by treatment with antineoplastic drugs often results in difficulties in obtaining venous blood samples from cancer patients. Capillary blood sampling can now be recommended for therapeutic drug monitoring and pharmacokinetic studies of doxorubicin. To minimize the dilution of the blood with the interstitial fluid, the capillary blood sampling must be conducted with free flowing blood with minimum squeezing of the finger.

The phenomenon and rationale of blood sampling site dependence on drug concentrations have been reviewed *(42,43)*. A careful examination of drug concentration differences in capillary and venous blood samples is necessary prior to change of sampling site. Even though concentrations of large numbers of drugs in capillary and venous blood samples have been compared, the results are in general difficult to interpret because of unsuitable treatment of data, that is, the use of scatter diagrams. A high correlation coefficient and/or a *p* value < 0.05 is often considered sufficient for conclusions of interchangeable sampling sites. Hence, it was concluded that methotrexate venous blood sampling can be substituted by capillary blood sampling, as a scatterplot of the concentration data showed a correlation coefficient of 0.934 *(44)*. A closer examination of the data showed that the capillary/venous concentration ratio ranged from 0.2 to 3.1, a fact that may have serious consequences when basing the leucovorin rescue on measured methotrexate concentrations.

9. CONCLUSIONS

Many of the anticancer drugs are demanding from an analytical point of view, for example, chemical instability, low blood/plasma concentrations, and sometimes also the need to quantify several chemically closely related compounds. To obtain optimal results in pharmacokinetic/pharmacodynamic studies and therapeutic drug monitoring, a close interaction among analytical chemists, pharmacokinetic expertise, clinicians, nurses, and experts working in other disciplines is mandatory.

REFERENCES

1. De Palo E, Deyl F. Anticancer and antiviral agents including theraphy monitoring and diagnostic marker aspects. J Chromatogr B Biomed Sci Appl 2001; 764:1–464.
2. Andersson A, Ehrsson H. Stability of cisplatin and its monohydrated complex in blood, plasma and ultrafiltrate—implications for quantitative analysis. J Pharmaceut Biomed Anal 1995; 13:639–644.
3. Jiang JD, Zhang H, Li JN, et al. High anticancer efficacy of L-proline-*m-bis* (2-chloroethyl)amino-L-phenylalanyl-L-norvaline ethyl ester hydrochloride (MF 13) in vivo. Anticancer Res 2001; 21: 1681–1689.
4. Ehrsson H, Lönroth U, Wallin I, Ehrnebo M, Nilsson SO. Degradation of chlorambucil in aqueous solution—influence of human albumin binding. J Pharm Pharmacol 1981; 33:313–315.
5. Eksborg S, Ehrsson H, Wallin I, Lindfors A. Quantitative determination of adriamycin and daunorubicin—handling of blood and plasma samples. Acta Pharmaceut Suec 1981; 18:215–220.
6. Eksborg S, Nilsson B. Reversed-phase liquid chromatographic determination of idarubicin and its 13-hydroxy metabolite in human plasma. J Chromatogr 1989; 488:427–434.
7. Graham MA, Lockwood GF, Greenslade D, Brienza S, Bayssas M, Gamelin E. Clinical pharmacokinetics of oxaliplatin: a critical review. Clin Cancer Res 2000; 6:1205–1218.
8. Ehrsson H, Wallin I, Yachnin J. Pharmacokinetics of oxaliplatin in humans. Med Oncol 2002; 19:261–265.
9. Eksborg S. Reversed-phase liquid chromatography of adriamycin and daunorubicin and their hydroxyl metabolites adriamycinol and daunorubicinol. J Chromatogr 1978; 149:225–232.
10. Eksborg S, Strandler HS, Edsmyr F, Näslund I, Tahvanainen P. Pharmacokinetic study of i.v. infusions of adriamycin. Eur J Clin Pharmacol 1985; 28:205–212.
11. Eksborg S, Cedermark BJ, Strandler HS. Intrahepatic and intravenous administration of adriamycin— a comparative pharmacokinetic study in patients with malignant liver tumours. Med Oncol Tumor Pharmacother 1985; 2:47–54.
12. Andersson A, Ehrsson H. Determination of cisplatin and *cis*-diammineaquachloroplatinum(II) ion by liquid chromatography using post-column derivatization with diethyldithiocarbamate. J Chromatogr B 1994; 652:203–210.
13. Hassan M, Ehrsson H. Gas chromatographic determination of busulfan in plasma with electron-capture detection. J Chromatogr B 1983; 277:374–380.
14. Theil H. A rank-invariant method of linear and polynomial regression analysis. I. Proc Ned Akad Wet Pt A 1950; 53:386–392.

15. Sen PK. Robust statistical procedures in problems of linear regression with special reference to quantitative bio-assays. Rev Int Stat Inst 1971; 39:1–38.
16. Hussain SS, Sprent P. Non-parametric regression. J R Statist Soc Pt 2 1983; 146:182–191.
17. Daniel WW. Applied nonparametric statistics. Boston, MA: Houghton Mifflin, 1978, pp. 343–359.
18. Woosley JT. Simple method for nonparametric linear regression analysis. Clin Chem 1986; 32:203.
19. Rousseeuw PJ. Least median of squares regression. J Am Stat Assoc 1984; 79:871–880.
20. Peck CC, Beal SL, Sheiner LB, Nichols AI. Extended least squares nonlinear regression: a possible solution to the "choice of weights" problem in analysis of individual pharmacokinetic data. J Pharmacokin Biopharm 1984; 12:545–558.
21. Eksborg S, Ehrsson H. Calibration curves—calculation and evaluation of accuracy. Ther Drug Monit 1994; 16:629–630.
22. Andersson A, Fagerberg J, Lewensohn R, Ehrsson H. Pharmacokinetics of cisplatin and its monohydrated complex in humans. J Pharmaceut Sci 1996; 85:824–827.
23. Andersson A, Hedenmalm H, Elfsson B, Ehrsson H. Determination of the acid dissociation constant for *cis*-dimmineaquachloroplatinum(II) ion. A hydrolysis product of cisplatin. J Pharmaceut Sci 1994; 83:859–862.
24. Ehrsson H, Wallin I, Andersson A, Edlund PO. Cisplatin, transplatin and their hydrated complexes: separation and identification using porous graphitic carbon and electrospray ionization mass spectrometry. Analyt Chem 1995; 67:3608–3611.
25. Yachnin JR, Wallin I, Lewensohn R, Sirzén F, Ehrsson H. The kinetics and cytotoxicity of cisplatin and its monohydrated complex. Cancer Lett 1998; 132:175–180.
26. Ekborn A, Lindberg A, Laurell G, Wallin I, Eksborg S, Ehrsson H. Ototoxicity, nephrotoxicity and pharmacokinetics of cisplatin and its monohydrated complex in the guinea pig. Cancer Chemother Pharmacol 2003; 51:36–42.
27. Campbell KCM, Rybak LP, Meech RP, Hughes L. D-Methionine provides excellent protection from cisplatin ototoxicity in the rat. Hear Res 1996; 102:90–98.
28. Reser D, Rho M, Dewan D, et al. L- and D-methionine provide equivalent long term protection against CDDP-induced ototoxicity in vivo, with partial in vitro and in vivo retention of antineoplastic activity. Neurotoxicology 1999; 20:731–748.
29. Ekborn A, Laurell G, Johnström P, Wallin I, Eksborg S, Ehrsson H. D-Methionine and cisplatin ototoxicity in the guinea pig: D-Methionine influences cisplatin pharmacokinetics. Hear Res 2002; 165:53–61.
30. Launchbury AP, Habboubi N. Epirubicin and doxorubicin: a comparison of their characteristics, therapeutic activity and toxicity. Cancer Treat Rev 1993; 19:197–228.
31. Weenen H, Lankelma J, Penders PG, et al. Pharmacokinetics of 4'-epi-doxorubicin in man. Invest New Drugs 1983; 1:59–64.
32. Eksborg S, Andersson M, Domellöf L, Lönroth U. A pharmacokinetic study of adriamycin and 4'epi-adriamycin after simultaneous intra-arterial liver administration. Med Oncol Tumor Pharmacother 1986; 3:105–110.
33. Eksborg S, Stendahl U, Lönroth U. Comparative pharmacokinetic study of adriamycin and 4'epi-adriamycin after their simultaneous intravenous administration. Eur J Clin Pharmacol 1986; 30:629–631.
34. Eksborg S, Palm C, Björk O. A comparative pharmacokinetic study of doxorubicin and 4'-epi-doxorubicin in children with acute lymphocytic leukemia using a limited sampling procedure. Anticancer Drugs 2000; 11:129–136.
35. Eksborg S. Anthracycline pharmacokinetics. Limited sampling model for plasma level monitoring with special reference to epirubicin (Farmorubicin). Acta Oncol 1990; 29:339–342.
36. Eksborg S, Hardell L, Bengtsson N-O, Sjödin M, Elfsson B. Epirubicin as a single agent therapy for the treatment of breast cancer—a pharmacokinetic and clinical study. Med Oncol Tumor Pharmacother 1992; 9:75–80.
37. Sandström M. Freijs A, Larsson R, et al. Lack of relationship between systemic exposure for the component drug of the fluorouracil, epirubicin, and 4-hydroxycyclophosphamide regimen in breast cancer patients. J Clin Oncol 1996; 14:1581–1588.
38. de Valeriola D. Dose optimization of anthracyclines. Anticancer Res 1994; 14:2307–2313.
39. Desoize B, Robert J. Individual dose adaptation of anticancer drugs. Eur J Cancer 1994; 30A:844–851.
40. Palm C, Björk O, Björkholm M, Eksborg S. Quantification of doxorubicin in plasma—a comparative study of capillary and venous blood sampling. Anticancer Drugs 2001; 12:859–864.
41. Eksborg, S. Evaluation of method-comparison data. Clin Chem 1981; 27:1311–1312.

42. Chiou WL. The phenomenon and rationale of marked dependence of drug concentration on blood sampling site. Implications in pharmacokinetics, pharmacodynamics, toxicology and therapeutics (part I). Clin Pharmcokinet 1989; 17:175–199.

43. Chiou WL. The phenomenon and rationale of marked dependence of drug concentration on blood sampling site. Implications in pharmacokinetics, pharmacodynamics, toxicology and therapeutics (part II). Clin Pharmcokinet 1989; 17:275–290.

44. Bomelburg T, Ritter J, Schellong G. Bestimmung der Methotrexatkonzentration im Serum: Vergleich zwischen Kapillar-und Venenblut. Klin Pädiat 1987; 199:230–232.

7
Validation and Control of Bioanalytical Methods in Clinical Drug Development

H. Thomas Karnes, PhD

CONTENTS

INTRODUCTION
METHOD DEVELOPMENT
METHOD VALIDATION
QUALITY CONTROL
CONCLUSION

1. INTRODUCTION

Validation and control of bioanalytical methods as practiced in U.S. Food and Drug Administration (FDA)-regulated drug development studies is the approach most often used for anticancer drugs. The discipline has progressed from one that was in its infancy a decade ago to a largely mature endeavor more recently. Validation and control procedures in other areas of bioanalysis such as clinical chemistry and forensic toxicology have been largely consistent for a number of decades. The primary difference between the drug development discipline and other areas of bioanalysis is the fact that drug development requires application of consistent standards for analytical methods that are investigational rather than routine. Validation and control attempts in drug development studies carried out prior to 1990 were the result of individual policies that varied a great deal from company to company. The importance of consistent procedures for validation and control in drug development was first outlined by Shah in 1987 *(1)* and specific procedures were proposed by Karnes in 1991 *(2)*. Since these two works on the subject, a number of reviews and research articles have been published along with two conferences that have led to the establishment of a "Guidance for Industry" on Bioanalytical Method Validation *(3)*. The first conference was held in 1990 with the results published in 1992 *(4)*. A draft guidance was also published as a result of this conference in 1999 *(5)*. Following an acknowledgment that small molecules should be treated differently than large molecules, two more conferences were held in 2000 and the proceedings published in 2000 and 2001 for small and large molecules, respectively *(6,7)*. All of this activity resulted in the final guidance that was approved by the Center for Drug Evaluation and Research (CDER) of FDA in cooperation with the Center for Veterinary Medicine (CVM) and published in May of 2001. The guidance has

Handbook of Anticancer Pharmacokinetics and Pharmacodynamics
Edited by: W. D. Figg and H. L. McLeod © Humana Press Inc., Totowa, NJ

regulatory implications for a variety of biological matrices analyzed in human and animal clinical and preclinical studies. The document applies to chromatographic, spectrometric, immunological, and microbiological procedures and was intended as a nonbinding general recommendation that can be adjusted depending on circumstances. The document outlines fundamental parameters for bioanalytical method validation that include accuracy, precision, selectivity, sensitivity, reproducibility, and stability. The document addresses situations in which a bioanalytical method may be modified and suggests different levels of validation to ensure that validity is maintained. The document also includes a glossary of terms. Although this document represents the current thinking of the FDA and is based on the conferences held, the procedures and criteria were primarily negotiated. They were based on an amalgam of procedures that existed within the industry prior to the conferences and are not necessarily based on the best scientific approach. This chapter endeavors to present the best scientific approaches based on the literature while considering them in the context of the FDA guidance.

There are two major divisions in the endeavor to ensure the quality of analytical results. The two divisions consist of method validation and method quality control. There are referred to as prestudy validation and during-study validation, respectively, in the draft FDA guidance (5) but no nominal distinction is made in the final FDA guidance (3). Another division that is used often in describing validation and control processes is a method development or establishment phase in which the method is not yet complete but some validation results may be collected in an effort to establish optimal conditions. As such, the method development or establishment phase should be free from regulatory scrutiny for the most part since the method is dynamic at this point. The validation phase represents the stage at which a method is complete but has not yet been used for analysis of "real samples." The question to be addressed at this phase is whether or not the method is good enough for an intended purpose. It could be argued that the criteria used here should be flexible so that methods used for critical purposes such as therapeutic monitoring of a narrow therapeutic index drug would require strict and tight guidelines, whereas other situations may not require such rigorous criteria. The approach of the FDA recommendations has been to apply a "one size fits all" approach without built in flexibility for a large variety of drug types and for a large number of different applications. The FDA guidance makes no distinction between the method development/establishment and validation phases. The quality control phase represents the period in which data are collected from quality control samples and exists to ensure the quality of "real sample" results. The question to be addressed in this phase is no longer related to how good a method is but to determining whether the method is performing according to specifications set during method validation. The procedures used for these three phases should reflect the goals to be achieved. The FDA guidance does this for the most part but fails to address some valid scientific issues related to these goals in some cases. The following sections presents approaches suggested in the guidance along with scientific justifications when appropriate. Other approaches are presented as alternatives to the guidance that may have more scientific validity or better address the individual goals of method development, validation, and quality control.

2. METHOD DEVELOPMENT

Two important factors in achieving good performance of bioanalytical methods in the method development phase are selective recovery from sample processing and calibration with appropriate primary standards. Selective recovery for a bioanalytical method refers to the provision of an analytical response for the entire amount of analyte contained in a sample without residual interferences or matrix effects from other sample components (2). Although selectivity must be dealt with in method development from the standpoint of achievement of selectivity, this is largely a validation parameter and is dealt with in that section. Recovery of a bioanalytical method most appropriately refers to analyte extraction efficiency and is termed absolute recovery. Absolute recovery may be measured in a number of ways and is calculated using the general formula below:

$$\frac{\text{Extracted response}}{\text{Unextracted response}} \times 100 = \% \text{ Recovery}$$

The extracted response is the quantitative instrumental measurement from a sample, spiked at a known concentration, into a blank matrix sample that is processed and measured. The unextracted sample may be represented by a number of response values depending on the particular situation. The simplest experiment is to measure the unextracted response from a nonmatrix solvent solution spiked at the same concentration. This provides absolute recovery, although the value may not be representative because of residual matrix effects in the extracted sample or poor reproducibility of the instrument response. Matrix effects can be compensated for by adding an appropriate amount of analyte to an extracted blank matrix and then measuring the unextracted response in the presence of the blank extract. Instrument response variability can be lessened by addition of an internal standard to both the extracted sample following the extraction process and at the same concentration to the unextracted sample. The measured response then becomes the response ratio of the analyte to that of the internal standard. Absolute recovery can also be easily estimated if radioactive analogs of the drug are available. In this experiment, radioactivity counts prior to extraction provide the unextracted response, whereas the radioactivity counts following extraction from the same spiked sample provide the extracted response. This procedure eliminates intersample variability and the possibility of a matrix effect with an isotopically labeled analog is remote. Sufficient replication needs to be employed to provide sufficient confidence in the calculated recovery and the more variable measurements (typically the extracted samples) require greater replication than the less variable measurements (typically the unextracted samples).

There are a number of experiments that have been referred to as recovery experiments that do not provide absolute recovery or an estimate of sample processing efficiency. They include experiments evaluating the measured response ratio of a sample extracted from the intended matrix to that extracted from a nonmatrix solution. This experiment provides information on the effect of components of the matrix on the measured signal and is an important experiment to evaluate method selectivity, but should not be confused with an experiment to measure absolute recovery. Another experiment that has been reported as a recovery experiment is the ratio of the assayed concentration to that of the prepared concentration. The is an accuracy experiment and again does not address recovery as is intended in the FDA guidance. One last example of an experiment that may be reported as recovery but does not address processing efficiency is the ratio of the internal standard compensated response that has been extracted to the corresponding response unextracted, provided the internal standard is added prior to processing. This experiment will evaluate how well the internal standard is functioning, but again provides no information on sample processing efficiency. The FDA guidance defines recovery as specifically pertaining to absolute recovery experiments that indicate extraction efficiency. The guidance suggests that recovery experiments should be conducted but that recovery need not be 100% *(3)*.

For chromatographic methods, another question to be addressed pertains to the use of an internal standard. As mentioned above the use of an internal standard involves adding a structural or isotopic analog to a sample prior to processing so that errors in sample processing can be corrected for by including a ratio of the response of the analyte to that of the analog.

It has been noted by a few authors that the use of an internal standard is not necessary in many cases *(8)* or can actually lead to a degradation of analytical results in the absence of systematic errors *(9)*. Method degradation from the use of an internal standard will occur if the following is true:

$$RSDb > r\, RSDa$$

where RSDb and RSDa are the relative standard deviations of the internal standard and analyte responses, respectively, and *r* represents the correlation coefficient for the responses of the analyte vs the internal standard. This relationship was derived mathematically and proven with experimental data by Haefelfinger et al. *(9)*. Even though there are good arguments for not using an internal standard for chromatographic procedures, they are based on random and not systematic error. It is well accepted that internal standards are essential for correcting technical systematic errors such as loss of sample caused by variable phase transfers or dilutions and allow for many volume transfers to be nonquantitative, thus increasing sample throughput. Correction of errors or shifts related to partition, chemical reactivity, and detector stability will depend on the characteristics of the internal standard relative to the analyte and the closer the chemical and physical properties of the analyte and internal standard are, the greater the probability that these errors will be accurately corrected for. Internal standards that are isotopes of the analyte have become popular for this reason although a mass detector is required to discriminate between responses. The FDA guidance does not specifically require the use of an internal standard, but it is generally expected for chromatographic procedures. Care must be taken, however, not to use an internal standard that is chemically inappropriate simply to address this expectation or the quality of results could suffer.

Calibration of an analytical method is an important consideration in method development. The concentration range for calibration must be established and an appropriate model applied to the data that will allow accurate calculation of unknown sample concentrations. The lower limit of calibration is usually established through a consideration of the lower limit of quantitation (LLOQ) and the point at which the data no longer fit the calibration model determines the upper limit. Practical considerations such as the concentration range expected for samples are also employed in setting up the calibration range. The choice of a calibration model should be determined by experimental concentration vs response data, and the model that best fits the data should be used. The FDA Guidance suggests that the simplest model that adequately describes the relationship be used, thus indicating a bias toward the linear model, but use of nonlinear functions is not prohibited. Determination of the appropriate range for calibration and application of the most appropriate model requires a consideration of the quality of fit of the experimental data and is intimately related to method validation, which is covered in the following section.

3. METHOD VALIDATION

3.1. Calibration

Method calibration is the crossover point between method development and method validation, as it involves both setting up procedures and also showing that they work well enough for a stated purpose. The quality of fit of the data to the selected calibration model will determine the allowable upper limit of calibration. This will be the highest concentration that will consistently provide an acceptable fit throughout the entire range of calibration. To establish the range and model for calibration it is most helpful to evaluate residual errors and to use the model that provides the lowest residual error. For example, residual error for the linear model can be calculated as follows:

$$e_i = y_i - a - bx_i$$

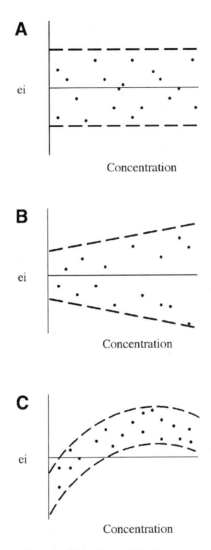

Fig. 1. Schematic representation of calibration residuals vs concentration. Homoscedastic data are represented in **A**, whereas heteroscedastic data are represented in **B** and **C**. **B** shows a proportional increase in the residuals that may be corrected by weighting. **C** represents a residuals pattern that is indicative of non-linear data for which an alternate non-linear calibration model should be used.

where e_i represents the residual error at a given concentration, y_i and x_i are the dependent and independent variables, respectively, and a and b are the best fit intercept and slope form a linear regression of the entire calibration range. These residuals are often expressed as a concentration by "backfitting" individual calibration data. Although the FDA guidance has a bias in favor of the simplest calibration model (linear), it does not prevent use of nonlinear calibration models that may provide a better fit to the data and allow more accurate calculation of unknown values over a wider concentration range. If residual values are plotted vs concentration, a pattern as shown in Fig. 1A will result for homoscedastic data and the use of a nonweighted linear calibration model can be considered appropriate. If the residuals demonstrate heteroscedastic data in which there is a proportional increase in the residuals as concentration increases, represented in Fig. 1B,

Table 1
Back-Calculated Standards (Range and Goodness of Fit)
Mean Deviation ($n = 5,\%$)

Conc. (ng/mL)	Power fit	Weighted 1/conc.	Unweighted
10	5.15	5.98	18.55
20	3.40	3.40	6.06
50	1.78	1.82	1.70
100	2.23	4.04	3.26
250	0.99	0.34	0.23
500	3.26	4.31	3.32

a weighted linear calibration is most appropriate. Figure 1C is representative of a residuals pattern that indicates the data to be nonlinear and the linear model is therefore inappropriate. Weighted linear calibration is carried out using a normal linear regression modified to include a weighting factor as a multiplier when calculating the sum of squared residuals (10). The most appropriate weighting factor is the inverse of the variance at each concentration; however, because this variance has been shown to be proportional to concentration, the inverse of concentration squared or simply the inverse of concentration can be used. These weighting factors can be used on a trial basis to determine which factor provides the lowest residual error throughout the concentration range. If a pattern of residuals emerges that is similar to the heteroscedastic pattern shown in Fig. 1C, then a systematic departure from the model is indicated and an alternative to the linear model such as a power or a polynomial fit should be investigated. Caution should be used in attempts to force truly nonlinear data to a linear calibration model in response to the FDA bias. Table 1 shows concentration residual data for linear, weighted linear, and a nonlinear power fit of real bioanalytical data. It can be seen from Table 1 that the linear calibration provides unacceptably high residuals at low concentration. These residuals are improved significantly by use of the weighted linear model. The function of the weighting factor is to increase the influence of the low concentration data on the best fit regression slope, and therefore the low concentration residuals are improved whereas the high concentration residuals are made worse. This occurs because forcing the line closer at the low concentrations acts as a fulcrum to force the inflexible linear calibration line away from the data at high concentrations. The solution to this problem is to allow some flex in the calibration curve and to use a nonlinear calibration model that will provide a better fit at both extremes of calibration for such data.

There are many approaches to assessment of the quality of fit for analytical calibration data in addition to an evaluation of residuals. These include but are not limited to correlation coefficients, sensitivity plots, polynomial fits, log–log plots, and the F-test for lack of fit (11). Sensitivity plots, polynomial fits, and log–log plots are limited to evaluation of the linear model and are not widely used in bioanalysis so they are not addressed in this chapter. Log–log plots have been shown to provide comparable results to the F-test for lack of fit and residuals analysis, whereas the polynomial fit approach was found to be more conservative (11). For linear analytical data, calculation of the correlation coefficient involves the false statistical assumption that the independent variable in regression analysis (concentration) is errorless. The correlation coefficient is essentially a measure of the amount of variation in the dependent variable (analytical response) that is accounted for by the independent variable (concentration). It does not distinguish random from systematic error well. Also, with regard to testing the linear model, correlation coefficients have been shown to produce good correlation for data that do not conform to the linear model *(12)* and have been shown to be a more liberal criteria than other approaches *(11)*. For these reasons, the correlation coefficient has been deemphasized as a method of evaluation for goodness of fit and is not mentioned in the final FDA guidance.

The *F*-test for lack of fit is a statistical test of whether or not the sum of the variances attributable to lack of fit (the differences between mean and fitted values for the analytical response at each calibrator concentration) is significantly different from the sum of the variances attributable to pure error (the differences of individual calibrators from the mean at a given concentration). The *F*-test for lack of fit has been shown to provide comparable results to residuals analysis and log–log plots. Although the *F*-test for lack of fit is the most appropriate test of goodness of fit statistically and can be used to evaluate both liner and nonlinear models, replication is required to obtain statistical significance and the test may not be easily understood at all levels of bioanalytical practice. The only specific criterion for calibration goodness of fit to the model offered by the FDA guidance is a criterion applied to concentration residuals *(3)*. This criterion states that all concentration residuals must be within 20% of the nominal value for the lower limit of quantitation and within 15% at all other concentrations. This criterion is easy to understand and does not require deviation from a set protocol to achieve statistical significance. A criticism of this criterion is that it is based on consensus opinion and does not possess a statistical foundation.

3.2. Selectivity

There has been confusion over the terms selectivity and specificity, and they are often used interchangeably. Specificity may be used appropriately to refer to an analytical method that provides a response for only a single analyte. The term has also been used appropriately to describe the absolute condition of selectivity. Selectivity is the more appropriate term for analytical purposes, as few if any analytical systems can be said to respond to only a single species without being affected by components of the matrix. In an analytical method in which concentration is determined as a function of response, the degree to which the response is unaffected by contributions from the matrix is referred to as the selectivity of the method. There are two independent components to selectivity referred to as matrix effects and interferences. Interferences are predeterminate errors caused most frequently in bioanalysis by a component of the matrix producing a measurable response. This causes an error in the intercept of the calibration curve, which is represented in Fig. 2A where the dotted line represents a calibration with the interference and the solid line represents the unaffected calibration curve. Interferences are best evaluated by analysis of the baseline from a blank measurement if a suitable blank exists. Interferences must be differentiated from contamination (a response from the intended analyte in the blank) by qualitative means when contamination is suspected. In biopharmaceutical analysis interferences are relatively easy to evaluate because the analyte is normally a xenobiotic and a blank is readily available for each biological source as a predose sample. Analysis of this predose sample by the method demonstrating a lack of significant response indicates good selectivity. The FDA guidance states that a lack of interferences needs to be demonstrated in six independent sources of blank matrix and that there should be evidence that the substance being quantified is the intended analyte. The guidance does not specify what constitutes a lack of interference or what evidence is needed for demonstration of qualitative identification of the analyte. Commonly used criteria for chromatographic procedures include a lack of interference of < 5% or 20% of

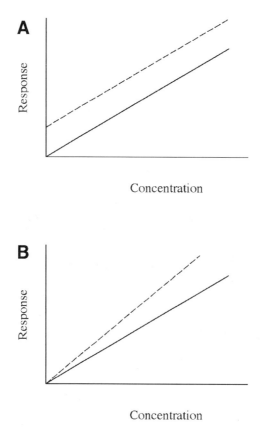

Fig. 2. Errors in selectivity caused by a predeterminant and constant shift in the calibration are referred to as interferences and are represented in **A**. Matrix effects are proportional errors of slope as shown in **B**. The dotted lines represent calibration with the error present and the solid line represents the unaffected calibration curve.

the limit of quantitation and a retention time match with a primary standard for qualitative identification.

The situations in which the predose blank matrix approach to interference evaluation does not prove adequate include instances in which interferences may appear over time because of lack of stability of the matrix or analyte, situations in which interferences are caused by metabolites of the drug that are not present in the predosed blank, and situations in which the analyte is an endogenous compound for which there is no predose sample. Stability issues are a separate concern and include a consideration of more than just the maintenance of the selectivity of the method with time under storage conditions and these will are dealt with later in this chapter. Interference from metabolites is a concern especially when using mass spectrometry (MS) as an analytical method, as the source of ions for MS is a reaction chamber where metabolites and other analogs of the analyte, most notably internal standards, can be fragmented into ions that are the same as those that originate from the analyte *(13)*. This phenomenon is referred to as "cross-talk." For this reason, it is necessary for evaluation of interferences by use of primary standards of the individual metabolites or by modification of chromatographic conditions to effect a separation of the analogue from the analyte. Once the modified chromatographic conditions have been shown to produce no differences in measured response, the original chromatographic conditions may be used.

This special precaution, which is important for MS, is less of a concern for other methods, as complete separation from components of the matrix is routinely carried out for these methods. No provision for this extra concern regarding interferences with MS methods is included in the FDA guidance. It is recommended practice, however, to evaluate "cross-talk" at high levels for potentially interfering internal standards and metabolites along with conducting experiments at altered retention times in dosed (ex vivo) samples.

Matrix effects are proportional errors of slope as shown in Fig. 2B, where the dotted line represents a calibration with the matrix effect and the solid line represents the unaffected calibration curve. Unlike interferences that are caused most often by components from the matrix that yield a response, matrix effects are generally caused by some interaction, either chemical or physical, of the analyte with some component of the matrix. An example of this is shown below for charge transfer and proton transfer reactions that occur in atmospheric pressure ionization (API) MS:

$$\text{Charge transfer:} \quad A^+ + M \rightarrow M^+ + A$$
$$\text{Proton transfer:} \quad AH^+ + M \rightarrow MH^+ + A$$

where A^+ and AH^+ represent charged and protonated analyte molecules, respectively, and M^+ and MH^+ represent the corresponding species for a matrix component. A and M represent the uncharged, unprotonated forms and negative charges may be involved as well as the positive charges pictured. These reactions both lead to ion suppression matrix effects that result in a decreased response for the analyte as compared to nonmatrix analysis. The proportional nature of the matrix effect error is a result of this type interaction because the effect is mediated through an interaction constant and is proportional to concentration in the simplest case.

Matrix effects can often be compensated for by duplication of the sample matrix in calibration standards. This will adjust the slope in calibration standards to match that of the sample matrix. The assumption involved is that the blank matrix used for calibration standards is sufficiently similar to that of the samples to yield accurate results. This assumption is generally valid for most bioanalytical methods that involve an extraction and chromatographic separation, as the factors that may affect extractability and separation such as pH and protein content are relatively constant in biological samples from the same origin. MS methods again require special attention because quantitation is often carried out without complete extraction and separation of the analyte from matrix components. Although the FDA guidance does not specify any test of matrix effects, it is recommended practice for MS methods. It is advisable to use an isotopically labeled internal standard if possible, to increase chromatographic retention times as a test to see if results change, and to evaluate instrument response in a variety of sources of biological matrix. A very useful experiment for validation of the lack of ion suppression or enhancement in MS is the post-column infusion experiment in which a steady infusion of the analyte is pumped into the system post-column generating a steady response from the analyte (Fig. 3). In this configuration, blank matrix is injected precolumn and the ion suppression or enhancement appears as a negative or positive deflection of the baseline response. This negative or positive deflection (Fig. 4B) in the baseline (Fig 4A) can be compared to where the analyte elutes if injected precolumn (Fig. 4C). The chromatography can then be modified so that the elution time of the analyte is not coincident with suppression or enhancement peaks.

3.3. Detectability

Detectability has been one of the most broadly interpreted parameters of validation. The term detectability is used here because it more accurately reflects the parameters used for

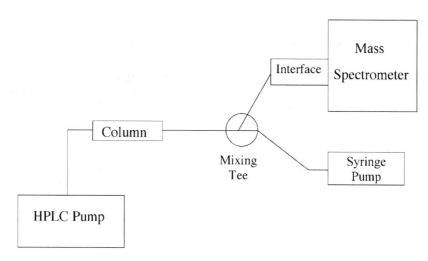

Fig. 3. A schematic representation of a post-column infusion hardware setup in which a steady infusion of the analyte is pumped into column elluent. Blank matrix can be injected pre-column in order to monitor ion suppression or enhancement.

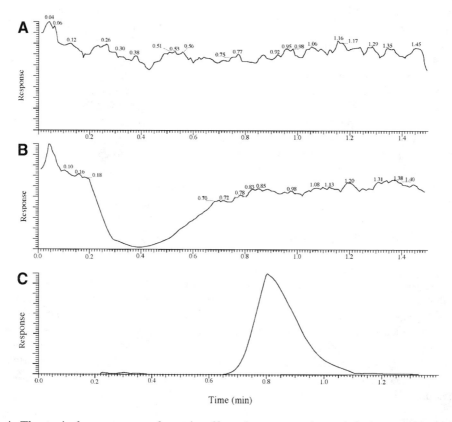

Fig. 4. The typical appearance of matrix effects in a post-column infusion experiment. Ion suppresssion or enhancement appears as negative infusion experiment. Ion suppression or enhancement appears as ngeative (**B**) or positive (**C**) deflections in the baseline (**A**), respectively.

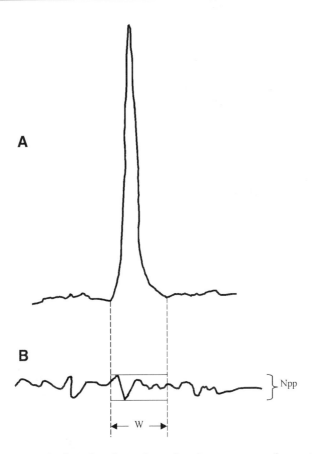

A

B

Npp

W

Fig. 5. A common way to calculate signal to noise ratios. **A** represents a chromatogram of standard material and **B** represents the baseline from a blank injection. Npp represents peak to peak noise and "w" indicates the elution window of the peak.

validation of the lowest concentrations to be measured. The term sensitivity is often used for this purpose. It is used in the literature to indicate the slope of the analytical calibration curve, however, and is not defined in the FDA glossary of terms, so it would seem inappropriate to use it to refer to detectability except in the most general sense. There are a number of different mathematical definitions for detectability that will yield different results and many of them are referred to by the same terminology *(10)*. Most often, detectability has been defined based on blank noise measurements. Valid statistical approaches have also been based on confidence limits associated with a calibration curve *(15)*. Discussion of detectability is limited to the blank noise approach here because this approach is more accepted in FDA-regulated drug development. Blank noise can be defined in a number of ways. For chromatographic methods this consists of measuring the biological analytical signal over the elution window of the peak of interest in a matrix blank sample. This is shown in Fig. 5, where Fig. 5A represents a chromatogram of standard material and Fig. 5B the baseline from a blank injection. The blank signal should be an average from a number of blank matrices. The most conservative estimates will be yielded by use of the peak-to-peak noise signal rather than the peak noise signal although both have been used. Root mean square (RMS) noise has also been used, although use of this noise estimate would provide a very liberal estimate of detectability relative to the others.

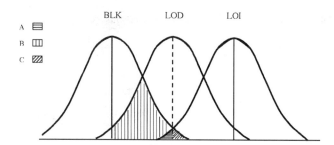

Fig. 6. A graphical representation of the probabilities related to various detectability parameters. Probability A represents the low probability of measurement made at the limit of identification (LOI) actually being blank (BLK). Probability B represents the probability that a measurement made at the limit of detection (LOD) will be indistinguishable from a measurment made from a blank. Probability C represents the the probability of a blank measurement yielding a reponse above the limit of detection.

The blank noise approach involves multiplication of some factor (K) times the standard deviation of the blank noise to yield a confidence interval. The confidence interval then allows prediction of an error probability associated with making an incorrect decision of detection for the analyte (16). This value is then divided by the slope of the calibration curve to yield results in concentration units as shown below:

$$K\, S_b/m = X_{LLOD}$$

where S_b represents the standard deviation of the blank noise measurement, m is the slope of the calibration curve near the limit and X_{LLOD} is the lower limit of detection. This limit represents the concentration that can be distinguished as nonzero with great probability or with low probability of actually being a blank (probability A in Fig. 6). The K factor used determines the width of the confidence interval and thus the probability of an incorrect decision, that is, the sample being measured as above the lower limit of detection (LLOD) but one that is truly blank. Typically used values for K are 2 and 3, representing error probabilities of 95.4% and 99.7%, respectively, 3 being the most conservative and most commonly used. The LLOD calculated in this way is not useful for the purpose of setting a parameter for quantification and should be used only to compare absolute detectability potentials of analytical systems. This is the case because an analytical measurement made at the LLOD would yield a high probability of being indistinguishable from a measurement made at zero. This is shown in Fig. 6 as the sum of probabilities $A + B + C$. To solve this problem, a new limit is defined as the lower limit of identification (LLOI), which uses a value for the K factor of 6 and defines the concentration at which there is a low probability (area C in Fig. 6) of being less than the defined LLOD. The lower limit of identification has a practical meaning as the threshold for presence of an analyte in a sample. It can be said with a defined level of confidence that if the measured concentration is above the lower limit of identification, then the analyte is present in a sample. The most useful application of this is in purity testing of chemical substances and dosage forms, but the parameter has little application in quantitative bioanalysis except for situations in which a method selectivity argument is made.

The most useful limit in quantitative bioanalysis is the LLOQ. The LLOQ represents the concentration above which accurate and precise quantification can be carried out. This limit can be traditionally estimated using the blank noise approach with a K factor of 10. This factor for K is intended to target a coefficient of variation (CV) of 10%, in the absence of systematic errors. An appropriate K factor for a desired level of precision can be arrived at through the following expression:

$$K = 1/CV$$

where CV is the coefficient of variation expressed as a decimal fraction. The above expression is derived through a combination of the general lower limit of detection equation and the expression for CV. A K factor of 5 as recommended in the FDA guidance would therefore predict a CV of 20% which is the precision limit at the LLOQ allowable in the FDA guidance *(3)*. The FDA guidance is therefore consistent with accepted theory although the approach does not account for the fact that this value is lower than the LLOI and is technically not present in the sample with great probability (99.7%). A slightly more conservative approach would be to use a K factor of 6 or 10 as an estimate of LLOQ.

LLOQs may be estimated with the blank noise approach but are established through actual testing of concentrations prepared at that level to ensure that precision and accuracy limits are met. The estimates provided by the blank noise approach should be used as a guide as to where to set concentrations for evaluation but should not be used as evidence for validation. The best approach to establishment of the LLOQ is to prepare several concentrations near the LLOQ estimate and to measure them in replicate. The lowest concentration to yield the desired acceptable level of accuracy and precision would therefore represent the LLOQ and should be established as the lowest concentration in the calibration curve. The greater the number of concentrations tested, the better will be the estimate for LLOQ. In practice, it is inefficient to measure a large number of low concentrations with sufficient replication to establish the LLOQ rigorously. Typically, the blank noise estimated LLOQ is used as a guide and a single LLOQ is tested. If the results of this test yield acceptable accuracy and precision (20% systematic error and 20% CV in the FDA guidance), then this single concentration is established as the LLOQ and used as the lowest calibrator. The question of whether or not there is a lower concentration that would yield acceptable results is often not addressed.

3.4. Accuracy and Precision

The accuracy and precision of an analytical method are by far the most important determinants of analytical method quality. The impact of these two parameters has already been discussed in establishment of the LLOQ and the acceptability of residuals in the evaluation of the quality of fit for calibration curves. They are considered together here, as they are often lumped together to represent the total error of a measurement and it is important to distinguish these three parameters. Accuracy and precision are interdependent in assessment of the acceptability of an analytical method. The FDA guidance defines accuracy as "the degree of closeness of the determined value to the nominal or known true value under prescribed conditions." The accuracy component of total error can be represented by the following:

$$\frac{u - \overline{x}}{u} \times 100 = \% \text{ Accuracy deviation}$$

where u is the "true" or "nominal" value and $\overline{x}$ is the average of measured values. It is important to make sure that the average has been calculated from enough measurements to allow for an adequate reduction in the random (imprecision) error so that only the systematic (inaccuracy) error is represented. It is therefore incorrect to represent accuracy for an individual measurement. This concept is illustrated in Fig. 7, where the Gaussian distribution shown represents a distribution around a measured average that determines an analytical method's precision. The difference between this average and the true value is the accuracy as described mathematically above, and the sum of the two errors is referred to as total error or bias. Both accuracy and precision are traditionally evaluated through control samples prepared at various concentrations to reflect the range of expected values and should be measured independent of the calibration standards. The "true value" for these control samples can be established either through comparison of results to a reference method or through assigning a known concentration from spiking of weighed standards into a blank matrix.

The imprecision or random error component of total error can be estimated from calculation of the percentage relative standard deviation (RSD), which is also referred to as the coefficient of variation (CV). This value is calculated as follows:

$$\frac{sd}{\overline{x}} \times 100 = \% \text{ RSD}$$

where sd represents the standard deviation of a group of multiple measurements of the same sample and $\overline{x}$ again represents the calculated average from the same group. Precision is often confused with reproducibility and repeatability, although these terms have distinctly different meanings. Reproducibility is the closeness of results measured under different conditions, such as different laboratories, and repeatability refers to the closeness of results from successive measurements of the same sample (2). Precision is normally assessed on a within-batch and a between-batch basis. The within-batch assessment is considered an estimate of the precision under optimal conditions without the variability associated with batch-to-batch results. It is for this reason that it is advisable to run unknown samples generated from the same subject but different legs of a clinical study in the same batch if possible. The between-batch assessment is a more realistic estimate of the precision of a method because it normally is subjected to a greater number of sources of variability.

The total error or "bias" of an analytical measurement is appropriately represented for individual measurements and it is not appropriate, therefore, to apply an accuracy criterion to a single measurement (2,17). Any criterion for individual measurements should be referred to as a total error criterion. The criterion should be broad enough to include both the random and the systematic error components of the total error. Total error for an individual measurement can be calculated as follows:

$$|x - u| + 2.58 \, sd = E$$

where x represents the individual measured value and E represents the total error or bias of that individual measurement. The random error component for the example above has been considered to be the width of a confidence interval specified at 99%. The random error component of an analytical measurement is a characteristic of the method and the primary measure of the method's performance. Systematic errors are theoretically correctable errors and are related more to calibration and the purity of primary standards. It may be desirable to determine if the observed error is due to random error alone so that systematic errors can be corrected if they exist. This is accomplished through application of a t-test to determine whether or not the average value of a set of measurements differs significantly from that of the true or nominal value (17). If the difference is significant, there is some correctable systematic error.

The FDA lists accuracy and precision criteria for acceptance of a method for the purpose of bioanalytical data submissions (3). It is recommended that four control concentrations spanning the range of calibration should be employed, one of which is no more than three times the LLOQ and one prepared at the LLOQ. The percentage accuracy deviation and percentage RSD must be within 15% for all controls except for the LLOQ, which is expected to be within 20% RSD and accuracy. This absolute approach taken by the FDA guidance is generally appropriate for validation of analytical methods, as the question addressed in validation is whether or not the method is good enough for the intended purpose. The fixed acceptance criteria for bioanalytical methods suggest that all data be at least as good as a minimal threshold value and that all methods should conform to this threshold. It could be argued that some methods that are very precise by nature or that measure relatively high concentrations should be held to a higher standard or conversely that very challenging methods should be given more flexibility. It also follows that certain applications such as very narrow therapeutic window drugs might require tighter control whereas other applications may not. These situations may be compensated for in application of the guidelines although deviations from the fixed recommendations will no doubt require rigorous scientific justification. If it is simply not possible for a given analytical method at a needed concentration to provide results within the fixed guidelines, the most straightforward solution to the problem is to conduct sample analysis and validation in replicate. The RSD of a method can be effectively reduced by a factor of $1/\sqrt{n}$, where represents the number of replicates assayed. In this way, the variability of both the sample measurement and the validation data will be lowered through use of an average value rather than the single individual measurement. This approach is recommended in the FDA guidance. In cases in which inaccuracy exceeds the threshold value, use of the average of replicate measurements may provide a better estimate of the true value but will not necessarily reduce inaccuracy. The systematic error may also be corrected through better calibration or standardization of the method or by limiting calibration to a smaller concentration range.

3.5. Stability Testing

Stability of an analyte in the matrix in question is an important part of the validation process. The stability of an analyte is not only a function of the chemical nature of the substance itself but also of the matrix and container in which it is stored. Instability can result from both chemical and physical processes and the most accepted way to show stability is to monitor the concentration of the analyte in question over a time period and under conditions set to reflect the handling of unknown samples. Although the FDA guidance suggests that stability should be evaluated during the sample collection process, there are few analytical laboratories that have control over this process. Stability studies that are normally carried out by analytical laboratories include:

1. Freeze/thaw stability testing in which three control samples are frozen at the storage temperature and thawed and refrozen a total of three times. The sample is then analyzed after the third cycle and the results are compared to results measured prior to the freezing cycles.
2. Short-term stability in which controls are stored at room temperature for 4–24 h (based on the expected time samples will be kept at room temperature), then analyzed and compared to results from samples not left at room temperature.
3. Long-term storage stability in which samples are stored under long-term storage conditions and analyzed after a time expected to be the longest storage time for samples. Results measured from freshly prepared controls are compared to the results from the stored samples to indicate storage stability or instability.
4. Stock solution stability in which standard solutions in the appropriate solvent and container are analyzed before and after a minimum of 6 h of storage, or the longest time expected for stock solution storage. The storage conditions should replicate that which is employed for normal conditions. The instrument responses of these samples should then be compared to those of freshly prepared solutions.
5. Prepared sample stability in which processed samples stored under the conditions needed for analysis such as on an autosampler tray are analyzed and compared to results obtained form samples not stored for the indicated period of time.

All of these stability studies involve comparison of results from stored samples to those freshly prepared or unstored. The guidance suggests that samples from dosed subjects may also be investigated for stability but stop short of requiring that this type of sample be tested.

There is no acceptance criterion established in the FDA guidance, although it is suggested that a statistical approach based on confidence limits may be employed. The guidance does not prevent employment of combined stability studies, and these may make sense in terms of preserving laboratory efficiency. For example, samples could be analyzed that not only have been frozen and thawed three times but have also been kept at room temperature and left prepared on an autosampler for a designated amount of time. In this way three stability studies are combined into one and if stability is indicated, nothing further needs to be done. If instability is indicated, however, individual studies should be carried out to determine the source of the instability.

In contrast to procedures for determination of accuracy and precision, the FDA guidance offers little information as to how to conduct stability studies. General principles for stability tests of drug products have been established and would apply to bioanalytical studies as well *(18)*. These include the following:

1. The method used for stability testing must be shown to be stability indicating. For bioanalytical methods, this should consist of making sure that degradation products, either known or created through forced degradation, do not interfere with quantitation of the analyte.
2. The time zero reference should be a measured (not nominal) value that has been rigorously established with sufficient replication.
3. Sufficient replication of the timed stability samples needs to be carried out to provide a reliable mean measured result.
4. The entire concentration range in question should be investigated, as significant differences in rated of degradation can occur at different concentrations.
5. Blank matrix samples should be run in conjunction with stability samples to ensure the absence of interferences that may appear with time.
6. Freshly prepared and matrix matched samples should be used.

The decision as to whether or not to conclude stability or instability should be based on the precision of the method and the acceptance criterion for validation. As the FDA guideline states that a method should be accurate to within 15 %, it would follow that an acceptance criterion for stability should be similar. This would result in a straightforward fixed threshold value that would be consistent with the accuracy criterion. Accuracy is based on a comparison to the nominal value and stability studies are more appropriately based on a measured mean reference value. If a criterion of 15 % is to be applied to stability testing in a matrix, then it should be measured relative to a mean time zero reference. A more statistically valid approach would be to compare the measured stability values via a confidence interval approach. This may involve the upper limit of the confidence interval of stability measurements being not less than some lower acceptable limit (usually 90% of the reference) or that the lower limit of the confidence interval be not greater than some higher acceptable limit (usually 110% of the reference). This approach ensures that a method does not fail the stability test unless there is a high level of confidence that the sample mean is outside the acceptance range. The level of confidence or probability that the sample is actually unstable when you have concluded that it is not, is determined by the size of the confidence interval chosen. Ninety-five percent and 90 % confidence intervals have both been used for this purpose.

4. QUALITY CONTROL

The goal of a good quality control program is to determine whether or not a method is performing up to specifications during the process of analyzing unknown samples. This is in contrast to the goal of validation, in which it is desired to show that a method is good enough for an intended purpose. For this reason, it is necessary to view the quality control process as more of a relative criterion than an absolute one. Relative assessment of quality control data from a sample run can be efficiently carried out employing the use of quality control charts (19). The control chart concept involves setting up an acceptance criterion based on the mean of quality control measurements at a given concentration plus and minus some factor, related to the desired level of confidence, times the standard deviation of the quality control measurements. For example, an acceptance range of 12.06–18.34 would result from a mean of 15.2 with a standard deviation of 1.22 if the level of confidence chosen were 99% (a factor of 2.58). The mean and standard deviation are established with the control results themselves as collected or based on validation data collected prior to the sample run. They can be updated with new data as quality control runs are carried out. The precision of the method itself therefore determines the acceptance criterion, and more precise methods would generate a narrower acceptance range whereas less precise methods would generate a broader acceptance range. This is appropriate if the established goal is to monitor whether or not a method is performing as well as it should be expected to perform. A fixed criterion applied to the same data set would not allow this kind of flexibility and the fixed criteria would inherently be too wide to be effective for precise methods and would be sufficiently narrow such that less precise methods would fail at a high rate, even though the method is performing as well as expected based on validation data (2).

The control chart approach is the standard in areas such as forensic science, clinical chemistry, and general manufacturing. There are a large number of scientific and statistical investigations and procedures to draw from that utilize the general control chart approach. These allow decision-making such as trend and shift analysis (10). Westgard's rules, which are based on control charts, have been shown to be optimal in terms of maximizing error detection while minimizing false rejection of data (20). Although control charts do a good job of monitoring method precision and consistency, they do not alone address accuracy of control data during the time samples are analyzed, and an additional accuracy criterion should be employed to make sure the mean value for the control data is accurate to within an established reasonable limit.

Questions to be addressed when setting up an analytical run incorporating quality control samples is the number and sequence of quality control samples and the way in which acceptance criteria will be applied. It is generally accepted that control samples should be prepared at three concentrations that are representative of the concentration range of the method. The number of replicates of these three concentrations will of course determine the total number of quality control samples run, which in turn will affect the error detection and false rejection probabilities as well as the sample throughput efficiency. The number of replicates is therefore an important consideration, and this number should be established as a percentage of the total number of samples in the run to preserve consistency in these critical parameters from run to run. It is also important to keep the number of replicates at each of the three concentrations consistent to preserve a balanced statistical design and to ensure the same decision-making power at each concentration level.

Quality control samples should be sequenced within the analytical run to maximize the degree of concentration coverage over the entire run and to minimize the number of samples run between each control. The best decision-making power would be derived from a run sequence that involves all three controls being run before and after each sample. In this way each sample would be controlled at each concentration just prior to and after it is run, minimizing any time delay before a control sample is run. Few industries can allow such inefficient sample throughput, however, and a good compromise would be to alternate high, medium, and low concentration controls each separated by an equal number of samples. Acceptance of the sample data can then be done according to criteria applied to the entire run or the run can be subdivided into "brackets." Samples that are contained between each control would constitute a bracket and whether or not the samples are acceptable depends on the acceptability of only the controls that bracket the samples. The advantages of the brackets approach are that acceptable samples are taken only from between acceptable controls and portions of a run may be preserved even if a significant portion of the run is out of specification. The brackets approach does a much better job of controlling for transient errors that may appear and disappear during the course of a run. In contrast, a criterion based on rejection of an entire run would result in data being rejected even though the problem had disappeared if rejection was due to a transient problem. The advantage of a criterion applied to the entire run is that the process is simpler and easier to manage.

The FDA guidance *(3)* favors a criterion applied to the entire run. The guidance further states that quality control samples should be run at three concentrations in duplicate but further stipulates that the number of quality control samples (run in multiples of the three concentrations to provide a balanced design) should be dependent on the number of samples in a run. The minimum percentage of quality controls to samples is specified as 5%. The FDA guidance offers no stipulation on the sequence of samples, calibration standards, and quality controls within an analytical run.

The primary acceptance criterion for the entire run is that at least four of six quality control samples must be within 15% of their respective nominal value although the two allowed outside this range cannot be the same concentration. This so-called 4/6/15 rule was modified from a draft version of the guidance that stipulated a 4/6/20 rule. The FDA Guidance also states that a confidence interval approach yielding comparable accuracy and precision is an appropriate alternative to the 4/6/15 rule but does not specify the level of confidence to be applied. The 4/6/15 rule is loosely based on a quality control procedure proposed by Causey et al. that used a 67% (1S) confidence interval to establish acceptance limits although their limit was 10% rather than 15% or 20% *(21)*. The FDA guidance contains further stipulations on the acceptance of concentration residuals from the calibration curve and implies that validation type criteria are applied to intrarun quality control data *(3)*.

The acceptance criterion proposed by Causey et al. is consistent with the criterion of 10% they proposed for validation of precision and is statistically valid. The 4/6/10 rule with a 10% acceptance criterion for the RSD (also based on 1S) is statistically valid, if applied relative to a mean measured value, as a 67% confidence interval around a mean would be predicted statistically to yield 67% of measurements within this interval. This is provided that the method demonstrated a precision of 1S (10% in this case) and there were no method errors beyond the level of error demonstrated during validation. These method errors that inflate the level of error beyond what has been determined to be acceptable during validation are what a quality control program is supposed to detect. The FDA guidance criterion of 4/6/15 would also be consistent with their validation criterion of 15% RSD if it were based on a mean measured value. The guidance states, however, that the criterion is to be applied to a "nominal" value, which is most often taken as the target value the quality control sample was prepared to be. This means that the FDA guidance criterion encompasses both random and systematic error. The validation criterion in the guidance for both random and systematic error (accuracy and precision) is 15%, and because these errors are additive, the criterion is actually a criterion for total error. The statistically valid criterion for quality control based on a nominal value would therefore be 30%, which is derived form the sum of the allowable accuracy and precision errors. This concept is again illustrated by Fig. 7. The allowable random error is determined in this case by the 1S interval (67% or 4 of 6) and is 15%

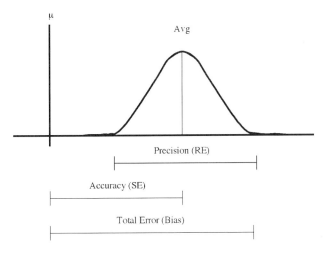

Fig. 7. The concept of total error. Imprecision or random error (RE) is related to the standard deviation of the set of measurements. The accuracy or systematic error (SE) of the measurements is shown as the difference between the measured average (AVG) and the true value (μ). Total error of bias of is shown as the sum of systematic and random errors.

according to the guidance on precision validation. The allowable systematic error is 15% also as determined by the accuracy criterion and the criteria for bias should therefore be 30% to be statistically valid. The FDA guidance could also be made statistically valid by application of the 4/6/15 rule to the mean of quality control values and with a separate accuracy criterion of 15%. The FDA guidance approach has been compared using real bioanalytical data for 10 analytical methods and found to be in disagreement with three statistically derived approaches involving confidence intervals, Westgard's rules, and a range chart approach *(22)*. The statistically valid approaches were all relatively consistent with one another. The danger that exists for the bioanalytical scientist is that methods that pass the FDA guidance validation criteria but are borderline in terms of accuracy and precision can be expected to incur a large number of quality control failures in routine analysis. To avoid this, a reasonable practice would be to proceed with routine analysis of samples only when methods demonstrate a total error (inaccuracy plus imprecision) of no more than 15%, even though the acceptance limit for total error in validation is 30% according to the FDA guidance. It is also important to be aware that the FDA criterion is not statistically valid, and although it is the standard of practice in drug development, can be challenged successfully on a scientific basis.

5. CONCLUSION

A scientific and statistically valid approach to validation and quality control is important to be consistent with the standard of practice outside of the drug development discipline. The science of validation and quality control is generally well developed and easily understood for those with a background in statistics. Standard operating procedures should be developed with this in mind and a balance should be found between what is perceived to be compliance and good science. It is inappropriate to sacrifice good science to comply with what are perceived to be regulatory preferences. This concept is strongly supported by the FDA guidance in its introduction, where it states that the guidance is intended to provide general recommendations for bioanalytical method validation that can be adjusted or modified.

There are a number of areas that are not well developed in the guidance such as acceptance criteria for stability investigations, repeat samples, ruggedness testing, selectivity in mass spectroscopy, and others. This would imply that the current FDA guidance is a work in progress and additional conferences may be held to refine and expand the current guidelines further.

REFERENCES

1. Shah VP. Analytical methods used in bioavailability studies: A regulatory viewpoint. Clin Res Pract Drug Reg Affairs 1987; 5:51–60.
2. Karnes HT, Shiu G, Shah VP. Validation of Bioanalytical Methods. Pharmaceut Res 1991; 8:421–426
3. US Dept of Health & Human Services. Guidance for Industry: Bioanalytical Method Validation. FDA,CDER, CVM, May 2001 BP.
4. Shah VP, Midha KK, Dighe S, et al. Conference Report. Analytical Methods Validation: Bioavailability, Bioequivalence and Pharmacokinetic Studies. Pharmaceut Res 1992; 9:249–258
5. US Dept of Health & Human Services. Guidance for Industry: Bioanalytical Methods Validation for Human Studies. FDA, CDER, Dec. 1998 BP.
6. Shah VP, Midha KK, Findlay JWA, et al. Bioanalytical methods validation—a revisit with a decade of progress. Pharmaceut Res 2000; 17:1551–1557.
7. Miller KJ, Bowsher RR, Celniker A, et al. Workshop on Bioanalytical Methods Validation for Macromolecules: Summary Report. Pharmaceut Res 2001; 18:1373–1383.
8. Curry SH, Whelpton R. Statistics of drug analysis, and the role of internal standards. In Reid E (ed), Blood Drugs and Other Analytical Challenges. Chichester, UK:Ellis Horwood, 1978, pp. 29–41.
9. Haefeltinger P. Limits of the internal standard technique in chromatography. J Chromatogr 1981; 218:73–81.
10. Massart DL, Andeginste BGM, Deming SN, Michotte Y, Kaufman L. Chemometrics a Textbook, New York, NY:Elsevier, 1988.
11. Karnes HT, March C. Calibration and Validation in Chromatographic Biopharmaceutical Analysis. J Pharmaceut Biomed Anal 1991; 9:911.
12. Cassidy R, Janoski M. Is Your Calibration Curve Linear? LD-GC 1992; 10:692.
13. Constanzer ML, Chavez CM, Matuszewski BK. Picogram determination of finasteride in human plasma and semen by high-performance liquid chromatography with atmosphere-pressure chemical-ionization tandem mass spectrometry. J Chromatogr B 1994; 658, 281–287.
14. Nelson MD, Dolan JW. Ion Suppression in LC-MS-MS–a case study. LCGC N Am 2002; 20(1).
15. Hubaux A, Vos G. Decision and detection limits for linear calibration curves. Anal Chem 1970; 42(8).
16. Long GL, Winefordner JD. Limit of detection—a closer look at the IUPAC definition. Analyt Chem 1983; 55:712A–722A.
17. Anderson RL. Practical Statistics for Analytical Chemists. New York, NY:Van Norstrand, 1987.
18. Trissel LA. Avoiding Common Flaws in Stability and Compatibility Studies of Injectable Drugs. American Society of Hospital Pharmacists, Inc. 1983; 0002-9289.83/0701-1159900.50.
19. Levey S, Jennings ER. The use of control charts in the clinical laboratory. Am J Clin Pathol 1950; 20:1059–1066.
20. Westgard JO, Barry PL. Cost-Effective Quality Control: Managing the Quality and Productivity of Analytical Processes. Washington, DC: AACC Press, 1986.
21. Causey AG, Hill HM, Phillips LJ. Evaluation of Criteria for the Acceptance of Bioanalytical Data. J Biomed Anal 1990; 8:625–628.
22. Karnes HT, March C. Precision Accuracy and Data Acceptance Criteria in Biopharmaceutical Analysis. Pharmaceut Res 1993; 10:1420.

8 Clinical Pharmacology Overview

Andrew P. Beelen, MD, BS Pharm
and Lionel D. Lewis, MB, BCh, MD, FRCP (London)

CONTENTS

1. INTRODUCTION

Clinical pharmacology is the branch of pharmacology that focuses on the study of drugs in humans. A comprehensive understanding of the principles of clinical pharmacology facilitates the clinician prescribing optimal therapy to an individual patient. Over the last 30 yr the clinical pharmacology of many drugs has been elucidated with advances in sophisticated, accurate, and precise analytical tools to determine plasma drug and/or metabolite concentrations in biological fluids. This has permitted a better understanding of the relationship between the pharmacokinetics (derived from the Greek *pharmakon* [drug] and *kinisis* [movement] and meaning drug concentration over time) and the pharmacodynamics (derived from the Greek *pharmakon* and *dynameos tis* [power], meaning drug action or power) for many drugs (Fig. 1). Oncology has, only somewhat belatedly, generated adequate data on these pharmacological properties of many widely used cytotoxic drugs. This is to some extent unfortunate, because cytotoxic drug therapy demands close attention to pharmacological principles as the therapeutic index of many anticancer agents is narrow, that is, $TD_{50}/ED_{50} \leq 2$ (see Fig. 2). To achieve the primary therapeutic endpoint (tumor cell death leading to tumor shrinkage), the limits of tolerable drug toxicity to normal tissues are often encroached. Importantly, adverse events, both anticipated and unexpected, must be integrated into therapeutic decisions to optimize patient outcome; thus ongoing assessment and reassessment of the cytotoxic drug effects on tumor and normal tissues are required. Drug–drug, drug–herb/food and drug–comorbid disease interactions, if not considered and anticipated, can have dire consequences for cancer patients. Furthermore, the rapidly increasing numbers of genetic polymorphisms in proteins involved either in the primary mechanism of a drug action and/or the processes that determine drug pharmacokinetics (absorption, distribution, metabolism, and excretion)

Handbook of Anticancer Pharmacokinetics and Pharmacodynamics
Edited by: W. D. Figg and H. L. McLeod © Humana Press Inc., Totowa, NJ

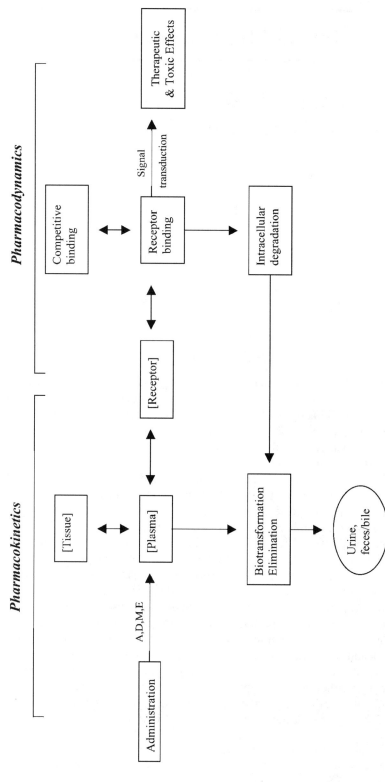

Fig. 1. Schematic representation of the physiologic processes determining drug disposition in the human body and the relationship of pharmacokinetics and pharmacodynamics to these processes.

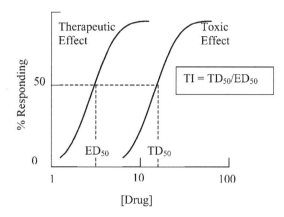

Fig. 2. Therapeutic index (TI): the ratio of the TD_{50} to the ED_{50} is an indicator of a drug's selectivity for producing the desired therapeutic effect in relation to its toxic effects.

further increase the complexity of optimal drug prescribing. This chapter focuses on the principles of clinical pharmacology applied to cytotoxic chemotherapy, and forms a basis as to why these principles assist the oncologist in optimizing the efficacy/toxicity ratio for cancer chemotherapeutic agents in individual patients.

2. MECHANISMS OF DRUG ACTION (PHARMACODYNAMICS)

The study of the effects of drugs on biologic and physiologic processes is termed pharmacodynamics. Most drug effects result from interactions with specific macromolecules or *targets* that induce a biochemical or physiologic change *(1–3)*. The target of the drug may be an enzyme found in the plasma or sited intracellularly; a cell-membrane-located protein; an ion channel protein or a structural protein; or DNA, RNA, or other macromolecules (e.g., microtubules). The site of action of many drugs is a *receptor* which normally binds an endogenous regulatory ligand (e.g., hormones, growth factors, neurotransmitters); the receptor function is modified on drug binding. Drugs that bind to receptors and mimic the endogenous ligand are termed *agonists* (e.g., recombinant human erythropoietin [rhEPO], granulocyte colony stimulating factor [G-CSF], opioids). When a drug binds to a receptor and blocks the effects of the endogenous ligand, the drug is termed an *antagonist* (e.g., flutamide, an androgen receptor antagonist; ondansetron, a 5-hydroxytryptamine type 3 [5-HT_3] antagonist, trastuzumab [Herceptin™] monoclonal antibody against HER-2 /neu). Certain agents have both agonist and antagonist properties at receptors and are termed partial agonists (e.g., tamoxifen-mixed estrogen receptor agonist/antagonist, nalbuphine-mixed μ/κ/δ opiate receptor agonist/antagonist). Many established and novel anticancer agents inhibit the function of endogenous enzymes by binding directly to an enzyme and are thus termed *enzyme inhibitors* (e.g., dihydrofolate reductase inhibitors—methotrexate; topisomerase I inhibitors, such as members of the camptothecin family; epidermal growth factor receptor [EGFR]-associated tyrosine kinase I inhibitors—OSI-774 [Tarceva™] and ZD1839 [Iressa™]; and the farnesyl transferase inhibitor trifarnib).

2.1. Drug Action

The binding of a drug to its target is often highly specific and dictated by the three-dimensional structure of both the ligand and target as well as electrostatic, dipole–dipole, ionic, van der Waals, hydrophobic, and hydrogen bond forces. The greater the net sum of

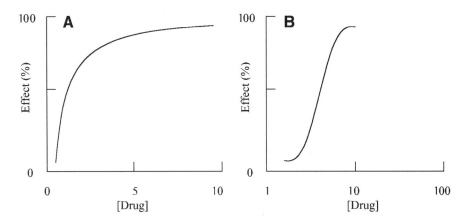

Fig. 3. Dose–response curves plotted (**A**) arithmetically and (**B**) semilogarithmically.

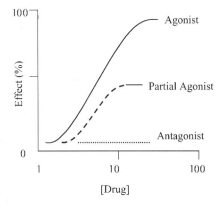

Fig. 4. Semilogarithmic plot of percent maximal effect vs drug concentration for an agonist, partial agonist, and antagonist.

these forces, the higher the binding affinity of the drug to its target *(1–3)*. Occasionally, a drug will form irreversible covalent bonds with its target, for example, alkylation of the 7-nitrogen and 6-oxygen atom in the guanine ring by ifosforamide mustard, the active metabolite of the ifosfamide. The pharmacologic effects of any drug most often occur in a graded, effect site concentration-dependent manner *(3–5)*. In many cases the plasma drug concentration is linearly related to the dose of the drug administered; the graphical representation of drug effect is thus often referred to as a *dose–response curve* (Figs. 3A, B). Agonist drugs produce a graded dose response up to a maximum value (E_{max}), above which increasing the drug concentration no longer produces a significant increase in effect. Antagonists produce no response and partial agonists have a reduced effect and reduced maximal effect–response (Fig. 4). Each drug has a specific shape to its dose (concentration)–response curve at its target site. In clinical therapy its importance underpins the need for dose titration of a drug to optimize the desired response *(6)*.

2.2. Receptor Pharmacology and Function

Molecular cloning techniques, along with advanced biochemical methods, have greatly enhanced our ability to discover and characterize physiological receptors, signal transduc-

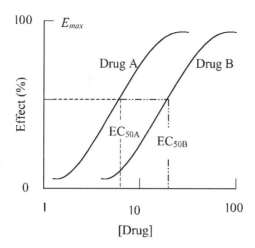

Fig. 5. Relative potency: semilogarithmic plot of percent maximal effect vs drug concentration for two drugs (A and B) with equal maximum pharmacologic effect (E_{max}). The relative potency can be estimated by the ratio of EC_{50B}/EC_{50A} (when measured in the same biologic system). EC_{50} = concentration of drug at which a 50% maximal response is observed.

tion pathways, and effector proteins. Receptors for endogenous ligands are classified into four "superfamilies" with distinct functional properties. Three families are localized to the cell membrane: ligand gated ion channel receptors (e.g., glutamate, nicotinic acetylcholine, and γ-aminobutyric acid receptors); G-protein coupled receptors (e.g., opiate receptors), and receptors with enzymatic activity (e.g., EGFR and platelet derived growth factor receptor [PDGFr]) *(7,8)*. A fourth family of receptors is located within the cell and is known as nuclear transcription factor receptors (e.g., steroid hormone receptors, retinoic acid [RA] receptors, and retinoid X receptors [RXR]). Agonist binding to any one of these receptors, regardless of family, activates a signal transduction pathway, for example, activation of a specific enzyme or cascade of enzymes, release of a second messenger(s), or transcription of a particular gene, and it is this intracellular physiologic change that mediates the effect of a ligand stimulating the receptor.

2.2.1. AGONISTS

Agonists (e.g. morphine, bromocriptine, lutenizing hormone-releasing hormone agonist, [leuprolide]) produce an effect by interacting with and activating specific receptors for endogenous ligands *(1,2,3,7)*. The particular signal transduction pathway linked to a receptor determines the process of receptor activation. Drugs that bind directly to and inhibit the activity of enzymes or proteins are not considered agonists because they do not first interact with an endogenous receptor. A useful parameter to compare drugs with equal maximal effect is EC_{50}, the concentration of drug at which a 50% maximal response is observed. Agonist properties can be quantified in terms of potency and magnitude of effect. Potency depends on four factors: receptor density, efficiency of receptor signal transduction, drug affinity for the receptor, and the degree of signal transduction induced by the drug binding to the receptor (*efficacy*). The latter two are properties of the drug itself and can be quantitated by plotting the percentage maximal effect vs log drug concentration for two comparison drugs, which will give relative potency (Fig. 5) or relative efficacy (Fig. 6).

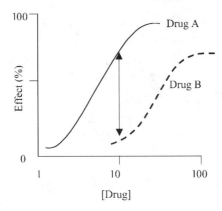

Fig. 6. Relative efficacy: semilogarithmic plot of percent maximal effect vs drug concentration for two drugs (A and B) with differing maximal effects. Drug A elicits a greater pharmacologic effect at the same concentrations and is therefore considered more potent and more effective than drug B (when measured in the same biologic system).

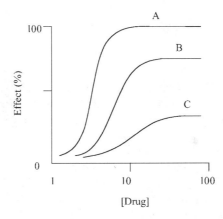

Fig. 7. Noncompetitive antagonism: The maximal effect of an agonist (line A) is attenuated by the addition of increasing concentrations of a noncompetitive antagonist (lines B and C).

2.2.2. COMPETITIVE ANTAGONISTS

Competitive antagonists (e.g., trastuzumab, alemtuzumab, rituximab) bind the same endogenous receptors as agonists, but they fail to induce a response (i.e., there is no receptor-mediated downstream signal transduction). Agonists in the presence of competitive antagonists simultaneously compete for the same receptors. The drug concentration in the effect compartment and receptor affinity determine the degree of receptor occupancy of each agent at any given moment in time. The effects of a competitive antagonist can be overcome by increasing the concentration of the agonist. Noncompetitive antagonists, on the other hand, in effect decrease the number of "effective" receptors and attenuate the maximal response to an agonist (Fig. 7). The effects of a noncompetitive antagonist cannot be overcome by increasing the agonist concentration *(1,2,4,6)*.

2.2.3. ENZYME INHIBITION

Similar concepts can be applied to drugs that are enzyme inhibitors (e.g., methotrexate, camptothecins, EGFR tyrosine kinase inhibitors). Thus the drug and the endogenous substrate compete for the same binding site on the enzyme. When the drug is bound, the enzyme can no longer bind substrate and the rate of the enzymatic reaction is reduced. One of the most successful molecularly targeted agents that possesses such a mechanism is imatinib mesylate (STI571/Gleevec™), which inhibits ATP binding to the tyrosine kinases activity of the protooncogene *KIT*, PDGFr, and BCR–ABL, inhibiting protein phosphorylation and signaling *(9–11)*. Alternatively, some drugs (e.g., chloradenosine as its anabolite chlorodeoxy ATP and the non-nucleoside reverse transcriptase inhibitors [NNRTI] of HIV-1, nevirapine, and efavirenz) bind to enzymes at sites other than the endogenous substrate-binding site and induce a conformational change in the enzyme structure *(12)*. This structural change modifies the three-dimensional shape of the endogenous substrate binding site so that the endogenous substrate is no longer recognized and is unable to bind. These drugs are termed allosteric or noncompetitive enzyme inhibitors.

2.2.4. PARTIAL AGONISTS

Partial agonists (e.g., tamoxifen [a partial agonist at the estrogen receptor] *[13]*, bryostatin [a partial agonist of protein kinase C] *[14]*, certain opioids [nalbuphine, buprenorphine]) stimulate endogenous receptors, but to a lesser degree than full agonists because of their intrinsically low efficacy. When an agonist is administered in the presence of a partial agonist, the maximal effect of the agonist is diminished because some receptors are occupied by the less effective partial agonist, which implies that partial agonists are also partial antagonists (Fig. 4). The partial agonist properties of a drug can be overcome by increasing the concentration of the pure agonist.

2.3. Non-Receptor-Mediated Drug Action

Some drugs exert their effects based solely on the physical or chemical nature of the drug. In cancer therapy, examples of drugs that work via this mechanism are purine analogs (e.g., 6-mercaptopurine and thioguanine) and certain pyrimidine analogs (e.g., fludaribine), which do not target specific endogenous receptors. They are incorporated into nucleic acids causing the impairment of DNA or RNA synthesis. This mechanism has been termed "counterfeit incorporation."

2.4. Pharmacodynamic Models

Pharmacodynamic models quantify the pharmacologic effect of a drug as it relates to the concentration of drug at its site of action (effect compartment concentration). These models are dependent on the assumptions of receptor *occupancy theory (1,3,7)*. This theory states that the intensity of the drug effect is proportional to the number of receptors bound by drug and that the maximum effect occurs when all receptors are occupied by the drug. The assumptions of the receptor occupancy theory are as follows: (1) drug--receptor association/dissociation is rapid and at equilibrium, (2) each receptor binds only one drug molecule at a time, (3) drug-receptor binding is reversible. The clinically most pertinent pharmacodynamic model is the E_{max} model, which is based on the hyperbolic relationship between pharmacologic effect and drug concentration (Fig. 8). The effect (E) can be quantitated by the following equation:

$$E = \left(E_{max} \times C \right) / \left(EC_{50} + C \right)$$

where E_{max} is the maximal effect, C is the plasma drug concentration, and EC_{50} is the concentration of drug at which a 50% maximal response is observed. If a receptor can bind

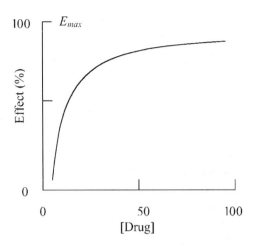

Fig. 8. E_{max} pharmacodynamic model. This is based on the equation:

$$\text{Effect} = \frac{E_{max} \times C}{EC_{50} + C}$$

where E_{max} is the maximal effect, EC_{50} is the drug concentration producing 50% of the maximal effect, and C is drug concentration.

more than one drug molecule simultaneously (e.g., oxygen binding to hemoglobin), then the sigmoid E_{max} model is used and the equation for effect becomes:

$$E = \left(E_{max} \times C^{\gamma}\right) / \left(EC_{50}^{\gamma} + C^{\gamma}\right)$$

where γ is the "Hill coefficient" and relates to the number of drug binding sites per receptor; it determines the slope of the curvilinear relationship (see Fig. 9) *(1–5)*.

3. PHARMACOKINETICS

The study of the time course of drug absorption, distribution, metabolism, and elimination by the human body is termed *pharmacokinetics (4,6,15,16)*. An adequate understanding of the basic principles of pharmacokinetics combined with the specific pharmacokinetic parameters for an individual drug enable the prescriber to choose the most appropriate route of administration, dose, and dosing frequency to obtain an optimal pharmacologic response while minimizing toxicity (see Fig. 1) *(15,16)*.

3.1. Absorption *(15–17)*

Most drugs must enter the systemic circulation to reach specific sites of action (usually intracellular targets for cancer drugs), which are often distant from the site of administration. Drug absorption is a highly variable process dependent on the physicochemical properties of the drug such as molecular size and shape, lipid solubility, degree of ionization, and protein and tissue binding characteristics. Passive diffusion is by far the most important process by which drugs move across cell membranes. The thickness of the cell membrane and the presence or absence of drug efflux pumps *(18)* (e.g., ATP binding cassette [ABC] transporters, e.g., ABCB1—also known as MDR-1 and P-glycoprotein)

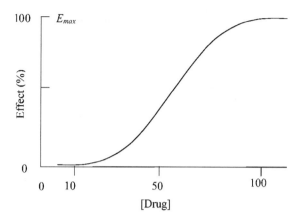

Fig. 9. Sigmoid E_{max} pharmacodynamic model. This is based on the equation:

$$\text{Effect} = \frac{E_{max} \times C^{\gamma}}{EC_{50}^{\gamma} + C^{\gamma}}$$

where E_{max} is the maximal effect, EC_{50} is the drug concentration producing 50% of the maximal effect and C is drug concentration, and where γ is the steepness of the slope.

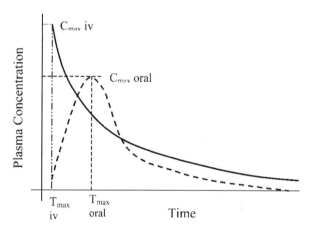

Fig. 10. Plasma drug concentration time curves following intravenous *(solid line)* and oral *(dashed line)* administration. C_{max} is the observed maximal plasma drug concentration and T_{max} is the time at which C_{max} is observed. The oral bioavailability *(F)* of a drug is determined from the ratio of AUC_{oral}/AUC_{iv}, where AUC is the area under the curve.

also determine the rate and extent of drug absorption. Oral (enteral) drug administration is the most common route of drug delivery because it is convenient, safe, and economical. The majority of cancer drugs, however, are either poorly absorbed from the gastrointestinal tract or undergo significant metabolism or excretion by the gastrointestinal mucosa and/or liver prior to entering the systemic circulation. This process is known as the *first-pass effect*. Drugs with a high first pass effect have low *bioavailability (F)*, a term used to describe the fractional extent to which a dose of drug reaches the systemic circulation (Fig. 10).

Examples of drugs with low oral bioavailability include morphine, many cytotoxics (e.g., paclitaxel, docetaxel, daunorubicin), and monoclonal antibodies (which are proteins and therefore degraded by acid in the stomach). Intravenous administration of drugs used in cancer chemotherapy circumvents the factors related to absorption and the first-pass effect, and by definition provides 100% bioavailability. Other routes of drug administration (e.g., subcutaneous, intramuscular, intra-arterial, intrathecal, and topical) are important in cancer therapeutics, but are not discussed in detail in this chapter.

3.2. Distribution (15–17)

Once a drug enters the systemic circulation, it begins to equilibrate (distribute) throughout the body. Many factors contribute to drug distribution including cardiac output, regional blood flow and blood flow within a tumor, pH of the local environment, presence of drug efflux pumps (especially ABCB1 [MDR-1 /P-glycoprotein] and other ABC transporters that are present in many tumors [19]), and the physicochemical properties of the drug, especially its lipid solubility. Binding to plasma proteins (mainly albumin for acidic drugs and α_1 acid glycoprotein for basic drugs) can limit the degree of drug distribution because only unbound (free) drug can passively diffuse through cell membranes. Some drugs accumulate in certain tissues preferentially, usually because they are highly lipophilic or secondary to tissue-specific binding (e.g., paclitaxel to beta-tubulin). Many chemotherapeutic agents have to enter tumor cells to produce a cytotoxic effect. Distribution into tumor cells can be facilitated by transport proteins (carriers) and may be energy dependent (i.e., active transport). Active transport moves drugs against electrochemical and concentration gradients, which can significantly increase drug concentration in tumor cells. Examples of drugs that are actively transported into cells in addition to their transmembrane flux by passive diffusion include fludarabine, gemcitabine, and methotrexate (20–22).

3.3. Metabolism (Biotransformation) (15–17)

Many drugs undergo enzymatic modification (metabolism), which most commonly reduces their pharmacological activity and enhances the body's ability to excrete the drug. In some instances, the metabolite is more pharmacologically active than the parent drug (e.g., conversion of ifosfamide to ifosforamide mustard; CPT-11 to SN-38) or an active metabolite may be cleared more slowly than the parent compound (e.g., CPT-11 metabolite SN 38, morphine metabolite, morphine-6-glucuronide [23]). Drug metabolism can be categorized into two phases: phase 1 reactions, which involve metabolic modifications of the drug (often oxidation, reduction, or hydrolysis), and phase 2 reactions, which are synthetic conjugation reactions involving the covalent linkage of a highly polar molecule (glucuronic acid, sulfate, amino acid, glutathione, acetate) to the drug or its metabolite. The products of phase 2 reactions have increased water solubility and are readily excreted in the urine (or bile).

The primary site of drug metabolism (both phase 1 and phase 2 reactions) is the liver, although the gastrointestinal tract, kidney, and lungs play important roles for some drugs. Within the liver, the cytochrome P450 (CYP450) monooxygenase system accounts for the vast majority of phase 1 drug metabolism. There are more than 50 known functionally active cytochrome P450's in humans, with only eight isoforms accounting for more than 90% of all drug metabolism. CYP 3A4 and CYP 3A5 (nearly identical isoforms and also expressed in the intestinal epithelium) metabolize approx 50% of all drugs; CYP 2D6 (20% of drugs) and CYP2C9/19 account for the metabolism of another 20–25% of drugs; all the other active isoforms (CYP1A1/2, CYP2B6, CYP2A6, CYP2E1) accounting for the remaining CYP450 metabolic activity *(15,16)*. Many drugs are substrates for (and thus metabolized by) more than a single member of the CYP450 enzyme family, having differing affinities for binding to the different CYP450s. Drugs can be both substrates for the CYP450 enzymes and inducers or inhibitors of these enzymes.

Concurrent use of drugs that interfere with the metabolism of another drug may result in significant toxicity or therapeutic failure. The recent identification of multiple genetic polymorphisms for many of the CYP450 enzymes *(24,25)* has in part allowed us further insight into the interindividual variability in drug metabolism. The best example of this is the four different CYP2D6 phenotypes; which yield poor, intermediate, extensive, and ultrarapid metabolism of drugs that are substrates for this enzyme.

Phase 2 conjugation reactions also take place in the liver, the most important of which is glucuronidation. This involves the addition of a glucuronide group to the drug by uridine diphosphate glucuronosyltransferase (UGT). More than 15 isoforms of UGTs have been identified, and as with the CYP450 system, functional polymorphisms have been identified (UGT1A1 catalyzes the glucuronidation of SN-38 to SN-38 glucuronide). The same holds true for *N*-acetyltransferase (NAT) and accounts for the "slow and fast acetylator" phenotypes, which affects the metabolism of amonafide to *N*-acetylamonafide (NAT2) and its toxicity profile (fast acetylators experience greater myelosuppression) *(26)*. Intracellular metabolism is another important mechanism of drug biotransformation. Many antimetabolite drugs are dependent on intracellular anabolism/metabolism to yield pharmacologically active entities (e.g., 5-fluorouracil, gemcitabine, 6-mercaptopurine).

3.4. Excretion (Elimination) (15–17)

Drugs can be eliminated from the body either in an unchanged form or as metabolites. Lipid-soluble drugs generally are metabolized (as described in Subheading 3.3.) to more polar compounds to facilitate their elimination from the body via the kidney. The kidneys are primarily responsible for the excretion of drugs and their metabolites while biliary excretion plays an important role for certain drugs (e.g., taxanes, SN-38 glucuronide). Elimination of drugs via the urine is dependent on three processes: glomerular filtration, active tubular secretion, and passive tubular reabsorption. The glomerular filtration rate is reduced in the elderly and many disease states and is dependent on cardiac output and intravascular volume. Drug molecules that are not protein bound ("free drug") can be filtered. Other physicochemical properties of drugs and metabolites that facilitate renal excretion include small molecular size (mol wt < 500 Da) and being un-ionized at physiological pH, which depends on the pK_a of the compound.

3.5. Pharmacokinetic Parameters (15–17)

A simple plot of plasma drug concentration vs time offers the prescriber useful pharmacokinetic data (Fig. 10). C_{max} is defined as the maximal plasma concentration following a specific dose and t_{max} is the time at which C_{max} is observed. The area under the plasma drug concentration vs time curve (AUC) is a useful measure of the body's total drug exposure.

3.5.1. VOLUME OF DISTRIBUTION *(15)*

The concept of volume of distribution can be demonstrated by the theoretical administration of a drug as a rapid intravenous bolus injection with sampling and measurement of plasma concentrations at specified time intervals. The resultant log plasma drug concentration vs time graph for a drug that rapidly distributes and equilibrates throughout the body (i.e., the one-compartment, well-stirred model with first-order elimination) will appear similar to the plot representing drug A in Fig. 11. Extrapolation of the line back to time zero gives a theoretical plasma drug concentration (C_0) that would have occurred if drug equilibration were instantaneous. This theoretical concentration results from the dilution of a known amount of drug (usually milligrams) into an unknown volume of the human body, which is known as the *apparent volume of distribution* or V_d. Dividing the dose (D) by C_0 gives the value for V_d (usually expressed in liters): $V_d = D/C_0$. Factors affecting the volume of distribution include the physicochemical properties of the drug (see Subheading 3.2.) and many patient-dependent factors such as body size, fat composition, water content, and plasma protein concentration. The V_d is often referred to as the "apparent" volume of distribution because it does not represent a true physiologic single space or compartment within the human body, but rather a theoretical composite value for all the compartments to which the drug distributes. The one-compartment model is a convenient mathematical representation of drug distribution and elimination for many, but not all drugs. More complex models are required for drugs that have protracted distribution times (e.g., paclitaxel, daunorubicin). In the two-compartment model represented for drug B in Fig. 11 (e.g., docetaxel), the body is divided into two theoretical spaces, a smaller central compartment (blood volume plus the extracellular space of highly perfused tissues; heart, lung, liver, kidneys) and a larger peripheral compartment, which represents all other tissues. A semilogarithmic plot of plasma drug B concentration vs time reveals a biphasic decline in plasma drug concentration over time (Fig. 11). The first phase, known as the alpha phase, represents redistribution of drug B out of the central (sampling) compartment and into the peripheral tissues. The beta phase, also known as the terminal elimination phase, occurs after drug B has equilibrated between the two compartments and primarily represents drug elimination. Three-compartment models are necessary to describe some drugs (e.g., paclitaxel, many anthracyclines) that have two distribution phases preceding the terminal elimination phase. The volume of distribution for drugs following a multicompartment model is conceptually the same as for one-compartment modeling, but calculated in a slightly different way.

3.5.2. CLEARANCE *(15,17)*

Clearance represents the rate at which a drug is eliminated from the body and is expressed in terms of volume per unit time for first-order elimination. The volume term represents the theoretical volume of blood (or more often plasma) totally cleared of drug during a given time interval, which remains constant and independent of plasma drug concentration. The amount or mass of drug removed from the body per unit time, however, is constantly changing (depending on plasma drug concentration) during first-order elimination and is therefore not a convenient means to express clearance. When clearance mechanisms are saturated (i.e., operating at full capacity), zero-order elimination kinetics is followed and a constant mass (milligrams) of drug is cleared from the body per unit time regardless of the plasma drug concentration.

Most drug pharmacokinetics fit a one-compartment, first-order elimination kinetics model with an elimination rate constant (k_e) equal to the slope of the line for the log plasma drug concentration vs time plot (drug A in Fig. 11). The total body clearance, Cl_T (which is a summation of all clearance mechanisms; renal, hepatic, and other) of a drug is directly proportional to k_e and V_d: $Cl_T = k_e \times V_d$. Another useful equation to calculate Cl_T for first order elimination is:

$$Cl_T = F \times \text{dose/AUC}$$

where F is the bioavailability and AUC is the area under the log plasma drug concentration time curve.

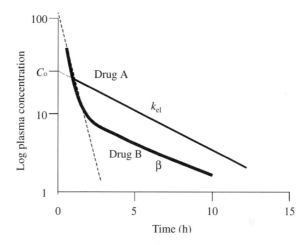

Fig. 11. One compartment model *(straight line)* vs two-compartment model *(curvilinear line)* following rapid intravenous administration. Drug A exhibits a monoexponential decay (one-compartment model). C_0 is the theoretical plasma concentration at time zero ad k_{el} is the elimination rate constant. Drug B exhibits a biexponential decay representing a two-compartment model α represents the redistribution phase rate constant, and β represents the terminal elimination phase rate constant.

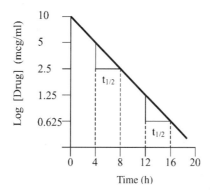

Fig. 12. Half-life: log plasma drug concentration vs time plot for a drug following first-order elimination kinetics and a half-life of 4 h.

3.5.3. ELIMINATION HALF-LIFE ($t_{1/2}$) (15,17)

The amount of time it takes for the plasma drug concentration to decline by 50% is defined as the half-life ($t_{1/2}$; see Fig. 12). Half-life is also related to the ke: $t_{1/2} = 0.693/k_e$. Substitution of Cl_T/V_d for k_e yields the equation: $t_{1/2} = 0.693 \times V_d/Cl_T$.

$$t_{1/2} = 0.693 \times V_d/Cl_T$$

Thus, $t_{1/2}$ changes as a function of both V_d and Cl_T (under steady-state conditions). The half-life of a drug is useful in determining the dosing interval for many drugs that are dosed to a steady state and the time required to reach steady-state plasma concentrations (i.e., four half-lives to reach 94% of steady state) as well as being useful for estimating the time for a specific percentage of administered drug to be removed from the body (i.e., on cessation of drug therapy, the plasma drug concentration will decrease by 50% for each $t_{1/2}$ time interval).

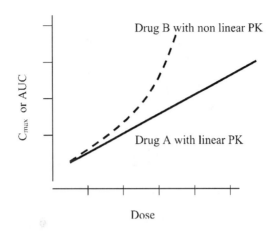

Fig. 13. Drug A has linear pharmacokinetics with dose proportional increases in $C_{\max}$ and AUC. Drug B exhibits nonlinear (dose-dependent) pharmacokinetics with nonlinear increases in $C_{\max}$ and AUC with dose. Drug B is said to obey Michaelis–Menton (or saturation) pharmacokinetics.

3.5.4 . NONCOMPARTMENTAL MODELING

Noncompartmental modeling uses statistical moment theory to derive the same pharmacokinetic parameters and provides the additional parameters of AUMC or area under the first-moment curve (analogous to AUC) and the mean residence time (MRT). The primary advantage of noncompartmental modeling is the requirement for fewer model specific assumptions.

3.5.5. NONLINEAR "DOSE-DEPENDENT" PHARMACOKINETICS *(27)*

Clearance, for most drugs, remains constant (proportional to plasma drug concentration) over the therapeutic dose range and as a result, first-order kinetics are obeyed. Occasionally, clearance mechanisms become overwhelmed (i.e., saturated) and there is no longer an exponential decline in plasma drug concentration over time (i.e., zero-order kinetics are followed). Under such circumstances in which clearance mechanisms are saturated (e.g., enzyme saturation, Michaelis–Menton kinetics apply), small increases in dose can dramatically increase plasma drug concentration or AUC (see Fig. 13). In such cases (e.g. paclitaxel at doses > 135 mg/m^2 administered over 3 h), the pharmacokinetics are considered "dose dependent" or "capacity-limited." This is also termed Michaelis–Menton pharmacokinetics as the nonlinear relationship of concentration and dose can be fitted to the classical enzyme kinetic model. The processes of drug absorption (e.g., oral methotrexate, melphalan), distribution, and excretion can also become saturated, which in turn leads to a drug exhibiting nonlinear pharmacokinetics.

4. POPULATION PHARMACOKINETICS *(28)*

Pharmacokinetic parameters can vary widely from one patient to the next, which may lead to significant toxicity in some patients and therapeutic failure in others. Population pharmacokinetic modeling of pharmacokinetic data from many different patients can help quantify some of this variability. This can be especially useful when the target population for the drug is heterogeneous or when the therapeutic window is narrow (i.e., effective plasma drug concentrations approach toxic concentrations). These models can simultaneously quantitate the effects of identifiable patient demographic variables (e.g., age, sex, weight, etc.), pathophysiological variables (e.g., renal or liver function, congestive heart failure, etc.), and therapeutic variables such as concomitant drug therapy on drug disposition. Another advantage is that the residual variability (the variability not accounted for by the other specified covariates) is quantitated, which includes intraindividual variability, model misspecification, and measurement error (see Chapter 9 for further discussion and details).

5. PHARMACOKINETIC–PHARMACODYNAMIC RELATIONSHIP (28,29)

Pharmacokinetic modeling describes the change of plasma drug concentration over time and pharmacodynamic modeling relates drug concentration to pharmacologic effect (without regard to time). Pharmacokinetic–pharmacodynamic (PK–PD) modeling relates pharmacologic effect to the change of plasma drug concentration over time. The goal is to predict not only the magnitude but also the duration of pharmacologic effect based on the pharmacokinetic parameters of a particular drug. PK–PD models are predicated on the assumption that the concentration of drug in the plasma (accessible compartment) is proportional to the drug concentration at the receptor site (effect compartment). There are some drugs for which there is no correlation between plasma concentration and pharmacologic effect; however, toxicity may be correlated to plasma concentration in some cases (e.g., methotrexate). Such models have perhaps been best used in oncology to predict drug toxicity rather than antitumor effect.

6. INTERPATIENT VARIABILITY

The pharmacokinetic parameters and the pharmacologic response from a specific dose of a drug may vary widely from patient to patient. There are multiple reasons for the observed interpatient variability in drug response that involves both pharmacokinetic (15,30) and pharmacodynamic processes (29,31,32). These include organ dysfunction, disease state, concurrent medications, receptor and metabolic enzyme phenotype, age, sex, and other demographic characteristics. Drug bioavailability may vary from patient to patient secondary to increased or decreased expression or activity of intestinal enzymes that metabolize drugs or varying expression of drug efflux pumps (i.e., ABCB1- MDR-1 or P-glycoprotein). ABCB1 (P-glycoprotein) also pumps drugs out of cells, thus lowering the intracellular drug concentration, its overexpression in tumor cells is a well-documented mechanism of tumor cell resistance. One of the primary causes of pharmacokinetic variability is interpatient differences in the rate of drug clearance. In the case of drugs (or drugs with active metabolites) that are primarily cleared by the kidney, decreased renal function will dictate the need for dose reduction to avoid excessive toxicity (e.g., methotrexate). Drugs that undergo extensive hepatic biotransformation and/or biliary excretion may require dose modification in patients with severely compromised hepatic function (e.g., taxanes, anthracyclines, vinca alkaloids). Genetic polymorphisms in the CYP450 enzyme and other phase 2 enzyme systems (e.g., *N*-acetylation transferase-2, glutathione -*S*-transferase, and uridine diphosphate glucuronosyltransferase) will also contribute to differences in an individual's ability to metabolize anti-cancer drugs (30). Another major reason for altered CYP450 activity is the use of concurrent medications that either inhibit or induce one or more isoforms, which may result in significant changes in the rate of drug clearance. Variability in the volume of distribution of a drug can also account for some of the observed interpatient variability. Age is particularly important for volume of distribution because infants have approx 70–80% total body water compared to 60% for adults. Elderly patients have relatively more adipose tissue and less water content as well as decreased muscle mass. Disease-related alterations in plasma protein concentrations in cancer patients can affect the volume of distribution of drugs that are highly protein bound (e.g., α_1-acid glycoprotein which binds docetaxel and UCN-01) influencing free drug concentrations and drug clearance.

Pharmacodynamic variability is produced not only by differences between patients in the concentration of drug at the effect site as a result of pharmacokinetic variation (Fig. 1) but also by receptor/target polymorphisms. Examples of these polymorphisms include cases in which a receptor is more or less responsive to a certain drug concentration, as is the case for opioid receptors (33,34), or where paclitaxel resistance is linked to variants in the β-tubulin (35).

7. CONCLUSION

In conclusion, it is very important for all physicians to have an understanding of the principles of clinical pharmacology to optimize drug dose and schedule for their patients, and to recognize the underlying reasons for variability in drug response.

REFERENCES

1. Ross EM, Kenakin TP. Pharmacodynamics: mechanisms of drug action and the relationship between drug concentration and effect. In: Hardman JG, Limbird LE (eds). Goodman & Gilman's The Pharmacological Basis of Therapeutics, 10th Edit. New York, NY: McGraw-Hill, 2001, pp. 31–43.
2. Nies AS. Principles of Therapeutics. In: Hardman JG, Limbird LE, (eds). Goodman & Gilman's The Pharmacological Basis of Therapeutics, 10th Edit. New York, NY: McGraw-Hill, 2001, pp. 45–66.
3. Lowe ES, Balis FM. Dose-effect and concentration-effect analysis. In: Atkinson AJ, Daniels CE, Dedrick RL, Grudzinskas CV, Markey SP (eds). Principles of Clinical Pharmacology. Boston, MA: Academic Press, 2001, pp. 235–244.
4. Ritter JM, Lewis LD, Mant TGK. A Textbook of Clinical Pharmacology, 4th Edit. London, UK: Arnold, 1999, pp. 8–58.
5. Atkinson AJ. Kinetic analysis of pharmacologic effect. In: Atkinson AJ, Daniels CE, Dedrick RL, Grudzinskas CV, Markey SP (eds). Principles of Clinical Pharmacology. Boston, MA: Academic Press, 2001, pp. 245–252.
6. Nierenberg DW, Melmon KL. Introduction to clinical pharmacology and rational therapeutics. In: Carruthers GS, Hoffman BB, Melmon KL, Nierenberg DW (eds). Melmon and Morrelli's Clinical Pharmacology, 4th Edit. New York, NY: McGraw-Hill, 2000, pp. 3–62.
7. TP Kenakin, RA Bond, TI Bonner. Definition of pharmacological receptors. Pharmacol Rev 1992; 44:351–362.
8. Christopoulos A, Kenakin T. G Protein-coupled receptor allosterism and complexing. Pharmacol Rev 2002; 54:323–374.
9. Capdeville R, Buchdunger E, Zimmermann J, Matter A. Glivec (STI571, imatinib), a rationally developed, targeted anticancer drug. Nat Rev Drug Discov 2002; 1:493–502.
10. Druker BJ, Talpaz M, Resta DJ, et al. Efficacy and safety of a specific inhibitor of the BCR-ABL tyrosine kinase in chronic myeloid leukemia. N Engl J Med 2001; 344:1031–1037.
11. van Oosterom AT, Judson I, Verweij J, et al. Safety and efficacy of imatinib (STI571) in metastatic gastrointestinal stromal tumours: a phase I study. Lancet 2001; 358:1421–1423.
12. Smith PF, DiCenzo R, Morse GD. Clinical pharmacokinetics of non-nucleoside reverse transcriptase inhibitors. Clin Pharmacokinet 2001; 40:893–905.
13. Macgregor JI, Jordan VC. Basic guide to the mechanisms of antiestrogen action. Pharmacol Rev 1998; 50:151–196.
14. Caponigro F, French RC, Kaye SB. Protein kinase C: a worthwhile target for anticancer drugs? Anticancer Drugs 1997; 8:26–33.

15. Wilkinson GR. Pharmacokinetics: the dynamics of drug absorption, distribution, and elimination. In: Hardman JG, Limbird LE (eds). Goodman & Gilman's The Pharmacological Basis of Therapeutics, 10th Edit. New York, NY: McGraw-Hill, 2001, pp. 3–29.
16. Boroujerdi M. Pharmacokinetics: Principles and Applications. New York, NY: McGraw-Hill, 2002, pp. 343–367.
17. Shargel L, Yu ABC. Applied Biopharmaceutics and Pharmacokinetics, 4th Edit. Norwalk, CT: Appleton & Lange, 1999, pp. 573–605.
18. Borst P, Elferink RO. Mammalian abc transporters in health and disease. Annu Rev Biochem 2002; 71:537–592.
19. Gottesman MM, Fojo T, Bates SE. Multidrug resistance in cancer: role of ATP-dependent transporters. Nat Rev Cancer 2002; 2:48–58.
20. Jamieson GP, Snook MB, Bradley TR, et al. Transport and metabolism of 1-beta-D-arabino-furanosylcytosine in human ovarian adenocarcinoma cells. Cancer Res 1989; 49:309–313.
21. Mackey JR, Yao SY, Smith KM, et al. Gemcitabine transport in *Xenopus* oocytes expressing recombinant plasma membrane mammalian nucleoside transporters. J Natl Cancer Inst 1999; 91:1876–1881.
22. Moscow JA. Methotrexate transport and resistance. Leuk Lymphoma 1998; 30:215–224.
23. Kalman S, Metcalf K, Eintrei C. Morphine, morphine-6-glucuronide, and morphine-3-glucuronide in cerebrospinal fluid and plasma after epidural administration of morphine. Reg Anesth 1997; 22:131–136.
24. Roden DM. Principles in pharmacogenetics. Epilepsia 2001; 42(Suppl 5):44–48.
25. Relling MV, Dervieux T. Pharmacogenetics and cancer therapy. Nat Rev Cancer 2001; 1:99–108.
26. Innocenti F, Iyer L, Ratain MJ. Pharmacogenetics of anticancer agents: lessons from amonafide and irinotecan. Drug Metab Dispos 2001; 29:596–600.
27. Bachmann KA, Belloto RJ Jr. Differential kinetics of phenytoin in elderly patients. Drugs Aging 1999; 15:235–250.
28. Bruno R, Vivier N, Veyrat-Follet C, Montay G, Rhodes GR. Population pharmacokinetics and pharmacokinetic–pharmacodynamic relationships for docetaxel. Invest New Drugs 2001; 19:163–169.
29. Meibohm B, Derendorf H. Basic concepts of pharmacokinetic/pharmacodynamic (PK/PD) modelling. Int J Clin Pharmacol Ther 1997; 35:401–413.
30. Sekine I, Saijo N. Polymorphisms of metabolizing enzymes and transporter proteins involved in the clearance of anticancer agents. Ann Oncol 2001; 12:1515–1525.
31. Roden DM, George AL Jr. The genetic basis of variability in drug responses. Nat Rev Drug Discov 2002; 1:37–44.
32. Evans WE, Johnson JA. Pharmacogenomics: the inherited basis for interindividual differences in drug response. Annu Rev Genom Hum Genet 2001; 2:9–39.
33. Lotsch J, Skarke C, Grosch S, Darimont J, Schmidt H, Geisslinger G. The polymorphism A118G of the human mu-opioid receptor gene decreases the pupil constrictory effect of morphine-6-glucuronide but not that of morphine. Pharmacogenetics 2002; 12:3–9.
34. Wand GS, McCaul M, Yang X, et al. The mu-opioid receptor gene polymorphism (A118G) alters HPA axis activation induced by opioid receptor blockade. Neuropsychopharmacology. 2002; 26:106–114.
35. Monzo M, Rosell R, Sanchez JJ, et al. Paclitaxel resistance in non-small-cell lung cancer associated with beta-tubulin gene mutations. J Clin Oncol 1999; 17:1786–1793.

9 Pharmacokinetic Modeling

Sharyn D. Baker, *Pharm D*
and Michelle A. Rudek, *Pharm D, PhD*

CONTENTS

1. INTRODUCTION

Pharmacokinetics is the study of absorption, distribution, metabolism, and excretion of a drug over a time course. Measurement of a drug in the body is usually limited to the blood or plasma. Pharmacokinetic data analysis consists of examining plasma concentration–time data and estimating pharmacokinetic parameters that describe drug disposition. Methods used for pharmacokinetic analysis include noncompartmental analysis or pharmacokinetic modeling. Noncompartmental analysis does not depend on fitting mathematical models to the drug disposition data. Compartmental analysis is the most often used pharmacokinetic modeling approach. This chapter discusses various aspects of compartmental modeling.

2. SAMPLING STRATEGIES

In Phase I studies, the number of blood specimens taken and their timing must allow for the accurate description of the plasma disposition of the drug in individual subjects and for the estimation of individual pharmacokinetic parameter values. Because at the time of Phase I drug testing, the disposition of a drug in humans is usually unknown, it is necessary to employ an intensive (frequent) and extensive (prolonged) blood sampling scheme. To maximize the chances that all the phases of drug disposition are identified and measured, the following steps are undertaken: (1) sample intensively during drug administration and immediately following the discontinuation of drug administration; (2) sample at time points as far out after drug administration as is feasible; and (3) utilize highly sensitive assay methods. Intensive and extensive sampling schemes provide enough plasma concentration data to select among alternative models that best describe all the plasma disposition

Handbook of Anticancer Pharmacokinetics and Pharmacodynamics
Edited by: W. D. Figg and H. L. McLeod © Humana Press Inc., Totowa, NJ

phases of the drug (e.g., biexponential vs triexponential behavior) and allow for the detection and characterization of unexpected dispositional phenomena, such as enterohepatic recirculation.

In later stages of drug development, limited-sampling strategies are employed to allow estimation of pharmacokinetic parameters using a small number of plasma samples (e.g., *1–3*). This is possible only when the pharmacokinetic behavior of an agent is known. One approach to designing a limited-sampling strategy is by combining D-optimality with a Bayesian algorithm *(1)*. D-optimality uses optimal design theory to select a limited number of sampling times. A Bayesian algorithm then combines information from the limited sampling scheme with prior information about the population pharmacokinetic parameter values (e.g., the average value and variance) to then estimate pharmacokinetic parameters for individual patients. A linear regression approach is another method to design limited sampling schemes. This latter method generally allows for estimation of only a single pharmacokinetic parameter such as clearance or area under the concentration–time curve (AUC).

Disadvantages of the linear regression approach include the requirement for consistent timing of infusion duration and blood sampling. All data points must be obtained; all conditions are required for calculation of the pharmacokinetic parameter. The Bayesian algorithm is usually more robust and flexible and allows the description of the full pharmacokinetic profile and estimation of more than one pharmacokinetic parameter *(2,3)*. The development of a limited-sampling strategy using a Bayesian algorithm may be approached in the following manner. First, a population pharmacokinetic model is developed and average values for each pharmacokinetic parameter and the variance about the pharmacokinetic parameter are determined. Next, the concentration–time data sets to be used for developing a limited sampling scheme are randomly divided into two equal subsets, a training data set and a validation data set. Using the sample module of the software program ADAPT II (which employs D-optimality), a limited sampling scheme is defined for the training data set. The validation data set is then used to validate the limited-sampling scheme. Individual plasma concentrations, at the selected time points, are fitted using a Bayesian algorithm as implemented in ADAPT II, where the Bayesian priors and covariance matrix are derived from the population pharmacokinetic model. Reference pharmacokinetic parameters for individual patients in the validation set are determined using the full pharmacokinetic profile and maximum likelihood estimation. The predictive performance of the limited-sampling strategy is evaluated by calculating the bias and precision of the Bayesian parameter estimates *(2,3)*.

3. NONCOMPARTMENTAL ANALYSIS

Noncompartmental analysis, which is based on the statistical moment theory *(4)*, is routinely performed to calculate pharmacokinetic parameters quickly and easily. Noncompartmental analysis does not require the assumption of a specific compartmental model for drug disposition, which for some drugs can be a complex and time-consuming process. An underlying assumption with noncompartmental analysis is pharmacokinetic linearity, in which the pharmacokinetic parameter values do not vary with dose and/or time. This assumption applies to all parameters describing drug absorption, distribution, metabolism, and elimination.

4. COMPARTMENTAL ANALYSIS

Compartmental analysis is useful to describe drug disposition, estimate pharmacokinetic parameters, and predict plasma concentrations utilizing various schedules and doses of

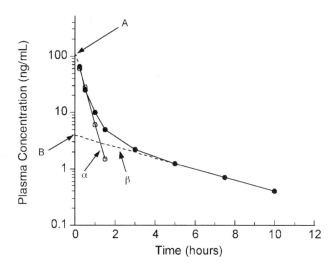

Fig. 1. Plasma concentration–time profile for a drug administered as an intravenous bolus dose and exhibiting a biexponential or two-compartment behavior. Residual values are denoted by the open circle symbol.

administration. During compartmental analysis, plasma disposition curves are fit by equations that describe the time course of plasma drug concentrations for the given mode of drug input. For example, the following equations describe a drug administered as an intravenous bolus that exhibits a mono- (Eq. 1) or bi-exponential (Eq. 2) decline:

$$C_t = C_0 e^{-Kt} \tag{1}$$

$$C_t = A e^{-\alpha t} + B e^{-\beta t} \tag{2}$$

where C_t represents the concentration at a particular time, C_0 is the concentration at time zero, A and B are macro-rate constants, K is the apparent first-order elimination rate constant, and α and β are macro-elimination rate constants. For a drug exhibiting a biexponential decline (Eq. 2), α and β correspond to the initial and terminal slopes, respectively. The method of residuals (5) can be applied to the concentration–time data to estimate A and B, which are zero-time intercepts for each disposition phase. Figure 1 depicts the fit of Eq. (2) to the concentration vs time values for a theoretical drug.

Plasma disposition curves can also be fit by equations that incorporate microconstants. For an open linear two-compartment model, the microconstants include the central volume of distribution (V_c), the elimination rate constant (k_{10}), and the intercompartment rate constants (k_{12}, k_{21}) (Fig. 2). For the model illustrated in Fig. 2, the microconstants are also known as the structural parameters of the model. Micro-constants can be estimated from macro-constants and vice-versa by the following equations (6):

$$A = \frac{D_{iv}}{V_c} \times \frac{(\alpha - k_{21})}{(\alpha - \beta)} \tag{3}$$

$$B = \frac{D_{iv}}{V_c} \times \frac{(\beta - k_{21})}{(\beta - \alpha)} \tag{4}$$

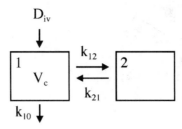

Fig. 2. Two-compartment model parameterized with microconstants.

$$\alpha = \frac{k_{21} \times k_{10}}{\beta} \tag{5}$$

$$\beta = \frac{1}{2} \times \left[\left(k_{12} + k_{21} + k_{10} \right) - \sqrt{\left(k_{12} + k_{21} + k_{10} \right)^2 - \left(4 \times k_{21} \times k_{10} \right)} \right] \tag{6}$$

$$k_{10} = \frac{\alpha \times \beta}{k_{21}} \tag{7}$$

$$k_{12} = \left(\alpha + \beta \right) - \left(k_{21} - k_{10} \right) \tag{8}$$

$$k_{21} = \frac{\left(A \times \beta \right) + \left(B \times \alpha \right)}{A + B} \tag{9}$$

$$V_c = \frac{D_{iv}}{A + B} \tag{10}$$

The following secondary parameters can be calculated from the model-estimated parameters using the equations listed below (6):

Half-life during the alpha (initial) disposition phase ($t_{1/2,}\alpha$):

$$t_{1/2, \alpha} = \frac{\alpha}{0.693} \tag{11}$$

Half-life during the beta (terminal) disposition phase ($t_{1/2,}\beta$)

$$t_{1/2, \beta} = \frac{0.693}{\beta} \tag{12}$$

Systemic clearance (Cl_s):

$$Cl_s = V_c \times k_{10} \tag{13}$$

$$Cl_s = \frac{D_{iv}}{AUC} \tag{14}$$

Area under the concentration–time curve (AUC):

$$AUC = \frac{A}{\alpha} + \frac{B}{\beta} \tag{15}$$

$$AUC = \frac{D_{iv}}{Cl_s} \tag{16}$$

Area under the first moment curve (AUMC)

$$\text{AUMC} = \frac{A}{\alpha^2} + \frac{B}{\beta^2} \tag{17}$$

Mean residence time (MRT):

$$\text{MRT} = \frac{\text{AUMC}}{\text{AUC}} \tag{18}$$

Volume of distribution at steady state (V_{ss}):

$$V_{ss} = Cl_s \times \text{MRT} = \frac{D_{iv} \times \text{AUMC}}{\text{AUC}^2} \tag{19}$$

Volume of distribution during the terminal disposition phase (V_β):

$$V_\beta = \frac{Cl_s}{\beta} \tag{20}$$

Bioavailability (F) can be estimated when a drug is given by both intravenous and an extravascular route (e.g., orally, subcutaneously, intramuscularly) route using eq. (21).

$$F = \frac{D_{iv} \times \text{AUC}_{oral}}{D_{oral} \times \text{AUC}_{iv}} \tag{21}$$

In addition, bioavailability can be estimated as a structural parameter of a pharmacokinetic model with simultaneous fit of the oral and intravenous plasma concentrations. This approach was applied to data for 5-fluorouracil (5-FU) given intravenously and orally with the oral dihydropyrimidine dehydrogenase inhibitor eniluracil *(7)*. As demonstrated for carboxyamidotriazole (CAI), relative bioavailability can be estimated as a structural parameter with simultaneous fit of plasma concentrations achieved following different oral formulations *(8)*.

When fitting a model to the concentration–time data, the model should fit the data to some degree of precision and accuracy, demonstrate no bias, and follow the rule of parsimony *(9–12)*. Generally, a coefficient of variation of up to 50% for clearance and half-life is deemed acceptable for most compounds. A large coefficient of variation for pharmacokinetic parameters may be due to insufficient (e.g., not extensive enough) or improper (e.g., poor time selection) sampling schema. Bias is determined by the inspection of the residual plot and determining whether the model consistently over- or underpredicts the actual concentration. When choosing between several models, the rule of parsimony is followed in that the simplest model that can adequately describe the data should be chosen. A model is validated when it has been demonstrated that extrapolation (e.g., single-dose to multiple-dose or a change in the dose or infusion duration) is accurate and if study conditions are adjusted (e.g., renal function changes) that the model accommodates the changes and maintains the robustness. The limitations of compartmental modeling potentially include the inability of a drug to be described by a single model (e.g., a two-compartment model at lower doses vs a three-compartment model at higher doses) and the oversimplification of body processes (e.g., multiple false assumptions regarding drug distribution). Some of the limitations are due to (1) sampling limited to plasma; (2) variability in the pharmacokinetics between patients; (3) lack of sensitive analytical techniques; (4) drug–drug and drug–formulation vehicle interactions *(13)*. An advantage of compartmental analysis is that pharmacokinetic linearity is not assumed and can be incorporated into a model during any of the pharmacokinetic processes (e.g., drug absorption, distribution, metabolism, and elimination).

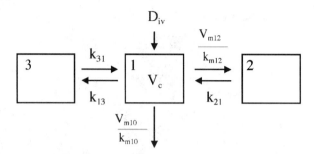

Fig. 3. Nonlinear three-compartment pharmacokinetic model that was fitted to docetaxel concentration-time profiles. (Modified from ref. *[15]*.)

5. NONLINEAR PHARMACOKINETIC MODELING

Nonlinear pharmacokinetic behavior can be a substantial source of variability in drug exposure and response. Linearity is evaluated by examining dose and time dependence. Dose dependence is assessed by normalizing plasma concentration–time profiles for dose and examining relationships between dose and exposure parameters such as maximum concentration (C_{max}), steady-state concentration (C_{ss}), and the area under the concentration–time curve (AUC). The average value for each exposure parameter is examined and a determination is made if they increase proportionally with increasing dose. Relationships between dose and clearance, half-life, and volume of distribution are also assessed.

Time dependence is evaluated when a drug is given by prolonged infusion or on multiple dosing schedules. During prolonged infusions, a change in C_{ss} over time suggests a change in drug clearance. With repetitive dosing schedules, an increase in pretreatment trough levels over time (in the absence of expected achievement of steady state based on the drugs half-life and dosing schedule) or a change in a pharmacokinetic parameter value suggests a change in drug clearance. For example, changes in AUC or half-life following the first and subsequent doses may suggest that clearance is changing with time.

If apparent nonlinearity is not felt to reflect the dosing schedule, assay sensitivity, or interpatient variability, sources for true nonlinearity should be evaluated. Sources for dose- or time-dependent pharmacokinetics following oral or intravenous administration may include saturable gut wall transport or first-pass hepatic metabolism, saturable plasma protein and tissue binding, concentration-dependent renal excretion, capacity-limited metabolism, and enzyme induction or inhibition *(14)*. In addition, formulation effects may affect the apparent nonlinear behavior of a drug *(13)*. Nonlinear pharmacokinetic models are employed to describe drug disposition. Figure 3 illustrates a three-compartment model that includes Michaelis–Menten saturable distribution into the second compartment and saturable elimination from the central compartment. This model was fit to docetaxel concentrations to explain an apparent nonlinear pharmacokinetic behavior of docetaxel administered at doses of 115 mg/m^2 *(15)*.

6. PARAMETER ESTIMATION AND MODEL ASSESSMENT

After the appropriate model has been identified (e.g., the model describes the concentration vs time data), pharmacokinetic parameters are calculated using pharmacokinetic modeling software (e.g., ADAPT II, WinNonlin, or other commercially available programs [http://www.boomer.org/pkin/soft.html]). The goodness of fit of the pharmacokinetic model is based on visual inspection of the observed and fitted concentration–time curve, minimization of the weighted sum of squares, examination of the dispersion of the weighted residuals, and inspection of the standard error, coefficients of variation (CV), and confidence intervals (CI) of each estimated pharmacokinetic parameters. In addition, discrimination between compartmental pharmacokinetic models is guided by minimization of the weighted least-squares, residuals, Akaike information criterion, Schwarz criteria, and the *F*-test *(9)*.

A main assumption made in pharmacokinetics is that the observations are independent and are measured with homoscedastic, random error. Because the error is normally heteroscedastic or evenly distributed, methods to correct the error are done with weighting and will normally correct the bias. Commonly used algorithms include the generalized least-squares regression, maximum likelihood, maximum *a posteriori* Bayesian (MAP-Bayesian), or weighted least-squares regression. The weighted least-squares regression approach finds the parameter values that will minimize the residuals. This can be accomplished with fixed variances of $1/y$ or $1/y^2$. The maximum likelihood approach determines the parameter values and variance parameters that most likely give rise to the observed value by maximizing this probability. The generalized least-squares regression is a combination of both the weighted least-squares regression and maximum likelihood approaches in a stepwise fashion. At first the variance parameters are fixed while the parameter values are optimized using weighted least-squares regression; then, the parameter values are fixed while the variance parameters are optimized using maximum likelihood; this stepwise approach occurs until the both the parameter values and variance parameters are stable. Finally, the MAP-Bayesian approach is used with sparse data sets or when there is large variance. MAP-Bayesian is a common approach in population pharmacokinetics. In this technique, the parameter values are determined by minimizing actual residuals for that patient and the difference between that patient's parameter values and the population's parameter values. Once the parameters are determined, one should verify that the true global minimum is found and not the local minimum. This is done by overestimating the parameters in the opposite direction from the initial parameter values and verifying that the same final parameter value is achieved upon convergence. For a more thorough review of the weighting techniques, please refer to refs. *(10–12)*.

The modeling of concentration–time profiles sometimes involves samples from sites other than or in addition to plasma. This may require the development of pharmacokinetic models that are more elaborate than standard compartmental pharmacokinetic models. A three-compartment open model that simultaneously described topotecan lactone and total concentrations in the plasma and cerebrospinal fluid has been described Fig. 4 *(16)*. However, one must always apply the rule of parsimony when distinguishing the model that best fits the data.

7. METABOLITE KINETICS

Many anticancer agents are extensively metabolized to inactive or active metabolites. Pharmacokinetic parameters for a drug metabolite are usually estimated using noncompartmental methods. The AUC ratio of metabolite to parent drug on a molar basis is then calculated to determine relative exposure of metabolite compared to parent compound. Pharmacokinetic parameters can also be estimated using compartmental models that describe the drug metabolite disposition. For example, the plasma disposition of temozolomide and its metabolites were characterized using a one-compartment linear model that had first-order absorption, first-order metabolite formation and elimination, and a peripheral distribution

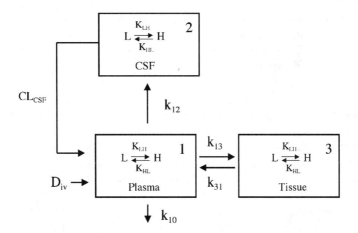

Fig. 4. Three-compartment model for topotecan lactone and total concentrations in the plasma and CSF. Cl_{CSF}, Clearance of drug from the cerebrospinal fluid (CSF); K_{LH} and K_{HL}, the forward and reverse rate constants for the lactone- to hydroxy-acid conversion, respectively. (Modified from ref. [16].)

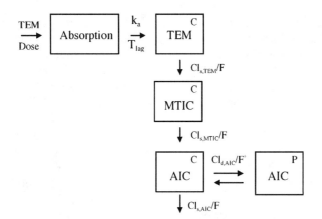

Fig. 5. Compartmental model for TEM, MTIC, and AIC concentrations in plasma. TEM, Temozolomide; MTIC, 5-(3-methyltriazen-1-yl)imidazole-4-carboxamide; AIC, 4-amino-5-imidazole-carboxamide; $Cl_{s,TEM}/F$, clearance for the conversion of TEM to MTIC; $Cl_{s,MTIC}/F$, clearance for the conversion of MTIC to AIC; $Cl_{s,AIC}/F$, AIC systemic clearance; $Cl_{d,AIC}/F$, AIC distribution clearance. (Modified from ref. [17].)

compartment for the metabolite, 4-amino-5-imidazole-carboxamide (Fig. 5) *(17)*. An alternative model for temozolomide has been described that incorporates clearance of parent drug via both chemical breakdown to 5-(3-methyltriazen-1-yl)imidazole-4-carboxamide and renal clearance *(18)*.

8. CONCLUSION

Pharmacokinetic modeling is a useful tool to be able to describe and predict concentration–time data. The sampling strategy is the most important first step to describing adequately the pharmacokinetics of a compound. If inadequate sampling occurs, various phenomena may be missed (e.g., a prolong elimination phase). Although noncompartmental analysis does provide a quick and easy determination of the pharmacokinetic parameters, it is based on the assumption that the pharmacokinetics is linear. This assumption can be remedied by analyzing the concentration–time profile with compartmental analysis. Various pharmacokinetic programs are commercially available that can aid in compartmental analysis of data. Compartmental analysis can involve a simple linear two-compartment model or more complicated models that incorporate nonlinear processes. As early clinical trials incorporate more pharmacokinetic and pharmacodynamic endpoints, the role of pharmacokinetic modeling will continue to grow.

REFERENCES

1. David O, Johnston A. Limited sampling strategies. Clin Pharmacokinet 2000; 39:311–3113.
2. van Kesteren C, Mathjt RA, Lopez-Lazaro L, et al, A comparison of limited sampling strategies for prediction of Ecteinascidin 743 clearance when administered as a 24-h infusion. Cancer Chemother Pharmacol 2001; 48:459–466.
3. McLeod HL, Graham MA, Aamdal S, Setanoians A, Groot Y, Lund B. Phase I pharmacokinetics and limited sampling strategies for the bioreductive alkylating drug EO9. EORTC Early Clinical Trials Group. Eur J Cancer 1996; 32A:1518–1522.
4. Noncompartmental Analysis Based on Statistical Moment Theory. In: Gibaldi M, Perrier D (eds). Pharmacokinetics, 2nd Edit., revised and expanded. New York, NY:Marcel Dekker 1982, pp. 409–417.
5. Appendix C: Methods of Residuals. In: Gibaldi M, Perrier D (eds). Pharmacokinetics, 2nd Edit., revised and expanded. New York, NY:Marcel Dekker 1982, pp. 433–444.
6. Pharmacokinetic concepts. In: Gabrielsson J, Weiner D (eds). Pharmacokinetic/Pharmacodynamic Data Analysis: Concepts and Applications, 2nd Edit., revised and expanded. Stockholm, Sweden: Apotekarsocieteten, 1997, pp. 58–171.
7. Baker SD, Khor SP, Adjei AA, et al. Pharmacokinetic, oral bioavailability, and safety study of fluorouracil in patients treated with 776C85, an inactivator of dihydropyrimidine dehydrogenase. J Clin Oncol 1996; 14:3085–3096.
8. Bauer KS, Kohn EC, Lush RM, et al. Pharmacokinetics and relative bioavailability of carboxyamidotriazole with respect to food and time of administration: use of a single model for simultaneous determination of changing parameters. J Pharmacokinet Biopharmacol 1998; 26:673–687.
9. Ludden TM, Beal SL, Sheiner LB. Comparison of the Akaike Information Criterion, the Schwarz criterion and the F test as guides to model selection. J Pharmacokinet Biopharmcol 1994; 22:431–445.
10. Peck CC, Beal SL, Sheiner LB, Nichols AI. Extended least squares nonlinear regression: a possible solution to the "choice of weights" problem in analysis of individual pharmacokinetic data. J Pharmacokinet Biopharm 1984; 12:545–558.
11. Sheiner LB. Analysis of pharmacokinetic data using parametric models—1: Regression models. J Pharmacokinet Biopharm 1984; 12:93–117.
12. Sheiner LB. Analysis of pharmacokinetic data using parametric models. II. Point estimates of an individual's parameters. J Pharmacokinet Biopharm 1985; 13:515–540.
13. Sparreboom A, van Zuylen L, Brouwer E, et al. Cremophor EL-mediated alteration of paclitaxel distribution in human blood: clinical pharmacokinetic implications. Cancer Res 1999; 59:1454–1457.
14. Jusko WJ. Pharmacokinetics of capacity-limited systems. J Clin Pharmacol 1989; 29:488–493.
15. McLeod HL, Kearns CM, Kuhn JG, et al. Evaluation of the linearity of docetaxel pharmacokinetics. Cancer Chemother Pharmacol 1998; 42:155–159.
16. Baker SD, Heideman RL, Crom WR, Kuttesch JF, Gajjar A, Stewart CF. Cerebrospinal fluid pharmacokinetics and penetration of continuous infusion topotecan in children with central nervous system tumors. Cancer Chemother Pharmacol 1996; 37:195–202.
17. Baker SD, Wirth M, Statkeveich P, et al. Absorption, metabolism, and excretion of 14C-temozolomide following oral administration to patients with advanced cancer. Clin Cancer Res 1999; 5:309–317.
18. Rudek MA, Donehower RC, Rowinsky EK, et al. Temozolomide in patients with advanced cancer: a phase I and pharmacokinetic study. Pharmacotherapy 2004; 24:16–25.

10   Pharmacodynamic Modeling

Kenneth S. Bauer, Pharm D, PhD
and William P. Petros, Pharm D, FCCP

CONTENTS

1. INTRODUCTION

Pharmacodynamics is the relationship between drug concentrations and pharmacologic response. Drug concentrations used for pharmacodynamic analysis are typically plasma or serum; however, analytes may be measured at other sites such as cerebrospinal fluid, ascitic fluid, or another easily accessible tissue or fluid. While pharmacokinetic modeling enables prediction of plasma drug concentrations following dose administration, application of a pharmacodynamic model alone or in combination with a pharmacokinetic model enables determination of drug response at a specified concentration, or at any time after the administered dose. With this knowledge we can determine the optimal dosage regimen of the drug to be given to a specific patient or patient population.

The pharmacodynamic study of anticancer agents is beset with several pitfalls and hurdles making the analysis more difficult. Among these is the fact that often these drugs have a very narrow or nonexistent therapeutic index, defined as the ratio of the concentration causing severe toxicity to the concentration at which the drug exhibits the desired pharmacological effect. Anticancer agents typically cause severe toxicities prior to reaching the concentration that would yield the desired effect of complete remission or "cure." In addition, the desired effect of tumor cell kill is often not easily measured and is delayed. Novel therapies targeting tumor angiogenesis, invasion, metastases, or signal transduction present the additional challenge that they are not necessarily meant to kill the tumor cell directly but alter the biologic process enabling tumor survival. Thus, contemporary studies of these agents frequently employ pharmacologic biomarkers or surrogate endpoints to assess pharmacodynamics. Finally, one of the goals of anticancer drug pharmacody-

Handbook of Anticancer Pharmacokinetics and Pharmacodynamics
Edited by: W. D. Figg and H. L. McLeod © Humana Press Inc., Totowa, NJ

namic modeling is to optimize the dose such that maximal benefit can be obtained with minimal toxicity. Currently drugs used to treat cancer are most often dosed on mass basis, either by mg, mg/kg, or mg/m^2 dose. Clearly this is not the safest and most effective way to dose cancer therapies. Clinical investigation of anticancer agents has shown that pharmacokinetically guided dosing (1–4) as well as pharmacodynamically guided dosing (5) are feasible strategies. These methods would represent an improvement if they were clinically possible and cost effective. Thus, guiding the regimen of an anticancer agent based on its individual pharmacodynamic parameters would represent the most efficient means to dose these therapies (6).

2. DETERMINANTS OF PHARMACODYNAMIC EFFECTS

The endpoints for pharmacodynamic assessments are typically determined by what is suspected to be the drug's primary target for effect. Broad classifications include receptor binding, alteration of enzymes and proteins, membrane interactions, and transport blockade. Target identification will allow for speculation as to the immediacy and duration of response. For example, if a drug is known to stimulate an α-adrenergic receptor, one may anticipate an immediate effect, but one that may display altered response over continuous exposure time. Tachyphylaxis and hypersensitivity reactions are good examples of time-dependent pharmacodynamic effects. Perhaps the most difficult to evaluate are chronic pharmacodynamic effects of cancer therapy. Examples of such chronic effects include delayed growth effects, impaired learning, cardiac toxicity, and secondary malignancies.

It is important to realize that pathophysiologic factors may also influence the pharmacodynamic effect in an individual patient. For instance, a person who has been previously exposed to multiple cycles of myelosuppressive chemotherapy is likely to experience a greater effect from subsequent myelosuppressive agents owing to depleted bone marrow reserves.

3. CLINICAL SETTINGS

Human pharmacodynamic modeling is most commonly conducted during clinical Phase I trials. The reasons for this are twofold: first, this is the most common setting to have extensive pharmacokinetic data and second, a wide range of doses is typically explored in Phase I. The doses administered in Phase I studies typically vary from ones not exerting any measurable biologic effect to those producing intolerable toxicity, thus providing a broad range of dose or systemic exposure vs response profile. If a relationship exists, it should be evident with such a strategy; however, this is not an optimal approach to validate associations between systemic exposure and outcome. The reason for this is because there is almost always a direct correlation between dose and systemic exposure, thus, associations of the latter term with pharmacodynamic measures may simply be a reflection of the dose–effect relationship. The optimal setting for evaluation of a correlation between systemic exposure and a pharmacodynamic parameter would be in situations in which the dose is fixed for all patients (or normalized to body size), for example, Phase II and III trials. Despite this issue, pharmacokinetic–pharmacodynamic associations are important in many contemporary Phase I studies, as surrogate markers may be used as the sole determinant of dose selection for Phase II studies. Later phase studies will typically evaluate relationships between targets demonstrating usefulness on earlier studies with tumor response and/or survival.

4. SAMPLING/MEASUREMENT ISSUES

Pharmacokinetic studies are typically designed with rigor to ensure adequate evaluation of patient-specific parameters such as systemic exposure. Such detail is not as exquisitely expressed with many pharmacodynamic endpoints; thus, their accuracy is not as well controlled. The reasons for this vary from lack of attention for adequate evaluation of such variability to dealing with logistical issues. A good example is modeling of pharmacokinetic data with the pharmacodynamic endpoint of chemotherapy-induced myelosuppression. Routine clinical practice would entail monitoring the white blood cell count (WBC) on approximately a weekly basis for many drugs; however, to establish a good association between the nadir WBC and chemotherapy systemic exposure one may need to monitor the WBC several times a week.

Routine laboratory tests conducted by accredited clinical laboratories have sufficient quality control such that their data could be utilized in pharmacodynamic studies. Tests being conducted for research purposes on pharmacodynamic endpoints may not have sufficiently stringent controls or tight test measurement variability to conduct pharmacodynamic modeling, either because of inexperience of the type of the laboratory conducting the testing or the nature of the test itself.

Key to the success of a pharmacodynamic model is the accurate assessment of effect. This is best accomplished if the measure of effect is made at the effect site. These measures can safely be performed for many diseases. For example, a pharmacodynamic study of a proton pump inhibitor may include direct measures of gastric pH by the placement of a nasogastric tube for sample collection of gastric fluids at appropriate time points. However, for the assessment of antitumor effect for patients with solid tumors, the risk of tumor biopsy often outweighs the benefit. Although bone marrow biopsy is more easily performed than a solid tumor biopsy, serial samples are typically not obtained. In addition, to perform a robust pharmacodynamic study, repeated measurements would be necessary. This is not an option either in patients with solid malignancies or in those with leukemias. Thus, the clinical pharmacologist must rely on surrogate measurements for pharmacologic response in patient plasma or circulating white blood cells. Changes in transcription or protein expression can be measured in peripheral lymphocytes, but do changes in normal circulating cells reflect the pharmacology at the tumor site? Preclinical correlative studies are required to validate these types of studies. In tumor xenograft models the pharmacologist can measure changes in proteins and/or messenger RNA at the tumor site and in the circulating lymphocytes simultaneously with plasma concentration determination. If properly controlled, these preclinical studies can identify the most appropriate surrogate biomarker for clinical pharmacodynamic studies.

5. PHARMACODYNAMIC MEASURES OF INTEREST

If the ultimate goal of pharmacodynamic study is to optimize the drug regimen, then the primary markers of effect representing this endpoint for anticancer agents would be absolute tumor burden. However, because this is a very difficult, if not impossible, measurement to make we are left using categorical measures of toxicity and response, easily obtainable continuous measures for toxicity, or surrogate markers and biomarkers for effect. The type of data obtained from the effect measures may be continuous, scalar, categorical, or discrete/binomial variables. The type of variable plays a major role in the choice of pharmacodynamic model that can be used. Thus, for any anticancer agent being studied the investigator must determine the best choice of endpoint to be measured based on sampling feasibility, fluid or anatomic site of sample acquisition, availability of resources for measurement determination, and cost, and, finally, how well it relates with actual clinical response.

The typically used categorical measures for toxicity are complete response (CR), partial response (PR), stable disease (SD), and progressive disease (PD). An additional parameter of minor response (MR) is also used on occasion. Clinical toxicity is a scalar

Table 1
Examples of Cytotoxic Chemotherapeutic Agents
and Reported Pharmacodynamic Measures

Drug	Pharmacodynamic measure	Reference
Carboplatin	Thrombocytopenia,	(7)
	leukopenia	(8)
Doxorubicin	Neutropenia	(9)
Etoposide	Leucopenia, neutropenia	(10)
Fluorouracil	Leucopenia, mucosytis	(11)
Ifosfamide	Neurotoxicity (orientational disorder)	(12)
Paclitaxel	Neutropenia, peripheral neuropathy	(13)
Topotecan	Neutropenia	(14)

variable with a value of 1–5 based on a predetermined grading scheme such as the National Cancer Institute (NCI) common toxicity criteria. Measures of toxicity often utilize hematological toxicity as a simple measure, while surrogate biomarkers must take into account the mechanism of action of the agent. As previously mentioned, one of the challenges in the study of pharmacodynamics of cancer therapy is the delayed measurable effect of decreased tumor burden (i.e., tumor shrinkage) or measurable toxicity (decreased blood cell counts). For classical cytotoxic chemotherapies, several relatively noninvasive easily measured indices have been established (Table 1). However, novel therapies targeting specific signal transduction pathways or cellular and molecular processes will require more complex measures to determine the early effects of the drug in the clinical setting. Because many of these new drugs are not directly cytotoxic and target aberrant cellular processes and pathways, they may not exhibit the hematologic toxicity seen with the classical cancer chemotherapies. Thus, identifying an easily obtainable marker for effect may present more of a challenge (Table 2). For agents targeting tumor angiogenesis, markers of angiogenic signaling might be measured in the plasma, in urine, or in biopsy tissues if available. For agents targeting specific signaling pathways a downstream protein or event might be measured in lymphocytes, skin, or tumor tissue. One approach currently under development for monitoring agents that are designed to stimulate apoptosis uses a radiolabeled annexin V product. Annexin V has been shown to bind to phosphatidylserine, an intracellular membrane-associated protein. During apoptosis phosphatidylserine is expressed on the external cell membrane. By labeling annexin V with a radioimaging agent such as ^{99}Tc, the rate of apoptosis can be measured (20). This approach may allow for quick, noninvasive, direct measures of tumor response in patients with a number of solid tumors. This technology could lead to the ideal pharmacodynamic marker, a means to determine directly tumor burden in real time. In addition to the mechanism of action of the agent providing the means for determining a biomarker, the disease itself may also produce a specific biomarker for tumor burden. In the cases of prostate cancer, and ovarian cancer, the biomarkers prostate-specific antigen (PSA) and CA-125 are commonly used as clinical markers for disease progression and can also be used as pharmacodynamic measures for drug response.

Once the optimal endpoint for the agent has been selected, practical issues involving the clinical setting and sampling issues are then addressed to fit the model appropriately to the data.

Table 2
Examples of Investigational Agents and Pharmacodynamic Measures Assessed

Drug	Pharmacodynamic measure	Reference
Antiangiogenesis agents		
Carboxyamido-triazole	Serum VEGF, serum bFGF	(4)
Col-3	Plasma MMP-2, plasma MMP-9, plasma VEGF	(15)
SU5416	Urine VEGF, urine bFGF	(16)
Signal transduction		
BAY 37-9751	Phosphorylated ERK1 and ERK2 (in lymphocytes)	(17)
R115777	Farnesyl protein transferase activity (bone marrow)	(18)
ZD1839 (iressa)	Activated EGFR, activated MAPK (skin biopsy)	(19)

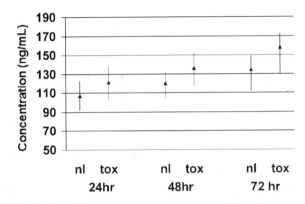

Fig. 1. Example of a pharmacodynamic segregation analysis. Patients were given a potentially nephrotoxic chemotherapeutic agent by continuous infusion over 3 d. Renal toxicity was assessed as a change from baseline. Daily, steady-state concentrations were segregated into groups based on the presence (tox) or absence (nl) of postexposure nephrotoxicity.

6. MODELING

Most clinical pharmacodynamic studies of anticancer therapies approach data analysis in a nonmodeling fashion. One typical approach utilizes segregation of patients by response, then statistical comparison of the difference in mean or median systemic exposure values (Fig. 1). Initial evaluation of an effect often can most efficiently be conducted by investigation of pharmacokinetics in groups with the largest differences in outcomes. For instance, it may be easier to see differences in the pharmacokinetics of a potential hepatotoxin when the assessed population contains groups of patients with either no hepatic toxicity or exorbitant toxicity compared to a population of patients with all degrees of toxicity. Obviously, later studies will need to determine the feasibility of identifying patients who will subsequently have only mild toxicity compared to morbid effects.

Given the limited nature of the Phase I study and the discontinuity of some of the pharmacodynamic measures the statistical approach may be the only practical method of pharmacodynamic assessment. Comparisons between pharmacologic response value and and drug concentration can be modeled using a cumulative linear logistic (logit) model.

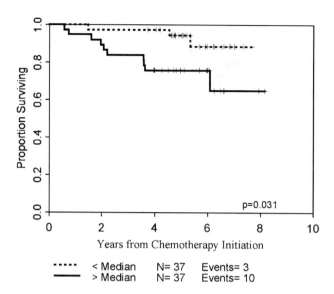

Fig. 2. Example of a pharmacokinetic segregation analysis. Kaplan–Meier survival analysis of patients who were segregated based on the median population systemic exposure to a prodrug (lower values = more exposure to active moiety).

For pharmacological response parameters described best by a binary function (i.e., Response [+] or No response [–]) a simple logit model or a Wilcoxin Rank Sum analysis may be the most appropriate methods to assess differences in response. A cumulative logit model analysis might be performed to assess the association between level of clinical response and pharmacologic response parameter. The ordinal data parameters of treatment response categorized as CR, PR, SD, and PD as previously defined would be used for this analysis. Similarly, a cumulative logit model might be used to assess the effect of plasma concentrations on the ordinal parameters of toxicity grade (NCI grade I–IV). If the toxicity data are better described by a binary function, the simple logit model can be used to assess the toxicity as a function of change pharmacologic parameter. If the data are continuous, a comparison of two or more groups using the paired t-test or analysis of variance (ANOVA) might be used assuming the data meet the criteria for parametric testing. An alternative method places patients into discrete groups based on their degree of systemic exposure (e.g., median value), then compares any difference in the pharmacodynamic response amplitude or duration between the groups (Fig. 2).

Determination of an appropriate approach to model an association with systemic exposure and pharmacodynamics is often initially conceived by the outcome measures and the mechanistic basis for the effect. Situations in which one has multiple response outcomes for one patient (e.g., daily change in gene expression based on changes in drug concentration) may lend themselves to evaluation of each patient's data set via a standard, two-stage approach. It is typical in oncology studies to have just one pharmacodynamic outcome for each patient, for example, survival. In the latter setting the approach would be to evaluate patients in a single-stage approach, that is, group all the systemic exposure, survival data points into one file and evaluate at the same time.

Selection of the model is often based on the mechanistic relationship expected. Many models used in oncology are based on receptor occupancy (Fig. 3). In these situations one

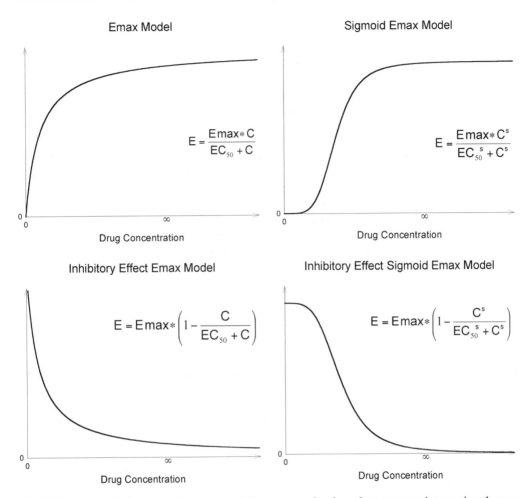

Fig. 3. Examples of pharmacodynamic modeling approaches based on receptor interaction theory.

expects no observable effect until a minimal exposure is achieved, followed by a nonlinear increase in effect, a linear portion of the curve, and finally a maximization of the effect, above which no significant increase in response is noted.

Despite the difficulties with pharmacodynamic measures for cancer therapy the Hill equation (Eq. 1) *(21)*, and the many variations thereof such as the Sigmoid E_{max} model, has been used to describe the pharmacodynamic relationship for many oncologic drugs:

$$E = \frac{E_{max} \times C^s}{EC_{50}^s + C^s} \qquad (1)$$

where E is the effect response, E_{max} is the maximum effect response, C is a measure of drug exposure/concentration, EC_{50} is the concentration/exposure producing one-half the maximum effect, and s is the Hill constant.

These relationships can take the form of direct or indirect response models and can relate various drug exposure parameters such as discrete concentration at the time of the response (C), maximum concentration (C_{max}), and area under the concentration–time curve (AUC) to the actual pharmacologic response. Pharmaologic response entails changes in circulating plasma proteins involved in tumor growth and metastases [e.g., vascular endothelial growth factor (VEGF), matrix metallo proteinase 2 (MMP-2)], toxicity measurements (absolute neutrophil count [ANC], nerve conduction parameters), radiologic response, or clinical response.

Another feasible method employs comparisons between pharmacologic response value and drug concentrations obtained from the various dose or exposure groups using a regression analysis to assess validity of a putative correlative marker.

Later phase evaluation of pharmacokinetic–pharmacodynamic effects may employ sparse pharmacokinetic sampling approaches. These could entail utilization of Bayesian algorithms or traditional population-based models such as those employed by NONMEM. Several contemporary, large studies have utilized this strategy to identify potentially important physiologic markers that are associated with interpatient variability in pharmacokinetics. The typical approach is to follow up this type of analysis with a study that then validates the relationships using traditional, full assessments of pharmacokinetics and pharmacodynamics.

7. IMPLEMENTATION AND ASSESSMENT

Attention to pharmacokinetic methods is vital to ensure that the parameters selected to evaluate relationships between pharmacokinetics and pharmacodynamics are adequately described. Typical parameters utilized in oncology studies include systemic exposure (AUC), maximal concentration, minimal concentration (for multidose), and concentration above a target value (especially for cycle-specific drugs). Preclinical data (both animal and cell culture) can often be useful to assist in determination of the optimal parameter. Most sample schemas will be adequately constructed to enable estimation of AUC; however, accurate determination of time above a target concentration mandates a degree of attention to terminal curve sampling.

A variety of pharmacokinetic programs are also utilized to conduct pharmacodynamic modeling. Many programs (e.g., WinNonlin, Pharsight, Inc.) have embedded the standard receptor-based equations in their model libraries. Pharmacodynamic measurements are often conducted based on changes from a baseline value. The latter can be affected by diurnal changes, day-to-day variability, and a variety of other factors. It is generally a good practice to obtain at least two baseline values for pharmacodynamic evaluations that involve continuous data. Initial model selection also involves determination whether the model will be based on a direct or an inverse (inhibitory) effect. Assessment of models is statistically based on approaches similar to those used in pharmacokinetic analyses.

Although it is relatively easy to identify relationships between pharmacokinetics and pharmacodynamics, the strength of the association is often not sufficient to justify utilization of the data for establishment of a therapeutic target.

8. DATA INTERPRETATION

Arguably, one of the most appropriate techniques for assessment of a model's utility is the evaluation of bias and precision *(22)*. The bias can be easily be calculated as the mean prediction error (me) (Eq. 2) and the precision measured as the root mean squared predicition error (rmse) (Eq. 3). Knowledge of these data will enable accurate assessment of how relevant the model will be for prospective clinical use.

$$me = \frac{1}{N} \sum_{i=1}^{N} pe_i \qquad (2)$$

$$rmse = \sqrt{\frac{1}{N} \sum_{i=1}^{N} pe_i^2} \tag{3}$$

where pe is the error of the predicted value.

Establishment of a relationship between pharmacokinetics and pharmacodynamics is typically used to justify investigation of therapeutic drug monitoring. Simply establishing the link does not mean that individualization of doses can be conducted feasibly and accurately.

Data may also be utilized to determine the optimal schedule of administration and provide clues toward the biologic mechanism of action. For example, if the time of plasma exposure experienced above a potentially cytotoxic concentration correlates to response better than the maximal observed concentration, then this would suggest a cycle-dependent mechanism. A prolonged exposure regimen may be preferred for future studies based on these data.

9. SUMMARY

Pharmacodynamic modeling of anticancer agents presents a unique set of challenges from measurement to model building. However, diligence has proven that appropriate models can be produced to predict accurately the pharmacologic effects of these drugs at given drug exposures and times. The real challenge remaining is the development of simple and cost-effective means to use these models to individualize cancer therapies for maximum benefit and minimal toxicity.

REFERENCES

1. Figg WD, Stevens JA, Cooper MR. Adaptive control with feedback of suramin using intermittent infusions. J Clin Oncol 1994; 12:1523–1524.
2. Lowis SP, Price L, Pearson AD, Newell DR, Cole M. A study of the feasibility and accuracy of pharmacokinetically guided etoposide dosing in children. Br J Cancer 1998; 77:2318–2323.
3. Ghazal-Aswad S, Tilby MJ, Lind M, et al. Pharmacokinetically guided dose escalation of carboplatin in epithelial ovarian cancer: effect on drug-plasma AUC and peripheral blood drug-DNA adduct levels. Ann Oncol 1999; 10:329–334.
4. Bauer KS, Figg WD, Hamilton JM, et al. A pharmacokinetically guided Phase II study of carboxyamido-triazole in androgen-independent prostate cancer. Clin Cancer Res 1999; 5:2324–2329.
5. Ratain MJ, Mick R, Janisch L, et al. Individualized dosing of amonafide based on a pharmacodynamic model incorporating acetylator phenotype and gender. Pharmacogenetics 1996; 6:93–101.
6. Burke GA, Estlin EJ, Lowis SP. The role of pharmacokinetic and pharmacodynamic studies in the planning of protocols for the treatment of childhood cancer. Cancer Treat Rev 1999; 25:13–27.
7. Egorin MJ, Van Echo DA, Tipping SJ, et al. Pharmacokinetics and dosage reduction of cis-diammine(1,1-cyclobutanedicarboxylato) platinum in patients with impaired renal function. Cancer Res 1984; 44:5432–5438.
8. Newell DR, Siddik ZH, Gumbrell LA, et al. Plasma free platinum pharmacokinetics in patients treated with high dose carboplatin. Eur J Cancer Clin Oncol 1987; 23:1399–1405.
9. Minami H, Ohtsu T, Fujii H, et al. Phase I study of intravenous PSC-833 and doxorubicin: reversal of multidrug resistance. Jpn J Cancer Res 2001; 92:220–230.
10. Ratain MJ, Schilsky RL, Choi KE, et al. Adaptive control of etoposide administration: impact of interpatient pharmacodynamic variability. Clin Pharmacol Ther 1989; 45:226–233.
11. Vokes EE, Mick R, Kies MS, et al. Pharmacodynamics of fluorouracil-based induction chemotherapy in advanced head and neck cancer. J Clin Oncol 1996; 14:1663–1671.
12. Kerbusch T, de Kraker J, Keizer HJ, et al. Clinical pharmacokinetics and pharmacodynamics of ifosfamide and its metabolites. Clin Pharmacokinet 2001; 40:41–62.
13. Gianni L, Kearns CM, Giani A, et al. Nonlinear pharmacokinetics and metabolism of paclitaxel and its pharmacokinetic/pharmacodynamic relationships in humans. J Clin Oncol 1995; 13:180–190.

14. Stewart CF, Baker SD, Heideman RL, Jones D, Crom WR, Pratt CB. Clinical pharmacodynamics of continuous infusion topotecan in children: systemic exposure predicts hematologic toxicity. J Clin Oncol 1994; 12:1946–1954.

15. Cianfrocca M, Cooley TP, Lee JY, et al. Matrix metalloproteinase inhibitor COL-3 in the treatment of AIDS-related Kaposi's sarcoma: a phase I AIDS malignancy consortium study. J Clin Oncol 2002; 20:153–159.

16. Stopeck A, Sheldon M, Vahedian M, Cropp G, Gosalia R, Hannah A. Results of a Phase I dose-escalating study of the antiangiogenic agent, SU5416, in patients with advanced malignancies. Clin Cancer Res 2002; 8:2798–2805.

17. Chow S, Patel H, Hedley DW. Measurement of MAP kinase activation by flow cytometry using phospho-specific antibodies to MEK and ERK: potential for pharmacodynamic monitoring of signal transduction inhibitors. Cytometry 2001; 46:72–78.

18. Karp JE, Lancet JE, Kaufmann SH, et al. Clinical and biologic activity of the farnesyltransferase inhibitor R115777 in adults with refractory and relapsed acute leukemias: a phase 1 clinical-laboratory correlative trial. Blood 2001; 97:3361–3369.

19. Baselga J, Rischin D, Ranson M, et al. Phase I safety, pharmacokinetic, and pharmacodynamic trial of ZD1839, a selective oral epidermal growth factor receptor tyrosine kinase inhibitor, in patients with five selected solid tumor types. J Clin Oncol 2002; 20:4292–4302.

20. Belhocine T, Steinmetz N, Hustinx R, et al. Increased uptake of the apoptosis-imaging agent (99m)Tc recombinant human Annexin V in human tumors after one course of chemotherapy as a predictor of tumor response and patient prognosis. Clin Cancer Res 2002; 8:2766–2774.

21. Wagner JG. Kinetics of pharmacologic response I. Proposed relationships between response and drug concentration in the intact animal and man. J Theoret Biol 1968; 20:173–201.

22. Sheiner LB, Beal SL. Some suggestions for measuring predictive performance. J Pharmacokinet Biopharm 1981; 4:503.

11 Pharmacometric Knowledge-Based Oncology Drug Development

Paul J. Williams, Pharm D, MS, FCCP,
James A. Uchizono, Pharm D, PhD,
and Ene I. Ette, Pharm D, PhD, FCP, FCCP

Contents

1. INTRODUCTION

Drug development and clinical trial structure functions most efficiently when based on pharmacometric (PM) knowledge. PM knowledge comes from outstanding data, and when it is interpreted in light of development goals and other knowledge, then an understanding is gained of the direction that future development ought to take. In the current drug development climate volumes of data are generated but little emphasis is placed on knowledge generation and therefore the direction that drug development should take is ambiguous. Poor decision-making is supported by the fact that the cost of introducing a drug to market in 2001 was $802 million and the time for a drug to reach market was 7–12 yr with the execution of more than 60 clinical trials *(1,2)*. The process of knowledge discovery when applied to PM model development ensures that information embedded in the data is thoroughly understood and apporopriately applied *(3)*. Modern data analysis methods and modern statistical software such as S-Plus® have revolutionized the manner in which PM analyses can be performed.

Handbook of Anticancer Pharmacokinetics and Pharmacodynamics
Edited by: W. D. Figg and H. L. McLeod © Humana Press Inc., Totowa, NJ

2. PM KNOWLEDGE DISCOVERY (PHARKNOWDISC)

PM knowledge is best extracted from data when the knowledge discovery process is applied to its generation. Knowledge discovery has been defined as the search for relationships and global patterns that exist in large data sets but are "hidden" among the vast amounts of data *(4)*. PM modeling, especially population PM modeling, is itself a process of knowledge discovery from the population PM data set. When applied to PM modeling, knowledge discovery incorporates all steps taken from data assembly to the development of the PM model to the reporting of the results.

Knowledge discovery exists at the intersection of computer science (database, artificial intelligence, graphics, and visualization), statistics, and several application domains such as clinical pharmacology in general and PM in particular. Some modern graphical and statistical procedures useful in PHARKNOWDISC include histograms with density plots, pairs plots, multiple linear regression (MLR), generalized additive modeling (GAM), box plots, nonparametric smooth plots, and tree models *(5,6)*. Knowledge discovery from a large PM data set is a process that can be formalized into a number of steps *(3)*. In brief, these steps are as follows:

1. Defining or stating the objective of the PHARKNOWDISC process.
2. Creating a data set on which PHARKNOWDISC will be performed. (Data preparation is a very critical in the PHARKNOWDISC. Sometimes more effort can be expended in preparing data than in analysis.)
3. Data quality analysis (i.e., cleaning and processing the data *(7–9)*.
4. Data structure analysis, exploratory examination of raw data (dose, exposure, response, and covariates) for hidden structure, and the reduction of the dimensionality of the covariate vector.
5. Determining the basic PM model that best describes the data and generating *post hoc* empiric individual Bayesian parameter estimates.
6. Searching for patterns and relationships between parameters and covariates through graphical displays and visualization.
7. Exploratory modeling using modern statistical modeling techniques such as MLR, GAM *(5,6)*, cluster analysis, and tree-based modeling (TBM) to reveal structure in the data and initially select explanatory covariates.
8. Consolidating the discovered knowledge in item 7 into an irreducible form, that is, developing a population pharmacokinetic/pharmacodynamic model, using the nonlinear mixed effects modeling approach.
9. Determining model robustness through sensitivity analysis, examination of parametric/ nonparametric standard errors, stability checking with or without predictive performance depending on the objective of the PHARKNOWDISC.
10. Interpreting the results: the PHARKNOWDISC process prescribes that the model developed is interpreted in a relational manner. That is, do the findings of the PHARKNOWDISC make sense in the domain in which they will be used? Can the results be communicated in a manner that they can be used? Only if they make sense can the results be considered as "knowledge" (which is viewed pragmatically here).
11. Applying (or utilizing) the discovered knowledge. The pragmatic view of knowledge implies that the results of the PHARKNOWDISC process must have some impact on the way individuals act. Thus, the discovered knowledge must be applied to demonstrate how it can be used.
12. Communicating the discovered knowledge.

The PM knowledge discovery process must be focused. Having a clearly defined objective for the process greatly influences the remainder of the steps. For instance, the choice of data set(s) to be used in the PM knowledge discovery process is determined by the objective that prompts the process.

3. LEARN: CONFIRM–LEARN APPROACH TO DRUG DEVELOPMENT

The drug development process is governed by one's philosophy of the process, which in turn will affect one's attitude and approach to both the macro-strategy and any individual study. A very useful and promising philosophy of drug development has been described by Sheiner *(10)*, termed the learn–confirm approach. Sheiner contends that drug development ought to consist of alternating elements of learning from experience and then confirming what has been learned. One ought always to be interested in learning, even when confirming is the primary objective of a study; therefore, we have modified the terminology slightly by naming the second phase confirm–learn.

The earliest parts of the process of clinical drug development ought to emphasize learning but later stages will, by their nature, emphasize the confirm–learn type of study and analysis. Thus, learning and confirming become a part of each clinical trial although their relative emphasis changes as the drug progresses toward approval. Although learning and confirming can be performed to varying degrees on the same data set, their goals are quite different. Clinical trial structures that optimize confirming often impair learning. The focus of commercial drug development on confirmation is understandable, as this immediately precedes and justifies regulatory approval. However, the focus on confirming has led to a low level of learning that has in turn resulted in drug development that is most often inefficient and inadequate.

Learning has as its objective answering many questions such as the relationship among dose, prognostic variables, and outcome. Learning is often model based and focuses on building a model between outcome and many variables such as dosing strategy, exposure, patient type, and prognostic variables. The model that is built here is the defining of the response surface. The response surface can be thought of as three-dimensional. On one axis are the input variables (controllable factors) such as dosage regimen and concurrent therapies. Another axis incorporates patient characteristics, which summarizes all the important ways patients can differ that affect the benefit to toxicity ratio. The final axis represents the benefit to toxicity ratio. Sheiner has stated, "... the real surface is neither static, nor is all information about a patient conveyed by his initial prognostic status, nor are exact predictions possible. A realistically useful response ... must include the elements of variability, uncertainty and time ..." *(10)*. The response surface deals with a complex of relationships to answer the question of what is the relationship between input profile and dose magnitude to beneficial and harmful pharmacological effects and how does this relationship vary with individual patient characteristics and time to explain tolerance or sensitivity? For rational drug development and the optimization of individual therapy, this response surface must be mapped for the target population. These models then allow extrapolation beyond the immediate study subjects to predict the effects of competing dosing strategies, patient type selection, competing study structures, and endpoints; they therefore aid in the construction of future studies. One important feature of model-based learning is that models increase the signal-to-noise ratio because they can translate some of the noise in a data set to signal. This is important because the information content of a data set is proportional to the signal-to-noise ratio. For the learning study, which attempts to define the dose–concentration–effect model, pharmacokinetics (PK) delineates the dose–concentration component and pharmacodynamics (PD) defines the concentration–effect component of the model.

In contrast, the goal of confirming is to falsify the hypothesis that efficacy is absent and the only question that it aims to answer is, Is the null hypothesis true or false? Therefore, factors that increase learning such as administering differing dose levels and enrolling subjects who differ with regard to demographics and disease state are often eliminated from confirming studies. Confirming studies proceed by contrasting the average outcomes between two study groups.

4. PHARMACOMETRICS

Pharmacometrics (PM) has been defined as the science of developing and applying mathematical and statistical methods to characterize, understand, and predict a drug's pharmacokinetic and pharmacodynamic behavior; quantify uncertainty of information about that behavior; and rationalize knowledge-driven decision-making in the drug development process. PM is dependent on knowledge discovery; the application of informative graphics; and an understanding of biomarkers/surrogate endpoints. When applied to drug development, PM often involves the development or estimation of pharmacokinetic, pharmacodynamic, pharmacodynamic-outcomes linking, and disease progression models. These models can be linked and applied to competing study designs to aid in understanding the impact of varying dosing strategies, patient selection criteria, different study endpoints, varying study structure, and so forth on the final study results.

4.1. Pharmacokinetics

Pharmacokinetics (PK) is the estimation and development of mathematical models that describe the time course of drug and metabolite levels in various regions of a subject's body as a function of some drug input function, most often route and dose. PK models can be characterized as compartmental, noncompartmental, linear, and nonlinear. PK models are often described with figures illustrating the location of each compartment, as a geometric shape, and drug movement between compartments represented by arrows. Most models are parametrized in terms of clearances, apparent volumes, and rate constants; other models may not be founded on compartments; and still others may be physiologically based. Once data are assembled, the PK modeler determines which model best describes the data, which may involve the determination of the number of compartments that should be applied to the model or whether the model follows dose-dependent PK. These models can then be used to estimate the expected drug levels that would be the result of competing dosing strategies. PK models have their greatest utility when they are employed in conjunction with pharmacodynamic models. Figure 1 shows a diagrammatic example of a pharmacokinetic model.

4.2. Pharmacodynamics

Pharmacodynamic (PD) models are mathematical representations of the relationship between either the drug input function (dose and route) or the measured drug concentration and time, and some response variable (biomarker or surrogate) such as granulocyte count or tumor load. When selecting a PD model one must address:

1. What shape is the drug level–response relationship?
2. What are the response kinetics?
   a. How long does the response take to develop (i.e., reach steady state for a given drug input/concentration); Is the PD effect immediate, delayed, or cumulative?
   b. How long does the response last after the drug is discontinued?
3. Should the response be related to drug dose or concentration?

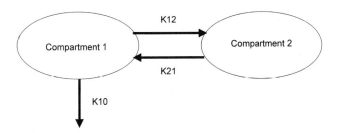

Fig. 1. A diagrammatic example of a two-compartment pharmacokinetic model.

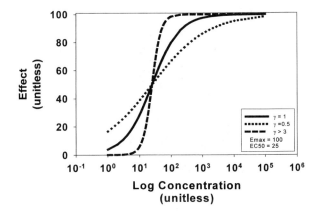

Fig. 2. Concentration (level) vs effect for a simple E_{max} model.

4. Which mathematical description best describes the relationship between the input function and the response variable?
5. Should the PD model be derived from known underlying mechanisms of action or estimated by empirical functions?
6. Are there time-varying (circadian) or state-varying (tolerance, induction) factors that affect the response?
7. Does the baseline effect need to be included in the model?

Commonly employed time-invariant PD models include the linear model (Eq. 1), the simple E_{max} model (Eq. 2), and the sigmoid E_{max} model (Hill equation, Eq. 3). More recently, indirect pharmacologic response models *(11–13)* have been popular for modeling state- or time-varying pharmacologic responses. For the E_{max} and Hill equation, E_{max} represents the maximum possible effect. That is, as the drug level approaches infinity, the effect asymptotically approaches E_{max}. EC_{50} is the drug level at which 50% of E_{max} is observed and is a measure of the sensitivity to the drug. The lower the EC_{50} the more sensitive the system. Figure 2 presents a plot of the level vs effect for this type of model.

$$\text{Effect} = \text{Constant} \times \text{conc.} \tag{1}$$

$$\text{Effect} = \frac{E_{max} \times \text{conc.}}{EC_{50} + \text{conc.}} \tag{2}$$

A modification of the simple E_{max} model is the sigmoid E_{max} model, which is sometimes referred to as the Hill equation. This model adds an exponential component to the drug level

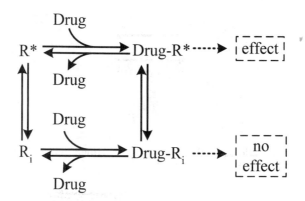

Fig. 3. The four-state receptor desensitization model. R^* and R_i are the receptors in the active and inactive states, respectively. Drug can bind to either the active or inactive form of the receptor. Drug-R^* and Drug-R_i are drug-bound–receptor complexes in the active and inactive forms, respectively. Drug bound to the active receptor causes the measured effect, and drug bound to the inactive receptor leads to no effect.

and the EC_{50} (Eq. 3). Figure 3 shows the shape of a model where the EC_{50} is 25, E_{max} is 100, and gamma (the exponential) is 3.5.

The sigmoid E_{max} (Hill equation) model is

$$\text{Effect} = \frac{E_{max} \times \text{conc.}^{\gamma}}{EC_{50}^{\gamma} + \text{conc.}^{\gamma}} \qquad (3)$$

Careful consideration must be given when selecting a PD model. Although the above approaches to modeling PD responses are appealing, real-life pharmacology is more complex than described by formulas. Additional factors that must be considered in the model are tolerance effects, placebo effects, circadian rhythms, and drug interactions (12–14).

In time-invariant or stationary PD systems, a one-to-one correspondence exists between drug level at the effect site (C_e) and the effect (E). Often drug effects can be adequately described by time-invariant PK/PD, however, there are many drug effects that cannot. Frequently, drugs used in the treatment of cancers fall into this category of state- or time-varying PD. State-varying PD refers to PD parameters that change as an explicit function of the state of another aspect of the system/cascade (e.g., amount of enzyme, receptor, precursor, cofactor, or transporter such as multidrug resistance [MDR, P-glycoprotein]), which means that the observed effect is not simply the result of drug concentration, but rather some combination of the drug concentration and one or more of these states). Typical examples of state-varying PK/PD include drug tolerance, drug resistance, and enzyme induction or inhibition. Time-varying PK/PD, chrono-PK/PD, simply refers to PK/PD parameters that change as an explicit function of time (e.g., baseline effect or drug metabolism changes as a function of circadian rhythms or cell cycle). Because circadian rhythms and cell-cycle changes are presumably related to underlying changes in a state or states of the system, they could be referred to as state-varying as well. State-varying changes are directly linked to drug action, whereas the states of time-varying systems are primarily driven by genetic or internal biological clocking mechanisms. Although some drugs can alter a system's internal biological clock, a discussion of this topic is beyond the scope of this chapter.

Although extensive literature exists describing the occurrence of drug tolerance, the literature contains significantly fewer references describing its quantitative time course

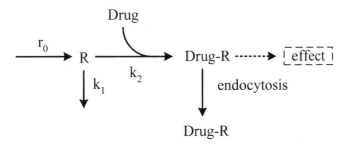

Fig. 4. The receptor down-regulation model. Drug binds to R, unbound cell surface receptor, and initiates the effect or a cascade leading to the effect. Down-regulation occurs when the drug-R complex is endocytosed into the cell.

(development [onset] and recovery [offset] kinetics). Drug tolerance is a reversible decrease in drug effect in the presence of constant drug level. The timely reversible aspect of drug tolerance distinguishes it from drug resistance. Reversible decreased effect means that within the normal time frame of therapy the effect returns toward the drug-naïve state on cessation of drug input, whereas drug resistance, for example multidrug resistance (MDR), is usually the result of genetically driven alterations to the cells that are more permanent relative to the duration of therapy. Although systems experiencing drug resistance may ultimately return to the naïve state, the length of time to do so generally makes dosing regimens based on these kinetics impractical and clinically irrelevant.

4.3. Drug Tolerance Models

The mathematical distinctions between various models provide insight into differentiating between underlying mechanisms of tolerance. For example, some models of tolerance are restricted to identical onset and recovery rates *(12)*, while others allow asymmetrical onset and recovery rates *(16,18,20,27)*. In this chapter, we present five general tolerance models. For a more complete comparison of current models, the reader is directed to Gardmark et al. *(21)*.

The first model is known as receptor desensitization *(14,20,22)*. This model, which has great modeling diversity, was first developed 1957 by Katz and Thessleff. Figure 3 shows the four different states of the drug receptor: (1) active with no drug bound, (2) active with drug bound, (3) desensitized with no drug bound, and (4) desensitized with drug bound. Although this model is capable of describing the kinetics of various tolerance mechanisms, pragmatically, its modeling robustness is tempered by its mathematical complexity *(20)*.

The second model is the receptor down-regulation model *(24,25)*. In this model, drug action is often initiated by the binding of drug to a cell surface receptor (see Fig. 4). On binding with cell surface receptors, the drug–receptor complexes are endocytosed into the cell, leaving fewer total receptors on the cell surface, thus leading to decreased sensitivity to the drug. Mathematically, this model can be expressed as

$$\frac{d[\text{R}]}{dt} = r_0 - \left(k_1 + k_2 [\text{drug}]\right)[\text{R}] \tag{4}$$

where R is the receptor, r_0 is the zero-order rate constant describing production, k_1 is a first-order rate constant describing constitutive receptor removal, and k_2 is the second-order rate constant describing receptor loss due to endocytosis-mediated down-regulation. In this model, the receptor concentration moves between two different steady-states $[\text{R}]_{ss(1)}$ = r_0 / k_1 and $[\text{R}]_{ss(2)} = r_0 / (k_1 + k_2 [\text{drug}])$, corresponding to the naïve state and tolerant state,

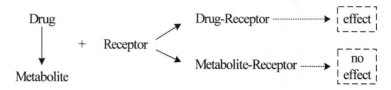

Fig. 5. Antagonistic activity model. In this model, the drug is converted to a metabolite that can also bind to the receptor. The drug–receptor complex produces an effect and the metabolite–receptor complex does not produce an effect. As more of the receptors are filled with metabolite, the extent of drug tolerance becomes greater.

respectively. Because [drug] $\geq$ 0, two constraints of this model are apparent: (1) the rate of tolerance development ($k_1 + k_2$ [drug]) will always be greater than the rate of recovery k_1; and (2) this model is asymmetrical with respect to tolerance development and recovery.

The third model (Fig. 5), which is mathematically a subset of the receptor desensitization model, is tolerance due to antagonistic activity. The antagonistic activity can be caused by one or more of the following: (1) one or more metabolites of the parent drug; (2) one or more metabolites of another drug, or even another drug, being used concomitantly; and (3) the production of some factor that leads to a decrease in the receptor binding affinity or the total amount of receptor protein. The antagonism can be competitive and/or non-competitive. This model requires symmetry between the onset and offset of tolerance, which is its most prominent constraint. The following two equations show competitive and noncompetitive antagonistic inhibition tolerance:

$$\text{Effect} = \frac{E_{max} C_e}{C_{50}\left(\dfrac{T_{50} + T}{T_{50}}\right) + C_e} \tag{5}$$

$$\text{Effect} = \frac{E_{max}\left(\dfrac{T_{50}}{T_{50} + T}\right) C_e}{C_{50} + C_e} \tag{6}$$

where E_{max} is the asymptotic maximal effect, C_e is the drug concentration at the effect site, C_{50} is the drug concentration leading to 50% of E_{max} in the absence of tolerance, T is the amount of tolerance, and T_{50} quantifies the relationship between C_e at steady-state and T.

A fourth model of tolerance (see Fig. 6) is embodied in the indirect PD response models proposed by Jusko *(16,17,19)*, specifically models I and IV, according to their nomenclature. Their four models are based upon the premise that "a measured response (R) to a drug may be produced by indirect mechanisms" *(16)*. The following two modified equations show the four possible models:

$$\frac{dR}{dt} = k_m V\left(S_{1..n}, t\right) - k_{out} R \tag{7}$$

$$\frac{dR}{dt} = k_m - k_{out} W\left(S_{1..n}, t\right) R \tag{8}$$

The functions $V(S_{1..n}, t)$ and $W(S_{1..n}, t)$ can be stimulatory or inhibitory, depending on the specific drug response. Only two of these four models describes drug tolerance: when V is inhibitory (model I) and/or W is stimulatory (model IV). Model 1 corresponds to a drug-

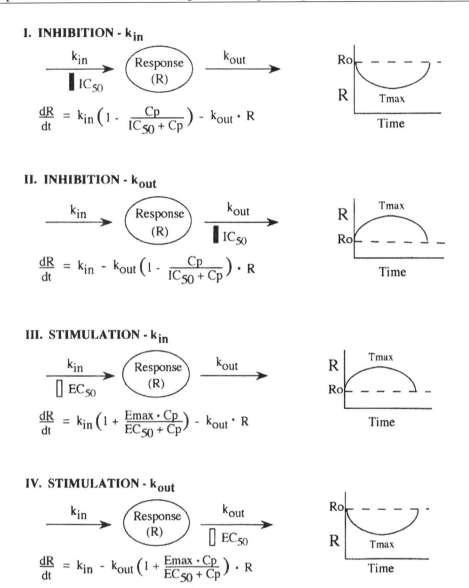

I. INHIBITION - k_{in}

$$\frac{dR}{dt} = k_{in}\left(1 - \frac{Cp}{IC_{50} + Cp}\right) - k_{out} \cdot R$$

II. INHIBITION - k_{out}

$$\frac{dR}{dt} = k_{in} - k_{out}\left(1 - \frac{Cp}{IC_{50} + Cp}\right) \cdot R$$

III. STIMULATION - k_{in}

$$\frac{dR}{dt} = k_{in}\left(1 + \frac{Emax \cdot Cp}{EC_{50} + Cp}\right) - k_{out} \cdot R$$

IV. STIMULATION - k_{out}

$$\frac{dR}{dt} = k_{in} - k_{out}\left(1 + \frac{Emax \cdot Cp}{EC_{50} + Cp}\right) \cdot R$$

Fig. 6. The four fundamental types of pharmacodynamic indirect response models.

related loss of a precursor necessary for the measured effect, while model IV corresponds to a system where the drug causes an increased removal rate of receptor, similar to the down-regulation model. This model has been used to model leukopenia secondary to cancer chemotherapy.

The fifth model of tolerance (Fig. 7) involves variations of an adaptive systems approach *(26,27)*, which is familiar to the engineering discipline. Despite some major differences between competing systems approach models, the primary assumption made in all models is that the body seeks to maintain homeostasis and drugs disturb that homeostasis or trigger counterregulatory mechanisms. Mandema and Wada proposed an elegant tolerance model

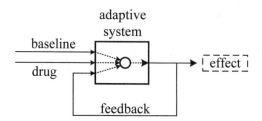

Fig. 7. Adaptive systems tolerance model. In this model, the baseline, disturbance (drug) and the output (effect) feedback combine together to produce an overall effect. In a simple model, the drug input would cause an increase in effect and the feedback input would cause a decrease in effect, thereby negating the drug's effect and causing drug tolerance.

based on physiological changes, both molecular and cellular *(27)*. Although their model is quite sophisticated, it appears to be the only model that can account for within-systems and between-systems adaptation and should have applicability for MDR models in the future.

When modeling drug tolerance, one of the above five general models should be sufficient to describe the kinetic onset and offset of tolerance. When choosing a tolerance model, one should ask several questions: (1) Is the pharmacological mechanism known for the drug being studied? (2) Is the rate of tolerance development and recovery symmetrical or asymmetrical with respect to time? (3) Does the drug of interest really undergo pharmacological tolerance or are the data simply the result of a tissue distribution artifact or PK sampling artifact? (4) Will an empirical model, not based on a specific mechanism, be sufficient for the intended purpose(s)? The answers to these questions will guide the choice of an appropriate drug-tolerance model.

Finally, two PK phenomena that can confound the interpretation of drug-tolerance data are (1) when the body establishes a steady state relationship between C_p and C_e more quickly than the establishment of a steady state between the site of drug administration and drug sampling site; and (2) when the drug causes an increase in its own clearance by inducing the enzyme responsible for the drug's metabolism, known as enzyme autoinduction.

5. OUTCOMES MODELS

An outcomes model relates some input function, biomarker, or surrogate endpoint (dose, drug serum concentration, tumor load, or lymphocyte count, MDR) to a terminal subject effect such as cure or no cure, improved vs worsened, survival, or disease progression. Outcomes models can be time to event models such as Kaplan–Meier curves for which hazard functions can be estimated. There are several hazard functions such as Weibull functions and Gompertz models that are differential equations that when integrated link the PD biomarker to the outcome in a time-dependent manner. Discrete outcomes can also be modeled as logistic regression or discriminant function models where the biomarker at some exact moment in time is related to an outcome. The disease progression model has recently been shown to be useful in relating drug administration to outcomes *(28)*. Other models that should be considered are disease tolerance models that can be applied to such outcomes as tumor or viral load.

MDR has a profound impact on outcomes because it is a major variable related to the failure of cancer chemotherapy. Recently, the presence of MDR-associated protein (MRP) was identified in resistant small-cell lung cancer cell lines. Several proteins have been associated with drug resistance including P-glycoprotein (Pgp) overexpression, p110 major vault protein, enzymes in the glutathione metabolic pathways, and DNA topoisomerases. The most common mechanism of MDR is the overexpression of Pgp and this is present in cancers with intrinsic resistance such as colon, renal, and pancreatic cancers. Pgp causes MDR by increasing the removal of chemotherapeutic agents from cancer cells. Drugs are being developed to inhibit the activity of Pgp. In the future it will be necessary to develop outcomes models that take into account the mechanism of MDR and the effect of those agents that counter the mechanisms of MDR and thus sensitize the cancer to drug.

Although outcomes models are important, they are less often available for use or application than are PK or PD models and therefore their development is one of the greatest areas of need in PM.

6. POPULATION MODELS

Population modeling is the study of sources and correlates of variability of dependent variables (drug concentration or biomarkers) among individuals who are the target patient population receiving clinically relevant doses of a drug of interest. Therefore, covariates such as demographic variables (size or gender) are related to either PK or PD parameters such as clearance or E_{max}. As with other models, typical values for subjects are estimated, but most significantly with population models the between- and within-subject random effects are also estimated. Three approaches to estimating population models have been described. In recent years population models have become popular because of their broad applicability to drug development *(7,29,30)* and a guidance on population pharmacokinetics has been issued by the Food and Drug Administration.

In the standard two-stage approach, one first estimates the individual model parameters for each subject *(7,31,32)*. To implement this approach several observations per subject (usually eight or more) must be obtained and the individual parameters of the model estimated in the first of the two stages. In the second stage, the population parameters are estimated as the mean of all the individual parameters; the dependencies of the parameters on covariates can also be estimated by standard statistical approaches such as regression and in the final step the between-subject variability is estimated. When this approach is taken, the typical population parameter estimates are usually without bias; however, the variance and covariance parameters are inflated *(31)*. The global two-stage approach has been proposed to improve the two-stage approach through bias correction for the random effects (covariance) and differential weighting of individual data according to the data's quality and quantity *(32)*.

The naïve pooled data (NPD) approach is simple and is executed by pooling all the data across individuals to estimate the population parameters *(33,34)*. This approach does not yield a characterization of the between-individual variability and therefore its ability to project the range of expected outcomes is limited. Although the NPD has worked well for population PK model estimation, it has not been valid for the E_{max} PD model because it does not account for the fact that different patients have different EC_{50}s and for the sigmoid E_{max} PD model, the estimate of γ is low *(35,36)*.

The nonlinear mixed effects modeling approach has great utility for population model estimation *(7,29,31,32)*. The nonlinear mixed-effects approach to population modeling can be used to obtain typical parameter estimates, between-subject variability, and unexplained residual variability, and relate PM parameters to covariates. It has great value when only sparse data have been or can be obtained, as for many pediatric studies, and the standard two-stage approach cannot be used because individual parameter estimates cannot be estimated directly. However, maximum *a posteriori* Bayesian (MAP Bayesian) estimates of individual subjects parameters can be generated from this approach. The nonlinear mixed effects approach was developed from the recognition that if PM models were to be developed in populations of investigated patients, practical considerations dictate that data should be collected under conditions that are not as restrictive as traditional study designs. This approach considers the study group as the unit of analysis rather than the individual and it functions even when data are sparse, fragmentary, and unbalanced. This approach has been used successfully to estimate PK, PD, and outcomes models of many different types. A general scheme for the implementation of this approach was presented Fig. 1 and explained, in detail, in the knowledge discovery section, Subheading 2 *(3)*.

Valid PM models developed from the nonlinear mixed-effects approach are especially useful for extrapolation to help understand the results of various competing study strategies. With these types of models the expected range of results of competing dosing strategies, differing patient populations, duration of study, and so forth can be investigated by Monte Carlo simulations.

7. THE ROLE OF REAL-TIME MODELING

For drug development there is always pressure to complete the process as expeditiously as possible. Real-time data collection and modeling can aid in lessening the time for drug development so that downstream segments can be impacted by the knowledge discovered from the PM models. Real-time data analysis and model development results in expeditious knowledge discovery, and can help identify potential problems in the analysis at an early stage of data collection *(7,8,37)*.

8. THE NECESSITY OF PLANNING

The complexities of drug development and the pivotal role of PM models point to the importance of planning *(7,8,37)*. Both a macro-plan for the entire drug development process and a micro-plan for individual projects or studies must be in place. The macro-plan identifies (1) important questions that need to be answered, (2) the application and intended use of the PM model, (3) which covariates need to be studied, and (4) and possible drug–drug interaction.

Micro-planning at the level of the individual project or study must also take place. Plans must be in place for data management, data collection, quality assurance of the data, and staff training for data collection. A plan for data analysis and model validation must also be in place.

9. THE USE OF SIMULATION

Monte Carlo simulation is a technique that is useful for the construction of clinical trials in the drug development process *(38)*. Recent advances in computational performance, the appearance of new simulation software targeting clinical trials, and improved methods for estimating PM models have streamlined the execution of Monte Carlo simulations. Monte Carlo simulation provides an excellent avenue for application of the developed PM models. Simulation of clinical trials provides a means of evaluation of the impact of various dosing strategies, various compliance patterns, patient selection strategies, competing trial structures, competing outcomes measures, and competing statistical methods with all stochastic elements in the trial execution model on power, informativeness, efficiency, and robustness of a clinical trial. One large pharmaceutical company has reported that the early integration of PM models via simulation resulted in development time-savings, regulatory concurrence, and a perceived value that outweighed costs *(39)*.

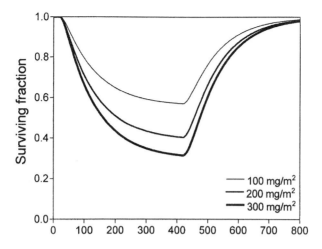

Fig. 8. Model projected time course of leukocyte survival after different doses of paclitaxel.

For a simulation, three types of models are defined: the covariate model, the input–output model, and the execution model. The covariate model creates simulated individuals after defining the distribution of variables such as age, gender, weight, renal function, and so forth. The input–output models are the main place where the PM models enter into the simulation process. Here the trial structure (refer to the following section), PK, PD, and outcomes models are defined in terms of both their typical parameter values and the variability of the parameters and also the residual random variability of the model. The execution model for a simulation deals with patient and practitioner behaviors during the execution of the trial, describing dropouts, compliance, and missing samples.

Simulation provides a powerful tool for evaluating a broad range of assumptions and clinical trial structures on the eventual power, efficiency, informativeness, and robustness or any proposed study.

10. DOSE RANGING TRIALS

For most therapeutic categories, dose-ranging studies have as their objective identifying a dose that is effective while avoiding toxicity or adverse effects. In contrast, for cancer chemotherapeutic agents dosing is limited by the maximum tolerated dose (MTD), because, for these agents, toxic and therapeutic effects cannot be separated by a dosing strategy. Targeting the MTD as the optimal dose in humans has implications for the dose ranging study. For efficiency it would be best if the initial dose in humans could begin at the highest yet safe dose with escalation occurring as rapidly as safety concerns will allow.

First time in man (FTIM) studies and early clinical studies are targeted at identifying the MTD, single- and multiple-dose pharmacokinetics, and gender plus food effects on drug disposition *(40–45)*. As such, these studies are initial attempts at dose ranging. Initially these FTIM studies require allometric scaling from animals to humans. Historically, this scaling has been on a mg/m^2 basis, but this can be improved on because of substantial interspecies differences in drug disposition and metabolism; and a stronger relationship between concentration and drug effect has been demonstrated when compared to dose alone. For example, it has been demonstrated that the MTD/LD$_{10}$ ratio ranged from 0.1 to 6, whereas the AUCMTD/LAUC$_{10}$ ranged from 0.1 to 3.3, where LD$_{10}$ is the lethal dose at

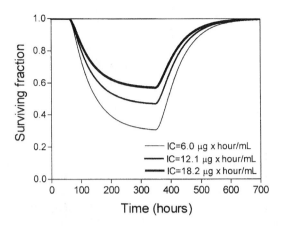

Fig. 9. Model based predictions of time course of leukocyte survival at different assumptions of IC (the AUC at which 50% of maximum effect occurs).

which 10% of the animals died, AUCMTD is the area under the concentration–time curve at the maximum tolerated dose for humans, and $LAUC_{10}$ is the AUC at which 10% of the animals died. When the highest and lowest extremes were eliminated from the data, it was demonstrated that the MTD/LD_{10} ratio ranged from 0.4 to 5, whereas the AUCMTD/ $LAUC_{10}$ ranged from 0.6 to 1.3 (36). Therefore, an exposure expressed as a function of concentration and time (e.g., the area under the concentration–time plot [AUC]) greatly improves on dose.

Early human trials for cancer chemotherapeutic agents have often been lengthy. The time taken to complete these trials is the number of dose escalations times the duration of each cycle. The typical drug here requires 12 cycles and 2 mo at each cycle; thus, 2 yr can be spent in this early clinical development stage. Collins et al. (40) have stated, "The primary disadvantages of these lengthy trials are readily appreciated. Not only are the trials very resource intensive, but most of the patients receive doses with no potential for biological activity. Consequently, these studies are discouraging to both the investigator and the patient."

Collins et al. (40) have proposed that murine and human biological effects occur at similar concentrations. Their proposed approach is based on exposure as a function of AUC rather than straight dose and is as follows:

1. Assume the murine $LAUC_{10}$ = human AUCMTD.
2. Determine the murine LD_{10} (current routinely done in toxicology protocols).
3. Determine the murine AUC at LD_{10}; this is the murine $LAUC_{10}$.
4. Begin human testing at a safe starting dose (1/10th the LD_{10}). This must be done because at the beginning of the FTIM study the pharmacokinetics in man are not yet known.
5. Estimate the AUC and pharmacokinetics at the starting dose in humans; this is routinely done for FTIM studies.
6. Set out an escalation strategy based on the initial AUC in humans and the target AUC, which in this case is the murine $LAUC_{10}$.

The above approach was applied to eight drugs. For four of the eight drugs, 2–12 cycles (average = 8 cycles) were eliminated, resulting in 4–24 mo time savings (average = 16 mo) in development while in no case was the time devoted to development increased. These studies not only result in time savings, but also fewer subjects are enrolled to complete early development. Thus there is a positive direct and indirect impact on expenditures.

Finally, delivery schedules must be considered when approaching early clinical development. There are some toxicities that are dependent on the maximum concentration (C_{max}) achieved during a dosing cycle. If a toxicity is C_{max} dependent, then a strategy must be laid out that takes this into account. It may be that a prolonged or continuous infusion could result in the desired AUC exposure and therefore efficacy while not exceeding the threshold C_{max} that would result in toxicity.

11. APPLYING PM MODELS

As PM knowledge is generated the intended use of the model must be kept in mind because the intended use of a model will influence the attitude and modeling approaches used by the pharmacometrician at the various stages of the modeling process. The intended use will determine what covariates are considered important and which parameters are of primary concern.

Models can be applied in several ways. Typical or average parameter estimates from models can be used to estimate typical values for dependent variables such as serum drug concentrations, typical exposures; typical biomarker effects such as tumor load or granulocyte count; or PK parameters such as area under the concentration–time curve. Issues that could be addressed with this type of model would be:

1. What would be the typical concentration–time profile for several different dosing approaches or for different types of patients?
2. What would be the typical biomarker as a function of patient type or differing dosing strategies?
3. What would be the expected concentration–time area under the curve for a capsule to be swallowed vs a buccal preparation design to avoid first-pass metabolism?

To estimate these types of variables from the model one simply applies the typical model parameters (clearance, apparent volume, etc.) and then inserts the missing elements such as dose and/or time to estimate the typical dependent variable.

Models characterized by only typical values and applications estimating only average outcomes lack broad applicability and result in suboptimal understanding of the variable being studied (e.g., dose). Models containing random effects in addition to typical values have broader applications when compared to the models without random effects. These are the population models mentioned previously that contain typical values, between-subject random effects, and residual random effects. With these models not only can the typical result be projected but also the range of expected outcomes. These projections require not only models but also the implementation of Monte Carlo simulations (38). Simulations can be implemented in any of a number of software programs such as the Pharsight Trial Simulator® or the NONMEM program with the simulation subroutine. These are implemented by supplying the software with the typical PM model values along with the random effects. In the end, a vector of concentrations or biomarkers' outcomes is generated, and at each time point these could be ranked as the 10th, median, and 90th percentile concentrations observed. Therefore rather than estimate the typical concentration as a function of dose, one could go further and suggest a dosing strategy, then estimate the typical concentration, the 90th percentile concentration, and the 10th percentile concentration and even plot these as a function of time after dose.

A powerful use of PM models is their application for evaluation of the structure and strategy of confirming clinical drug trials. The PK, PD, and outcomes links models can be applied to understand the implications of various dosing strategies, patient compliance, patient population selection, dropout rates, duration of the study, and so forth on the power, robustness, efficiency, and informativeness of the trial. One may be interested in a strategy with four dosing levels for a pivotal confirming study. We would now wish to address the effect on power that would occur by adopting such a strategy. Adopting four levels of dosing has the advantage of adding a learning element to the confirming study. This may be valuable as one would not like the dose to be lowered after the drug has already entered the marketplace, and studying several levels of dosing ought to result in choosing an optimal dose. If the lower dose is equally effective as the higher dose, then it would be chosen as the standard of care. If the lower dose is less effective than the high dose, the administration of the low dose would be unethical, as the documentation of the inappropriateness of the lower dose has occurred. In the simulation one would specify in the software program the typical and random effects for the PK, PD, and linking parameters; an execution model would be employed by specifying the number of subject, patient compliance, dropout rates, duration of the study, and so forth; and finally a covariate model (distribution of gender, weights, etc.) would be specified. Power would then be calculated by determining how often the treatment was superior to the placebo after running 200 simulations. That is, if for these simulations the drug effect was greater than the placebo effect in 192 of the 200 simulations, then the power was estimated to be 0.96.

The cost of drug development has continued to escalate and is currently very high with no prospect of decreasing. PM offers an opportunity for knowledge-based drug development by developing models and applying them to clinical trial construction via Monte Carlo simulation. Application of knowledge-based PM models will result in powerful, efficient, informative, and robust clinical trials.

11.1. An Example of PM Model Application

Bruno et al. *(46)* have provided an example of population pharmacokinetic (PPK) model application to clinical oncology drug development. The study was done in patients with non-small-cell cancer. In this example PPK was prospectively integrated into the clinical development of docetaxel. The integration was done so that exposure to the drug could be estimated and related to clinical outcome and adverse events. A PPK model was estimated from data obtained in 24 Phase II studies and MAP-Bayesian estimates of drug clearance and exposure were obtained for each subject.

Once the clearance and exposure was estimated for each subject, several PK parameters were estimated for each subject. A high AUC was noted to be a significant predictor of clinical response (time to progression [TTP]), where patients with the higher exposures had a prolonged TTP even after adjustment for other covariates. AUC was also noted to be a predictor of febrile and grade 4 neutropenia. However, the most significant predictor of febrile neutropenia was clearance, so that a 50% decrease in the clearance (CL) increased the odds by threefold.

It was noted further that patients with liver disease had a 27% lower CL than subjects without liver disease. This fact, combined with the association of low CL with febrile neutropenia, motivated a further analysis. Of the 1366 patients in the entire clinical database, 54 were noted to have elevated liver function tests. These 54 patients were further documented to have a threefold increase in the incidence of febrile neutropenia when compared with patients who had normal liver function tests.

The results of the PM analysis influenced the European Summary of Product Characteristics. On the basis of the PM analysis, a 25% decrease in dosing was recommended. Interestingly, in the US package insert there is no downward adjustment in this patient subgroup, but rather a complete avoidance is recommended in patients with liver function tests > 1.5 times the upper limit of normal. In contrast, the European guideline recommends that "Dosage should be reduced in hepatic impairment and hepatic function should be monitored." The docetaxel PM model development and application showed how the identification of subgroup differences led to a further analysis that when interpreted in light of the PPK model resulted in dosage modification in a subgroup. These findings were carried forward and recommended to the regulatory authorities. Thus, the analysis and application of these results impacted the safety, efficacy, and drug labeling.

12. SUMMARY

Drug development has become unacceptably costly both in terms of money and in time expended. Most of the expenditures (both time and money) are applied to clinical development. It has been reported that increasing the approval rate from 21% to 25% and the efficiency of drug development by 19% would decrease the cost from $802 million to $560 million for each drug entering the marketplace (1). One important tool that will aid in decreasing the cost of development is changing from empirical boiler plate development to knowledge-based development. Without thoroughly applying PM, knowledge-driven drug development is not possible. The essential elements of PM have been presented so that they can be applied to knowledge-driven drug development in the oncology drug therapeutic arena or any therapeutic class in general.

REFERENCES

1. Tufts Center for the Study of Drug Development. Press release November 30, 2001.
2. Peck CC. Drug development: improving the process. Food Drug Law J 1997; 52:163–167.
3. Ette EI, Williams PJ, Sun H, et al. The process of knowledge discovery from large pharmacokinetic data sets. J Clin Pharmacol 2001; 41:25–34.
4. Fayyad U, Piatetsky-Shapiro G, Smyth P. From data mining to knowledge discovery: an overview. In: Fayyad U, Piatetsky-Shapiro G, Smyth P, Uthursamy R (eds). Advances in Knowledge Discovery and Data Mining, Menlo Park, CA: AIII Press/MIT Press, 1996, pp. 1–34.
5. Ette EI, Ludden TM. Population pharmacokinetic modeling: the importance of informative graphics. Pharmaceut Res 1995; 12:1845–1855.
6. Ette EI. Statistical graphics in pharmacokinetics and pharmacodynamics: a tutorial. Ann Pharmacother 1998; 32:818–828.
7. Guidance for Industry: Population Pharmacokinetics. Rockville, MD: US Food and Drug Administration, Department of Health and Human Services, 1999.
8. Grasela TH, Antal EJ, Fiedler-Kelley J, et al. An automated drug concentration screening and quality assurance program for clinical trials. Drug Inform J 1999; 33:273–279.
9. Williams PJ, Ette EI. The role of population pharmacokinetics in drug development in light of the food and drug administration's 'Guidance for Industry: Population Pharmacokinetics.' Clin Pharmcokinet 2001; 39:385–395.
10. Sheiner LB. Learning versus confirming in clinical drug development. Clin Pharmacol Ther 1997; 61:275–291.
11. Holford NH, Sheiner LB. Understanding the dose–effect relationship: clinical application of pharmacokinetic-pharmacodynamic models. Clin Pharmacokinet 1981; 6:429–453.
12. Porchet HC, Benowitz NL, Sheiner LB. Pharmacodynamic model of tolerance: application to nicotine. J Pharmacol Exp Ther 1988; 244:231–236.
13. Derendorf H, Mollman H, Hochhaus G, Meibohm B, Barth J. Clinical PK/PD modeling as a tool in drug development of cortecosteroids. Int J Clin Pharmacol Ther 1997; 35:481–488.
14. Katz B, Thesleff S. A study of the 'desensitization' produced by acetylcholine at motor end-plate. J Physiol 1957; 138:63–80.
15. Williams PJ, Lane JR, Turkel C, Capparelli EV, Dzewanowska Z, Fox A. Dichloroacetate: population pharmacokinetics with a pharmacodynamic sequential link model. J Clin Pharmacol 2001; 41:259–267.

16. Dyneka NL, Garg V, Jusko WJ. Comparison of four basic models of indirect pharmacodynamic responses. J Pharmacokinet Biopharm 1993; 21:457–478.
17. Jusko WJ, Ko HC. Physiologic indirect response models characterize diverse types of pharmacodynamic effects. Clin Pharmacol Ther 1994; 56:406–419.
18. Rang HP, Ritter JM. On the mechanism of desensitization at cholinergic receptors. Mol Pharmacol 1970; 6:357–382.
19. Sharma A, Ebling WF, Jusko WJ. Precursor-dependent indirect pharmacodynamic response model for tolerance and rebound phenomena. J Pharmaceut Sci 1998; 87:1577–1584.
20. Segel LA, Goldbeter A, Devreotes PN, Knox BE. A mechanism for exact sensory adaptation based on receptor modification. J Theor Biol 1986; 120:151–179.
21. Gardmark ML, Brynne L, Hammarlund-Udenaes M, Karlsson MO. Interchangeability and predictive performance of empirical tolerance models. Clin Pharmacokinet 1999; 36:145–167.
22. Weiland G, Georgia B, Lappi S, Chignell CF, Taylor P. Kinetics of agonist-mediated transitions in state of the cholinergic receptor. J Biologic Chem 1977; 252:7648–7656.
23. Riccobene TA, Omann GM, Linderman JJ. Modeling activation and desensitization of g-protein coupled receptors provides insight into ligand efficacy. J Theor Biol 1999; 200:207–222.
24. Kenakin TP, Beek D. Measurement of antagonist affinity for purine receptors of drugs producing concomitant phosphodiesterase blockade: the use of pharmacologic resultant analysis. J Pharmacol Exp Ther 1987; 243:482–486.
25. Licko V. Drugs, receptors and tolerance. In: Barnett G, Chary CN (eds). Pharmacokinetics and Pharmacodynamics of Psychoactive Drugs. Foster City, CA: Biomedical Publications, 1985, pp. 311–322.
26. Veng-Pedersen P, Modi NB. A system approach to pharmacodynamics. Input–effect control system analysis of central nervous system effect of alfentanil. J Pharmaceut Sci 1993; 82:266–272.
27. Mandema JW, Wada DR. Pharmacodynamic model for acute tolerance development to electroencephalographic effects of alfentanil in rat. J Pharmacol Exp Ther 1995; 275:1185–1194.
28. Holford NHG, Peace KE. Results and validation of a population pharmacodynamic model for cognitive effects in Alzheimer patients with tacrine. Proc Natl Acad Sci USA 1992; 89:11471–11475.
29. Sheiner LB, Rosenberg B, Marathe V. Estimation of population characteristics of pharmacokinetic parameters from routine clinical data. J Pharmacokinet Biopharm 1977; 5:445–479.
30. Mandema JW, Verotta D, Sheiner LB. Building population pharmacokinetic pharmacodynamic models. J Pharmacokinet Biopharm 1992; 20:511–528.
31. Sheiner LB, Beal SL. Evaluation of methods for estimating population pharmacokinetic parameters. J Clin Pharmacokinet 1980; 9:635–651.
32. Steimer JL, Mallet A, Golmard JL. Alternative approaches to the estimation of population pharmacokinetic parameters: comparison with the nonlinear mixed effects model. Drug Metab Rev 1984; 15:265–292.
33. Egan TD, Lemmens HJ, Fiset P, et al. The pharmacokinetics of a new short-acting opioid remifentanil (G187084B) in healthy adult male volunteers. Anesthesiol 1993; 79:881–892.
34. Kataria BK, Ved SA, Nicodemus HF, et al. The Pharmacokinetics of propofol in children using three different analysis approaches. Anesthesiology 1994; 80:104–122.
35. Sheiner LB, Beal SL, Sambol NC. Study designs for dose-ranging. Clin Pharmacol Ther 1989; 46:63–77.
36. Sheiner LB, Hashimoto Y, Beal SL. A simulation study comparing designs for dose ranging. Stats Med 1991; 10:303–321.
37. Rombout F. Good pharmacokinetic practice (GPP) and logistics: a continuing challenge: In: Aarons L, Balant LP, Gundert-Remy UA, et al. (eds). The Population Approach: Measuring and Managing Variability in Response, Concentration and Dose. Office for Official Publications of the European Communities, Luxemborg, 1997, pp. 183–193.
38. Holford NH, Kimko HC, Monteleone JP, Peck CC. Simulation of clinical trials. Ann Rev Pharmacol Toxicol 2000; 40:209–234.
39. Reigner BG, Williams PEO, Patel IH, et al. Integration of PK/PD has improved recent Roche drug development. Clin Pharmacol Ther 1996; 51:191.
40. Collins JM, Greishaber DK, Chabner BA. Pharmacologically guided Phase I clinical trials based upon preclinical drug development. J Natl Cancer Inst 1990; 82:1321–1326.
41. Collins JM. Pharmacology and drug development. J Natl Cancer Inst 1988, 80:790–792.
42. Collins JM. Inproving the use of anticancer drugs: clinical pharmacokinetic approaches. Isr J Med Sci 1988; 24:483–487.
43. Collins JM, Zaharko DS, Dedrick RL, Chabner BA. Potential roles for preclinical pharmacology in Phase I clinical trials. Cancer Treat Rep 1986; 70:73–80.

44. Gianni L, Vigano L, Surbone A, et al. Pharmacology and clinical toxicity of 4-iodo4-deoxydoxorubicin: an example of successful application of pharmacokinetics to dose escalation in phase I trials. J Natl Cancer Inst 1990; 82:469–477.
45. Sulkes A, Collins JM. Reappraisal of some dosage adjustments guidelines. Cancer Treat Rep 1987; 71:229–232.
46. Bruno R, Vivier N, Vergniol JC, et al. A population pharmacokinetic model for docetaxel (taxotere): model building and validation. J Pharmacokinet Biopharm 1996; 24:153–172.

12 Protein Binding of Anticancer Drugs

Alex Sparreboom, PhD and Walter J. Loos, PhD

"Dismiss the idea that protein binding is a major influence of elimination."
—SH Curry, "Drug Disposition and Metabolism," Blackwell, Oxford, 1980

"Changes in plasma protein binding have little clinical relevance."
—LZ Benet, BA Hoener. Clin Pharmacol Ther 2002; 71:115–121

1. INTRODUCTION

During the last few decades, the value to clinical practice of determining plasma concentrations of chemotherapeutic agents has been demonstrated convincingly for several important drugs (1). Such tests generally are not appropriate for drugs of limited effectiveness and potency and in patients who respond well to the usual dosage regimen of a drug. They are also superfluous for drugs whose intensity of action can be judged accurately during their clinical use and whose dosage can be adjusted on that basis. Nevertheless, a broad area of clinical usefulness remains. Measurement of plasma concentrations generally clarifies the picture when usual doses of a drug fail to produce therapeutic benefits or result in unexpected toxicity. It has been proven particularly helpful in patients with hepatic or renal function disorders in whom the relationship between dosage and plasma concentration may be grossly abnormal, or when drugs are being administered concomitantly and may be altering each other's metabolic fate (2,3). Clearly, determinations of drug concentrations in plasma will become more widely applicable as we expand our knowledge of the pharmacologic correlates of plasma levels to clinical outcome for more drugs. One problem in achieving individual dose adjustment is identifying and interpreting what constitutes the therapeutic concentration of a drug in plasma. The intensity of effect is usually related to the concentra-

Handbook of Anticancer Pharmacokinetics and Pharmacodynamics
Edited by: W. D. Figg and H. L. McLeod © Humana Press Inc., Totowa, NJ

tion of the drug in the plasma water phase, as this establishes the diffusion gradient for the drug to reach its site of action *(4)*. The relationships of drug–plasma protein binding to the process that establishes the concentration of drug at the active site are shown in Fig. 1. Surprisingly, only in a few instances, plasma protein binding can significantly affect pharmacokinetic processes, such as distribution and elimination by renal and/or hepatic mechanisms, and thus have important pharmacodynamic implications *(5)*. Here, we discuss (1) the methodological aspects of protein–ligand interactions, (2) the relationship between protein binding and drug disposition, and (3) the clinical relevance of free drug monitoring in cancer patients.

2. DRUG–PROTEIN INTERACTIONS: GENERAL CONSIDERATIONS

Within blood, drugs can bind to many components including blood cells, particularly erythrocytes and platelets, and plasma proteins. As a consequence of the binding, the concentration of drug in whole blood, in plasma (C_p), and unbound drug in plasma water (C_u) can differ greatly. Binding of drugs to proteins is usually instantaneous and reversible so rapid that an equilibrium is established within milliseconds. Consequently, the associated (bound) and dissociated (unbound) forms of a drug can be assumed to be at equilibrium at all times and under virtually all circumstances. If there is a perfusion limitation, dissociation of the unbound drug and diffusion of this species across membranes occur so rapidly that delivery of drug, rather than protein binding itself, limits the transport.

The degree of drug binding to plasma proteins is frequently expressed as the ratio of the bound concentration to the total concentration. This ratio has limiting values of 0–1. Drugs with values > 0.9 are said to be highly bound, and those with values < 0.2 are said to show little or no plasma protein binding. However, the value of the fraction of drug in plasma that is bound to proteins (f_u) is usually considered of greater utility in therapeutics than is that for bound drug:

$$f_u = C_u / C_p \tag{1}$$

Binding is a function of the affinity of the protein for the drug. Because of the limited number of binding sites of a protein, binding also depends on the molar concentrations of both drug and protein. Assuming a single binding site of the protein, the association is summarized simply by the following reaction:

$$[\text{Drug}] + [\text{Protein}] \leftrightarrow [\text{Drug–Protein complex}] \tag{2}$$

From mass law considerations, the equilibrium is expressed in terms of the concentrations of unbound drug, unoccupied protein, and bound drug (C_{bd}) by the association constant K_a, which is a direct measure of the affinity of the protein for a given drug. It is possible from binding data to obtain information of K_a by fitting observed data to the following equations for saturable (Eq. 3) and nonsaturable binding (Eq. 4):

$$C_{bd} = \sum_{i=1}^{m} \left(n_i P \times K_i \times C_u \right) / \left(1 + K_1 \times C_u \right) \tag{3}$$

$$C_{bd} = \left(nK \right) \times C_u \tag{4}$$

where C_{bd} and C_u are expressed as molar concentrations, m is the number of binding site classes, n the number of saturable binding sites per mole of protein in the ith class, P the molar concentration of protein, K the association constant, and nK the contribution constant of nonspecific, nonsaturable binding on one site.

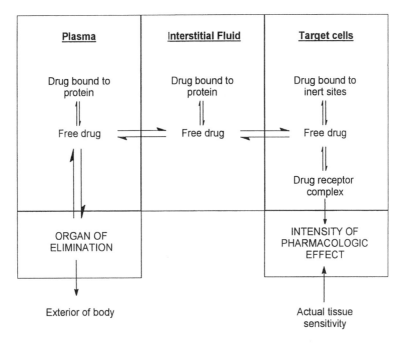

Fig. 1. Representation of the diffusion equilibria that occur to relate the concentration of drug in plasma to the drug concentration at the site of action and subsequent intensity of drug effect. (After MM Reidenberg.)

The usual approach of drug–protein binding studies is to fit experimental data to Eq. (4), and to plot them as linear regression to C_{bd} vs C_u or in a transformed representation in the form of C_{bd}/C_u versus C_{bd} (i.e., the Scatchard plot) (6). Both approaches have specific limitations, including the oversimplification of ligand attachment to the binding site(s) by fitting of curvilinear plots with straight lines or, conversely, the detection of visionary, biochemically, or pharmacologically not interpretable acceptor heterogeneity (7–11). In addition, experimental artifacts may cause curvilinearity of the Scatchard plot, and low-affinity binding components might be overlooked by an incorrect data analysis. Although the Scatchard plot is likely to be used further for quantitative evaluation purposes in the future, a number of alternative graphical representations has been proposed, including the Bjerrum plot (8,9).

3. METHODOLOGICAL ASPECTS

3.1. General Considerations

The various techniques available for quantitation of protein–ligand interactions are usually based on one of the following procedures: (1) separation of free and protein-bound fraction of ligand (i.e., determination of the free drug concentration); (2) detection of a change in a physicochemical property of the complexed ligand; or (3) detection of a change in a physicochemical behavior of the binding protein (12). In contrast to nonseparation methods, the separation methods allow the study and description of not only the characteristics of primary high-affinity sites, but also the concomitant presence of secondary low-affinity binding sites (13). Although the identification of binding structures and the calculation of binding structures and the calculation of binding parameters in vitro can provide very useful quantitative or qualitative information, only combined in vitro and in vivo data can give a comprehensive picture of the impact of binding on a drug's overall pharmacokinetic profile.

3.2. Conventional Methods

Protein binding of anticancer drugs is most commonly determined by equilibrium dialysis, ultrafiltration, or ultracentrifugation. All of these methods are based on the separation of free drug from bound drug under equilibrium conditions and have their own merits and disadvantages (13). Equilibrium dialysis is based on establishment of an equilibrium state between a protein-containing compartment and a buffer compartment, which are separated by a semipermeable membrane. Although this technique is often regarded as the reference method for protein–ligand interactions, no available experimental data support this supposed superiority. In particular, the method has a number of problems, including the long time needed to attain equilibrium (e.g., more than 24 h) (14,15), volume shifts (16,17), and nonspecific adsorption to the test device (13). Several simple and inexpensive dialysis systems employing small volumes have been developed employing microtubes, which can be constructed in any laboratory at a minimal cost and discarded after use (18).

Ultrafiltration has been introduced widely for routine monitoring of free drug, as it offers significant advantages over equilibrium dialysis, including short analysis time, ease of use, and lack of dilution effects and volume shifts, although a major controversy involves the stability of the binding equilibrium during the separation process (19). Ultracentrifugation is an alternative to both equilibrium dialysis and ultrafiltration, as it eliminates the problems associated with membrane effects and enables the separation of the free and protein-bound fraction without addition of buffer systems and dilution problems. Discrepant results have been reported between equilibrium dialysis and ultracentrifugation related to sedimentation, back diffusion, viscosity, and binding to lipoproteins in the supernatant fluid (20–22).

3.3. Other Methods

The progress in chromatographic technology, particularly affinity chromatography (23) and micellar chromatography (24), has led to the development of various automated systems for routine monitoring of free fractions of drugs in biological fluids. Although these procedures have received only limited attention in cancer pharmacology, binding data obtained by such methodologies offer much higher precision and reproducibility than those measured using conventional techniques (13). Because of its speed, efficiency, and selectivity, capillary electrophoresis is currently the most dynamically growing analytical technique in this area, and applications include affinity capillary electrophoresis (25), capillary affinity gel electrophoresis (26), and packed-capillary electrochromatography with immobilized protein-stationary phase (27).

Despite reports from some authors of a good correlation between binding parameters obtained by separation methods as compared to spectroscopic methods (13), this approach is successful mainly for high-affinity binding sites and is poorly sensitive to low-affinity interactions. Nevertheless, these methods facilitate insight into three-dimensional protein structure and conformational variations of a protein molecule resulting from ligand attachment. The most widely used methods for the purpose of studying protein–ligand interactions in this group are those based on fluorescence spectroscopy (28–30) and nuclear magnetic resonance (NMR) spectroscopy (31), as well as a number of chiroptical methods such as optical rotary dispersion or circular dichroism (32–34). Rather exceptionally, some other methods have been used for protein binding studies, with respect to unique features of the ligand or to reveal specific qualititative or quantitative aspects of the interaction. Examples include the use of polarography *(35)*, calorimetry *(36)*, stopped-flow analysis *(37)*, fluorescence-polarization immunoassay *(38)*, biomolecular interaction analysis mass spectrometry *(39)*, or (dextran-coated) charcoal adsorption-based procedures *(40,41)*. Several physiologically based approaches have also been put forward for the determination of the non-protein-bound fraction of drugs in dynamically functioning living biological systems. However, these kinds of measurements, which include analysis of saliva *(42)*, cerebrospinal fluid *(43)*, red-cell partitioning *(44,45)*, and capillary ultrafiltration *(46)* are only of limited general utility for therapeutic monitoring of free drug levels. Because of its experimental versatility, techniques based on microdialysis *(47,48)* offer at present the most promising methodological alternative for monitoring of dynamic changes of free drug in vivo in different body compartments.

4. BINDING AS A DISPOSITION FACTOR

Variability in systemic drug binding has frequently been demonstrated in humans *(5,49–51)*. However, the significance of this variability to drug disposition and pharmacodynamics depends largely on the drug's pharmacokinetic characteristics. The impression gained from the literature is a tendency to overemphasize the general importance of the binding phenomenon. However, only in cases of highly protein-bound agents, that is, > 90%, binding might be important in a practical sense. Many investigators, in attempting to extrapolate from in vitro to in vivo, lose sight of the fact that the plasma compartment comprises a relatively small fraction of the total volume available for drug distribution, and that protein–drug complexes of rather extraordinary stability must be formed to reduce substantially the amount of active, diffusible, unbound drug. To elaborate on this, a simple calculation taken from Wagner *(52)* is highly illustrative to show the relationship between protein binding and the volume of distribution. Total serum and interstitial albumin for a 70-kg male is about 276 g, or about 0.4% of body weight. Because total body water is about 60% of body weight, one can assume that the remainder (40% of body weight) is "dry tissue." Thus, the "dry tissue" mass is about $0.4 \times 70 = 28$ kg, and, hence, the ratio of "dry tissue"/total albumin = $28 / 0.276 = \sim 100$. Because there is about 100 times more "dry weight" than albumin, one would expect that the binding of drugs to tissues in the body would affect drug distribution and elimination more than binding of drugs to plasma proteins.

Many authors have reported a correlation between the elimination rate of a drug and the percentage bound to plasma proteins, and that individual differences in plasma binding were associated with pronounced variations in the elimination rate constant *(5)*. In comparing different drugs, however, there may be a pitfall. One cannot assume that just because a drug is highly bound to plasma proteins it will have a long half-life. For example, the anticancer agent chlorambucil is 99% bound to albumin and yet the median half-life is only 1.3 ± 0.90 h *(53)*. Such a short half-life, for such a highly bound drug, has not been explained, but makes one wary about making predictions about other drugs. It is also noteworthy that if a drug is bound to only one class of binding sites on a protein molecule, the carrying capacity of the plasma for the drug is limited to one times the molar equivalent of the plasma's protein content. For albumin, this is on the order of $6–7 \times 10^{-4}$ M, which for a compound with a molecular weight of 300 (such as cisplatin) is equivalent to a plasma concentration of 200,000 ng/mL. Although, theoretically, at higher concentrations the unbound fraction would increase very rapidly above this threshold, the expected plasma levels after therapeutically relevant doses are several orders of magnitude lower than this. Indeed, for almost all drugs the total plasma concentration required for a clinical effect is much less than 0.6 mM, so that albumin binding sites are far from saturation. It is important to realize, however, that some

Table 1
Major Plasma Protein Fractions[a]

Protein	Amount (mg/dL)	Molecular weight
Serum albumin[b]	3500–4500	67,000
α_1-Globulins	300–600	40,000–60,000
α_2-Globulins	400–900	100,000–400,000
β-Globulins	600–1100	110,000–120,000
γ-Globulins	700–1500	150,000–200,000
Lipoproteins	Variable	200,000–2,400,000
Fibrinogen	3000	340,000
Prothrombin	100	69,000
Transcortin	3.0–7.0	53,000
α_1-Acid glycoprotein[c]	40–100	42,000

[a] The total plasma protein content is 7000–7500 mg/dL. Many different proteins are found in blood plasma; only the major classes are listed.
[b] Might be decreased in cancer patients.
[c] Might be increased in cancer patients.

drugs, including tolbutamide and some sulfonamides, induce their effects at plasma concentrations at which the binding to protein is approaching saturation (52). On the other hand, saturable binding might occur if drugs are mainly bound to proteins other than albumin, such as α_1-acid glycoprotein.

5. BINDING PROTEINS

Apart from neutral, lipid-soluble drugs, that can be associated with the globulins of lipoprotein complexes by solution in the lipid component, plasma protein binding consists usually in the interaction of ionized polar or nonpolar groups of a drug with corresponding groups of a protein (Table 1 and Fig. 2). Most anticancer drugs are organic chemicals that are either weak acids or weak bases. The demonstration that plasma from uremic patients had markedly decreased binding of organic acids but not of organic bases has led to grouping drugs into one or the other of these classes for the purpose of drug binding studies and analysis (54). Most of the binding of acidic drugs is to human serum albumin (HSA), and multiple binding sites for drugs have been identified (55,56). Agents that compete for binding at one of these sites do not necessarily change the binding properties of any of the other sites. In contrast, basic drugs bind to HSA to only a small extent but to other plasma proteins to a much greater extent. α_1-Acid glycoprotein (AAG; orosomucoid), an acute phase reactant, is a major binder for many basic drugs. This was first recognized by Fremstad et al. (57) when they observed an increase in the plasma protein binding of quinidine in patients following surgery. Other plasma proteins, including γ-globulin and lipoproteins, also bind some basic drugs, although, overall, their relative importance is low.

Besides changes in drug binding connected with structural alteration of a protein molecule, the most important changes in the free fraction of a drug are related particularly to disease-induced variations in plasma protein levels. For example, significantly and clinically important changes in binding have been demonstrated for drugs with hepatic flow-dependent extraction (58,59). In addition, it has been demonstrated that the plasma protein

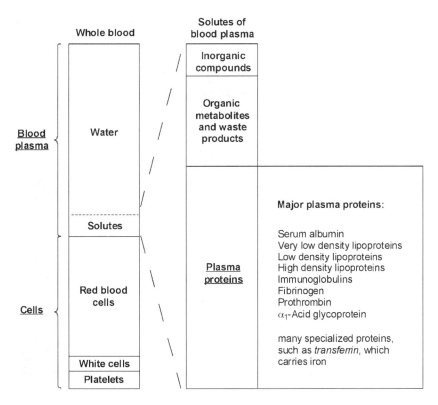

Fig. 2. Composition of human blood. The plasma fractions contain about 10% of dissolved solids, of which about 70% consists of plasma proteins. (After AL Lehninger.)

binding of several anticancer drugs is altered in patients with cancer. The primary changes in drug binding proteins seen in these patients are an increase in AAG *(60,61)* and a decrease in HSA concentration *(62)*. The physiologic role of AAG is not clear, although it is elevated in several degenerative and malignant conditions *(63)*. In addition, the plasma levels of AAG vary widely in healthy individuals, and females seem to have a slightly lower AAG level than males. Interestingly, the affinity of lidocaine for the presumed AAG binding site was higher in plasma from cancer patients compared with healthy controls *(64)*. Although the amino acid composition was similar to normal human AAG, the carbohydrate side chains were different, possibly accounting for the difference in affinity. Although it seems likely that aging does not have a clinically remarkable impact on protein binding of drugs *(65)*, the genetically determined modifications of proteins exhibit dramatically altered binding behavior. This has been observed in vitro for genetic variants of AAG interacting with various drugs, including tricyclic antidepressives *(66)* and quinidine *(67)*. Diurnal variations in AAG concentration may also contribute to inter- and intraindividual variability in binding characteristics and should be considered for their accurate interpretation *(68)*.

In contrast to AAG, HSA levels vary less than twofold in healthy individuals, although in cancer patients, this range may be substantially larger. Hence, a decrease in HSA may lead to an increase in the unbound fraction for drugs normally highly bound to this protein. In patients with cancer, the HSA levels may be decreased because of decreased synthesis, increased plasma volume, and increased catabolic rate *(62)*. Other pathophysiologic processes can also lead to a decrease in plasma protein binding and an increased fraction unbound. Specifically, hyperbilirubinemia can displace drugs from binding sites on HSA *(69)*, and lead to an increase in unbound drug concentrations, although this appears to be clinically relevant only at bilirubin concentrations above 10 mg/dL *(70)*. Similar to the observed variants of AAG, a large number of alloalbumins has been discovered *(71–73)*, which exhibit either no change in binding properties *(74)* or reduced binding affinity owing to slight variations in protein conformation *(75)*.

6. BINDING OF ANTICANCER DRUGS

The degree of binding of anticancer drugs can vary over the entire range from essentially no binding for drugs such as bleomycin and thiotepa to almost all of the drug present in plasma being bound to proteins, as in the case of teniposide and vinblastine (Table 2). The interindividual variation in plasma protein binding of anticancer drugs is usually quite small in metabolically normal individuals. Therefore, protein binding is not an important consideration in therapeutic drug monitoring. It is also important to realize that the clinical significance of protein binding displacement interactions has been severely overstated, and based largely on in vitro interaction data *(115,116)*. In addition, when drugs are not highly protein bound or when the more easily measured total drug concentration provides a consistent and accurate reflection of the free concentrations with little interpatient variability, monitoring the unbound drug concentration is not necessary. Drugs that are highly protein bound are most likely to show wide variations among patients in the unbound drug concentration and are the most likely candidates for monitoring unbound drug concentrations. In very few instances, the total concentration is not reflective of the unbound drug level. For some anticancer agents, this situation arises if (1) the agent demonstrates protein concentration-dependent binding, (2) irreversible or near-covalent binding occurs after therapeutic doses of an anticancer drug, (3) formulation vehicles (e.g., liposomes and nonionic surfactants) change the binding characteristics of the formulated agent, and (4) the agent demonstrates metabolic interconversion.

6.1. Protein Concentration-Dependent Binding

The epipodophyllotoxins etoposide and teniposide are both extensively bound to plasma proteins (Table 2). Whereas etoposide is approx 95% bound in patients with normal serum albumin and bilirubin, an even higher extent of binding has been observed for teniposide, with >98% bound to plasma proteins *(89,105)*. Interestingly, wide interindividual variability in the percentage-unbound etoposide has been reported in patients with cancer (range, 5–45%) *(117)*. In addition, a significant interaction between both HSA and, to a lesser degree, total bilirubin with the free fraction was identified *(2,118)*. Although concentration-dependent binding of etoposide was not observed in vitro, the binding ratio was significantly correlated with HSA levels *(119,120)*. The addition of exogenous bilirubin to donor plasma supported competitive binding to HSA as the mechanism for the effect of bilirubin on etoposide protein binding. A pharmacokinetic model for prediction of etoposide plasma protein binding in humans, based on HSA and total bilirubin levels, has been prospectively validated in cancer patients, with only slight bias toward overestimation of the free fraction in patients with normal bilirubin or low HSA levels *(99)*. The clinical implications of the variable etoposide protein binding were illustrated recently in a study of 28 adult cancer patients *(121)*. The systemic exposure to unbound etoposide more precisely correlated with measures of hematologic toxicity than total drug levels. In addition, patients with HSA levels <35 mg/dL had substantially larger area under the curves of unbound etoposide than patients

Table 2
Plasma Protein Binding of Anticancer Agents

Agent	% Unbound	Binding matrix	V (L/kg)^a	t$_{1/2}$ (h)^b	References
Amsacrine	3	HSA, AAG, γ-GL	~2.5	2.6	(76)
Bleomycin	>99	Plasma	0.27 ± 0.09	3.1 ± 1.7	(77)
Brequinar	2	HSA	0.11–0.27	13–18	(78)
Busulfan	72	HSA	0.99 ± 0.23^c	2.6 ± 0.5	(79)
Carboplatin	10	HSA	0.24 ± 0.03	2.0 ± 0.2	(80)
Chlorambucil	1	plasma	0.29 ± 0.21	1.3 ± 0.9	(81)
Cisplatin	<5	HSA, TF, γ-GL	0.28 ± 0.07	0.5 ± 0.1	(82)
Cyclophosphamide	87	Plasma	0.78 ± 0.57	7.5 ± 4.0	(83)
Cytarabine	87	Plasma	3.0 ± 1.9	2.6 ± 0.6	(84,85)
Docetaxel	<2	HSA, AAG, HDL	1.8 ± 1.2	14 ± 7.5	(86)
Doxorubicin	15–25	HSA	17 ± 11	26 ± 17	(87,88)
Etoposide	4	HSA	0.36 ± 0.15	8.1 ± 4.3	(89)
5-Fluorouracil	>95	HSA, α,β,γ-GL	0.25 ± 0.12	0.2 ± 0.07	(90)
Ifosfamide	45	Plasma	0.50 ± 0.20	3.8–8.6	(91)
Irinotecan	65	HSA	3.4–6.4	12 ± 3.0	(92)
Melphalan	71–80	HSA, AAG	0.45 ± 0.15	1.4 ± 0.2	(93,94)
6-Mercaptopurine	81	HSA, AAG	0.56 ± 0.38	0.9 ± 0.4	(95)
Methotrexate	54	HSA	0.55 ± 0.19	7.2 ± 2.1	(96,97)
Oxaliplatin	13–21	HSA, γ-GL	5.0 ± 1.9	240 ± 54	(98)
Paclitaxel	2–8	HSA, AAG, HDL	2.0 ± 1.2	16 ± 8.9	(99,100)
SN-38	2	HSA, AAG	NA	24 ± 6.0	(92,101,102)
Tamoxifen	<2	HSA, β-GL	50–60^c	96–264	(103,104)
Teniposide	<1	HSA	0.22 ± 0.05	9.0 ± 3.0	(105)
Thiotepa	90	HSA,HDL	0.71 ± 0.18	2.1 ± 0.4	(106)
Topotecan	79	HSA	0.40–2.45	3.5 ± 1.5	(107,108)
Trimetrexate	2	HSA, AAG	0.33 ± 0.18	13.0 ± 5.0	(109)
UCN-01	<0.02	AAG	0.11 ± 0.08	1370 ± 280	(110,111)
Vinblastine	<1	AAG	1.4–27	29 ± 12	(112,113)
Vinorelbine	12	AAG	51–76	45 ± 12	(114)

HSA, Human serum albumin; AAG, α$_1$-acid glycoprotein; HDL, high-density lipoprotein; GL, globulin; TF, transferrin; NA, not available.

^{a} Mean distribution volume.

^{b} Terminal disposition half-life.

^{c} Distribution volume divided by oral bioavailability.

with normal HSA, bilirubin, and serum creatinine values (122). Because this increase in systemic exposure was associated with more severe neutropenia, these findings suggest that unbound etoposide concentrations might be indicated for therapeutic drug monitoring, particularly in patients with aberrant binding (e.g., in case of hypoalbuminemia). Similarly to what has been observed for etoposide, the percentage-unbound teniposide is highly variable among patients, and has a strong inverse linear relationship with HSA levels (123). Furthermore, systemic exposure to unbound teniposide correlated significantly with hematologic toxicity, whereas exposure measures based on total drug were not as well correlated (123). Thus, it is likely that prospective monitoring of epipodophyllotoxins as a selective approach to therapy optimization might be useful. However, additional studies are required to further define relationships between exposure to unbound etoposide and pharmacodynamic outcome of treatment (i.e., side effects and antitumor efficacy).

6.2. Irreversible Binding

Platinum-containing anticancer drugs, including cisplatin, carboplatin, and oxaliplatin, are currently the only agents for which unbound concentrations are routinely measured and for which the relationship between unbound drug and therapeutic effects has been studied extensively. In body fluids, these agents are readily attacked by nucleophiles with exchange of one or both chloride ligands to form high and low molecular weight complexes. For example, one day after intravenous administration of cisplatin, 65–98% of platinum in plasma is protein bound *(124,125)*, while no unbound platinum has been detected at any time in plasma of patients after slow 20-h infusions *(125)*. The extent of protein binding also results in significantly lower urinary excretion and an increased tissue deposition of platinum *(125)*. It has been demonstrated that the unbound fraction is affected by many factors. Plasma components such as HSA, hemoglobin, transferrin, and γ-globulin were previously suggested to be the main ligands for cisplatin *(126)*, and the binding of cisplatin to HSA was considered to be essentially irreversible, although this has recently been questioned *(127)*. Nevertheless, the concentration–time curves of unbound cisplatin in plasma and total cisplatin (bound to plasma proteins plus unbound) do not run in parallel (Fig. 3). This suggests that the clearance of cisplatin is restrictive, and that for a representative calculation of the area under the curve and clearance, the unbound cisplatin concentrations should be used.

In contrast to cisplatin, the concentration–time profiles of unbound and total carboplatin are similar over the first 6 h after drug administration, with the distribution half-life being similar for the different species (approx 1 h) *(128)*. Thereafter, the concentrations of total platinum remain higher, indicating that protein binding is relatively slow. Indeed, the protein binding of carboplatin averaged 10% at the end of the administration and increased progressively to reach more than 90% at 24 h after the end of infusion. The extent of binding of related platinum analogue, oxaliplatin, to plasma proteins in cancer patients has also confirmed these results, and showed that at 5 d posttreatment, plasma protein binding was estimated to be >95% *(98)*. Overall, these results suggest that plasma protein binding and the pharmacokinetic behavior of platinum analogs is determined by (1) the stability of the leaving ligand, and thereby the chemical reactivity and intrinsic cytotoxicity of the complex, and (2) the nature of the carrier ligand that influences the binding and distribution characteristics of the molecule. Regardless of the exact nature of these processes, the protein binding studies conducted with platinum-containing anticancer agents may provide a firm scientific basis for the safe and effective use of these agents in the clinic.

A striking example of very extensive binding of an agent to human plasma proteins has been UCN-01 (7-hydroxystaurosporine), a protein kinase C inhibitor, which is presently under clinical investigation as an anticancer drug. The clinical pharmacokinetic behavior of UCN-01 after administration as a 3- or 72-h infusion to cancer patients in initial Phase I trials displayed distinctive features that could not have been predicted from preclinical data *(110)*. Specifically, the distribution volume (0.08–0.16 L/kg) and the systemic clearance (0.05–0.25 mL/h/kg) were extremely low, in contrast to the large distribution volume and rapid clearance in experimental animals. In vitro protein binding experiments have demonstrated that these discrepant findings were directly attributable to a near-covalent binding of UCN-01 to human AAG, with an association constant in the order of $8 \times 10^8 M^{-1}$ *(111)*. Clearly, the implication of such pharmacological features of UCN-01, that is, the extremely low unbound concentrations and long exposure in cancer patients following its administration, will need to be evaluated further in both preclinical and clinical studies to find exposure measures that can be linked to treatment outcome.

6.3. Drug Formulation Interference

The use of liposomes (i.e., microparticulate carriers that consist of one or more lipid bilayer membranes enclosing an internal aqueous phase) as a drug delivery system has been an area of increasing interest in anticancer drug development, and has significant implications for pharmacokinetic monitoring. Over the last decade, the use of anticancer agents encapsulated in liposomes has proven useful in attenuating toxicity while maintaining or increasing efficacy of certain compounds, thus enhancing the therapeutic index *(129–131)*. A complete evaluation of such trials will require a comprehensive plasma pharmacokinetic analysis. There are several factors contributing to the complexity of the pharmacologic handling of drugs delivered by liposomes after intravenous administration: (1) circulating drug is present in three distinguishable forms (i.e., liposomal associated, protein bound, and unbound), and (2) plasma clearance occurs as a result of various processes with different elimination rates (i.e., tissue uptake of liposomes carrying the drug, leakage of drug from liposomes, and clearance of unbound drug). It has been argued that pharmacokinetic studies with such agents limited to the analysis of total drug concentrations in plasma is not informative enough and may even be misleading, as pharmacological effects are related mainly to the level of free drug in plasma. A small number of reports have addressed this issue for liposomal formulated anticancer agents (e.g., doxorubicin and vincristine), and have demonstrated that the vast majority of drug present in the circulation after injection of liposomal preparations remains entrapped with the lipid carrier *(132,133)*. At present, various reliable analytical procedures based on high-performance liquid chromatography preceded by ultrafiltration or solid-phase extraction have been reported to separate unbound from liposome-associated drug *(134–137)*. Clearly, implementation of such techniques in the future would significantly increase the capability to evaluate rigorously the complete pharmacokinetic behavior of liposomal anticancer drugs in a clinical setting.

Similar to liposomal entrapment, anticancer drugs can also be sequestered by other formulation excipients, such as micelles composed of nonionic surfactants used in pharmaceutical preparations of intravenous dosage forms. The most extensively studied example of this kind is encapsulation of the antimicrotubule agent paclitaxel (Taxol) with its formulation vehicle, Cremophor EL, a polyoxyethylated castor oil. Initially, it was found that paclitaxel binds extensively (~ 95%) to human plasma in vitro at clinically relevant concentrations (0.1–6 μM) in a concentration-independent manner *(99)*. These studies also indicated that HSA and AAG contributed about equally to overall binding, with a minor contribution from lipoproteins. Subsequently, it was demonstrated that this in vitro protein-binding phenomenon was substantially altered in the presence of Cremophor EL *(100)*. Furthermore, a recent clinical pharmacokinetic study with paclitaxel has shown that after intravenous drug administration over 3 h (at the recommended dose of 175 mg/m^2), the principal fraction of the agent in blood is associated with the hydrophobic interior space of Cremophor EL micelles *(138)*. Because the clearance of this formulation vehicle itself is schedule dependent (with a significant increase in its clearance with prolongation of the infusion duration from 1–3 to 24 h), this type of drug sequestration is likely to affect paclitaxel pharmacokinetics with alternative infusion duration *(139)*. An assay method for separation of unbound and bound (i.e., Cremophor EL plus protein associated) drug based on equilibrium dialysis with a tracer of tritiated paclitaxel followed by liquid-scintillation counting has become available recently, and implemented in retrospective analysis of clinical samples from patients treated with paclitaxel *(140)*. A population pharmacokinetic model for unbound paclitaxel following its administration after 1-, 3-, and 24-h infusions has demonstrated that systemic exposure to unbound drug correlated significantly with neutropenia and could explain the schedule-dependent hematological pharmacodynamics of this agent (i.e., more severe bone marrow suppression with prolongation of infusion duration) *(141)*.

6.4. Metabolic Interconversion

Another aspect of the relevance of anticancer drug plasma protein binding is seen with agents that are enzymatically or chemically converted back and forth from metabolites or degradants to the administered drugs (i.e., interconversion) (Fig. 4). Usually, irrespective of which form of such agent is administered, both the parent and interconversion product are present in plasma. How quickly the equilibrium is established and where the ratio lies depends not only on the kinetics of interconversion but also on the irreversible loss of each species from the body, as well as on the binding to plasma proteins. One example of an anticancer agent undergoing interconversion is camptothecin, a pentacyclic structure with a lactone functionality that is not only essential for antitumor efficacy, but also confers a degree of instability in aqueous solutions *(142)*. This agent, as well as its analogues, can undergo a pH-dependent reversible interconversion between the lactone form and a ring-opened carboxylate form *(143)*. The equilibrium between the lactone and carboxylate forms of camptothecins is not solely dependent on pH, but also on the presence of specific binding proteins, notably HSA *(144)*. Investigations have shown that HSA had a significant preference for the carboxylate form of camptothecin compared with albumin from five other animal species *(145)*. However, structural modification to the camptothecin ring structure seen with irinotecan, its metabolite SN-38, and topotecan diminished interspecies differences in stabilization of the carboxylate forms *(145–147)*. In the case of the related agent, 9-aminocamptothecin, the lactone moiety appears to be stabilized by murine serum albumin but not by HSA, with $35 \pm 6.2\%$ being present in the pharmacologically active lactone forms in the presence of murine serum albumin, and only $0.63 \pm 0.10\%$ in the presence of HSA *(146)*. Because the lactone and carboxylate forms of these various analogues have very distinct pharmacokinetic profiles as a result of variable binding to HSA *(142)*, it has been proposed that separate measurement of both drug forms has clinical importance *(148)*. To ensure adequate measurements of the pharmacologically active lactone forms of the camptothecin analogues in pharmacokinetic studies, blood samples have to be processed directly after sampling at the site of the patient either by (1) direct analysis of the samples, (2) direct extraction of the lactone form from the plasma, or (3) stabilizing the lactone to carboxylate ratio. This latter procedure is clearly preferable, as it is the least laborious approach *(148)*.

7. OVERALL SIGNIFICANCE

Knowledge of the protein binding of anticancer drugs may have significant clinical relevance in a very limited number of cases. In general, plasma protein binding is unimportant for monitoring levels of poorly bound drugs (i.e., < 90%), and when the total drug concentrations reflect the unbound levels (i.e., when binding is concentration independent and reversible). In these circumstances, the practicing physician should regard protein binding of any drug with the minor degree of attention it deserves. For highly protein-bound drugs, knowledge of the parameters that influence the binding is important in interpreting the plasma concentrations of such agents. For some anticancer drugs, including epipodophyllotoxins, platinum analogues, paclitaxel, and liposomal formulated agents, the therapeutic implications of binding to proteins (or other macromolecules) seem to be clearly defined. However, with the exception of some very interesting clinical data regarding etoposide and a few studies with paclitaxel, it seems that we have learned relatively

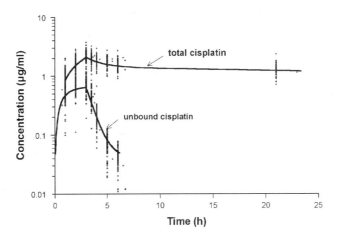

Fig. 3. Representative plasma concentration–time profiles of unbound and total cisplatin in patients treated with a 3-h intravenous infusion of cisplatin at a dose of 70 mg/m². (Unpublished data, Erasmus MC—Daniel den Hoed Cancer Center, Rotterdam, The Netherlands.)

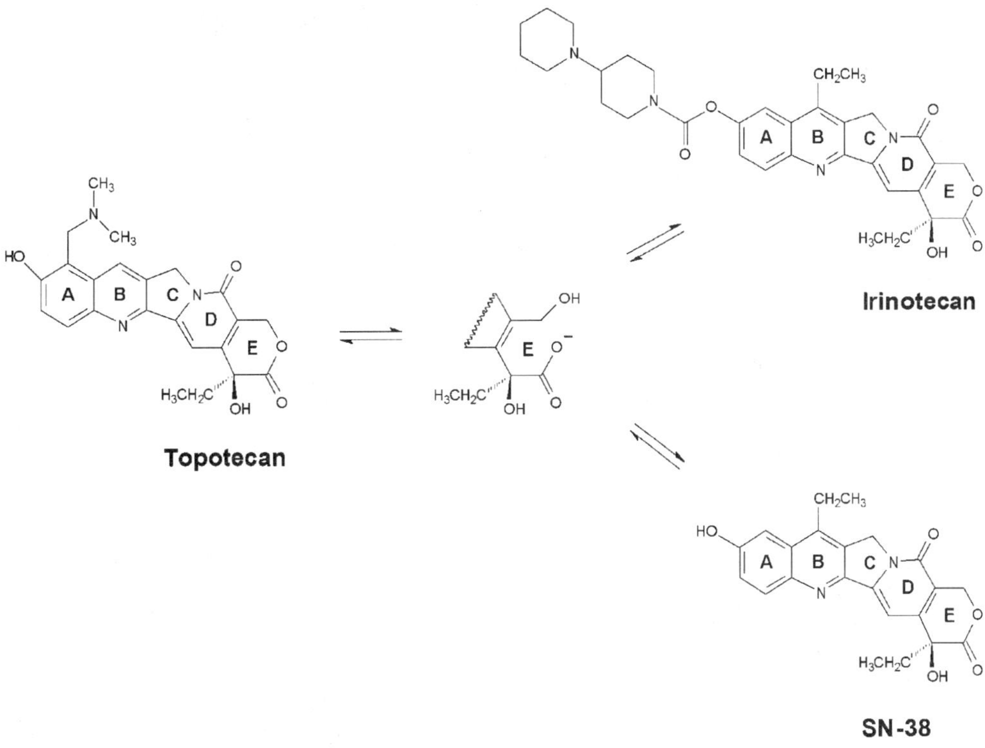

Fig. 4. The concept of metabolic interconversion, exemplified by the lactone and carboxylate forms of topotecan, irinotecan (CPT-11), and its pharmacologically active metabolite SN-38.

little regarding unbound drug concentration–effect relationships. Although available evidence suggests that unbound concentrations correlate better with clinical effects than total plasma concentrations, there are insufficient data to justify the recommendation of the routine use of unbound drug concentration monitoring for any of these agents at present.

Nonetheless, for new anticancer agents, as well as their (active) metabolites, it will be imperative that the extent and variability of protein binding be documented in an early phase of drug development to allow, if indicated, accurate determination of the relationship between unbound drug exposure and pharmacodynamic effect (i.e., toxicity and efficacy). Recent advances in techniques to determine unbound drug concentration have greatly simplified the task of monitoring this parameter in clinical practice (reviewed in *[149,150]*). Eventually, the utility of such monitoring must be carefully considered in the environment of cost containment in which clinicians must currently function.

8. SUMMARY

The major purpose of therapeutic drug monitoring is to enable drug dosage individualization for differences among patients in rates of drug metabolism and/or excretion. Most standard analytical methods for measuring concentrations of drugs in plasma determine drug bound to plasma proteins as well as free drug dissolved in plasma water. For this reason, the relationship between total drug concentration in plasma and treatment outcome (i.e., toxicity and efficacy) will be good only if the degree of plasma protein binding of the agent is constant, or if so little drug is protein bound that changes in binding make insignificant changes in unbound concentration. Available literature data indicate that, in general, protein binding of anticancer drugs is not of principal clinical relevance. However, there are several instances in which monitoring of unbound concentrations might be useful: (1) agents demonstrating protein concentration dependent binding, (2) agents that bind irreversibly or near covalently, (3) when formulation excipients modulate unbound drug levels, and (4) metabolically interconvertible agents. While available evidence suggests that for these agents unbound drug levels correlate better with clinical effects than total plasma concentrations, there are insufficient data to justify the recommendation of the routine use of unbound drug concentration monitoring for any of these agents at present.

REFERENCES

1. Van den Bongerd HJ, Mathot RA, Beijnen JH, Schellens JHM. Pharmacokinetically guided administration of chemotherapeutic agents. Clin Pharmacokinet 2000; 39:345–367.
2. Kintzel PE, Dorr RT. Anticancer drug renal toxicity and elimination: dosing guidelines for altered renal function. Cancer Treat Rev 1995; 21:33–64.
3. Donelli MG, Zucchetti M, Munzone E, D'Incalci M, Crosignani A. Pharmacokinetics of anticancer agents in patients with impaired liver function. Eur J Cancer 1998; 34:33–46.
4. Rowland M, Tozer TN. Clinical pharmacokinetics; concepts and applications. Philadelphia, PA: Lea & Febiger, 1989.
5. Rowland M. Protein binding and drug clearance. Clin Pharmacokinet 1984; 9:10–17.
6. Monot C, Lapicque F, Benamghar L, Muller N, Payan E, Netter P. Representation of affinity in the case of co-operativity in protein-ligand binding. Fundam Clin Pharmacol 1994; 8:18–25.
7. Pedersen JB, Lindup WE. Interpretation and analysis of receptor binding experiments which yield nonlinear Scatchard plots and binding constants dependent upon receptor concentration. Biochem Pharmacol 1994; 47:179–185.
8. Klotz IM. Numbers of receptor sites from Scatchard graphs: facts and fantasies. Science 1982; 217: 1247–1249.
9. Munson PJ, Rodbard D. Number of receptor sites from Scatchard and Klotz graphs: a constructive critique. Science 1983 220:979–981.
10. Zierler K. Misuse of nonlinear Scatchard plots. Trends Biochem Sci 1989; 14:314–317.
11. Kermode JC. The curvilinear Scatchard plot. Experimental artifact or receptor heterogeneity? Biochem Pharmacol 1989; 38:2053–2060.
12. Klotz IM. Physiochemical aspects of drug–protein interactions: a general perspective. Ann NY Acad Sci 1973; 226:18–35.

13. Oravcová J, Böhs B, Lindner W. Drug–protein binding studies. New trends in analytical and experimental methodology. J Chromatogr B 1996; 677:1–28.

14. Kurz H, Trunk H, Weitz B. Evaluation of methods to determine protein-binding of drugs. Equilibrium dialysis, ultrafiltration, ultracentrifugation, gel filtration. Arzneimittelforsch 1997; 27:1373–1380.

15. Bowers WF, Fulton S, Thompson J. Ultrafiltration vs equilibrium dialysis for determination of free fraction. Clin Pharmacokinet 1984; S1:49–60.

16. Huang JD. Errors in estimating the unbound fraction of drugs due to the volume shift in equilibrium dialysis. J Pharmaceut Sci 1983; 72:1368–1369.

17. Mapleson WW. Computation of the effect of Donnan equilibrium on pH in equilibrium dialysis. J Pharmacol Methods 1987; 17:231–242.

18. Reinard T, Jacobsen HJ. An inexpensive small volume equilibrium dialysis system for protein-ligand binding assays. Analyt Biochem 1989; 176:157–160.

19. Parsons DL, Fan HF. Loss of propranolol during ultrafiltration in plasma protein binding studies. Res Commun Chem Pathol Pharmacol 1986; 54:405–408.

20. Oellerich M, Mnuller-Vahl H. The EMIT FreeLevel ultrafiltration technique compared with equilibrium dialysis and ultracentrifugation to determine protein binding of phenytoin. Clin Pharmacokinet 1984; S1:61–70.

21. Verbeeck RK, Cardinal JA. Plasma protein binding of salicylic acid, phenytoin, chlorpromazine, propranolol and pethidine using equilibrium dialysis and ultracentrifugation. Arzneimittelforsch 1985; 35:903–906.

22. Barre J, Chamouard JM, Houin G, Tillement JP. Equilibrium dialysis, ultrafiltration, and ultracentrifugation compared for determining the plasma–protein-binding characteristics of valproic acid. Clin Chem 1985; 31:60–64.

23. Hage DS. High-performance affinity chromatography: a powerful tool for studying serum protein binding. J Chromatogr B 2002; 768:3–30.

24. Garcia Alvarez-Coque MC, Carda Broch S. Direct injection of physiological fluids in micellar liquid chromatography. J Chromatogr B 1999; 736:1–18.

25. Heegaard NH. Capillary electrophoresis for the study of affinity interactions. J Mol Recogn 1998; 11: 141–148.

26. Hage DS, Tweed SA. Recent advances in chromatographic and electrophoretic methods for the study of drug–protein interactions. J Chromatogr B 1997; 699:499–525.

27. Gomez FA, Avila LZ, Chu YH, Whitesides GM. Determination of binding constants of ligands to proteins by affinity capillary electrophoresis: compensation for electroosmotic flow. Analyt Chem 1994; 66:1785–1791.

28. Sugiyama Y, Suzuki Y, Sawada Y, et al. Auramine O as a fluorescent probe for the binding of basis drugs to human alpha 1-acid glycoprotein (alpha 1-AG). The development of simple fluorometric method for the determination of alpha 1-AG in human serum. Biochem Pharmacol 1985; 34:821–829.

29. Rahman MH, Maruyama T, Okada T, Yamasaki K, Otagiri M. Study of interaction of carprofen and its enantiomers with human serum albumin—I. Mechanism of binding studied by dialysis and spectroscopic methods. Biochem Pharmacol 1993; 46:1721–1731.

30. Morin D, Zini R, Ledewyn S, Tillement JP. Inhibition of binedaline binding to human alpha 1-acid glycoprotein and other serum proteins by chlorpromazine, imipramine, and propranolol. J Pharmaceut Sci 1986; 75:883–885.

31. Chen A, Shapiro MJ. Affinity NMR. Analyt Chem 1999; 71:669A–675A.

32. Chignell CF. Optical studies of drug–protein complexes. II. Interaction of phenylbutazone and its analogues with human serum albumin. Mol Pharmacol 1969; 5:244–252.

33. Chignell CF. Optical studies of drug–protein complexes. 3. Interaction of flufenamic acid and other N-arylanthranilates with serum albumin. Mol Pharmacol 1969; 5:455–462.

34. Chignell CF, Starkwheather DK. Optical studies of drug–protein complexes. V. The interaction of phenylbutazone, flufenamic acid, and dicoumarol with acetylsalicylic acid-treated human serum albumin. Mol Pharmacol 1971; 7:229–237.

35. Squella JA, Becerra R, Nunez-Vergara LJ. Polarography: a new toll in the elucidation of drug–albumin interactions. Biochem Pharmacol 1987; 36:3531–3533.

36. Aki H, Yamamoto M. Thermodynamics of the binding of phenothiazines to human plasma, human serum albumin and alpha 1-acid glycoprotein: a calorimetric study. J Pharmaceut Pharmacol 1989; 41:674–679.

37. Shaklai N, Garlick RL, Bunn HF. Nonenzymatic glycosylation of human serum albumin alters its conformation and function. J Biol Chem 1984; 259:3812–3817.

38. Chen BH, Taylor EH, Pappas AA. Total and free dispyramide by fluorescence polarization immunoassay and relationship between free fraction and alpha-1 acid glycoprotein. Clin Chim Acta 1987; 163:75–80.
39. Nelson RW, Krone JR. Advances in surface plasmon resonance biomolecular interaction analysis mass spectrometry (BIA/MS). J Mol Recogn 1999; 12:77–93.
40. Sablonniere B, Dallery N, Griller I, Formstecher P, Dautrevaux M. Physicochemical parameters affecting the charcoal adsorption assay for quantitative retinoid-binding measurement. Analyt Biochem 1994; 217:110–118.
41. Yuan J, Yang DC, Birkmeier J, Stolzenbach J. Determination of protein binding by in vitro charcoal adsorption. J Pharmacokinet Biopharmacol 1995; 23:41–55.
42. Svensson CK, Woodruff MN, Baxter JG, Lalka D. Free drug concentration monitoring in clinical practice. Rationale and current status. Clin Pharmacokinet 1986; 11:450–469.
43. Drobitch RK, Svensson CK. Therapeutic drug monitoring in saliva. An update. Clin Pharmacokinet 1992; 23:365–379.
44. Highley MS, de Bruijn EA. Erythrocytes and the transport of drugs and endogenous compounds. Pharmaceut Res 1996; 13:186–195.
45. Hinderling PH. Red blood cells: a neglected compartment in pharmacokinetics and pharmacodynamics. Pharmacol Rev 1997; 49:279–295.
46. Linhares MC, Kissinger PT. Capillary ultrafiltration: in vivo sampling probes for small molecules. Analyt Chem 1992; 64:2831–2835.
47. Scott DO, Sorenson LR, Steele KL, Punckett DL, Lunte CE. In vivo microdialysis sampling for pharmacokinetic investigations. Pharmaceut Res 1991; 8:389–392.
48. Muller M. Science, medicine, and the future: microdialysis. Br Med J 2002; 324:588–591.
49. Wilkinson GR. Plasma and tissue binding considerations in drug disposition. Drug Metab Rev 1985; 151:193–203.
50. Meijer DKF, Van der Sluijs P. Covalent and noncovalent binding of drugs: implications for hepatic clearance, storage, and cell-specific drug delivery. Pharmaceut Res 1989; 6:105–118.
51. Stewart CF, Zamboni WC. Plasma protein binding of chemotherapeutic agents. In: Grochow LB, Ames MM (eds). A Clinician's Guide to Chemotherapy Pharmacokinetics and Pharmacodynamics. Baltimore, MD: Williams & Williams, 1998, pp. 55–66.
52. Wagner JG. Fundamentals of Clinical Pharmacokinetics. Hamilton, IL: Drug Intelligence Publications, 1979.
53. Lind MJ, Ardiet C. Pharmacokinetics of alkylating agents. Cancer Surv 1993; 17:157–188.
54. Reidenberg MM, Odar-Ceederlof I, von Bahr C, Borga O, Sjoqvist F. Protein binding of diphenylhydantoin and demethylimipramide in plasma from patients with poor renal function. N Engl J Med 1971; 285:264–267.
55. Kragh-Hansen U. Structure and ligand binding properties of human serum albumin. Dan Med Bull 1990; 37:57–84.
56. Grandison MK, Boudinot FD. Age-related changes in protein binding of drugs: implications for therapy. Clin Pharmacokinet 2000; 38:271–290.
57. Fremstad D, Bergerud K, Haffner JF, Lunde PK. Increased plasma binding of quinidine after surgery: a preliminary report. Eur J Clin Pharmacol 1976; 10:441–444.
58. Zini R, Riant P, Barre J, Tillement JP. Disease-induced variations in plasma protein levels. Implications for drug dosage regimens (Part I). Clin Pharmacokinet 1990; 19:147–159.
59. Zini R, Riant P, Barre J, Tillement JP. Disease-induced variations in plasma protein levels. Implications for drug dosage regimens (Part II). Clin Pharmacokinet 1990; 19:218–229.
60. Bacchus H. Serum glycoproteins and malignant neoplastic diseases. Prog Clin Pathol 1977; 6:111–135.
61. Bacchus H. Serum glycoproteins in cancer. Prog Clin Pathol 1975; 6:111–135.
62. Rossing N. Albumin metabolism in neoplastic diseases. Scand J Clin Lab Invest 1968; 22:211–216.
63. MacKichan JJ. Influence of protein binding and use of unbound (free) drug concentrations. In: Evans WE, Shentag JJ, Jusko WJ (eds). Applied Pharmacokinetics: Principles and Therapeutic Drug Monitoring. Vancouver, Canada: Applied Therapeutics, 1992, pp. 1–48.
64. Rudman D, Treadwell PE, Vogler WR, et al. An abnormal orosomucoid in the plasma of patients with neoplastic disease. Cancer Res 1972; 32:1951–1952.
65. Wallace SM, Verbeeck RK. Plasma protein binding in the elderly. Clin Pharmacokinet 1987; 12:41–72.
66. Tinguely D, Baumann P, Conti M, Jonzier-Perey M, Schopf J. Interindividual differences in the binding of antidepressives to plasma proteins: the role of the variants of alpha 1-acid glycoprotein. Eur J Clin Pharmacol 1985; 27:661–666.

67. Li JH, Xu, JQ, Cao XM, Ni L, Li Y, Zhuang YY, Gong JB. Influence of the ORM1 phenotypes on serum unbound concentration and protein binding of quinidine. Clin Chim Acta 2002; 317:85–92.

68. Yost RL, DeVane CL. Diurnal variation of alpha 1-acid glycoprotein concentration in normal volunteers. J Pharmaceut Sci 1985; 74:777–779.

69. Van Breemen RB, Fenselau C, Mogilevsky W, Odell GB. Reaction of bilirubin glucuronides with serum albumin. J Chromatogr 1986; 383:387–392.

70. Tozer TN. Concepts basic to pharmacokinetics. Pharmacol Ther 1981; 12:109–1311.

71. Takahashi N, Takahashi Y, Isobe T, et al. Amino acid substitutions in inherited albumin variants from Amerindian and Japanese populations. Proc Natl Acad Sci USA 1987; 84:8001–8005.

72. Arai K, Ishioka N, Huss K, Madison J, Putnam FW. Identical structural changes in inherited albumin variants from different populations. Proc Natl Acad Sci USA 1989; 86:434–438.

73. Galliano M, Minchiotti L, Porta F, et al. Mutations in genetic variants of human serum albumin found in Italy. Proc Natl Acad Sci USA 1990; 87:8721–8725.

74. Reed RG. Ligand-binding properties of albumin Parklands: Asp365—His. Biochim Biophys Acta 1988; 965:114–117.

75. Vestberg K, Galliano M, Minchiotti L, Kragh-Hansen U. High-affinity binding of warfarin, salicylate and diazepam to natural mutants of human serum albumin modified in the C-terminal end. Biochem Pharmacol 1992; 44:1515–1521.

76. Paxton JW, Jurlina JL, Foote SE. The binding of amsacrine to human plasma proteins. J Pharmaceut Pharmacol 1986; 38:432–438.

77. Crooke ST, Luft F, Broughton A, Strong J, Casson K, Einhorn L. Bleomycin serum pharmacokinetics as determined by a radioimmunoassay and a microbiologic assay in a patient with compromised renal function. Cancer 1977; 39:1430–1434.

78. King SY, Agra AM, Shen HS, et al. Protein binding of brequinar in the plasma of healthy donors and cancer patients and analysis of the relationship between protein binding and pharmacokinetics in cancer patients. Cancer Chemother Pharmacol 1994; 35:101–108.

79. Ehrsson H, Hassan M. Binding of busulfan to plasma proteins and blood cells. J Pharmaceut Pharmacol 1984; 36:694–696.

80. Go RS, Adjei AA. Review of the comparative pharmacology and clinical activity of cisplatin and carboplatin. J Clin Oncol 1999; 17:409–422.

81. Newell DR, Calvert AH, Harrap KR, McElwain TJ. Studies on the pharmacokinetics of chlorambucil and prednimustine in man. Br J Clin Pharmacol 1983; 15:253–258.

82. Ivanov AI, Chrostodoulou J, Parkinson JA, et al. Cisplatin binding sites on human albumin. J Biol Chem 1998; 273:14,721–14,730.

83. Boddy AV, Yule SM. Metabolism and pharmacokinetics of oxazaphosphorines. Clin Pharmacokinet 2000; 38:291–304.

84. Van Prooijen HC, Vierwinden G, Wessels J, Haanen C. Cytosine arabinoside binding to human plasma proteins. Arch Int Pharmacodyn Ther 1977; 229:199–205.

85. Slevin ML, Johnston A, Woollard RC, Piall EM, Lister TA, Turner P. Relationship between protein binding and extravascular drug concentrations of a water-soluble drug, cytosine arabinoside. J R Soc Med 1983; 76:365–368.

86. Urien S, Barré J, Morin C, Paccaly A, Montay G, Tillement JP. Docetaxel serum protein binding with high affinity to alpha$_1$-acid glycoprotein. Invest New Drugs 1996; 14:147–151.

87. Eksborg S, Ehrsson H, Ekqvist B. Protein binding of anthraquinone glycosides, with special reference to adriamycin. Cancer Chemother Pharmacol 1982; 10:7–10.

88. Demant EJ, Friche E. Equilibrium binding of anthracycline cytostatics to serum albumin and small unilamellar phospholipid vesicles as measured by gel filtration. Biochem Pharmacol 1998; 55:27–32.

89. Stewart CF, Pieper JA, Arbuck SG, Evans WE. Altered protein binding of etoposide in patients with cancer. Clin Pharmacol Ther 1989; 45:49–55.

90. Czejka M, Schuller J. [The binding of 5-fluorouracil to serum protein fractions, erythrocytes and ghosts under in vitro conditions]. Arch Pharm (Wienheim) 1992; 325:69–71.

91. Zheng JJ, Chan KK, Muggia F. Preclinical pharmacokinetics and stability of isophosphoramide mustard. Cancer Chemother Pharmacol 1994; 33:391–398.

92. Combes O, Barré J, Duche JC, et al. In vitro binding and partitioning of irinotecan (CPT-11) and its metabolite, SN-38, in human blood. Invest New Drugs 2000; 18:1–5.

93. Reece PA, Hill HS, Green RM, et al. Renal clearance and protein binding of melphalan in patients with cancer. Cancer Chemother Pharmacol 1988; 22:348–352.

94. Gera S, Musch E, Osterheld HK, Loos U. Relevance of the hydrolysis and protein binding of melphalan to the treatment of multiple myeloma. Cancer Chemother Pharmacol 1989; 23:76–80.

95. Sjoholm I, Stjerna B. Binding of drugs to human serum albumin XVII: irreversible binding of mercaptopurine to human serum proteins. J Pharmaceut Sci 1981; 70:1290–1291.

96. Maia MB, Saivin S, Chatelut E, Malmary MF, Houin G. In vitro and in vivo protein binding of methotrexate assessed by microdialysis. Int J Clin Pharmacol Ther 1996; 34:335–341.

97. Skibinska L, Ramlau C, Zaluski J, Olejniczak B. Methotrexate binding to human plasma proteins. Pol J Pharmacol Pharmaceut 1990; 42:151–157.

98. Graham MA, Lockwood GF, Greenslade D, Brienza S, Baysaas M, Gamelin E. Clinical pharmacokinetics of oxaliplatin: a critical review. Clin Cancer Res 2000; 6:1205–1218.

99. Kumar GN, Walle UK, Bhalla KN, Walle T. Binding of taxol to human plasma, albumin, and alpha 1-acid glycoprotein. Res Commun Chem Pathol Pharmacol 1993; 80:337–344.

100. Sparreboom A, Van Zuylen L, Brouwer E, et al. Cremophor EL-mediated alteration of paclitaxel distribution in human blood: clinical pharmacokinetic implications. Cancer Res 1999; 59:1454–1457.

101. Burke TG, Zoorob G, Slatter JG, Schaaf LF. In vitro protein binding of CPT-11 metabolites SN-38, SN-38 glucuronide (SN-38G), and APC and possible displacement by commonly used co-medications. Proc Am Soc Clin Oncol 1998; 17:195a (Abstr).

102. Ma M, Zamboni WC, Radomski KM, et al. Pharmacokinetics of irinotecan and its metabolites SN-38 and APC in children with recurrent solid tumors after protracted low-dose irinotecan. Clin Cancer Res 2000; 6:813–819.

103. Spila H, Nanto V, Kangas L, Anttila M, Halme T. Binding of toremifene to human serum proteins. Pharmacol Toxicol 1988; 63:62–64.

104. Shah IG, Parsons DL. Human albumin binding of tamoxifen in the presence of a perfluorochemical erythrocyte substitute. J Pharmaceut Pharmacol 1991; 43:790–793.

105. Petros WP, Rodman JH, Relling MV, et al. Variability in teniposide plasma protein binding is correlated with serum albumin concentrations. Pharmacotherapy 1992; 12:273–277.

106. Hagen B, Nilsen OG. The binding of thio-TEPA in human serum and to isolated serum protein fractions. Cancer Chemother Pharmacol 1987; 20:319–323.

107. Burke TG, Mi Z. The structural basis of camptothecin interactions with human serum albumin: impact on drug stability. J Med Chem 1994; 37:40–46.

108. Wall JG, Burris HA 3d, Von Hoff DD, et al. A phase I clinical and pharmacokinetic study of the topoisomerase I inhibitor topotecan (SK&F 104864) given as an intravenous bolus every 21 days. Anticancer Drugs 1992; 3:337–345.

109. Fanucchi MP, Walsh TD, Fleisher M, et al. Phase I and clinical pharmacology study of trimetrexate administered weekly for three weeks. Cancer Res 1987; 47:3303–3308.

110. Fuse E, Tanii H, Kurata N, et al. Unpredicted clinical pharmacology of UCN-01 caused by specific binding to human α_1-acid glycoprotein. Cancer Res 1998; 58:3248–3253.

111. Fuse E, Tanii H, Takai K, et al. Altered pharmacokinetics of a novel anticancer drug, UCN-01, caused by specific high affinity binding to α_1-acid glycoprotein in humans. Cancer Res 1999; 59:1054–1060.

112. Steele WH, Haughton DJ, Barber HE. Binding of vinblastine to recrystallized human alpha 1-acid glycoprotein. Cancer Chemother Pharmacol 1982; 10:40–42.

113. Steele WH, King DJ, Barber HE, Hawksworth GM, Dawson AA, Petrie JC. The protein binding of vinblastine in the serum of normal subjects and patients with Hodgkin's disease. Eur J Clin Pharmacol 1983; 24:683–687.

114. Urien S, Bree F, Breillout F, Bastian G, Krikorian A, Tillement JP. Vinorelbine high-affinity binding to human platelets and lymphocytes: distribution in human blood. Cancer Chemother Pharmacol 1993; 32:231–234.

115. Rolan PE. Plasma protein binding displacement interactions—why are they still regarded as clinically important? Br J Clin Pharmacol 1994; 37:125–128.

116. Sansom LN, Evans AM. What is the true clinical significance of plasma protein binding displacement interactions? Drugs Safety 1995; 12:227–233.

117. Schwinghammer TL, Fleming RA, Rosenfeld CS, et al. Disposition of total and unbound etoposide following high-dose therapy. Cancer Chemother Pharmacol 1993; 32:273–276.

118. Stewart CF, Arbuck SG, Fleming RA, et al. Changes in the clearance of total and unbound etoposide in patients with liver dysfunction. J Clin Oncol 1990; 8:1874–1879.

119. Fleming RA, Evans WE, Arbuck SG, et al. Factors affecting in vitro protein binding of etoposide in humans. J Pharmaceut Sci 1992; 81:259–263.

120. Stewart CF, Fleming RA, Arbuck SG, et al. Prospective evaluation of a model for predicting etoposide plasma protein binding in cancer patients. Cancer Res 1990; 50:6854–6857.

121. Stewart CF, Arbuck SG, Fleming RA, et al. Relation of systemic exposure to unbound etoposide and hematologic toxicity. Clin Pharmacol Ther 1991; 50:385–390.

122. Joel SP, Shah R, Slevin ML. Etoposide dosage and pharmacodynamics. Cancer Chemother Pharmacol 1994; 34:69–75.

123. Evans WE, Rodman JH, Relling MV, et al. Differences in teniposide disposition and pharmacodynamics in patients with newly diagnosed and relapsed acute lymphoblastic leukemia. J Pharmacol Exp Ther 1992; 260:71–79.

124. DeConti RC, Toftness BR, Lange RC, Creasey WA. Clinical and pharmacological studies with *cis*-diamminedichloroplatinum (II). Cancer Res 1973; 333:1310–1315.

125. Gullo JJ, Litterst CL, Maguire PJ, Sikic BI, Hoth DF, Woolley PV. Pharmacokinetics and protein binding of *cis*-dichlorodiammine platinum (II) administered as a one hour or as a twenty hour infusion. Cancer Chemother Pharmacol 1980; 5:21–26.

126. Perera F, Fischman HK, Hemminki K, et al. Protein binding, sister chromatid exchange and expression of oncogene proteins in patients treated with cisplatinum (cisDDP)-based chemotherapy. Arch Toxicol 1990; 64:401–406.

127. Takada K, Kawamura T, Inai M, et al. Irreversible binding of cisplatin in rat serum. Pharmaceut Pharmacol Commun 1999; 5:449–453.

128. Canal P. Platinum compounds: pharmacokinetics and pharmacodynamics. In: Grochow LB, Ames MM (eds). A Clinician's Guide to Chemotherapy Pharmacokinetics and Pharmacodynamics. Baltimore: Williams & Williams, 1998, pp. 345–374.

129. Rahman A, Treat J, Roh JK, et al. A phase I clinical trial and pharmacokinetic evaluation of liposome-encapsulated doxorubicin. J Clin Oncol 1990; 8:1093–1100.

130. Cowens JW, Creaven PJ, Greco WR, et al. Initial clinical (phase I) trial of TLC D-99 (doxorubicin encapsulated in liposomes). Cancer Res 1993; 53:2796–2802.

131. Gelmon KA, Tolcher A, Diab AR, et al. Phase I study of liposomal vincristine. J Clin Oncol 1999; 17:697–705.

132. Druckmann S, Gabizon A, Barenholtz Y. Separation of liposome-associated doxorubicin from non-liposome-associated doxorubicin in human plasma: implications for pharmacokinetic studies. Biochim Biophys Acta 1989; 980:381–384.

133. Gabizon A, Catane R, Uziely B, et al. Prolonged circulation time and enhanced accumulation in malignant exudates of doxorubicin encapsulated in polyethylene-glycol coated liposomes. Cancer Res 1994; 54:987–992.

134. Thies RL, Cowens DW, Cullis PR, Bally MB, Mayer LD. Method for rapid separation of liposome-associated doxorubicin from free doxorubicin in plasma. Analyt Biochem 1990; 188:65–71.

135. Mayer LD, St.-Onge G. Determination of free and liposome-associated doxorubicin and vincristine levels in plasma under equilibrium conditions employing ultrafiltration techniques. Analyt Biochem 1995; 232:149–157.

136. Srigritsanapol AA, Chan KK. A rapid method for the separation and analysis of leaked and liposomal entrapped phosphoramide mustard in plasma J Pharmaceut Biomed Anal 1994; 12:961–968.

137. Dipali SR, Kulkarni SB, Betageri GV. Comparative study of separation of non-encapsulated drug from unilamellar liposomes by various methods. J Pharmaceut Pharmacol 1996; 48:1112–1115.

138. Van Zuylen L, Karlsson MO, Verweij J, et al. Pharmacokinetic modeling of paclitaxel encapsulation in Cremophor EL micelles. Cancer Chemother Pharmacol 2001; 47:309–318.

139. Van Zuylen L, Gianni L, Verweij J, et al. Interrelationships of paclitaxel disposition, infusion duration and Cremophor EL kinetics in cancer patients. Anticancer Drugs 2000; 11:331–337.

140. Brouwer E, Verweij J, De Bruijn P, et al. Measurement of fraction unbound paclitaxel in human plasma. Drug Metab Dispos 2000; 28:1141–1145.

141. Henningsson A, Karlsson MO, Vigano L, et al. Mechanism based pharmacokinetic model for paclitaxel. J Clin Oncol 2001; 19:4065–4073.

142. Kehrer DFS, Soepenberg O, Loos WJ, Verweij J, Sparreboom A. Modulation of camptothecin analogues in the treatment of cancer: a review. Anticancer Drugs 2001; 12:89–106.

143. Mi Z, Burke TG. Differential interactions of camptothecin lactone and carboxylate forms with human blood components. Biochemistry 1994; 33:10,325–10,326.

144. Mi Z, Malak H, Burke TG. Reduced albumin binding promotes the stability and activity of topotecan in human blood. Biochemistry 1995; 34:13,722–13,728.

145. Mi Z, Burke TG. Marked interspecies variations concerning the interactions of camptothecin with serum albumins: a frequency-domain fluorescence spectroscopic study. Biochemistry 1994; 33: 12,540–12,545.

146. Loos WJ, Verweij J, Gelderblom AJ, et al. Role of erythrocytes and serum proteins in the kinetic profiles of total 9-amino-20(S)-camptothecin in humans. Anticancer Drugs 1999; 10:705–710.

147. De Jonge MJA, Verweij J, Loos WJ, Dallaire BK, Sparreboom A. Clinical pharmacokinetics of oral 9-aminocamptothecin in plasma and saliva. Clin Pharmacol Ther 1999; 65:491–499.

148. Loos WJ, De Bruijn P, Verweij J, Sparreboom A. Determination of camptothecin analogues in biological matrices by high-performance liquid chromatography. Anticancer Drugs 2000; 11:315–324.

149. Hervé F, Urien S, Albengres E, Duché JC, Tillement JP. Drug binding in plasma. A summary of recent trends in the study of drug and hormone binding. Clin Pharmacokinet 1994; 26:44–58.

150. Roberts SA. High-throughput screening approaches for investigating drug metabolism and pharmacokinetics. Xenobiotica 2001; 31:557–589.

13 Metabolism (Non-CYP Enzymes)

Sally A. Coulthard, PhD and Alan V. Boddy, PhD

CONTENTS

INTRODUCTION
PHASE I REACTIONS
PHASE II REACTIONS
CONCLUSIONS

1. INTRODUCTION

1.1. Scope

Drug metabolism is relevant to the pharmacology of anticancer drugs to the extent that it influences the delivery of active drug species to the tumor or to sites of potential toxicity (Fig. 1). The chemical modification of xenobiotics may be viewed as a means to increase the hydrophilic nature of the substrate molecule or to introduce chemical substituent moieties, which are then better substrates for subsequent conjugation. Although the division is not absolute, these reactions may be characterized as chemical modification (phase I) or conjugation reactions (phase II). A significant proportion of phase I reactions are oxidative, and the majority of oxidative metabolic reactions are mediated by the cytochrome P450 (CYP) superfamily of enzymes. The CYP enzymes are the subject of the next chapter.

A number of phase I metabolic reactions, both oxidative and nonoxidative, are mediated by enzymes other than those in the P450 family. These include oxidases, reductases, dehydrogenases, methyltransferases, and esterases. The phase II conjugation reactions are catalyzed by transferase enzymes that attach glucuronyl, glutathione, sulfonyl, or acetyl groups to suitable substrate sites on the drug molecule. These enzymes are named for their function, rather than for their membership in a genetically homologous family of proteins. For a given reaction, there do exist different genetically related isoforms, such as the UGT family of UDP-glucuronlytransferases.

1.2. Potential Influence

Drug metabolism is primarily a process of drug inactivation, the resulting metabolites being both less active than the parent compound and more rapidly eliminated from the body. The implication for metabolic reactions of this type is that individuals who have low or absent enzyme activity for a particular reaction will be at increased risk of unacceptable toxicity. Conversely, individuals in whom the relevant enzyme is highly active or induced will inactivate the drug faster, and so will have a lower probability of responding to treatment.

Handbook of Anticancer Pharmacokinetics and Pharmacodynamics
Edited by: W. D. Figg and H. L. McLeod © Humana Press Inc., Totowa, NJ

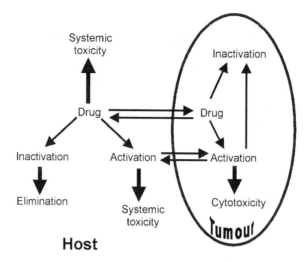

Fig. 1. Potential role for non-CYP metabolism in the pharmacology of chemotherapeutic agents. Pathways for drug activation and inactivation in the host and tumor tissues.

Exceptions to this general rule of inactivating metabolism include prodrugs, such as irinotecan, which is cleaved by esterases to yield an active metabolite. There are also examples of drugs whose metabolites have clinically significant potency, or where metabolites are more toxic than the parent drug. These exceptions will be discussed in detail where appropriate.

The chapter is organized according to the division between phase I and phase II reactions, with subsections on enzymes classified by the type of reaction catalyzed or on specific enzymes with a limited or exclusive substrate specificity. Issues of drug inhibition and induction and the genetics of each of the enzymes will be discussed where relevant and where sufficient characterization of the enzyme has been performed.

2. PHASE I REACTIONS

2.1. Non-CYP Oxidation

2.1.2. ALDEHYDE DEHYDROGENASE

The ALDH family of enzymes comprises more than 15 members, with a number of associated pseudogenes (1). The primary function of ALDH is to oxidize potentially toxic aldehydes to carboxylic acids, which are either excreted directly or are substrates for phase II conjugation reactions. ALDH enzymes can be either cytosolic or mitochondrial, and can use NAD or NADP as cofactors. Expression of ALDH varies for the different isoforms, but ALDH1A1 and ALDH3A1 are expressed mainly in the brain, heart, liver, kidney, and lung. ALDH expression and activity has also been found in tumors.

The most significant role for ALDH enzymes in the pharmacology of chemotherapeutic agents is probably interruption of the activation pathway of cyclophosphamide and ifosfamide. The activation of these oxazaphosphorines is initiated by CYP450-mediated 4-hydroxylation, tautomerization to an aldehyde intermediate, and spontaneous release of DNA-alkylating species (Fig. 2). The aldehyde intermediate is oxidized by ALDH enzymes to an inactive carboxylic acid.

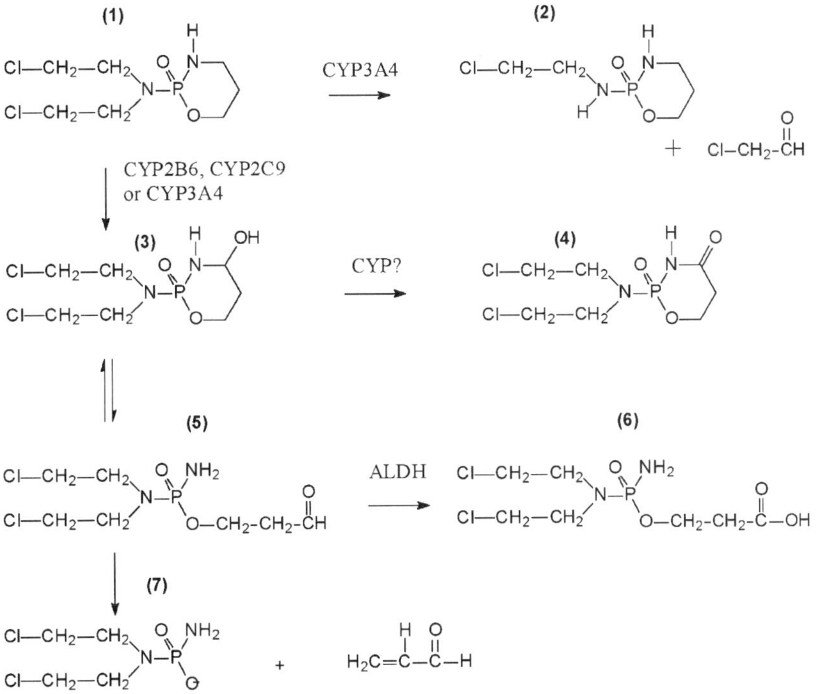

Fig. 2. Metabolism of cyclophosphamide (1), showing inactivation of aldophosphamide (5) by ALDH enzymes to the inactive carboxy form (6). Oxidation to inactive dechloroethyl (2) and keto (4) metabolites and to active 4-hydroxy (3) and phosphoramide mustard (7) forms mediated by cytochrome P450 enzymes.

The role of ALDH in inactivating the intermediate aldophosphamide was identified 10 yr ago (2,3), leading to the identification of ALDH expression in tumors (4) and erythrocytes (5) and the suggestion that ALDH might confer protection to bone marrow following gene transfection (6). ALDH1 and ALDH3 isoforms are primarily responsible for resistance to oxazaphosphorines, which may be reversed by the ALDH inhibitor disulfiram. Antisense oligonucleotides to ALDH1 suppress enzyme activity and increase sensitivity of K562 or A549 cells to 4-hydroxycyclophosphamide (7). Prediction of tumor sensitivity, according to expression of ALDH1A1 and ALDH3A1 in primary breast tumor, has been suggested as a means to individualize therapy (8). In addition to regulation by a number of exogenous factors, treatment with cyclophosphamide has been shown to decrease ALDH1 activity in erythrocytes (9).

Another DNA-alkylating drug, procarbazine, is activated to azoxy-intermediate metabolites. These azoxy compounds are substrates for and are inactivated by both ALDH and xanthine oxidase (XO) (10).

The role of ALDH1A isoforms enzyme in the synthesis of retinoic acids (11) is intriguing, given the differentiating and even cytotoxic effects of retinoids against some tumors. In turn, retinoic acid receptors regulate the expression of ALDH (12), and so retinoid levels in tumors may influence the degree of inactivation of oxazaphosphorines.

A genetic polymorphism in ALDH3A1 has been described (13). The relevance of this for cyclophosphamide or procarbazine inactivation has not been fully elucidated.

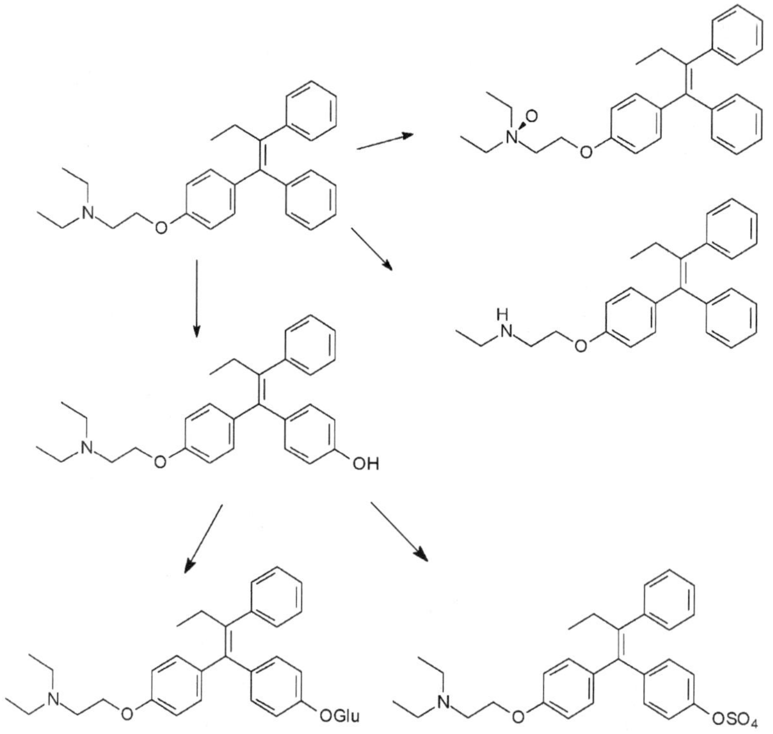

Fig. 3. Metabolism of tamoxifen, including *N*-oxidation by FMO. Competing reactions include CYP-mediated *N*-demethylation and 4-hydroxylation. The latter is followed by phase II conjugation by either glucuronsyl (UGT) or sulfonyl (SULT) transferases.

2.1.2. FLAVIN-CONTAINING MONO-OXYGENASES

These enzymes are involved in a number of oxidation reactions, and have some overlap in terms of substrate specificity with CYP isoforms. The only significant action of flavin-containing mono-oxygenases (FMOs) with relevance to the pharmacology of cancer treatment is the N-oxidation of tamoxifen (Fig. 3) *(14,15)*, which is associated with activation to a reactive carcinogen. This reaction is mediated principally by FMO3 *(16)*, which is highly expressed in the liver *(17)*. Genetic variants of FMO3 with reduced oxidation activity have been reported *(18)*.

2.1.3. XANTHINE OXIDOREDUCTASE (XOR)

XOR is a collective term for two forms of the same gene product. *Xanthine dehydrogenase* exists as a homodimer, and can readily be converted to *xanthine oxidase* by oxidation of essential thiol residues, followed by protease cleavage of a 20 kDa subunit from each monomer *(19)*. The endogenous substrate for XOR is xanthine, resulting ultimately in oxidation to uric acid, with corresponding reduction of NAD+. Xenobiotic substrates include purines, pyrimidines, heterocycles, and aldehydes *(20)*.

XOR can activate the bioreductive class of drugs, the prototype of which is mitomycin C (Fig. 4) *(21)*. This area is discussed in more detail in the section on NQO1. Other cancer chemotherapy agents that are substrates for XOR include doxorubicin, which may be activated to reactive oxygen species under aerobic conditions *(22)* or inactivated to an aglycone, under hypoxic conditions (Fig. 5) *(23)*.

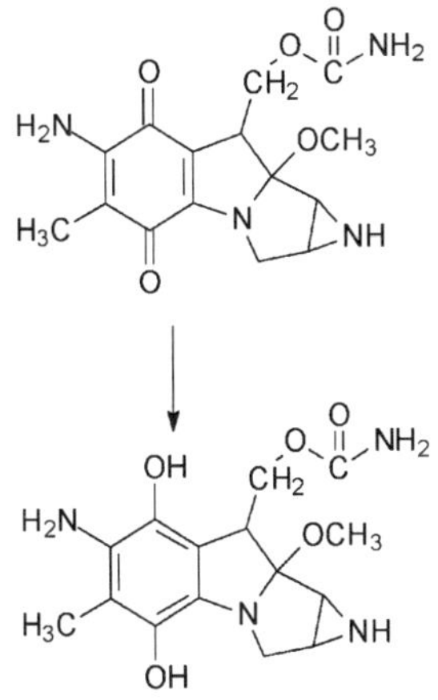

Fig. 4. Activation of mitomycin C by two-electron redution.

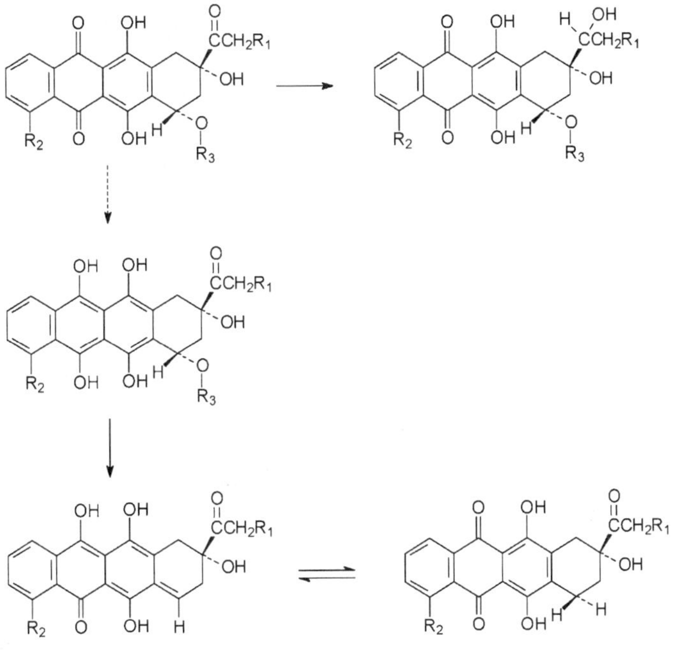

	R_1	R_2	R_3
Doxorubicin	—CH$_2$OH	—OCH$_3$	
Daunorubicin	—CH$_3$	—OCH$_3$	
Idarubicin	—CH$_3$	—H	
Epirubicin	—CH$_2$OH	—OCH$_3$	

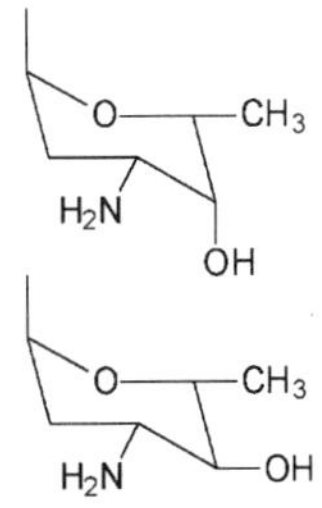

Fig. 5. Metabolism of anthracyclines. Illustrated are both ketone reduction by carbonylreductase enzymes and quinone reduction to hydroquinones by reductase enzymes.

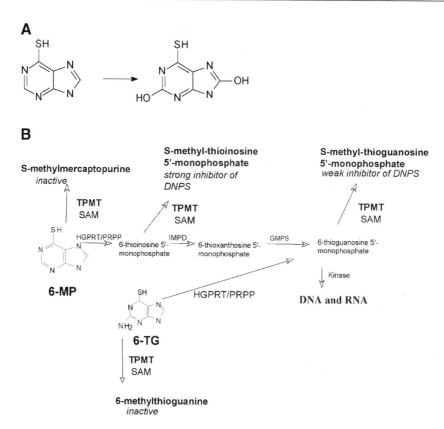

Fig. 6. (**A**) Metabolism of 6-mercaptopurine by xanthine oxidase to thiouric acid. (**B**) Metabolism of 6-MP and 6-TG in human ALL cells. PRPP, 5'-Phosphoribosyl-l-pyrophosphate; GMPS, guanosine monophosphate synthase; HGPRT, hypoxanthine guanine phosphoribosyltransferase; IMPD, inosine monophosphate dehydrogenase; SAM, S-adenosine-L-methionine; TPMT, thiopurine methyltransferase; AO, aldehyde oxidase; 8-OHTG, 8-hydroxythioguanine; XO, xanthine oxidase, TGN, thioguanine nucleotides; TIMP, thioinosine 5'-monophosphate; TXMP, thioxanthine monophosphate; TGMP, thioguanine monophosphate; MeTG methylthioguanine; MeMP, methylmercaptopurine.

For purine analogs, which are cytotoxic by incorporation into DNA or by inhibition of *de novo* purine synthesis, xanthine oxidase (XO) may mediate an important inactivating pathway of metabolism. For 6-mercaptopurine (6-MP) (see Subheading 2.3. on TPMT), XO catalyzes the formation of thioxanthine and thiouric acid (Fig. 6). Coadministration of the XO inhibitor allopurinol, which may be clinically indicated in lymphomas, results in impaired metabolism of 6-MP *(24)*. Also, the activity of XO may be linked to the degree of leukopenia observed after 6-MP treatment *(25)*. An additional consideration for XO metabolism of 6-MP is that concurrent treatment with methotrexate increases the plasma concentration of 6-MP after oral dosing *(26)*. Methotrexate 7-hydroxylation is mediated by XO *(27)*, which may explain the interaction with 6-MP. Activity of XO is low in extrahepatic tissues including circulating blood cells and in the bone marrow and is therefore unlikely to affect the activity of the thiopurine drugs in the lymphocytes *(28–30)*.

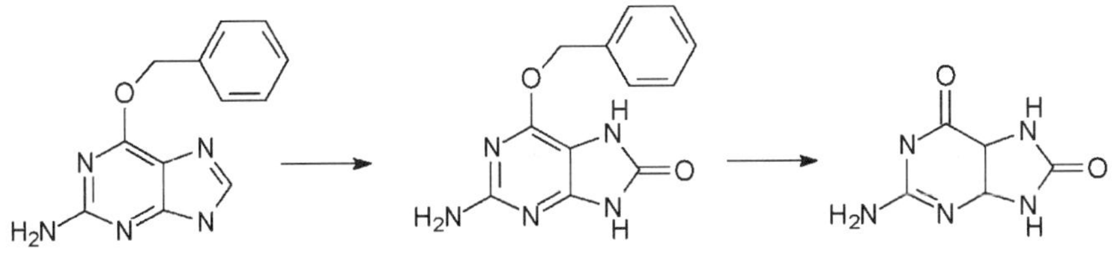

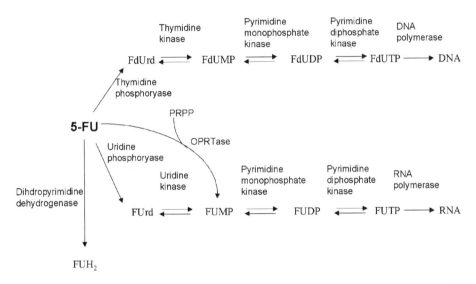

Fig. 7. Formation of 8-oxo-6-benzyl-guanine from O^6-benzylguanine by aldehyde oxidase and subsequent debenzylation.

Fig. 8. Intracellular activation of 5-FU, 5-fluorouracil, FdUrd, 5-fluorouridine; FdUMP, fluorodeoxyuridylate; FdUDP, fluorodeoxyuridine diphosphate; FdUTP, fluorodeoxyuridine triphosphate; FUrd, 5-fluoro-2'deoxyuridine; FUMP, fluorouridine monophosphate; FUDP, fluorouridine diphosphate; FUTP, fluorouridine triphosphate; FUH_2, dihydrofluorouridine; PPRP, phosphoribosyl phosphate.

2.1.4. ALDEHYDE OXIDASE

This enzyme may play a role in the formation of 7-hydroxymethotrexate *(27)* or of *O*-6-benzyl-8-oxoguanine (Fig. 7) *(31)*. The latter is the major metabolite of *O*-6-benzylguanine, an inhibitor of methylguanine methyltransferase which is responsible for the repair of DNA alkylation *(32)*.

2.2. Dihydropyrimidine Dehydrogenase

Dihydropyrimidine dehydrogenase (also known as dihydrouracil dehydrogenase, dihydrothymine dehydrogenase, uracil reductase, DPD, or DYPD; EC. 1.3.1.2) is the initial and rate-limiting enzyme in the three-step pathway of uracil and thymidine catabolism, leading to the formation of β-alanine *(33)*. Individuals who are deficient in this enzyme present with a nonspecific clinical picture of cerebral dysfunction and persistent urinary excretion of excessive uracil, thymine, and 5-hydroxymethyluracil. DPD is also the principal enzyme involved in the degradation of the chemotherapeutic agent 5-fluorouracil (5-FU or 5-FUra) *(34)*. DPD converts over 80–85% of 5-FU to dihydro-5-fluorouracil (5-FUH_2), an inactive metabolite (Fig. 8).

5-FU undergoes anabolism to cytotoxic nucleotides, 5-fluoro-2'-deoxyuridine 5'-mono-phosphate (FdUMP), fluorouridine triphosphate (FUTP), and fluorodeoxyuridine triphos-phate (FdUTP). FdUMP forms a stable covalent complex with 5,10-methylenetetrahydrofolate and thymidylate synthase (TS), thereby blocking the formation of dTMP (35). Consequently, there is depletion of dTTP, which is needed for both DNA synthesis and repair. FUTP and FdUTP are misincorporated into RNA or DNA respectively.

The liver has the highest DPD activity (mean, 705 n*M*/g tissue/h using 5-FU as the substrate), with minimal activity found in the kidneys, spleen, lung, colon, colon tumors, pancreas, breast tissue, breast tumors, bone marrow cells, and peripheral leukemic cells (36). DPD activity has also been reported in a significant proportion of malignant cells (37). DPD activity in both peripheral blood mononuclear cells and liver from normal individuals shows no significant difference with respect to age, gender, or race (38). In blood the highest level of DPD is found in monocytes, followed by that of lymphocytes, granulocytes, and platelets, whereas no activity could be found in erythrocytes (39).

Within both healthy populations and cancer patients a large degree of variation (8- to 21-fold) in peripheral blood mononuclear cell DPD activity has been observed (38,40–42). The frequencies of low and deficient DPD activity in the general population are estimated to be 3–5% and 0.1%, respectively (38,40). Family studies conducted with one of the initial patients with DPD deficiency suggested an autosomal-recessive pattern of inheritance (43). With the availability of genotyping tests, it has now been confirmed that DPD has an auto-somal codominant pattern of inheritance.

The *DPD* gene is over 950 kb containing 23 exons with about 3 kb of coding region (44–46) and has been located to chromosome 1p22 (47). To date at least 21 variant alleles have been describe in the gene coding for *DPD* (48–54). *DPYD*∗2A, a G to A mutation in the 5' splicing recognition sequence of intron 14, results in a 165 bp deletion of exon 14 and translation to a truncated protein. This is the most widely reported mutation associated with DPD deficiency (54).

5-FU was introduced as a chemotherapeutic agent over 40 yr ago and remains one of the most widely prescribed cancer chemotherapy drugs for the treatment of cancers of the digestive tract, breast, and head and neck (55). Following administration, about 85% of it undergoes catabolism via DPD into biologically inactive metabolites that are excreted in the urine and the bile (56,57). Plasma clearance of 5-FU is directly proportional to activity of DPD in peripheral blood lymphocytes (58). This is likely to be of clinical significance, as plasma 5-FU levels have been related to clinical outcome in patients with head and neck cancer (59). In addition, tumor DPD activity has been shown to influence response to treat-ment in this tumor type (60).

As the liver is the major site for catabolism of 5-FU by DPD, the majority of an oral dose of 5-FU is subject to first-pass metabolism reducing its bioavailability. After intravenous administration, 5-FU is rapidly eliminated with a half-life of 8–14 min. Administration protocols that use continuous infusion provide consistent exposure to 5-FU and continuous inhibition of the target enzyme TS (61). Continuous infusion schedules, with chronomodulation of infusion rate, may also overcome diurnal variation in DPD activity (62).

Strategies to modulate the anabolic and catabolic metabolism of 5-FU have been devel-oped. These treatment strategies fall into three main categories:

1. 5-FU prodrugs.
2. 5-FU combined with a DPD inhibitor.
3. 5-FU pro-drugs combined with a DPD inhibitor.

These approaches allow oral dosing, as 5-FU is then eliminated almost entirely by renal excretion, and plasma concentrations may be more consistent than with intravenous 5-FU

(63,64). 5-FU prodrugs include ftorafur (Tegafur) *(R,S*-1-1[tetrahydrofuran-2-yl]-5-FU) and capecitabine (*N*-4-pentyloxycarbonyl-5'-deoxy-5-fluorocytidine; Xeloda). DPD inhibitors include eniluracil or 5-ethynyluracil (5-EU) (a uracil analogue) which increases the bioavailability of 5-FU to approx 100% *(65–67)*.

S-1 is a combination of ftorafur and two 5-FU modulators, 3-cyano-2,6-dihydroxy-pyridine (CDHP) and oxonic acid, in a molar ratio1:0.4:1. CDHP is a competitive, reversible DPD inhibitor that prolongs the half-life of 5-FU. Oxonic acid is a pyrimidine phosphoribosyltransferase inhibitor that is intended to mitigate 5-FU-related gastrointestinal toxicity by preventing the phosphorylation of 5-FU in the digestive tract. Pharmacokinetic studies with S-1 have shown consistent release of 5-FU *(68,69)*, and demonstrated clinical activity *(70)*.

BOF A-2 (Emitefur) and UFT are examples of a 5-FU prodrug combined with a DPD inhibitor. In the case of BOF A-2, the 5-FU prodrug is 1-ethoxymethyl 5-FU and the DPD inhibitor is CDHP (combined in a molar ratio of 1:1). UFT comprises the prodrug of 5-FU, ftorafur and the DPD inhibitor uracil in a molar ratio of 1:4. Both of these approaches produce consistent 5-FU concentrations in plasma *(71–73)*.

The fluorinated pyrimidines have played a major role in the treatment of many common tumors since the introduction of 5-FU almost 40 yr ago. Understanding of the pharmacogenetics and enzymology of DPD has permitted the development of strategies to improve the efficacy of 5-FU. These have included the use of biochemical modulators such as folinic acid and the use of either administration of oral inactive 5-FU prodrugs or the administration of 5-FU with inhibitors of the enzyme DPD.

2.3. Thiopurine Methyltransferase

Thiopurine methyltransferase (TPMT) (EC 2.1.1.67) is an enzyme that is found in red blood cell (RBC) lysate, lymphocytes, kidney, liver, lung, and intestine *(74)*. TPMT catalyses the methylation of aromatic heterocyclic sulfydryl compounds including the thiopurine drugs, 6-mercaptopurine (6-MP), its prodrug azathioprine, and 6-thioguanine (6-TG), which are commonly used cytotoxic agents and immunosuppressants *(75,76)*. TPMT shows a trimodal activity pattern with about one in 300 individuals having no TPMT activity at all. Deficiency of TPMT does not have any impact in a healthy individual, which makes its normal function hard to discern.

The importance of understanding the role of TPMT in drug metabolism is that 6-MP has, since the early 1950s, been used extensively in the continuing treatment of childhood leukemia. 6-MP and 6-TG were first synthesized by Gertrude Elion and George Hitchins, who found that the substitution of oxygen by sulfur at the 6-position of guanine and hypoxanthine produced inhibitors of purine utilization. 6-MP and 6-TG were found to be active against a wide spectrum of rodent tumors and in children with acute lymphoblastic leukemia (ALL). At that time, children with ALL had a life expectancy of only a few months. 6-MP could produce temporary complete remission of ALL, leading the Food and Drug Administration (USA) to approve the drug for use in 1953. 6-TG and 6-MP are still used today in the treatment of leukemia, and azathioprine is still used as an immunosupressant in transplant therapy.

TPMT activity was first described in 1963 *(75)*, but it was not until 1980 that the first report on the trimodal distribution pattern of red blood cell TPMT activity was published *(77)*. TPMT activity has since been shown to be the same in both RBC lysate and lymphoblasts *(78–80)*. Kidney TPMT levels also reflect RBC lysate activity *(81,82)*. Adult liver TPMT activity (105 ± 57 pmol/min/mg of protein) is twofold higher than in the intestine and the kidney, threefold higher than in the lungs, and about fivefold higher than in the brain *(74)*.

In the human fetus, liver TPMT activity has been found to be about one-third that of adult liver and is similar to that of fetal kidney, lung, and intestine *(74)*. TPMT activity in RBC in neonates is about 50% higher than that of adults, although the trimodal distribution pattern seen in adults is still apparent *(83)*. From the age of 2, children have TPMT activities very similar to those of adults *(84)*.

The *TPMT* gene, which is situated on chromosome 6p22.3, encodes a 245-amino-acid protein with a predicted molecular mass of 35 kDa. The gene was originally reported to be approx 34 kb in length *(85)*; this has since been modified to 25 kb with minor sequence differences *(86)*. The underlying genetic reason for the variation in enzyme activity is the presence of single nucleotide polymorphisms (SNPs) in the *TPMT* gene (*87* and references cited therein).

The frequency of SNPs is related to ethnicity, with the most common being *TPMT*∗3A in Caucasians. *TPMT*∗3A is characterized by a G to A transition at position 460 with a substitution of alanine for tyrosine at amino acid 154 (A154Y) and a transition of A to G at nucleotide 719 resulting in a change of tyrosine to cysteine at position 240 (Y240C) *(85,88)*. Individuals who are heterozygous for *TPMT*∗3A have intermediate TPMT activity, but if base changes are present on both alleles no TPMT activity is detected (reviewed in *89*). Polymorphisms have also been identified within the 5' flanking promoter region of the *TPMT* gene due to a variable number of tandem repeats (VNTR∗3–∗8) *(85,86,90)*.

In addition to *S*-methylation by TPMT, 6-MP and 6-TG are also metabolized by xanthine oxidase (XO), hypoxanthine-guanine phosphoribosyl transferase (HGPRT), and aldehyde oxidase (AO) (Fig. 6A, B).

Together with the immunosupressant azathioprine, these three drugs were designed as purine analogs to disrupt normal DNA synthesis and as such are metabolized by the same pathways that control normal nucleotide homeostasis. They are administered orally and undergo first-pass metabolism in the liver. Azathioprine is rapidly converted to 6-MP. 6-MP and 6-TG are both oxidized by XO in the intestinal mucosa and in the liver, where XO activity is high. Also, 6-TG methylation by TPMT produces an inactive metabolite *S*-methylthioguanosine, whereas metabolism of 6-MP by TPMT also produces the inactive compound *S*-methylmercaptopurine. TPMT is subject to non-competitive inhibition by sulfasalazine and its metabolite 5-aminosalicylic acid (ASA), olsalzine and olsalazine-O-sulfate, drugs that are used in the treatment of inflammatory bowel disease *(91)*.

In order to exert a cytotoxic effect, both 6-MP and 6-TG require activation by HGPRT and/or TPMT (Fig. 6B). Metabolism of 6-TG by HGPRT produces 6-thioguanosine 5'-monophosphate (6-TGMP), which is further metabolized by a series of kinases and reductases to produce deoxy-6-thioguanosine 5'-triphosphate (dTGTP). Incorporation of dTGTP into DNA has been shown to be recognized by the mismatch repair pathway *(92)*. 6-MP is metabolized by HGPRT to 6-thio-inosine monophosphate (TIMP), which is converted by guanosine monophosphate synthetase to thioguanosine 5'-monophosphate (TGMP). TGMP is subsequently incorporated into the DNA as a fraudulent base.

As discussed above, TPMT shows a high degree of variation in activity and therefore has a direct impact on the cytotoxicity of these drugs. Thioguanine nucleotides (TGNs), and their subsequent incorporation into DNA and RNA, have been thought to be the main cause of cytotoxicity in patients treated with 6-MP and 6-TG *(93)*. Formation of TGNs in the RBC of patients treated with 6-MP is related to myelosuppression *(94)* and the level of TGN production is inversely proportional to TPMT activity *(84,95,96)*. In children with ALL, the TPMT activity in RBC lysate at diagnosis reflects that of the lymphoblasts *(79,80)*, and is increased during treatment, reverting to pretreatment levels after 6-MP therapy is stopped *(84,95)*. As yet the significance of this and the mechanism by which it occurs is not known.

Patients with low TPMT activity may be treated using individualized doses of 6-MP, for example, at 10% of the normal dose on alternate days *(97–101)*. Continuity of treatment, even at low doses, is most important for treatment outcome *(102)*.

Recently, evidence has emerged to suggest that TGN incorporation into the DNA is not the sole cause of cell death after 6-MP. In two papers a role for inhibition of de novo purine synthesis (DNPS) has been demonstrated, as higher TPMT levels were associated with a greater degree of cytotoxicity *(87,103)*. With 6-TG, the chief mode of cytotoxic action was found to be incorporation of TGNs into DNA. Thus, the modes of cell death with 6-MP and 6-TG are not entirely the same and may be dependent on an individual's TPMT activity. This hypothesis is supported by other observations on the cellular pharmacology of 6-MP and 6-TG *(99,104–106)*.

In most cases the thiopurine drugs are extremely well tolerated, although it is frequently difficult to maintain patients on a stable dose. This is partly because the normal route of administration is by mouth, and this introduces the variables of compliance and absorption *(107,108)*. The pharmacogenetics of TPMT introduces a further source of variability and indicates a need for dose individualization. Some centers now routinely assess RBC TPMT activity, and pretreatment assessment has become mandatory in some instances. Elsewhere, physicians have preferred to rely on the monitoring of the white cell count after initiation of therapy *(109)*. However, the onset of neutropenia can be very swift and life threatening in patients homozygous for inactivating alleles of TPMT. Assessment of TPMT status prior to treatment could save unnecessary toxicity, which would otherwise compromise successful treatment of leukemia.

2.4. Epoxide Hydrolase

Microsomal epoxide hydrolase (mEH or EPX1) is a member of a class of hydrolytic enzymes, many of which act on endogenous substrates such as leukotrienes and fatty acids. They may also metabolize carcinogens or procarcinogens *(110)*. A cytosolic form of epoxide hydrolase, EPX2, has also been described *(111)*. Variations in exon 3 of the *EPX1* gene may result in an increased susceptibility to lymphoma *(112)*, and variant forms of *EPX1* and *EPX2* have been described *(113)*.

There are few examples of EPX1 substrates among chemotherapeutic drugs, but one recently introduced agent is epothilone B. The metabolic pathways of epothilone have mainly focused on the hydrolysis of the ring ester (Fig. 9), but hydrolysis of the epoxide is always seen in the metabolites identified to date *(114)*.

Expression of EPX1 in tumors, including breast *(115)* and prostate *(116)*, has been reported, but may be no higher than that seen in peritumoral tissues *(117)*.

2.5. Reductases

2.5.1. CARBONYL REDUCTASE

The major pathway of metabolism for the anthracycline class of topoisomerase II poisons is via reduction of the keto group on carbon 13 (Fig. 5). This reaction is mediated by a carbonyl reductase member of the short-chain dehydrogenase/reductase (SDR) family of enzymes. CBR1 is a monomeric, cytosolic protein, expressed in a variety of tissues, including liver, GI tract, epidermis, CNS, kidney, and cardiac muscle *(118)*. A variant form, from the same chromosomal location (21q22.13) is CBR3 *(119)*.

Doxorubicinol, the alcohol metabolite of doxorubicin, is relatively inactive compared to the parent compound. Nevertheless, doxorubicinol concentrations in plasma can exceed those of doxorubicin, and the metabolite has a half-life similar to that of the parent *(120)*. The situation is similar for daunorubicin *(121)*. Epirubicin is a substrate for CBR *(122,123)*,

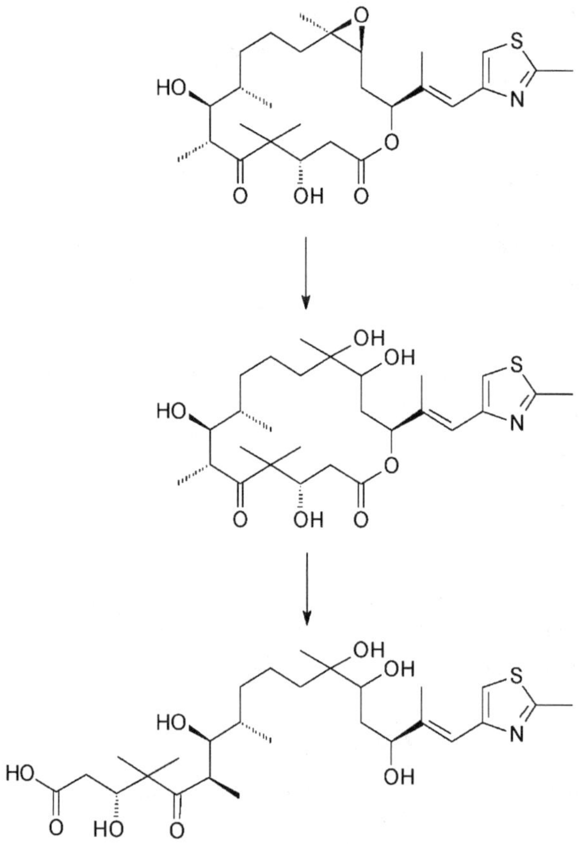

Fig. 9. Metabolism of epothilone B by epoxide hydrolase and by esterases. It is possible that esterase cleavage occurs prior to epoxide hydrolysis.

but epirubicinol is rapidly glucuronidated (see below). The concentrations of idarubicinol after administration of idarubicin are relatively high *(124)*, and idarubicinol retains equivalent or greater pharmacological potency than the parent *(125)*.

Tumor activity of CBR has been associated with resistance to anthracyclines treatment *(126–128)*. Conversely, formation of alcohol metabolites of anthracyclines has been associated with cumulative anthracycline-induced cardiotoxicity *(129)*.

2.5.2. NQO1

Also known as DT-diaphorase, NQO1 is an obligate two-electron reductase that can use either NADH or NADPH as cofactor. The gene encoding NQO1 is situated on chromosome 16, and a polymorphism resulting in a proline to serine amino acid substitution has been described *(130)*. This results in a protein that is more rapidly degraded via polyubiquitination *(131)*.

In reducing quinones to hydroquinones, NQO1 primarily acts to inactivate potential carcinogens. However, some hydroquinones are reactive, alkylating nucleophilic sites such as those on DNA *(132)*. The bioreductive class of alkylating agents exploits this mechanism to deliver alkylating species to tissues, such as tumor cells, where hypoxia and expression of NQO1 favor this pathway. Mitomycin C (Fig. 4) is the prototype drug of this class *(133)*. Other reductive enzymes, including xanthine oxidoreductase (see above), and cytochrome

P450 reductase *(134)* have been suggested to play a role in mitomycin C activation, but NQO1 appears to play a dominant role. Other drugs that have been designed specifically to be activated by bioreduction include EO9 *(135,136)* and RH1 *(137)*.

In terms of the pharmacokinetics of bioreductive agents, the rapid elimination of EO9 in humans *(138)* may be related to metabolism by NQO1. The pharmacokinetics of mitomycin C have not been extensively investigated after systemic administration. More information is available for intravesical administration of mitomycin C *(139)*, but the influence of NQO1 expression has not been determined. A genetic polymorphism has been described for NQO1, with those individuals homozygous for the variant form having low or absent NQO1 activity owing to more rapid protein degradation *(140)*. Whether this pharmacogenetic influence affects the systemic pharmacology of mitomycin C is unknown, however, the activity of NQO1 in peritoneal tumors was lower in individuals heterozygous or homozygous mutant for this polymorphism *(141)*. This reduction in tumor enzyme activity resulted in a worse response to hyperthermic intraperitoneal mitomycin C treatment *(141)*.

Recently, NQO1 has been found to influence the systemic and cellular pharmacology of 17-acetylamino-17-demethoxygeldanomycin (17AAG) *(142)*, which binds to HSP90 and disrupts the function of ErbB2 pathways, although studies in vitro suggest that the role for NQO1 may be limited *(143)*.

2.6. Esterases

Esterases are ubiquitous enzymes that hydrolyze ester linkages. The main relevance of this class of enzymes for chemotherapeutic drugs is in the release of active agents from ester prodrugs *(144)*. The evaluation of the contribution of ester hydrolysis to overall metabolism is complicated by the higher activity of these enzymes in rodent plasma compared to that in humans.

The primary example of an ester prodrug in cancer chemotherapy is that of irinotecan. This comprises a camptothecin, topoisomerase I binding moiety (SN-38), coupled to a piperidinopiperidine via an ester link. This ester is a substrate for carboxylesterase enzymes present in the plasma in rodents *(145)* and in the liver in humans *(146)*. The microsomal carboxylesterase CES2 or hCE2 has most activity toward irinotecan *(147,148)*, and is present in normal and tumor tissues *(147)*. The active SN-38 metabolite is subject to glucuronidation (see below), the extent of which determines the severity of diarrhea *(149)*.

3. PHASE II REACTIONS

3.1. Glucuronidation

Glucuronidation may occur at any suitable hydroxyl, carboxyl, or primary or secondary amine *(150)*. N-glucuronides are less common than O-glucuronides, but are more stable to enzymatic hydrolysis. The increase in molecular weight and in hydrophilicity following glucuronidation aids the elimination of xenobiotics by either biliary or renal excretion. Cleavage of glucuronides in the intestine, often by bacterial glucuronidase enzymes, may result in reabsorption of free drug and enterohepatic recycling. Because glucuronide conjugates are cleared from the body so rapidly, plasma concentrations are often undetectable.

In terms of chemotherapeutic agents, any drug with a suitable hydroxy, amine, or carboxylic acid function, or a drug metabolized to introduce such a function, may be a substrate for glucuronidation. Examples include epirubicin *(151,152)*, flavopiridol *(153)*, hydroxy metabolites of tamoxifen *(154,155)*, SN38 (activated form of irinotecan) *(156)*, topotecan, retinoic acids *(157)*, perillyl alcohol *(158)*, and DMXAA *(159)*.

Table 1
Classification of Glutathione S-Transferase Enzymes

Family	Genes	Chromosome	Reference
Alpha	GSTA1–GSTA4	6p12.2	169
Mu	GSTM1–GSTM5	1p13.3	171,174
Pi	GSTP1	11q13	167,168
Sigma	GSTS	4q	
Theta	GSTT1–GSTT2	22q11.2	172
Kappa	GSTK	Unknown	
Omega or chi	GSTO1	10q	170,175
Zeta	GSTZ1	14q24.3	173

A superfamily of genes encoding for UDP-glucuronosyltransferase enzymes has now been characterized (160). Individual isoforms associated with the glucuronidation of specific substrates have been identified. For instance, SN38 is glucuronidated by UGT1A1 (156), and genotypic variation in UGT activity relates to toxicity following irinotecan administration (161). UGT2B7 plays a role in the glucuronidation of retinoic acid metabolites (157) and also contributes to the formation of morphine glucuronide (162) and that of epirubicin (152). Polymorphisms have been identified in a number of these genes (163), including UGT1A1 (156), UGT2B7 (164), and UGT1A8 (165).

3.2. Sulfation

The conjugation of aryl drugs and their primary oxidation metabolites with sulfate is catalyzed by the sulfotransferase enzymes. SULT1A1 is the predominant form, a cytoplasmic enzyme that uses 3'-phosphoadenylsulfate as a sulfate donor. SULT1A1 is expressed mainly in the liver, lung, and kidney, and catalyzes the sulfation of tamoxifen metabolites (155) and the putative chemoprevention agent curcumin (166).

3.3. Glutathione S-Transferases

Glutathione S-transferases (GSTs) are a family of soluble, dimeric enzymes (EC 2.5.1.18) that play an important role in the cellular detoxification system and are thought to have evolved to protect cells against reactive oxygen metabolites.

The GSTs are comprised of two distinct supergene families that catalyze the conjugation of the tripeptide glutathione (γ-glu-cys-gly) (GSH) to a variety of electrophiles including arene oxides, unsaturated carbonyls, organic halides, and other substrates. A wide variety of endogenous (e.g., byproducts of reactive oxygen species action) and exogenous (e.g., polycyclic aromatic hydrocarbons) electrophilic substrates have been identified.

The genetic loci encoding the GSTs are located on seven chromosomes, and to date 16 different isoforms have been identified (167–175). Ten of these genes encode proteins expressed in tissue cytosol, with six being in membranes (176,177). Based on their substrate specificity, chemical affinity, amino acid sequence kinetic behavior, and structural properties, the soluble human GSTs are categorized into eight main classes (Table 1): alpha, mu, pi, sigma, theta, kappa, omega (or chi) (170–175), and zeta (GSTZ1) (176,178,179). SNPs have been described in many genes in these families; however most emphasis focuses on allelism in the mu, theta, and pi families (176,180).

GST proteins are expressed at high levels in mammalian liver and comprise up to 4% of the total soluble proteins *(181)*. Detailed patterns of expression of the GSTs in fetal and adult tissue have been investigated extensively. GSTA1, GSTA2, GSTM1, and GSTP1 have been detected in fetal tissues *(182*, and reviewed in *179)* hematopoietic cell lines *(183)*, hematopoietic cells *(184)*, and adult brain *(182)*. GSTO1-1 expression has been reported in a wide range of adult, fetal, and placental tissues *(185)*.

Expression of GST proteins is controlled by regulatory elements such as the glucocorticoid response element (GRE), antioxidant (or electrophile) response element (ARE), and the xenobiotic response element (XRE). However, GST expression also seems to be induced by compounds such as the isothiocyanates and alpha–beta unsaturated ketones *(186*, and references therein).

The GSTs, which exist mainly as dimers each monomer having a molecular weight of 25000 Da, catalyze the nucleophilic attack of GSH on electrophilic substrates, thus forming an important line of defence, protecting various cell components from reactive molecules *(181,187)*. There are many examples of chemotherapeutic agents that undergo GSH conjugation, including the electrophilic alkylating agents such as busulfan *(181,186)*, melphalan, and chlorambucil *(188,189)*. Detoxification involves the binding of GSH to electrophilic chemicals and the export of the resulting GSH S-conjugates from the cell.

Glutathione conjugates are excreted immediately via the bile or transported to the kidney where the gamma-glutamyl moiety is split off via gamma-glutamyl transpeptidase, the glycine via a dipeptidase, and the remaining cysteine is *N*-acetylated to be excreted as a mercapturic acid. Instead of *N*-acetylation, the cysteine conjugate can undergo several other metabolic reactions that can lead to bioactivation *(190)*.

Overexpression of some GSTs is implicated in resistance to several anticancer drugs and genetically determined GST deficiencies are risk factors for several forms of cancer (reviewed in ref. *178)*. A null allele at the *GSTM*1 locus is found in 40–45% of Caucasians and GSTT1 null is found in approx 20% of Caucasians *(191,192)*. *GSTM*1 deficiency may be a risk factor for cancer by providing increased sensitivity to particular chemical carcinogens *(193,194)* and, in smokers, is associated with susceptibility to lung cancer *(180,195)* and colorectal cancer *(196)*.

Null genotypes for both *GSTM*1 and *GSTT*1 have also been linked to a poorer survival of patients with ovarian cancer *(197)*. GST polymorphisms have been associated with basal cell carcinoma, asthma *(177)*, astrocytoma *(198)*, bladder cancer *(199)*, prostate cancer *(200)*, squamous cell carcinoma *(201)*, testicular cancer *(202)*, and leukemias *(203,204)*. In the case of childhood leukemia the *GSTM*1 null was associated with a better chance of remission, possibly due to less effective metabolism of drugs used in induction or continuing therapies *(205)*. In the case of breast cancer, however, the evidence for *GSTM*1 null genotype being linked to risk of disease is not so clear-cut *(206)*.

The influence of GST genotype on susceptibility to particular diseases, prognosis, and drug resistance has been extensively investigated over the past 30 yr. However, although some issues seem clear, the role of GSTs is still not completely understood. Drug treatments used in cancer vary considerably, such that a particular genotype may be an advantage in one instance and not in another. It is important to emphasize the different influences of particular GST genotypes on individual disease types and how the interindividual differences between people may affect regulation of GST expression *(193)*.

3.4. N-Acetyltransferase

The acetylation of aromatic and heterocyclic amines is mediated by two enzymes, NAT1 and NAT2. NAT1 is expressed in a variety of tissues, whereas NAT2 is confined to the liver.

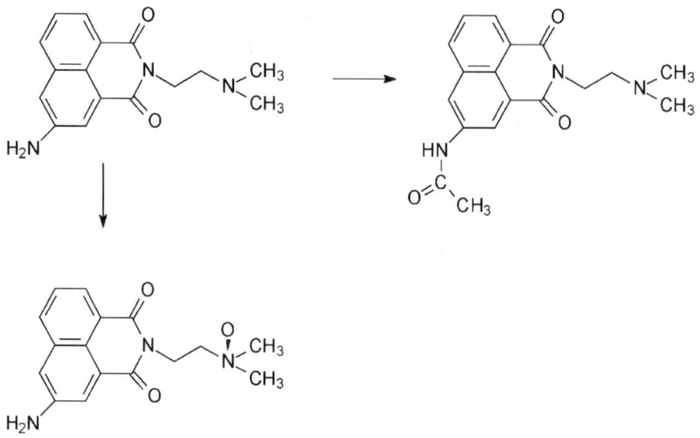

Fig. 10. Metabolism of amonafide by NAT2 and by CYP1A2. The N-acetyl metabolite of amonafide is also a substrate for CYP1A2 and inhibits the metabolism of the parent compound.

A genetic polymorphism in NAT2 was initially characterized with regard to slow and fast acetylators of isoniazid. Polymorphisms in NAT1 have also now been identified, with functional significance in terms of lower enzyme activity (207). The pharmacogenetics of NAT1 and NAT2 have been extensively investigated with regard to their role in the metabolism of carcinogenic arylamines (208).

In terms of the pharmacology of chemotherapeutic agents, amonafide is the best example of a drug subject to N-acetylation (Fig. 10). With regard to antitumor effect and toxicity, the interpretation of the influence of N-acetylation on clinical outcome is complicated by the fact that the metabolite inhibits the oxidative inactivation of the parent compound (209). Thus, plasma clearance of amonafide was lower and hematological toxicity was significantly greater in fast acetylators. Subsequent studies of this compound used a dosing scheme based on caffeine acetylation phenotype (210), and NAT status was incorporated into pharmacokinetic and pharmacodynamic models (211).

4. CONCLUSIONS

Although the study of drug metabolism often focuses on oxidation reactions mediated by cytochrome P450 enzymes, there is a significant role for other pathways of metabolism for many drugs used in cancer chemotherapy. In part this is inherent in the way that many antimetabolites mimic endogenous substrates, which have their own anabolic and catabolic pathways. Non-CYP mediated metabolism dominates the pharmacology of a number of these drugs (e.g., 6-mercaptopurine and 5-fluorouracil), such that understanding of the genetics and enzymology of the enzymes involved (TPMT and DPD, respectively) is essential for the safe use of the drug. In other examples, metabolism may be involved in inactivation of a reactive intermediate or activation of a prodrug, which may have implications for tumor sensitivity or host toxicity. As our knowledge of the genetics of the enzymes involved in these reactions increases, the classification of enzymes is changing. Identification of an enzyme by its substrate or co-factor specificity has been replaced by a classification system based on gene sequence homology. This process has been applied successfully to the CYP family of enzymes, and now extends to ALDH, UGT, NAT, and other non-CYP enzyme superfamilies. The genetic tools that accompany this evolution of nomenclature should also provide techniques for the further understanding and characterization of enzymes and their role in the pharmacology of chemotherapeutic agents.

ACKNOWLEDGMENTS

SAC is supported by the Leukaemia Research Fund, UK. AVB is supported by Cancer Research UK.

REFERENCES

1. Vasilou V, Pappa A, Petersen DR. Role of aldehyde dehydrogenases in endogenous and xenobiotic metabolism. Chem-Biol Interact 2000; 129:1–19.
2. Dockham PA, Lee M-O, Sladek NE. Identification of human liver aldehyde dehydrogenases that catalyze the oxidation of aldophosphamide and retinaldehyde. Biochem Pharmacol 1992; 43:2453–2469.
3. Sladek NE. Aldehyde dehydrogenase-mediated cellular relative insensitivity to the oxazaphosphorines. Curr Pharmaceut Design 1999; 5:607–625.
4. Sreerama L, Sladek NE. Identification and characterization of a novel class 3 aldehyde dehydrogenase overexpressed in a human breast adenocarcinoma cell line exhibiting oxazaphosphorine-specific acquired resistance. Biochem Pharmacol 1993; 45:2487–2505.
5. Dockam PA, Sreerama L, Sladek NE. Relative contribution of human erythrocyte aldehyde dehydrogenase to the systemic detoxicification of the oxazaphosphorines. Drug Metab Dispos 1997; 25: 1436–1441.
6. Magni M, Shammah S, Schiro R, et al. Induction of cyclophosphamide-resistance by aldehyde-dehydrogenase gene transfer. Blood 1996; 87:1097–1103.
7. Moreb JS, Maccow C, Schweder M, Hecomovich J. Expression of antisense RNA to aldehyde dehydrogenase class-1 sensitizes tumor cells to 4-hydroperoxycyclophosphamide in vitro. J Pharmacol Exp Ther 2000; 293:390–396.
8. Sreerama L, Sladek NE. Primary breast tumor levels of suspected molecular determinants of cellular sensitivity to cyclophosphamide, ifosfamide, and certain other anticancer agents as predictors of paired metastatic tumor levels of these determinants—rational individualization of cancer chemotherapeutic regimens. Cancer Chemother Pharmacol 2001; 47:255–262.
9. Ren S, Kalhorn TF, McDonald GB, Anasetti C, Appelbaum FR, Slattery JT. Pharmacokinetics of cyclophosphamide and its metabolites in bone marrow transplantation patients. Clin Pharmacol Ther 1998; 64:289–301.
10. Tweedie DJ, Fernandez D, Spearman ME, Feldhoff RC, Prough RA. Metabolism of azoxy derivatives of procarbazine by aldehyde dehydrogenase and xanthine-oxidase. Drug Metab Dispos 1991; 19:793–803.
11. Yoshida A, Rzhetsky A, Hsu LC, Chang C. Human aldehyde dehydrogenase gene family. Eur J Biochem 1998; 251:549–557.
12. Napoli JL. Interactions of retinoid binding proteins and enzymes in retinoid metabolism. Biochim Biophys Acta 1999; 1440:139–162.
13. Tsukamoto N, Chang C, Yoshida A. Mutations associated with Sjogren-Larsson syndrome. Annals Human Gen 1997; 61:235.
14. Mani C, Kupfer D. Cytochrome-P-450-mediated activation and irreversible binding of the antiestrogen tamoxifen to proteins in rat and human liver—possible involvement of flavin-containing monooxygenases in tamoxifen activation. Cancer Res 1991; 51:6052–6058.
15. Mani C, Hodgson E, Kupfer D. Metabolism of the antimammary cancer antiestrogenic agent tamoxifen. 2. flavin-containing monooxygenase-mediated N-oxidation. Drug Metab Disp 1993; 21:657–661.
16. Hodgson E, Rose RL, Cao Y, Dehal SS, Kupfer D. Flavin-containing monooxygenase isoform specificity for the N-oxidation of tamoxifen determined by product measurement and NADPH oxidation. J Biochem Mol Toxicol 2000; 14:118–120.
17. Overby LH, Carver GC, Philpot RM. Quantitation and kinetic properties of hepatic microsomal and recombinant flavin-containing monooxygenases 3 and 5 from humans. Chem-Biol Interact 1997; 106: 29–45.
18. Cashman JR, Akerman BR, Forrest SM, Treacy EP. Population-specific polymorphisms of the human FMO3 gene: significance for detoxication. Drug Metab Disp 2000; 28:169–173.

19. Pritsos CA. Cellular distribution, metabolism and regulation of the xanthine oxidoreductase enzyme system. Chem-Biol Interact 2000; 129:195–208.
20. Morpeth FF. Studies on the specificity toward aldehyde substrates and steady-state kinetics of xanthine oxidase. Biochim Biophys Acta 1982; 744:328–334.
21. Gustafson DL, Pritsos CA. Bioactivation of Mitomycin-C by xanthine dehydrogenase from Emt6 mouse mammary-carcinoma tumors. J Natl Cancer Inst 1992; 84:1180–1185.
22. Yee SB, Pritsos CA. Comparison of oxygen radical generation from the reductive activation of doxorubicin, streptonigrin, and menadione by xanthine oxidase and xanthine dehydrogenase. Arch Biochem Biophys 1997; 347:235–241.
23. Yee SB, Pritsos CA. Reductive activation of doxorubicin by xanthine dehydrogenase from EMT6 mouse mammary carcinoma tumors. Chem-Biol Interact 1997; 104:87–101.
24. Keuzenkamp-Jansen CW, DeAbreu RA, Bokkerink JPM, Lambooy MAH, Trijbels JMF. Metabolism of intravenously administered high-dose 6-mercaptopurine with and without allopurinol treatment in patients with non-Hodgkin lymphoma. J Pediatr Hematol Oncol 1996; 18:145–150.
25. Goadsby PJ, Day RO, Kwan YL, Miners J, Birkett DJ. 6-Mercaptopurine-related leukopenia and in vivo xanthine-oxidase activity. Lancet 1986; 2:869–870.
26. Innocenti F, Danesi R, DiPaolo A, et al. Clinical and experimental pharmacokinetic interaction between 6-mercaptopurine and methotrexate. Cancer Chemother Pharmacol 1996; 37:409–414.
27. Jordan CGM, Rashidi MR, Laljee H, Clarke SE, Brown JE, Beedham C. Aldehyde oxidase-catalysed oxidation of methotrexate in the liver of guinea-pig, rabbit and man. J Pharm Pharmacol 1999; 51:411–418.
28. Parks DA, Granger DN. Xanthine oxidase: biochemistry, distribution and physiology. Acta Physiol Scand 1986; 126.
29. Lennard L. The clinical pharmacology of 6-mercaptopurine. Eur J Clin Pharmacol 1992; 43:329–339.
30. Sarnesto A, Linder N, Raivio KO. Organ distribution and molecular forms of human xanthine dehydrogenase/xanthine oxidase protein. Lab Invest 1996; 74:48–56.
31. Roy SK, Korzekwa KR, Gonzalez FJ, Moschel RC, Dolan ME. Human liver oxidative-metabolism of O-6-benzylguanine. Biochem Pharmacol 1995; 50:1385–1389.
32. Bobola MS, Tseng SH, Blank A, Berger MS, Silber JR. Role of O-6-methylguanine-DNA methyltransferase in resistance of human brain-tumor cell-lines to the clinically relevant methylating agents temozolomide and streptozotocin. Clin Cancer Res 1996; 2:735–741.
33. Berger R, Stoker-de Vries SA, Wadman SK, et al. Dihydropyrimidine dehydrogenase deficiency leading to thymine-uraciluria. An inborn error of pyrimidine metabolism. Clin Chim Acta 1984; 141:227–234.
34. Lu ZH, Zhang R, Diasio RB. Purification and characterization of dihydropyrimidine dehydrogenase from human liver. J Biol Chem 1992; 267:17,102–17,109.
35. Montfort WR, Weichsel A. Thymidylate synthase: structure, inhibition, and strained conformations during catalysis. Pharmacol Ther 1997; 76:29–43.
36. Ho DH, Townsend L, Luna MA, Bodey GP. Distribution and inhibition of dihydrouracil dehydrogenase activities in human tissues using 5-fluorouracil as a substrate. Anticancer Res 1986; 6:781–784.
37. Naguib FN, el Kouni MH, Cha S. Enzymes of uracil catabolism in normal and neoplastic human tissues. Cancer Res 1985; 45:5405–5412.
38. Lu Z, Zhang R, Diasio RB. Dihydropyrimidine dehydrogenase activity in human peripheral blood mononuclear cells and liver: population characteristics, newly identified deficient patients, and clinical implication in 5-fluorouracil chemotherapy. Cancer Res 1993; 53:5433–5438.
39. Van Kuilenburg AB, van Lenthe H, Blom MJ, Mul EP, Van Gennip AH. Profound variation in dihydropyrimidine dehydrogenase activity in human blood cells: major implications for the detection of partly deficient patients. Br J Cancer 1999; 79:620–626.
40. Etienne MC, Lagrange JL, Dassonville O, et al. Population study of dihydropyrimidine dehydrogenase in cancer patients. J Clin Oncol 1994; 12:2248–2253.
41. Ridge SA, Sludden J, Brown O, et al. Dihydropyrimidine dehydrogenase pharmacogenetics in Caucasian subjects. Br J Clin Pharmacol 1998; 46:151–156.
42. Ridge SA, Sludden J, Wei X, et al. Dihydropyrimidine dehydrogenase pharmacogenetics in patients with colorectal cancer. Br J Cancer 1998; 77:497–500.
43. Diasio RB, Beavers TL, Carpenter JT. Familial deficiency of dihydropyrimidine dehydrogenase. Biochemical basis for familial pyrimidinemia and severe 5-fluorouracil-induced toxicity. J Clin Invest 1988; 81:47–51.
44. Johnson MR, Wang K, Tillmanns S, Albin N, Diasio RB. Structural organization of the human dihydropyrimidine dehydrogenase gene. Cancer Res 1997; 57:1660–1663.

45. Wei X, Elizondo G, Sapone A, et al. Characterization of the human dihydropyrimidine dehydrogenase gene. Genomics 1998; 51:391–400.
46. Shestopal SA, Johnson MR, Diasio RB. Molecular cloning and characterization of the human dihydropyrimidine dehydrogenase promoter. Biochim Biophys Acta 2000; 1494:162–169.
47. Takai S, Fernandez-Salguero P, Kimura S, Gonzalez FJ, Yamada K. Assignment of the human dihydropyrimidine dehydrogenase gene (DPYD) to chromosome region 1p22 by fluorescence in situ hybridization. Genomics 1994; 24:613–614.
48. Vreken P, Van Kuilenburg AB, Meinsma R, et al. A point mutation in an invariant splice donor site leads to exon skipping in two unrelated Dutch patients with dihydropyrimidine dehydrogenase deficiency. J. Inherit Metab Dis 1996; 19:645–654.
49. Vreken P, Van Kuilenburg AB, Meinsma R, Van Gennip AH. Dihydropyrimidine dehydrogenase (DPD) deficiency: identification and expression of missense mutations C29R, R886H and R235W. Human Genet 1997; 101:333–338.
50. Vreken P, Van Kuilenburg AB, Meinsma R, Van Gennip AH. Identification of novel point mutations in the dihydropyrimidine dehydrogenase gene. J Inherit Metab Dis 1997; 20:335–338.
51. McLeod HL, Collie-Duguid ES, Vreken P, et al. Nomenclature for human DPYD alleles. Pharmacogenetics 1998; 8:455–459.
52. Collie-Duguid ES, Etienne MC, Milano G, McLeod HL. Known variant DPYD alleles do not explain DPD deficiency in cancer patients. Pharmacogenetics 2000; 10:217–223.
53. Johnson MR, Wang K, Diasio RB. Profound dihydropyrimidine dehydrogenase deficiency resulting from a novel compound heterozygote genotype. Clin Cancer Res 2002; 8:768–774.
54. Mattison LK, Johnson MR, Diasio RB. A comparative analysis of translated dihydropyrimidine dehydrogenase cDNA; conservation of functional domains and relevance to genetic polymorphisms. Pharmacogenetics 2002; 12:133–144.
55. Grem JL. 5-Fluoropyrimidines. In: Chabner BA, Longo DL (eds). Cancer Chemotherapy and Biotherapy. Vol. 2, Philadelphia, PA: Lippincott-Raven, 2002, pp. 149–211.
56. Heggie GD, Sommadossi JP, Cross DS, Huster WJ, Diasio RB. Clinical pharmacokinetics of 5-fluorouracil and its metabolites in plasma, urine, and bile. Cancer Res 1987; 47:2203–2206.
57. Diasio RB. The role of dihydropyrimidine dehydrogenase (DPD) modulation in 5-FU pharmacology. Oncology 1998; 12:23–27.
58. Fleming RA, Milano G, Thyss A, et al. Correlation between dihydropyrimidine dehydrogenase-activity in peripheral mononuclear-cells and systemic clearance of fluorouracil in cancer-patients. Cancer Res 1992; 52:2899–2902.
59. Milano G, Etienne M, Renee N, et al. Relationship between fluorouracil systemic exposure and tumor response and patient survival. J Clin Oncol 1994; 12:1291–1295.
60. Etienne MC, Cheradame S, Fischel JL, et al. Response to fluorouracil therapy in cancer patients: The role of tumoral dihydropyrimidine dehydrogenase. J Clin Oncol 1995; 13:1663–1670.
61. Zhang R, Lu Z, Liu T, Soong SJ, Diasio RB. Relationship between circadian-dependent toxicity of 5-fluorodeoxyuridine and circadian rhythms of pyrimidine enzymes: possible relevance to fluoropyrimidine chemotherapy. Cancer Res 1993; 53:2816–2822.
62. Harris BE, Song R, Soong SJ, Diasio RB. Relationship between dihydropyrimidine dehydrogenase activity and plasma 5-fluorouracil levels with evidence for circadian variation of enzyme activity and plasma drug levels in cancer patients receiving 5-fluorouracil by protracted continuous infusion. Cancer Res 1990; 50:197–201.
63. Lamont EB, Schilsky RL. The oral fluoropyrimidines in cancer chemotherapy. Clin Cancer Res 1999; 5:2289–2296.
64. de Bono JS, Twelves CJ. The oral fluorinated pyrimidines. Invest New Drugs 2001; 19:41–59.
65. Baccanari DP, Davis ST, Knick VC, Spector T. 5-Ethynyluracil (776C85): a potent modulator of the pharmacokinetics and antitumor efficacy of 5-fluorouracil. Proc Natl Acad Sci 1993; 90:11,064–11,068.
66. Grem JL, Harold N, Shapiro J, et al. Phase I and pharmacokinetic trial of weekly oral fluorouracil given with eniluracil and low-dose leucovorin to patients with solid tumors. J Clin Oncol 2000; 18: 3952–3963.
67. Adjei AA, Reid JM, Diasio RB, et al. Comparative pharmacokinetic study of continuous venous infusion fluorouracil and oral fluorouracil with eniluracil in patients with advanced solid tumors. J Clin Oncol 2002; 20:1683–1691.
68. van Groeningen CJ, Peters GJ, Schornagel JH, et al. Phase I clinical and pharmacokinetic study of oral S-1 in patients with advanced solid tumors. J Clin Oncol 2000; 18:2772–2779.

69. Cohen SJ, Leichman CG, Yeslow G, et al. Phase I and pharmacokinetic study of once daily oral administration of S-1 in patients with advanced cancer. Clin Cancer Res 2002; 8:2116–2122.

70. Sulkes A, Benner SE, Canetta RM. Uracil-ftorafur: An oral fluoropyrimidine active in colorectal cancer. J Clin Oncol 1998; 16:3461–3475.

71. Nemunaitis J, Eager R, Twaddell T, et al. Phase I assessment of the pharmacokinetics, metabolism, and safety of emitefur in patients with refractory solid tumors. J Clin Oncol 2000; 18:3423–3434.

72. Sadahiro S, Suzuki T, Kameya T, Iwase H, Tajima T, Makuuchi H. A pharmacological study of the weekday-on/weekend-off oral UFT schedule in colorectal cancer patients. Cancer Chemother Pharmacol 2001; 47:457–460.

73. Damle B, Ravandi F, Kaul S, et al. Effect of food on the oral bioavailability of UFT and leucovorin in cancer patients. Clin Cancer Res 2001; 7:517–523.

74. Pacifici GM, Romiti P, Giuliani L, Rane A. Thiopurine methyltransferase in humans: development and tissue distribution. Dev Pharmacol Ther 1991; 17:16–23.

75. Remy CN. Metabolism of thiopyrimidines and thiopurines: S-methylation with S-adenosylmethionine transmethylase and catabolism in mammalian tissue. J Biol Chem 1963; 238:1078–1084.

76. Elion GB. Symposium on immunosuppressive drugs. Biochemistry and pharmacology of purine analogues. Fed Proc 1967; 26:898–904.

77. Weinshilboum RM, Sladek SL. Mercaptopurine pharmacogenetics: monogenic inheritance of erythrocyte thiopurine methyltransferase activity. Am J Human Genet 1980; 32:651–662.

78. Van Loon JA, Weinshilboum RM. Thiopurine methyltransferase biochemical genetics: human lymphocyte activity. Biochem Genet 1982; 20:637–658.

79. McLeod HL, Relling MV, Liu Q, Pui C-H, Evans WE. Polymorphic thiopurine methyltransferase in erythrocytes is indicative of activity in leukemic blasts from children with acute lymphoblastic leukemia. Blood 1995; 85:1897–1902.

80. Coulthard SA, Howell C, Robson J, Hall AG. The relationship between thiopurine methyltransferase activity and genotype in blasts from patients with acute leukemia. Blood 1998; 92:2856–2862.

81. Van Loon JA, Weinshilboum RM. Thiopurine methyltransferase isozymes in human renal tissue. Drug Metab Dispos 1990; 18:632–638.

82. Woodson LC, Dunnette JH, Weinshilboum RM. Pharmacogenetics of human thiopurine methyltransferase: kidney-erythrocyte correlation and immunotitration studies. J Pharmacol Exp Ther 1982; 222:174–181.

83. McLeod HL, Krynetski EY, Wilimas JA, Evans WE. Higher activity of polymorphic thiopurine S-methyltransferase in erythrocytes from neonates compared to adults. Pharmacogenetics 1995; 5:281–286.

84. Lennard L, Lilleyman JS, Van Loon J, Weinshilboum RM. Genetic variation in response to 6-mercaptopurine for childhood acute lymphoblastic leukaemia. Lancet 1990; 336:225–229.

85. Szumlanski C, Otterness D, Her C, et al. Thiopurine methyltransferase pharmacogenetics: Human gene cloning and characterization of a common polymorphism. DNA Cell Biol 1996; 15:17–30.

86. Krynetski EY, Fessing MY, Yates CR, Sun D, Schuetz JD, Evans WE. Promoter and intronic sequences of the human thiopurine S- methyltransferase (TPMT) gene isolated from a human Pac1 genomic library. Pharm Res 1997; 14:1672–1678.

87. Coulthard SA, Hogarth LA, Little M, et al. The effect of thiopurine methyltransferase expression on sensitivity to thiopurine drugs. Mol Pharmacol 2002; 62:102–109.

88. Tai HL, Krynetski EY, Yates CR, et al. Thiopurine S-methyltransferase deficiency: Two nucleotide transitions define the most prevalent mutant allele associated with loss of catalytic activity in Caucasians. Am J Human Genet 1996; 58:694–702.

89. McLeod HL, Krynetski EY, Relling MV, Evans WE. Genetic polymorphism of thiopurine methyltransferase and its clinical relevance for childhood acute lymphoblastic leukemia. Leukemia 2000; 14:567–572.

90. Spire-Vayron dlM, Debuysere H, Fazio F, et al. Characterization of a variable number tandem repeat region in the thiopurine S-methyltransferase gene promoter. Pharmacogenetics 1999; 9:189–198.

91. Lowry PW, Franklin CL, Weaver AL, et al. Leucopenia resulting from a drug interaction between azathioprine or 6-mercaptopurine and mesalamine, sulphasalazine, or balsalazide. Gut 2001; 49:656–664.

92. Swann PF, Waters TR, Moulton DC, et al. Role of postreplicative DNA mismatch repair in the cytotoxic action of thioguanine. Science 1996; 273:1109–1112.

93. Maddocks JL, Lennard L, Amess J, Amos R, Thomas RM. Azathioprine and severe bone marrow depression [letter]. Lancet 1986; 1:156.

94. Lennard L, Rees CA, Lilleyman JS, Maddocks JL. Childhood leukaemia: A relationship between intracellular 6-mercaptopurine metabolites and neutropenia. Br J Clin Pharmacol 1983; 16:359–363.

95. Lennard L, Van Loon JA, Lilleyman JS, Weinshilboum RM. Thiopurine pharmacogenetics in leukemia: Correlation of erythrocyte thiopurine methyltransferase activity and 6-thioguanine nucleotide concentrations. Clin Pharmacol Ther 1987; 41:18–25.

96. Lennard L, Davies HA, Lilleyman JS. Is 6-thioguanine more appropriate than 6-mercaptopurine for children with acute lymphoblastic leukaemia? Br J Cancer 1993; 68:186–190.

97. McLeod HL, Miller DR, Evans WE. Azathioprine-induced myelosuppression in thiopurine methyltransferase deficient heart transplant recipient. Lancet 1993; 341:1151.

98. Lennard L, Gibson BES, Nicole T, Lilleyman JS. Congenital thiopurine methyltransferase deficiency and 6-mercaptopurine toxicity during treatment for acute lymphoblastic leukaemia. Arch Dis Childh 1993; 69:577–579.

99. Evans WE, Horner M, Chu YQ, Kalwinsky D, Roberts WM. Altered mercaptopurine metabolism, toxic effects, and dosage requirement in a thiopurine methyltransferase-deficient child with acute lymphocytic leukemia. J Pediatr 1991; 119:985–989.

100. Lennard L, Lewis IJ, Michelagnoli M, Lilleyman JS. Thiopurine methyltransferase deficiency in childhood lymphoblastic leukaemia: 6-mercaptopurine dosage strategies. Med Ped Oncol 1997; 29: 252–255.

101. Andersen JB, Szumlanski C, Weinshilboum RM, Schmiegelow K. Pharmacokinetics, dose adjustments, and 6-mercaptopurine/methotrexate drug interactions in two patients with thiopurine methyltransferase deficiency. Acta Paediatr 1998; 87:108–111.

102. Relling MV, Hancock ML, Boyett JM, Pui CH, Evans WE. Prognostic importance of 6-mercaptopurine dose intensity in acute lymphoblastic leukemia. Blood 1999; 93:2817–2823.

103. Dervieux T, Blanco JG, Krynetski EY, Vanin EF, Roussel MF, Relling MV. Differing contribution of thiopurine methyltransferase to mercaptopurine versus thioguanine effects in human leukemic cells. Cancer Res 2001; 61:5810–5816.

104. Vogt MH, Stet EH, De Abreu RA, Bokkerink JP, Lambooy LHJ, Trijbels FJ. The importance of methylthio-IMP for methylmercaptopurine ribonucleoside (Me-MPR) cytotoxicity in Molt F4 human malignant T-lymphoblasts. Biochim Biophys Acta 1993; 1181:189–194.

105. Lancaster DL, Lennard L, Rowland K, Vora AJ, Lilleyman JS. Thioguanine versus mercaptopurine for therapy of childhood lymphoblastic leukaemia: a comparison of haematological toxicity and drug metabolite concentrations. Br J Haematol 1998; 102:439–443.

106. Erb N, Harms DO, Janka-Schaub G. Pharmacokinetics and metabolism of thiopurines in children with acute lymphoblastic leukemia receiving 6-thioguanine versus 6-mercaptopurine. Cancer Chemother Pharmacol 1998; 42:266–272.

107. Adamson PC, Poplack DG, Balis FM. The cytotoxicity of thioguanine vs mercaptopurine in acute lymphoblastic leukemia. Luekemia Res 1994; 18:805–810.

108. Lilleyman JS, Lennard L. Non-compliance with oral chemotherapy in childhood leukaemia [editorial]. Brit Med J 1996; 313:1219–1220.

109. Tan BB, Lear JT, Gawkrodger DJ, English JS. Azathioprine in dermatology: a survey of current practice in the U.K. Brit J Dermatol 1997; 136:351–355.

110. Fretland AJ, Omiecinski CJ. Epoxide hydrolases: biochemistry and molecular biology. Chem-Biol Interact 2000; 129:41–59.

111. Beetham JK, Tian T, Hammock BD. cDNA cloning and expression of a soluble epoxide hydrolase from human liver. Arch Biochem Biophys 1993; 305:197–201.

112. Sarmanova J, Benesova K, Gut I, Nedelcheva-Kristensen V, Tynkova L, Soucek P. Genetic polymorphisms of biotransformation enzymes in patients with Hodgkin's and non-Hodgkin's lymphomas. Human Mol Genet 2001; 10:1265–1273.

113. Farin FM, Janssen P, Quigley S, et al. Genetic polymorphisms of microsomal and soluble epoxide hydrolase and the risk of Parkinson's disease. Pharmacogenetics 2001; 11:703–708.

114. Blum W, Aichholz R, Ramstein P, et al. In vivo metabolism of epothilone B in tumor-bearing nude mice: identification of three new epothilone B metabolites by capillary high-pressure liquid chromatography/mass spectrometry/tandem mass spectrometry. Rapid Comm Mass Spectrom 2001; 15:41–49.

115. Murray GI, Weaver RJ, Paterson PJ, Ewen SWB, Melvin WT, Burke MD. Expression of xenobiotic metabolizing enzymes in breast-cancer. J Path 1993; 169:347–353.

116. Murray GI, Taylor VE, McKay JA, et al. The immunohistochemical localization of drug-metabolizing-enzymes in prostate-cancer. J Path 1995; 177:147–152.

117. Albin N, Massaad L, Toussaint C, et al. Main drug-metabolizing enzyme-systems in human breast-tumors and peritumoral tissues. Cancer Res 1993; 53:3541–3546.

118. Forrest GL, Gonzalez B. Carbonyl reductase. Chem-Biol Interact 2000; 129:21–40.
119. Watanabe K, Sugawara C, Ono A, et al. Mapping of a novel human carbonyl reductase, CBR3, and ribosomal pseudogenes to human chromosome 21q22.2. Genomics 1998; 52:95–100.
120. Jacquet J-M, Vressolle F, Galtier M, et al. Doxorubicin and doxorubicinol: intra- and inter-individual variations of pharmacokinetic parameters. Cancer Chemother Pharmacol 1990; 27:219–225.
121. Kokenberg E, Sonneveld P, Sizoo W, Hagenbeek A, Lowenberg B. Cellular pharmacokinetics of daunorubicin: relationships with the response to treatment in patients with acute myeloid leukemia. J Clin Oncol 1998; 6:802–812.
122. Mross K, Maessen P, Vandervijgh W, Gall H, Boven E, Pinedo HM. Pharmacokinetics and metabolism of epidoxorubicin and doxorubicin in humans. J Clin Oncol 1988; 6:517–526.
123. Morris RG, Kotasek D, Paltridge G. Disposition of epirubicin and metabolites with repeated courses to cancer-patients. Eur J Clin Pharmacol 1991; 40:481–487.
124. Robert J, Rigal-Huguet F, Harousseau JL, et al. Pharmacokinetics of idarubicin after daily intravenous administration in leukemia patients. Leukemia Res 1987; 11:961–964.
125. Tidefelt U, Prenkert M, Paul C. Comparison of idarubicin and daunorubicin and their main metabolites regarding intracellular uptake and effect on sensitive and multidrug-resistant HL60 cells. Cancer Chemother Pharmacol 1996; 38:476–480.
126. Ax W, Soldan M, Koch L, Maser E. Development of daunorubicin resistance in tumour cells by induction of carbonyl reduction. Biochem Pharmacol 2000; 59:293–300.
127. Soldan M, Ax W, Plebuch M, Koch L, Maser E. Cytostatic drug resistance—role of phase-I daunorubicin metabolism in cancer cells. Enzymol Mol Biol Carbonyl Metab 1999; 463:529–538.
128. Gonzalez B, Akman S, Doroshow J, Rivera H, Kaplan WD, Forrest GL. Protection against daunorubicin cytotoxicity by expression of a cloned human carbonyl reductase cDNA in K562 leukemia-cells. Cancer Res 1995; 55:4646–4650.
129. Forrest GL, Gonzalez B, Tseng W, Li XL, Mann J. Human carbonyl reductase overexpression in the heart advances the development of doxorubicin-induced cardiotoxicity in transgenic mice. Cancer Res 2000; 60:5158–5164.
130. Traver RD, Horikoshi T, Danenberg KD, et al. NAD(P)H:quinone oxidoreductase gene expression in human colon carcinoma cells: characterization of a mutation which modulates DT-diaphorase activity and mitomycin sensitivity. Cancer Res 1992; 52:797–802.
131. Siegel D, Anwar A, Winski SL, Kepa JK, Zolman KL, Ross D. Rapid polyubiquitination and proteasomal degradation of a mutant form of NAD(P)H:quinone oxidoreductase 1. Mol Pharmacol 2001; 59:263–268.
132. Ross D, Kepa JK, Winski SL, Beall HD, Anwar A, Siegel D. NAD(P)H:quinone oxidoreductase 1 (NQO1): chemoprotection, bioactivation, gene regulation and genetic polymorphisms. Chem-Biol Interact 2000; 129:77–97.
133. Siegel D, Gibson NW, Preusch PC, Ross D. Metabolism of mitomycin C by DT-diaphorase: role in mitomycin C-induced DNA damage and cytotoxicity in human colon carcinoma cells. Cancer Res 1990; 50:7483–7489.
134. Gan YB, Mo YQ, Kalns JE, et al. Expression of DT-diaphorase and cytochrome P450 reductase correlates with mitomycin c activity in human bladder tumors. Clin Cancer Res 2001; 7:1313–1319.
135. Fitzsimmons SA, Workman P, Grever M, Paull K, Camalier R, Lewis AD. Reductase enzyme expression across the National Cancer Institute tumour cell line panel: Correlation with sensitivity to mitomycin C and EO9. J Natl Cancer Inst 1996; 88:259–269.
136. Bailey SM, Lewis AD, Patterson LH, Fisher GR, Knox RJ, Workman P. Involvement of NADPH: cytochrome P450 reductase in the activation of indoloquinone EO9 to free radical and DNA damaging species. Biochem Pharmacol 2001; 62:461–468.
137. Loadman PM, Phillips RM, Lim LE, Bibby MC. Pharmacological properties of a new aziridinylbenzoquinone, RH1 (2,5-diaziridinyl-3-(hydroxymethyl)-6-methyl-1,4-benzoquinone), in mice. Biochem Pharmacol 2000; 59:831–837.
138. Schellens JHM, Planting AST, Vanacker BAC, et al. Phase-I and pharmacological study of the novel indoloquinone bioreductive alkylating cytotoxic drug E09. J Natl Cancer Inst 1994; 86:906–912.
139. Dalton JT, Wientjes MG, Badalament RA, Drago JR, Au JL-S. Pharmacokinetics of intravesical mitomycin C in superficial bladder cancer patients. Cancer Res 1991; 51:5144–5152.
140. Siegel D, McGuinnness SM, Winski SL, Ross D. Genotype-phenotype relationships in studies of a polymorphism in NAD(P)H:quinone oxidoreductase 1. Pharmacogenetics 1999; 9:113–121.
141. Fleming RA, Drees J, Loggie BW, et al. Clinical significance of a NAD(P)H: quinone oxidoreductase 1 polymorphism in patients with disseminated peritoneal cancer receiving intraperitoneal hyperthermic chemotherapy with mitomycin C. Pharmacogenetics 2002; 12:31–37.

142. Kelland LR, Sharp SY, Rogers PM, Myers TG, Workman P. DT-diaphorase expression and tumor cell sensitivity to 17-allylamino,17-demethoxygeldanamycin, an inhibitor of heat shock protein 90. J Natl Cancer Inst 1999; 91:1940–1949.

143. Brunton VG, Steele G, Lewis AD, Workman P. Geldanamycin-induced cytotoxicity in human colon-cancer cell lines: evidence against the involvement of c-Src or DT- diaphorase. Cancer Chemother Pharmacol 1998; 41:417–422.

144. Senter PD, Marquardt H, Thomas BA, Hammock BD, Frank IS, Svensson HP. The role of rat serum carboxylesterase in the activation of paclitaxel and camptothecin prodrugs. Cancer Res 1996; 56: 1471–1474.

145. Morton CL, Wierdl M, Oliver L, et al. Activation of CPT-11 in mice: identification and analysis of a highly effective plasma esterase. Cancer Res 2000; 60:4206–4210.

146. Slatter JG, Su P, Sams JP, Schaaf LJ, Wienkers LC. Bioactivation of the anticancer agent CPT-11 to SN-38 by human hepatic microsomal carboxylesterases and the in vitro assessment of potential drug interactions. Drug Metab Dispos 1997; 25:1157–1164.

147. Xu G, Zhang W, Ma MK, McLeod HL. Human carboxylesterase 2 is commonly expressed in tumor tissue and is correlated with activation of irinotecan. Clin Cancer Res 2002; 8:2605–2611.

148. Wu MH, Yan B, Humerickhouse R, Dolan ME. Irinotecan activation by human carboxylesterases in colorectal adenocarcinoma cells. Clin Cancer Res 2002; 8:2696–2700.

149. Gupta F, Lestingi TM, Mick R, Ramirez J, Vokes EE, Ratain MJ. Metabolic-fate of:rinotecan in humans—correlation of glucuronidation with diarrhea. Cancer Res 1994; 54:3723–3725.

150. Tukey RH, Strassburg CP. Human UDP-glucuronosyltransferases metabolism, expression and disease. Annu Rev Pharmacol Toxicol 2000; 40:581–616.

151. Camaggi CM, Strocchi E, Carisi P, Martoni A, Melotti B, Pannuti F. Epirubicin metabolism and pharmacokinetics after conventional-dose and high-dose intravenous administration—a cross-over study. Cancer Chemother Pharmacol 1993; 32:301–309.

152. Innocenti F, Iyer L, Ramirez J, Green MD, Ratain MJ. Epirubicin glucuronidation is catalyzed by human UDP-glucuronosyltransferase 2B7. Drug Metab Dispos 2001; 29:686–692.

153. Innocenti F, Stadler WM, Iyer L, Ramirez J, Vokes EE, Ratain MJ. Flavopiridol metabolism in cancer patients is associated with the occurrence of diarrhea. Clin Cancer Res 2000; 6:3400–3405.

154. Poon GK, Chui YC, McCague R, et al. Analysis of Phase-I and Phase-II metabolites of tamoxifen in breast-cancer patients. Drug Metab Disp 1993; 21:1119–1124.

155. Nishiyama T, Ogura K, Nakano H, et al. Reverse geometrical selectivity in glucuronidation and sulfation of cis- and trans-4-hydroxytamoxifens by human liver UDP-glucuronosyltransferases and sulfotransferases. Biochem Pharmacol 2002; 63:1817–1830.

156. Ando Y, Saka H, Asai G, Sugiura S, Shimokata K, Kamataki T. UGT1A1 genotypes and glucuronidation of SN-38, the active metabolite of irinotecan. Ann Oncol 1998; 9:845–847.

157. Samokyszyn VM, Gall WE, Zawada G, et al. 4-Hydroxyretinoic acid, a novel substrate for human liver microsomal UDP-glucuronosyltransferase(s) and recombinant UGT2B7. J Biol Chem 2000; 275:6908–6914.

158. Boon PJM, van der Boon D, Mulder GJ. Cytotoxicity and biotransformation of the anticancer drug perillyl alcohol in PC12 cells and in the rat. Toxicol Applied Pharmacol 2000; 167:55–62.

159. Zhou SF, Paxton JW, Tingle ID, et al. Identification and reactivity of the major metabolite (beta-1-glucuronide) of the anti-tumour agent 5,6-dimethylxanthenone-4- acetic acid (DMXAA) in humans. Xenobiotica 2001; 31:277–293.

160. Tukey R, Strassburg CP. Genetic multiplicity of the human UDP-glucuronosyltransferases and regulation in the gastrointestinal tract. Mol Pharmacol 2001; 59:405–414.

161. Ando Y, Saka H, Ando M, et al. Polymorphisms of UDP-glucuronosyltransferase gene and irinotecan toxicity: A pharmacogenetic analysis. Cancer Res 2000; 60:6921–6926.

162. Sawyer MB, Das S, Cheng C, et al. Identification of a polymorphism in the UGT2B7 promoter: Association with morphine glucuronidation in patients. Clin Pharmacol Ther 2002; 71:P40–P40.

163. Mackenzie PI, Miners JO, McKinnon RA. Polymorphisms in UDP glucuronosyltransferase genes: Functional consequences and clinical relevance. Clin Chem Lab Med 2000; 38:889–892.

164. Bhasker CR, McKinnon W, Stone A, et al. Genetic polymorphism of UDP-glucuronosyltransferase 2B7 (UGT2B7) at amino acid 268: ethnic diversity of alleles and potential clinical significance. Pharmacogenetics 2000; 10:679–685.

165. Huang YH, Galijatovic A, Nguyen N, et al. Identification and functional characterization of UDP-glucuronosyltransferases UGT1A8*1, UGT1A8*2 and UGT1A8*3. Pharmacogenetics 2002; 12:287–297.

166. Ireson CR, Jones DJL, Orr S, et al. Metabolism of the cancer chemopreventive agent curcumin in human and rat intestine. Cancer Epidemiol Biomarkers Prev 2002; 11:105–111.
167. Silberstein DL, Shows TB. Gene for glutathione *S*-transferase-1 (GST1) is on human chromosome 11. Somatic Cell Mol Genet 1982; 8:667–675.
168. Suzuki T, Board P. Glutathione-*S*-transferase gene mapped to chromosome 11 is GST3 not GST1. Somatic Cell Mol Genet 1984; 10:319–320.
169. Board PG, Webb GC. Isolation of a cDNA clone and localization of human glutathione *S*-transferase 2 genes to chromosome band 6p12. Proc Nat Acad Sci USA 1987; 84:2377–2381.
170. Singhal SS, Gupta S, Ahmad H, Sharma R, Awasthi YC. Characterization of a novel alpha-class anionic glutathione *S*-transferase isozyme from human liver. Arch Biochem Biophys 1990; 279:45–53.
171. Pearson WR, Vorachek WR, Xu SJ, et al. Identification of class-mu glutathione transferase genes GSTM1-GSTM5 on human chromosome 1p13. Am J Hum Genet 1993; 53:220–233.
172. Webb G, Vaska V, Coggan M, Board P. Chromosomal localization of the gene for the human theta class glutathione transferase (*GSTT1*). Genomics 1996; 33:121–123.
173. Blackburn AC, Woollatt E, Sutherland GR, Board PG. Characterization and chromosome location of the gene *GSTZ1* encoding the human zeta class glutathione transferase and maleylacetoacetate isomerase. Cytogenet Cell Genet 1998; 83:109–114.
174. Xu S, Wang Y, Roe B, Pearson WR. Characterization of the human class mu glutathione *S*-transferase gene cluster and the *GSTM1* deletion. J Biol Chem 1998; 273:3517–3527.
175. Board PG, Coggan M, Chelvanayagam G, et al. Identification, characterization, and crystal structure of the omega class glutathione transferases. J Biol Chem 2000; 275:24,798–24,806.
176. Hayes JD, Strange RC. Glutathione *S*-transferase polymorphisms and their biological consequences. Pharmacology 2000; 61:154–166.
177. Strange RC, Spiteri MA, Ramachandran S, Fryer AA. Glutathione-*S*-transferase family of enzymes. Mutat Res 2001; 482:21–26.
178. Hayes JD, Pulford DJ. The glutathione *S*-Transferase supergene family: Regulation of GST and the contribution of the isoenzymes to cancer chemoprotection and drug resistance. Crit Rev Biochem Mol Biol 1995; 30:445–600.
179. McCarver DG, Hines RN. The ontogeny of human drug-metabolizing enzymes: phase II conjugation enzymes and regulatory mechanisms. J Pharmacol Exp Ther 2002; 300:361–366.
180. Rebbeck TR. Molecular epidemiology of the human glutathione *S*-transferase genotypes GSTM1 and GSTT1 in cancer susceptibility. Cancer Epidemiol Biomarkers Prev 1997; 6:733–743.
181. Eaton DL, Bammler TK. Concise review of the glutathione *S*-transferases and their significance to toxicology. Toxicol Sci 1999; 49:156–164.
182. Carder PJ, Hume R, Fryer AA, Strange RC, Lauder J, Bell JE. Glutathione *S*-transferase in human brain. Neuropath Appl Neurobiol 1990; 16:293–303.
183. Wang L, Groves MJ, Hepburn MD, Bowen DT. Glutathione *S*-transferase enzyme expression in hematopoietic cell lines implies a differential protective role for T1 and A1 isoenzymes in erythroid and for M1 in lymphoid lineages. Haematologica 2000; 85:573–579.
184. Den Boer ML, Pieters R, Kazemier KM, et al. Different expression of glutathione *S*-transferase alpha, mu and pi in childhood acute lymphoblastic and myeloid leukaemia. Brit J Haematol 1999; 104:321–327.
185. Yin ZL, Dahlstrom JE, Le Couteur DG, Board PG. Immunohistochemistry of omega class glutathione *S*-transferase in human tissues. J Histochem Cytochem 2001; 49:983–987.
186. van Bladeren PJ. Glutathione conjugation as a bioactivation reaction. Chem-Biol Interact 2000; 129:61–76.
187. Mannervik B, Danielson UH. Glutathione transferases—structure and catalytic activity. CRC Crit Rev Biochem 1988; 23:283–337.
188. Hall AG, Tilby MJ. Mechanisms of action of, and modes of resistance to, alkylating agents used in the treatment of haematological malignancies. Blood Reviews 1992; 6:163–173.
189. Panasci L, Paiement JP, Christodoulopoulos G, Belenkov A, Malapetsa A, Aloyz R. Chlorambucil drug resistance in chronic lymphocytic leukemia: the emerging role of DNA repair. Clin Cancer Res 2001; 7:454–461.
190. Armstrong RN. Structure, catalytic mechanism, and evolution of the glutathione transferases. Chem Res Toxicol 1997; 10:2–18.
191. Seidegard J, Pero RW. The genetic variation and the expression of human glutathione transferase mu. Klin Wochenschr 1988; 66(Suppl 11):125–126.
192. Kote-Jarai Z, Easton D, Edwards SM, et al. Relationship between glutathione *S*-transferase M1, P1 and T1 polymorphisms and early onset prostate cancer. Pharmacogenetics 2001; 11:325–330.

193. Strange RC, Matharoo B, Faulder GC, et al. The human glutathione *S*-transferases: a case-control study of the incidence of the GST1 0 phenotype in patients with adenocarcinoma. Carcinogenesis 1991; 12: 25–28.
194. van Poppel G, de Vogel N, van Balderen PJ, Kok FJ. Increased cytogenetic damage in smokers deficient in glutathione *S*-transferase isozyme mu. Carcinogenesis 1992; 13:303–305.
195. Benhamou S, Lee WJ, Alexandrie AK, et al. Meta- and pooled analyses of the effects of glutathione *S*-transferase M1 polymorphisms and smoking on lung cancer risk. Carcinogenesis 2002; 23:1343–1350.
196. Houlston RS, Tomlinson IP. Polymorphisms and colorectal tumor risk. Gastroenterology 2001; 121: 282–301.
197. Howells RE, Redman CW, Dhar KK, et al. Association of glutathione *S*-transferase GSTM1 and GSTT1 null genotypes with clinical outcome in epithelial ovarian cancer. Clin Cancer Res 1998; 4: 2439–2445.
198. Strange RC, Lear JT, Fryer AA. Polymorphism in glutathione *S*-transferase loci as a risk factor for common cancers. Arch Toxicol 1998; 20:419–428.
199. Engel LS, Taioli E, Pfeiffer R, et al. Pooled analysis and meta-analysis of glutathione *S*-transferase M1 and bladder cancer: a HuGE review. Am J Epidemiol 2002; 156:95–109.
200. Elo JP, Visakorpi T. Molecular genetics of prostate cancer. Ann Med 2001; 33:130–141.
201. Geisler SA, Olshan AF. GSTM1, GSTT1, and the risk of squamous cell carcinoma of the head and neck: a mini-HuGE review. Am J Epidemiol 2001; 154:95–105.
202. Henderson CJ, McLaren AW, Moffat GJ, Bacon EJ, Wolf CR. Pi-class glutathione *S*-transferase: regulation and function. Chem-Biol Interact 1998; 111–112:69–82.
203. Iyer L, Ratain MJ. Pharmacogenetics and cancer chemotherapy. Eur J Cancer 1998; 34:1493–1499.
204. Perentesis JP. Genetic predisposition and treatment-related leukemia. Med Ped Oncol 2001; 36:541–548.
205. Hall AG, Autzen P, Cattan AR, et al. Expression of mu class glutathione *S*-transferase correlates with event-free survival in childhood acute lymphoblastic leukemia. Cancer Res 1994; 54:5251–5254.
206. Williams JA, Phillips DH. Mammary expression of xenobiotic metabolizing enzymes and their potential role in breast cancer. Cancer Res 2000; 60:4667–4677.
207. Hein DW, Doll MA, Fretland AJ, et al. Molecular genetics and epidemiology of the NAT1 and NAT2 acetylation polymorphisms. Cancer Epidemiol Biomarkers Prev 2000; 9:29–42.
208. Wikman H, Thiel S, Jager B, et al. Relevance of *N*-acetyltransferase 1 and 2 (NAT1, NAT2) genetic polymorphisms in non-small cell lung cancer susceptibility. Pharmacogenetics 2001; 11:157–168.
209. Ratain MJ, Mick R, Berezin F, et al. Paradoxical relationship between acetylator phenotype and amonafide toxicity. Clin Pharmacol Ther 1991; 50:573–579.
210. Ratain MJ, Mick R, Berezin F, et al. Phase-I study of amonafide dosing based on acetylator phenotype. Cancer Res 1993; 53:2304–2308.
211. Ratain MJ, Mick R, Janisch L, et al. Individualized dosing of amonafide based on a pharmacodynamic model incorporating acetylator phenotype and gender. Pharmacogenetics 1996; 6:93–101.

14 Cytochrome P450 and Anticancer Drugs

Yuichi Ando, MD, PhD

CONTENTS

1. OVERVIEW

1.1. P450 and Drug Metabolizing Enzymes

Drug metabolism is an enzymatic biotransformation of drugs. The early stage of drug metabolism generally consists of phase I reactions such as oxidation, reduction, and hydrolysis, effected by introducing a polar group into the parent molecule. The phase I reactions are followed by conjugations with hydrophilic compounds such as glucuronic acid and glutathione, to yield a more hydrophilic metabolite (phase II reactions). Cytochrome P450 (P450 or CYP) represents the enzyme that metabolizes drugs with various manners of oxidation as the phase I reaction. P450 is comprised of a large superfamily of heme-containing membrane-binding proteins that are classified into families and subfamilies. Most of the P450 related to drug metabolisms belong to CYP1, CYP2, or CYP3 families that are known as "drug metabolizing enzymes." Two or more P450 isoforms are frequently involved in the metabolism of the same drug, suggesting broad substrate specificity. P450 exists mainly in the liver, but may also exist in various organs such as the brain, lung, gastrointestinal tract, kidneys, and gonads. CYP3A4 is the most abundant isoform, occupying approx 30% of the total P450 amount in the human liver *(1)*. Because many therapeutic drugs are metabolized by CYP3A4, drug interactions related to the isoform occur frequently and interindividual variation of CYP3A4 activity is sometimes clinically significant via altering pharmacokinetics and pharmacodynamic actions. Furthermore, when a drug substrate of CYP3A4 is administered orally, the CYP3A4 activity in the intestine has a clinically significant effect on the bioavailability of the drug.

1.2. Nomenclature of P450

When a cytochrome P450 gene is described, cytochrome P450 is abbreviated as *CYP* or *Cyp* (*cy*tochrome *P*450), where all the letters are italicized. If all the letters are capitalized

Handbook of Anticancer Pharmacokinetics and Pharmacodynamics
Edited by: W. D. Figg and H. L. McLeod © Humana Press Inc., Totowa, NJ

as *CYP*, it represents a human gene, whereas if the latter two are lowercase *Cyp*, then it represents an animal model (mouse and *Drosophila*). The *CYP* or *Cyp* are usually followed by an Arabic number that designates the P450 family (amino acid homology >40%), a letter indicating the subfamily (homology >55%), and an Arabic numeral representing the individual gene. *P* (*ps* in mouse and *Drosophila*) after the gene number denotes a pseudogene. The cDNAs, mRNAs, and enzymes in all species (including mouse) should include all capital letters.

Recommendations for naming P450 have been publish by the Nomenclature Committee *(2)*. The updated information on the P450 nomenclatures is available through the Web (http://drnelson.utmem.edulcytochromeP450.html).

2. DRUG METABOLISM BY P450 AND CANCER CHEMOTHERAPY

2.1. Drug Metabolism in Cancer Chemotherapy

Normally, differences in the drug absorption, distribution, metabolism, and excretion cause interindividual variation in the pharmacokinetics of a drug when patients receive it at a uniform dose. Small changes in drug metabolism and/or pharmacokinetics of drugs commonly used for benign diseases are negligible because of the wide therapeutic windows. However, with cancer chemotherapy, serious clinical consequences may be triggered by the small changes of drug metabolism and those of pharmacokinetics. For example, interindividual variation of UDP-glucuronosyltransferase (UGT) activity is related to severe diarrhea of irinotecan *(3)*. Irinotecan is a prodrug that is hydrolyzed by carboxylesterase in vivo to form an active metabolite, SN-38. SN-38 is further conjugated and detoxified by UGT to yield β-glucuronide. The variation of sensitivity to irinotecan is related to large variations of biotransformation of the active metabolite SN-38, some of which are attributable to genetic polymorphism of UGT enzyme *(4)*.

Dosing of anticancer drugs is based on a Phase I study in which the dose is escalated up to a "maximum-tolerated dose." Inevitably, these drugs are administered to patients at toxic doses, and the therapeutic windows become narrower compared to other drugs used for benign diseases. Patients who are considered poor drug metabolizers usually exhibit low in vivo metabolic clearance thus increase the area under the concentration–time curve (AUC). Therefore, the patients would be exposed to the toxic compound and likely experience severe toxicity. Simultaneously, as the AUC would be decreased in patients who are extensive metabolizers, the same dose may be under-dosed. When a drug is activated after in vivo biotransformation (prodrug), patients with poor or extensive metabolic ability may not expect sufficient therapeutic benefits or may experience undesired severe toxicity, respectively.

2.2. Factors Affecting P450 Activity

Several factors may cause interindividual variations of P450 activity. These factors include genetic polymorphisms; changes in physiological conditions such as age, disease states, or intake of certain foods or drugs; or environmental factors such as smoking. Intuitively, liver dysfunction seems to decrease P450 contents, thereby impairing drug metabolism. As a matter of fact, cancer patients with severe liver dysfunction are not offered cytotoxic chemotherapy because of an empirical suspicion that they may experience severe toxicity. Based on several published pharmacokinetic data of anticancer drugs *(5)*, patients with severe or moderate liver impairment treated with vinca alkaloids or taxanes require dosage adjustments to prevent neutropenia and neurotoxicity. However, dosage reductions are unnecessary for patients with moderate liver impairment, although this information was obtained from studies with small sample sizes and nonhomogeneous patient groups *(5)*.

It is difficult to recognize specific factor(s) that may alter the P450 activity and pharmacokinetics/pharmacodynamics profile of chemotherapeutic drugs in individual cancer patients. The reason is that patients with cancer have heterogeneous backgrounds and complex physiological changes that may be caused by concomitant diseases states, organ dysfunction secondary to previous treatments, tumor invasions, malnutrition, and polypharmacy. Thus, when treating these patients, health care providers should determine whether their patients have any potential "factors," and if so, dosage modifications are required to minimize chemotherapy-induced toxicities.

2.3. Induction and Inhibition of P450

Concomitant drug combinations may affect drug metabolism, which may change the pharmacokinetics of the drugs and their clinical effects. Because induction and inhibition of drug-metabolizing enzymes have been regarded as the major mechanisms that may cause drug interactions, it is important to understand the metabolic pathway of each drug to explain and predict drug interactions. Series of in vitro metabolism experiments using human liver microsomes coupled with recombinant human liver P450 isoforms are powerful tools to characterize metabolic pathway and to identify the specific isoforms involved in the metabolism of the relevant drug. When drugs with a high affinity bind to a P450 isoform and are administered to a patient with other drugs that are metabolized by the same isoform, the former drug inhibits the metabolism of the latter. As a result, the pharmacological effects of the latter drug may be potentiated by increasing the amount of drug exposure.

An example of this is ZD1839 (Iressa), which is an epidermal growth factor receptor tyrosine kinase inhibitor that is metabolized by CYP3A4 (6). The pharmacokinetics of orally administered ZD1839 with or without rifampicin (a potent CYP3A4 inducer) was evaluated in a crossover study involving 18 healthy volunteers. When ZD1839 was administered with rifampicin (600 mg/d), the mean peak concentrations and AUC of 500 mg of ZD1839 were 65% and 83% lower, respectively, than without rifampicin. Furthermore, the CYP3A4 inhibitory effects of itraconazole (a potent CYP3A4 inhibitor) were explored in 24 volunteers receiving ZD1839. When ZD1839 was administered with itraconazole (200 mg/d), the mean peak concentrations and AUC of ZD1839 were increased by 32% and 58% at a dose of 500 mg, respectively. These two parameters were also increased by 51% and 80% at a dose of 250 mg. Although the clinical significance of these observations should be examined further, the study suggested possible drug interaction between ZD1839 and CYP3A4 inducers or inhibitors.

Some drugs are known to inhibit P450 activity nonspecifically, such as cimetidine (7) and ketoconazole (8), which may increase exposure and pharmacological activity of other drugs that are metabolized by some of the P450 isoforms. Satraplatin (JM216), the first orally available platinum-containing anticancer drug, also inhibits prototype reactions by P450 isoforms nonspecifically in vitro (9,10). The mechanism of the inhibition remains to be elucidated, but satraplatin may interact with the heme moiety of P450, which is critical to the activation of molecular oxygen to oxidize substrates. When satraplatin was given with etoposide in mice with murine tumors, a great dosage reduction was required when compared to monotherapy (11). Considering the results of the in vitro study, satraplatin might inhibit the in vivo metabolism of etoposide (by CYP3A4), thereby enhancing toxicity through increased exposure to etoposide. One should be cautious when treating patients on satraplatin with other drugs, as the correlation between in vivo and in vitro studies of this drug interaction has not been investigated.

2.4. Genetic Polymorphism

Genetic variations of the P450 gene, as well as some drug metabolizing enzymes, are known to cause phenotypic variability in the enzymatic process and alter drug pharmacoki-

Table 1
Anticancer Drugs Metabolized by Cytochrome P450

CYP	Drug (references)	Metabolic pathway
2A6	Tegafur (16,18)	5'-Hydroxylation
2B6	Cyclophosphamide (20)	4-Hydroxylation
	Ifosfamide (20,21)	4-Hydroxylation (minor) N-Dechloroethylation (major)
2C8	Paclitaxel (71)	6-α-Hydroxylation
2C9	Cyclophosphamide (22)	4-Hydroxylation
2C19	Thalidomide (52)	5- and 5'-Hydroxylation
2D6	Tamoxifen (31)	4-Hydroxylation
3A4	Cyclophosphamide (20)	4-Hydroxylation (minor) N-Dechloroethylation (major)
	Ifosfamide (20,21)	4-Hydroxylation N-Dechloroethylation
	Etoposide (63)	O-Demethylation
	Tamoxifen (30)	N-Demethylation
	Docetaxel (57)	Hydroxylation of the tert-butyl ester group
	Paclitaxel (71)	3'-p-Hydroxylation
	Vinca alkaloids (35)	Unidentified

netics (12). Accordingly, genetic variations may be the reason for the variable susceptibility to a drug. When there is a genotype–phenotype relationship, the probability of response or severe toxicity to the drug could be forecasted by analyzing the genotype of the relevant enzyme prior to therapy.

Typically, genetic polymorphism is a dominant factor to determine enzyme activity of drug metabolism. However, because drug effect is a sum of complex gene–environmental interactions, other factors may affect the phenotypic activity more than the genetic status, such as physiological condition and therapeutic drug use. The genetic polymorphism of the *CYP2C19* gene has been studied extensively (12). Subjects with a variant allele of the gene have poor drug metabolism catalyzed by CYP2C19 (poor metabolizer), and these subjects have an increased risk of an undesired drug effects because of low metabolic clearance. However, Williams et al. reported a decrease of CYP2C19 activity in patients with advanced cancer that resulted in discordance between the *CYP2C19* genotype and phenotype (13). In this case, patients with lower CYP2C19 activity could not be identified by genotyping alone.

2.5. Metabolisms of Anticancer Drugs by P450

A variety of anticancer drugs are metabolized by P450 (Table 1). Specific isoforms involved in the metabolism of each drug can be identified through comprehensive in vitro experiments using human liver microsomes and recombinant P450 isoforms. Quantitative estimation of in vivo drug metabolism from in vitro data is sometimes difficult and erroneous because various factors may cause discrepancies between in vitro and in vivo metabolisms, such as drug concentrations in liver tissue and interindividual variability in enzyme activity (14).

When there is a recognized interspecies difference in the metabolism of a drug, careful attention should be paid in interpreting results of animal experiments for the drug. For example, paclitaxel undergoes extensive P450 metabolisms by both human and rat liver microsomes. However, according to an in vitro study reported by Jamis-Dow et al., paclitaxel was catalyzed by rat liver microsomes into several metabolites, none of which had an identical peak of 6-α-hydroxypaclitaxel, a major metabolite of paclitaxel in humans *(15)*.

3. ANTICANCER DRUGS METABOLIZED BY P450

3.1. Tegafur

Tegafur is a prodrug of 5-fluorouracil (5-FU), which exerts its cytotoxic effects through the inhibition of thymidylate synthase and/or by its incorporation into RNA. 5-FU is then further biotransformed to an inactive molecule by dihydropyrimidine dehydrogenase. Tegafur is converted to 5-FU mainly by the liver via an unstable metabolic intermediate, 5'-hydroxytegafur. The 5'-hydroxylation of tegafur is mediated primarily by CYP2A6, followed by spontaneous decomposition of 5'-hydroxytegafur to 5-FU. In an in vitro study using a panel of 10 human microsomes (16), formation rates of 5-FU showed a significant correlation with activities of coumarin 7-hydroxylation, a prototype reaction of CYP2A6. The activity of 5-FU formation by recombinant CYP2A6 isoform was the highest among 10 other expressed P450 isoforms. Furthermore, specific chemical inhibitors and antiserum against CYP2A6 inhibited 5-FU formation. Therefore, it can be speculated that CYP2A6 may have an effect on the in vivo activation of tegafur. For instance, a patient who has lower activity of CYP2A6 may have little benefit from tegafur because of an insufficient exposure to 5-FU. As genetic polymorphism of the *CYP2A6* gene has been recognized to cause a decreased or absent activity of CYP2A6 *(17)*, a patient having the variant allele of the *CYP2A 6* gene would also be included in those who have little benefit from tegafur. 5-FU is also formed from tegafur by liver cytosolic thymidine phosphorylase *(18)*, which might harbor the clinical significance of CYP2A6 activity. Further clinical studies are required to determine how CYP2A6 activity may have an effect on the in vivo bioactivation of tegafur.

3.2. Oxazaphosphorine

Cyclophosphamide and ifosfamide are oxazaphosphorine-alkylating agents that require metabolic activation to exert their pharmacological activity. The metabolism and activation of these agents have been reviewed elsewhere *(19)*. There are two distinct metabolic pathways of these drugs: 4-hydroxylation as an activating pathway and *N*-dechloroethylation as an inactivating one. The active metabolites, 4-hydroxycyclophosphamide, and 4-hydroxyifosfamide are produced in the human body mainly by CYP2B6 and CYP3A4, respectively *(20,21)*. CYP2C9 has also been reported in 4-hydroxylation of cyclophosphamide *(22)*. These 4-hydroxy metabolites subsequently generate the alkylating species mustards to show antitumor activity, and together with a toxic byproduct, acrolein, may cause urotoxicity. The other pathway of *N*-dechloroethylation generates inactive metabolites and a toxic byproduct, chloroacetaldehyde. The pathway of *N*-dechloroethylation is catalyzed by CYP3A4 for cyclophosphamide and is catalyzed by both CYP3A4 and CYP2B6 for ifosfamide *(23)*. As an important difference in drug metabolism between cyclophosphamide and ifosfamide, the *N*-dechloroethylation accounts for approx 50% of the total administered dose of ifosfamide, but only 10% of cyclophosphamide *(24)*. Therefore, patients treated with ifosfamide are more exposed to toxic chloroacetaldehyde and are more likely to experience nephrotoxicity or neurotoxicity than those treated with cyclophosphamide.

P450 activity may alter the balance between the activating (4-hydroxylation) and inactivating (*N*-dechloroethylation) metabolic pathways, leading to variations in the pharmacokinetics and pharmacodynamics profile of oxazaphosphorine. In a clinical trial with 11 cancer patients, cyclophosphamide was administered weekly as single intravenous doses of 500 mg/kg *(25)*. The patients were pretreated with 200 mg of phenobarbital as a P450 inducer for three consecutive days prior to the second administration of the drug. Pharmacokinetic analysis of the study showed that blood levels of the parent drug were decreased and normustard-like metabolites were increased. This finding suggested that phenobarbital induced CYP2B6 and CYP3A4 activities, resulting in an enhanced metabolism of cyclophosphamide. With regard to ifosfamide, CYP2B6 is the dominant isoform in inactivating the *N*-dechloroethylation pathway and, furthermore, it plays a minor role in activating the 4-hydroxylation pathway. Thus, selective inhibition of CYP2B6 could improve therapeutic efficacy of ifosfamide theoretically, albeit definite clinical evidence has not been demonstrated. In animal models, retrovirus-mediated expressions of CYP2B6 in tumor cells have been reported to enhance the efficacy of cyclophosphamide by increasing metabolic activation *(26)*.

The oxazaphosphorines contain a chiral phosphorus atom, and therefore they are usually used as racemic mixtures of (+)-*R* and (−)-*S* enantiomers. According to an in vitro study on stereoselective metabolism of ifosfamide, *R*-ifosfamide has more favorable properties than *S*-ifosfamide with respect to less extensive *N*-dechloroethylation and more rapid 4-hydroxylation *(27)*. It has been reported that phenytoin would induce the enantioselective metabolism of cyclophosphamide *(28)*, in which inactivating *N*-dechloroethylation was induced to a greater extent in the *S*-enantiomer than the *R*-enantiomer. However, the clinical significance of stereoselective difference in the drug metabolism remains to be determined.

Cyclophosphamide is occasionally used in high-dose chemotherapy with bone marrow supports. Oncologists have a plausible concern that the drug metabolism by CYP2B6 might be saturated at high doses because CYP2B6 is one of the minor P450 isoforms *(1)*. The saturation may cause a greater proportion of the inactive or toxic metabolites generated by *N*-dechloroethylation pathway by CYP3A4. Therefore, a continuous infusion or divided doses over several days are usually preferred in high-dose chemotherapy of cyclophosphamide to avoid the saturation of the drug metabolism *(29)*. In addition, cyclophosphamide and ifosfamide can induce their own metabolism (autoinduction) with prolonged use of the drugs. Thus, saturation of the drug metabolism would be compensated to some extent *(19)*. However, the clinical significance of the prolonged use of cyclophosphamide and ifosfamide has not been well investigated.

3.3. Tamoxifen

Tamoxifen, a synthetic antiestrogen, has been used for many years to treat breast cancer. This drug requires metabolic activation by the P450 system to generate adducts of tamoxifen with DNA and protein *(30)*. The major metabolites of tamoxifen are *N*-desmethyltamoxifen that is formed by CYP3A4, 4-hydroxytamoxifen by CYP2D6, and tamoxifen *N*-oxide by flavin-containing monooxygenase *(30,31)*. The *N*-desmethyl and 4-hydroxy derivatives have several hundred times more and equal affinity toward the estrogen receptor α, respectively, as compared with the parent drug *(32)*. Recently, involvement of CYP2B6 has also been suggested in the metabolic activation of tamoxifen *(33)*. Thus, activities of these P450 isoforms may affect the pharmacological effects of tamoxifen, and, accordingly, drug interactions would occur when tamoxifen is combined with other drugs that can affect the activities of these P450 isoforms. As for pharmacogenetic consideration of tamoxifen, patients with a variant *CYP2D6* allele (poor metabolizers) may have less benefit from tamoxifen therapy than others because of less exposure to the active metabolite 4-hydroxytamoxifen. So far, the relationships between these enzymatic activities and clinical outcomes of tamoxifen therapy have not been identified.

3.4. Vinca Alkaloids

Vinca alkaloids belong to microtubule inhibitors and they receive drug metabolism mainly by CYP3A4 into unidentified metabolites. Vinorelbine, a semisynthetic vinca alkaloid used to treat non-small-cell cancer and metastatic breast cancer, has a high therapeutic index and less neurotoxicity than other vinca alkaloids (34). Drug metabolism of vinorelbine by CYP3A4 appears to cause large interpatient pharmacokinetic variability. According to an in vitro study using human liver microsomes, 50% inhibitory concentration (IC_{50}) of vinorelbine for testosterone 6-β-hydroxylase activity (catalyzed by CYP3A4) was estimated to be 155 μM (35). Although plasma concentrations of vinorelbine are much lower than the IC_{50} value, drug combinations that could inhibit or induce CYP3A4 activity may alter drug metabolism and pharmacological effects of vinorelbine.

There are several clinical reports of drug interactions with vinca alkaloids. Among 14 patients with acute lymphoblastic leukemia (ALL) receiving induction chemotherapy consisting of vincristine and itraconazole, four patients experienced severe neuropathy (paresthesia, muscle weakness, and paralytic ileus) after the first or second dose of vincristine (36). Increased neurotoxicity of vinca alkaloid-containing chemotherapy has also been reported in patients who simultaneously received cyclosporine (37,38) or in combination with erythromycin (39). As regards to anticancer agents, etoposide and teniposide have been reported to enhance vincristine-induced neurotoxicity, albeit other studies found no evidence of the interaction (40–42). The exact mechanism(s) of the drug interactions remains unclear. However, drugs that increase the toxicity of vinca alkaloids have been known to inhibit CYP3A4-mediated metabolism in a competitive or noncompetitive manner. Thus, it is possible that the inhibition of the detoxifying pathway by CYP3A4 would cause an increase in exposure to the drug, leading to unexpected toxicity. In addition, because cyclosporine and itraconazole also inhibit P-glycoprotein, the modulation of the P-glycoprotein would be another mechanism of the drug interaction.

3.5. Thalidomide

Thalidomide was originally developed as a sedative and was eventually removed from the market because of significant teratogenic effects (43). Recently, it has been reintroduced for the treatment of leprosy, multiple myeloma, and prostate cancer (44,45). While the true mechanism(s) of action still remains controversial, it has been suggested that thalidomide requires P450-catalyzed biotransformation to exert its pharmacological activities, including antiangiogenesis (46–48). Indeed, the main transformation of thalidomide is considered as a spontaneous nonenzymatic hydrolysis; however, these breakdown products are not responsible for this activity (49). At least two hydroxylated metabolites have been found in patients' plasma or urine: 5-hydroxythalidomide, formed by hydroxylation of the phthalimide ring, and cis- and trans-5'-hydroxythalidomide, by hydroxylation of the glutarimide ring (50,51).

Recently, it has been reported that the polymorphic enzyme CYP2C19 is primarily responsible for 5- and 5'-hydroxylation of thalidomide in humans (52). The interindividual variation of the CYP2C19 activity caused by its genetic polymorphism may attribute to the efficacy and toxicity profile of thalidomide. For instance, the biotransformation is impaired in patients who are poor metabolizers, resulting in very low or absent amount of these metabolites. A patient who is a normal "extensive" metabolizer is likely to have a therapeutic response to thalidomide; however, it will increase one's risk of adverse effects. In a case-control study conducted in 63 patients with prostate cancer, the associations of the CYP2C19 genotype with clinical events and formations of the hydroxylated metabolite were explored (53). Monotherapy thalidomide was administered at doses of 200–1200 mg/d, most of which (88%) received 200 mg/d. Results demonstrated that two patients were homozygous for the variant *CYP2CJ9*2* allele, The two patients were included in the 25 patients whose prostate-specific antigen (PSA) failed to demonstrate a decline (nonresponder), and the metabolite concentrations in plasma from both patients were below quantification. No apparent association was found between the 14 heterozygotes (extensive metabolizer) and PSA changes. These findings are consistent with the hypothesis that patients with poor metabolizing phenotype of CYP2C19 receive little benefit from thalidomide treatment and that the poor metabolizer genotype is associated with a lower ability to form the metabolites. A correlation between *CYP2CI9* genotype and clinical outcomes requires further investigation.

4. INTERINDIVIDUAL VARIATION OF CYP3A4 ACTIVITY

CYP3A4 exists most abundantly among human P450 isoforms. The enzymatic activity of CYP3A4 exhibits a remarkable interindividual variation as high as 20-fold *(1)*, which can be induced by glucocorticoids, rifampicin, and phenobarbital. Antifungal azole derivatives, such as ketoconazole itraconazole, inhibit CYP3A4, and 14-member macrolides also inhibit the isoform irreversibly by its active metabolites binding to the heme portion of P450 (mechanism-based inhibition). It has been known that CYP3A4 is responsible for the metabolism of many anticancer drugs (Table 1). Extensive attempts have been made to manipulate the large variation of CYP3A4 activity and to reduce pharmacokinetic variability of the relevant drugs, which includes genotyping of the *CYP3A4* gene, quantification and modulation of the phenotypic activity, and dose adaptation during a protracted treatment. However, the clinical significance of these attempts should be carefully evaluated in view of clinical practice.

4.1. Genetic Polymorphism of the CYP3A4 Gene

Despite attempts to explore genetic variations causing wide variability of CYP3A4, identifying genetic variants have minimal contribution to the interindividual variability *(54)*. Eiselt et al. investigated 18 variant alleles of the *CYP3A4* gene, including eight protein variants in 213 DNA samples from Caucasians. A total of 7.5% of the population studied had one of these variants heterozygously, and four of the eight protein variants exhibited some alteration in the enzymatic activity in their in vitro expression systems. However, most (15/18) of the variants had allele frequencies below 1%, and obviously the protein variants did not fully explain the observed large variability of CYP3A4 expression and activity. This implies that most functionally relevant genetic variance should be located in the regulatory region, if any, rather than a protein-coding region of the gene. As for the promoter region of the *CYP3A4* gene, an association of decreased risk for treatment-related leukemia with a variant sequence in the nifedipine-specific response element (*CYP3A4*1B*) has been reported (55). When CYP3A4 metabolizes certain drugs used for the treatment of leukemia (i.e., etoposide), catechol and quinone metabolites are formed, leading to DNA damage. Therefore, frequencies of the *CYP3A4 *1B* allele were investigated using genomic DNA from 99 patients with *de novo* leukemia and 30 with treatment related leukemia who had been treated with anticancer drugs metabolized by CYP3A4. The results revealed that a frequency of patients carrying the *CYP3A4*1B* allele was significantly lower (3%) among the treatment-related cases compared to the *de novo* cases (19%). It was speculated that the decreased activity of CYP3A4 would contribute to the reduced risk of leukemia because there is less exposure to the leukemogenic metabolites. To the contrary, in vitro experiments failed to yield a genotype–phenotype association of the *CYP3A4*1B* allele *(56)*. Neither nifedipine oxidation activity (a prototype reaction of CYP3A4) nor its protein levels were related to the genetic status of the *CYP3A4*1B* allele in the 15 human liver samples. The reason for this disagreement is unclear; however, the increased risk of leukemia by the variant *CYP3A4* gene may be due to linkage disequilibrium of the distinct variants or genes with a more potent leukemogenic effect. In addition, numerous environmental factors affecting in vivo CYP3A4 activity and physiologic conditions may contribute to the discordance. It seems that genetic status of the *CYP3A4* gene would have a smaller impact on its enzymatic activity than other P450 isoforms.

4.2. Quantification of CYP3A4 *Activity: Docetaxel*

4.2.1. PHENOTYPING CYP3A4 ACTIVITY

Docetaxel is primarily metabolized by CYP3A4 and CYP3A5 in humans, which causes a large interindividual variability in a pharmacokinetic/pharmacodynamic profile of the drug *(57,58)*. The in vivo effects of induction and inhibition of the CYP3A enzyme on docetaxel pharmacokinetics was studied in mice *(59)*. The results revealed that pretreatment with ketoconazole (CYP3A inhibitor) increased the AUC of docetaxel. On the other hand, dexamethasone (CYP3A inducer) decreased the AUC. These findings showed that enzymatic induction and inhibition of CYP3A would also have an effect on the docetaxel pharmacokinetics in humans and potentially on the antitumor potency of this drug.

Body surface area has been used for an individual dosing of anticancer agents including docetaxel. However, because of the large variability of the CYP3A4 activity, guidance by CYP3A4 activity appears to be a better way to determine a dose of docetaxel. Attempts have been made to quantify a phenotypic activity of CYP3A4 and to explore a correlation between the activity and the pharmacokinetic parameters of docetaxel. In a study with 21 sarcoma patients who were treated with docetaxel at a dose of 100 mg/m^2, [^{14}C-*N*-methyl] erythromycin breath test (ERMBT) was used to measure hepatic CYP3A4 activity in vivo *(60)*. The results of log-transformed ERMBT values accounted for 67% of the interpatient variation in the docetaxel clearance, and severe toxicity was seen in the patients with the lowest ERMBT values. In another study, Yamamoto et al. measured urinary 6-β-hydroxycortisol in 29 patients with non-small-cell lung cancer after receiving 300 mg of hydrocortisone intravenously, followed by a treatment with docetaxel of 60 mg/m^2 *(61)*. Multivariate analysis revealed that the total amount of 24-h urinary 6-β-hydroxycortisol was the strongest factor to predict docetaxel clearance. These studies suggested that CYP3A4 activity would be a useful indicator to predict in vivo docetaxel clearance and potentially its toxicity; thus, the CYP3A4-guided dosing would be a promising method for docetaxel dosing.

4.2.2. CYP3A4 GENE EXPRESSION

Fujitaka et al. reported induced expression of the CYP3A4 gene in peripheral mononuclear cells in lung cancer patients who received docetaxel *(62)*. Assuming that the level of the gene expression correlates between peripheral mononuclear cells and hepatocytes, it would be a convenient marker for docetaxel metabolism in the total body and may be used as a predictor for toxicity and response.

4.3. Modulation of CYP3A4 *Activity*

When an anticancer drug is mainly metabolized and detoxified by CYP3A4, the elimination pathway of the drug is slowed down and its pharmacological effects are potentiated by combining with other drugs that inhibit the CYP3A4. Particularly, inhibition of the CYP3A4 enzyme in the intestine and liver boosts the bioavailability of orally administered drugs that are substrates of CYP3A4. On the other hand, it has been known that CYP3A4 and P-glycoprotein, a multidrug transporter encoded by the *MDR1* gene, have many common substrates such as cyclosporin, calcium blockers, and azole compounds. Thus, some drugs that inhibit CYP3A4 would inhibit P-glycoprotein function simultaneously. Inhibition of P-glycoprotein may increase drug retention in normal tissues and delay elimination from the body of the substrate drugs, resulting in alterations of its pharmacological effects. Generally, the relative contribution of CYP3A4 and P-glycoprotein inhibitions by the same drug would be too complicated to be assessed independently.

4.3.1. ETOPOSIDE AND KETOCONAZOLE

Etoposide is a substrate of CYP3A4 and its pharmacokinetic parameters have a large interpatient variability *(63,64)*. A wide variability in oral etoposide bioavailability has also been known *(65)*. Kobayashi et al. conducted a pharmacokinetic study of oral etoposide with ketoconazole (200 mg), an inhibitor of CYP3A4 and P-glycoprotein *(66)*. In this study, 13 cancer patients received etoposide at a dose of 50 mg every other day or daily over 21 d. When etoposide was administered with ketoconazole, a median increase of AUC values was 44% (range, 14–50%) as compared to the AUC without ketoconazole. Although it was unclear if interpatient variability in the pharmacokinetic parameters decreased, the results implied that equivalent therapeutic efficacy could be expected with smaller doses of oral etoposide by combined use with ketoconazole. Unfortunately, the clinical significance of this foresighted study is limited owing to lack of an advantage of oral etoposide over conventional intravenous administration *(67)*.

4.3.2. DOCETAXEL AND CYCLOSPORINE

Fourteen patients with solid tumor received oral docetaxel at a dose of 75 mg/m^2 with or without a single oral dose of cyclosporine of 15 mg/kg *(68)*. The AUC of docetaxel was remarkably increased by the coadministration of cyclosporine from 0.37 ± 0.33 mg·h/L to 2.71 ± 1.81 mg·h/L (mean ± standard deviation). The AUC of oral docetaxel with cyclosporine was equivalent to $90\% \pm 44\%$ of AUC after intravenous docetaxel normalized to the same dose level. The interpatient variability of the AUC values was comparable between oral docetaxel with cyclosporine (67%) and intravenous docetaxel (53%). Interestingly, metabolites of docetaxel were detected in plasma only when docetaxel was administered with cyclosporine. The mechanism of emergence of the metabolites was unclear; however, it would be possible that elimination of the metabolites was delayed by the use of cyclosporine. The data suggested that oral formulation of docetaxel might be a possible dosing route in the future for cancer chemotherapy.

4.3.3. PACLITAXEL AND VALSPODAR (PSC 833)

Valspodar (PSC 833), a cyclosporine derivative, is a second-generation nonnephrotoxic and nonimmunosuppressive P-glycoprotein antagonist. Biotransformation of valspodar is CYP3A dependent. A Phase I study of paclitaxel over 4 d and oral valspodar (5 mg/kg administered every 6 h over 7 d) was conducted in patients with refractory cancer, where valspodar was primarily used to reverse multidrug resistance *(69)*. When patients received paclitaxel doses of 13.1 or 17.5 mg/m^2 per day with valspodar, the mean steady-state concentrations and AUC of paclitaxel were similar to those when they received paclitaxel at a dose of 35 mg/m^2 per day. Inhibition of rhodamine efflux from CD56+ cells was used as a surrogate marker for P-glycoprotein inhibition in this study. Despite of complete inhibition of P-glycoprotein in the surrogate assay, the large variability in paclitaxel pharmacokinetics was still observed, suggesting that it may be due to the variation in the P450 activity. The use of valspodar not only increased plasma concentrations of paclitaxel but also produced metabolites of the drug, similar to the case of docetaxel and cyclosporine *(70)*. Plasma concentrations of 6-α-hydroxypaclitaxel, a major metabolite of paclitaxel

(71), were increased to measurable levels in 21 of 22 patients in this trial. The metabolite was not detectable in plasma when paclitaxel was administered without valspodar in the same patients. There are several possible explanations for the clinical presence of the metabolite, albeit none of which are mutually exclusive. First, paclitaxel also undergoes 3'-*p*-hydroxylation by CYP3A4. Thus, it is possible that the pathway of 3'-*p*-hydroxylation may be inhibited competitively by valspodar, and, consequently, the metabolism of paclitaxel might shift from producing 3'-*p*-hydroxypaclitaxel to producing 6-α-hydroxypaclitaxel. Second, reabsorption of the excreted metabolites is increased through the inhibition of intestinal P-glycoprotein. Finally, valspodar might promote cholestasis and enhance the enterohepatic circulation, increasing plasma concentrations of the metabolite. Although the clinical significance of this metabolite remains unclear, this study emphasized that the concurrent use of an agent such as valspodar could considerably alter the drug metabolism and disposition.

4.4. Dose Adaptation During a Protracted Chemotherapy: Etoposide

When pharmacokinetic/pharmacodynamic relationships are recognized in a protracted use of a drug, therapeutic drug monitoring (TDM) may be a potential approach to improve therapeutic efficacy and toxicity. Chronic use of a chemotherapy agent of an oral drug is the best candidate due to its wide range of bioavailability. Etoposide undergoes CYP3A4-mediated metabolism of *O*-demethylation, forming a catechol *(63)*. Thus, in vivo clearance of etoposide depends on CYP3A4 activity, which would be one of the reasons for the large pharmacokinetic variability of the drug. Indeed, drugs that induce CYP3A4 used concomitantly may increase the clearance of etoposide *(72)*. According to pharmacokinetic studies of a protracted use of intravenous etoposide, it has been suggested that maintaining a plasma level (>1 μg/mL) of the drug would enhance the antitumor effect, whereas high peak levels (>2 μg/mL) may cause severe myelotoxicity *(64)*. Subsequent studies were conducted to utilize TDM for the protracted etoposide *(73,74)*. First, etoposide was infused for 14 d at 40 mg/m^2 per day initially in 21 courses of 12 patients with non-small-cell lung cancer *(73)*. The infusion rate (dose) was modified based on plasma concentration at 24 h following the initiation of the infusion to achieve a target concentration of 1.5 μg/mL. The range of the concentration became narrower after the dose adjustment: 1.1 μg/mL to 2.9 μg/mL at 24 h and 1.2 μg/mL to 2.0 μg/mL at steady state. Interpatient coefficient variations (CV = standard deviation/mean × 100) were significantly decreased from 22% to 14% and 13% at 96 h and 192 h, respectively. Interestingly, the CV values became larger as the time increased after the adjustment, 19% at 288 h and 19% at 336 h, suggesting that metabolism/disposition of etoposide would be changing during the treatment. In another study, TDM was applied to a 21-d therapy of oral etoposide for patients with lung cancer *(74)*. As a starting dose, a 25-mg capsule of etoposide was taken orally three times daily (75 mg/d). The target range of plasma concentration was 1.0 μg/mL to 1.5 μg/mL. The dose was adapted to 50 or 100 mg per day on and after d 5 to achieve the target range, according to the concentration on d 3 and 4. These studies demonstrated that TDM would be applicable for cancer chemotherapy to reduce the pharmacokinetic variability. The impact of the TDM on clinical outcomes, such as reduced incidence of adverse effects or improved survival, requires further studies.

5. SUMMARY

A variety of anticancer drugs are metabolized by P450, including tegafur cyclophosphamide, ifosfamide, paclitaxel, thalidomide, tamoxifen, etoposide, docetaxel, and vinca alkaloids. The variation in drug metabolism causes pharmacokinetic variability and may influence drug efficacy and toxicity. Drug metabolism depends on both genetic and environmental factors, which include genetic polymorphism and drug interactions (induction or inhibition of P450 activity). CYP3A4 is the major human P450 isoform with a remarkable interindividual variation in its activity. With regard to CYP3A4, environmental factors appear to influence its activity more than genetic status. The challenges have been made to control the phenotypic CYP3A4 activity and to reduce pharmacokinetic variability of the relevant drugs. However, the clinical advantages obtained from these efforts should be carefully evaluated in view of clinical practice.

REFERENCES

1. Shimada T, Yamazaki H, Mimura M, Inui Y, Guengerich FP. Interindividual variations in human liver cytochrome P-450 enzymes involved in the oxidation of drugs, carcinogens and toxic chemicals: studies with liver microsomes of 30 Japanese and 30 Caucasians. J Pharmacol Exp Ther 1994; 270:414–423.
2. Nelson DR, Koymans L, Kamataki T, et al. P450 superfamily: update on new sequences, gene mapping, accession numbers and nomenclature. Pharmacogenetics 1996; 6:1–42.
3. Gupta E, Lestingi TM, Mick R, Ramirez J, Vokes EE, Ratain MJ. Metabolic fate of irinotecan in humans: correlation of glucuronidation with diarrhea. Cancer Res 1994; 54:3723–3725.
4. Ando Y, Saka H, Ando M, et al. Polymorphisms of UDP-glucuronosyltransferase gene and irinotecan toxicity: a pharmacogenetic analysis. Cancer Res 2000; 60:6921–6926.
5. Donelli MG, Zucchetti M, Munzone E, D'Incalci M, Crosignani A. Pharmacokinetics of anticancer agents in patients with impaired liver function. Eur J Cancer 1998; 34:33–46.
6. Swaisland H, Smith RP, Farebrother J, Laight A. The effect of the induction and inhibition of CY3A4 on the pharmacokinetics of single oral doses of ZD1839 ('Iressa'), a selective epidermal growth factor receptor tyrosine kinase inhibitor (EGFR-TKI), in healthy male volunteers. Proc Am Soc Clin Oncol 2002; 21:83a.
7. Winzor DJ, Ioannoni B, Reilly PB. The nature of microsomal monooxygenase inhibition by cimetidine. Biochem Pharmacol 1986; 35:2157–2161.
8. Pasanen M, Taskinen T, Iscan M, Sotaniemi EA, Kairaluoma M, Pelkonen O. Inhibition of human hepatic and placental xenobiotic monooxygenases by imidazole antimycotics. Biochem Pharmacol 1988; 37:3861–3866.
9. Kelland LR. An update on satraplatin: the first orally available platinum anticancer drug. Exp Opin Invest Drugs 2000; 9:1373–1382.
10. Ando Y, Shimizu T, Mushiroda T, Nakagawa T, Kodama T, Kamataki T. Potent and nonspecific inhibition of cytochrome P450 by JM216, a new oral platinum agent. Br J Cancer 1998; 89:1170–1174.
11. Rose WC. Combination chemotherapy involving orally administered etoposide and JM-216 in murine tumor models. Cancer Chemother Pharmacol 1997; 40:51–56.
12. Meyer UA. Pharmacogenetics. In: Carruthers SG, Hoffman BB, Melmon KL, Nierenberg DW, (eds). Melmon and Morrelli's Clinical Pharmacology, 4th Edit. New York, NY: McGraw-Hill, 2000, pp. 1191–1192.
13. Williams ML, Bhargava P, Cherrouk I, Marshall JL, Flockhart DA, Wainer IW. A discordance of the cytochrome P450 2C19 genotype and phenotype in patients with advanced cancer. Br J Clin Pharmacol 2000; 49:485–488.
14. Iwatsubo T, Hirota N, Ooie T, et al. Prediction of *in vivo* drug metabolism in the human live from *in vitro* metabolism data. Pharmacol Ther 1997; 73:147–171.
15. Jamis-Dow CA, Klecker RW, Katki AG, Collins JM. Metabolism of Taxol by human and rat liver in vitro: a screen for drug interactions and interspecies differences. Cancer Chemother Pharmacol 1995; 36:107–114.
16. Ikeda K, Yoshisue K, Matsushima E, et al. Bioactivation of tegafur to 5-fluorouracil is catalyzed by cytochrome P-450 2A6 in human liver microsomes *in vitro*. Clin Cancer Res 2000; 6:4409–4415.
17. Nunoya K, Yokoi T, Kimura K, et al. A new deleted allele in the human cytochrome P450 2A6 (*CYP2A6*) gene found in individuals showing poor metabolic capacity to coumarin and (+)-*cis*-3,5-dimethyl-2-(3-pyridyl)thiazolidin-4-one hydrochloride (SM-12502). Pharmacogenetics 1998; 8:239–249.
18. Komatsu T, Yamazaki H, Shimada N, et al. Involvement of microsomal cytochrome P450 and cytosolic thymidine phosphorylase in 5-fluorouracil formation from tegafur in human liver. Clin Cancer Res 2001; 7:675–681.

19. Boddy AV, Yule SM. Metabolism and pharmacokinetics of oxazaphosphorines. Clin Pharmacokinet 2000; 38:291–304.
20. Chang TKH, Weber GF, Crespi CL, Waxman DJ. Differential activation of cyclophosphamide and ifosphamide by cytochromes P-450 2B and 3A in human liver microsomes. Cancer Res 1993; 53: 5629–5637.
21. Walker D, Flinois JP, Monkman SC, et al. Identification of the major human hepatic cytochrome P450 involved in activation and N-dechloroethylation of ifosfamide. Biochem Pharmacol 1994; 47:1157–1163.
22. Ren S, Yang JS, Kalhorn TF, Slattery JT. Oxidation of cyclophosphamide to 4-hydroxycyclo-phosphamide and deschloroethylcyclophosphamide in human liver microsomes. Cancer Res 1997; 57: 4229–4235.
23. Huang Z, Roy P, Waxman DJ. Role of human liver microsomal CYP3A4 and CYP2B6 in catalyzing N-dechloroethylation of cyclophosphamide and ifosfamide. Biochem Pharmacol 2000; 59:961–972.
24. Kaijser GP, Korst A, Beijnen JH, Bult A, Underberg WJ. The analysis of ifosfamide and its metabolites (review). Anticancer Res 1993; 13:1311–1324.
25. Maezawa S, Ohira S, Sakuma M, Matsuoka S, Wakui A, Saito T. Effects of inducer of liver drug-metabolizing enzyme on blood level of active metabolites of cyclophosphamide in rats and in cancer patients. Tohoku J Exp Med 1981; 134:45–53.
26. Jounaidi Y, Hecht JE, Waxman DJ. Retroviral transfer of human cytochrome P450 genes for oxaza-phosphorine-based cancer gene therapy. Cancer Res 1998; 58:4391–4401.
27. Roy P, Tretyakov O, Wright J, Waxman DJ. Stereoselective metabolism of ifosfamide by human P-450s 3A4 and 2B6. Favorable metabolic properties of R-enantiomer. Drug Metab Dispos 1999; 27:1309–1318.
28. Williams ML, Wainer IW, Embree L, Barnett M, Granvil CL, Ducharme MP. Enantioselective induction of cyclophosphamide metabolism by phenytoin. Chirality 1999; 11:569–574.
29. Busse D, Busch FW, Schweizer E, et al. Fractionated administration of high-dose cyclophosphamide: influence on dose-dependent changes in pharmacokinetics and metabolism. Cancer Chemother Pharmacol 1999; 43:263–268.
30. Mani C, Gelboin HV, Park SS, Pearce R, Parkinson A, Kupfer D. Metabolism of the antimammary cancer antiestrogenic agent tamoxifen. I. Cytochrome P-450-catalyzed N-demethylation and 4-hydroxylation. Drug Metab Dispos 1993; 21:645–656.
31. Dehal S, Kupfer D. CYP2D6 catalyzes tamoxifen 4-hydroxylation in human liver. Cancer Res 1997; 57:3402–3406.
32. Coezy E, Borgna JL, Rochefort H. Tamoxifen and metabolites in MCF7 cells: correlation between binding to estrogen receptor and inhibition of cell growth. Cancer Res 1982; 42:317–323.
33. Sridar C, Kent UM, Notley LM, Gillam EM, Hollenberg PF. Effect of tamoxifen on the enzymatic activity of human cytochrome CYP2B6. J Pharmacol Exp Ther 2002; 301:945–952.
34. Zhou XJ, Rahmani R. Preclinical can clinical pharmacology of vinca alkaloids. Drugs 1992: 44 (Suppl 4): 1–16; discussion 66–69.
35. Kajita J, Kuwabara T, Kobayashi H, Kobayashi S. CYP3A4 is mainly responsible for the metabolism of a new vinca alkaloid, vinorelbine, in human liver microsomes. Drug Metab Dispos 2000; 28:1121–1127.
36. Böhme A, Ganser A, Hoelzer D. Aggravation of vincristine-induced neurotoxicity by itraconazole in the treatment of adult ALL. Ann Hematol 1995; 71:311–312.
37. Weber DM, Dimopoulos MA, Alexanian R. Increased neurotoxicity with VAD-cyclosporin in multiple myeloma. Lancet 1993; 341:558–559.
38. Bertrand Y, Capdeville R, Balduck N, Philippe N. Cyclosporin A used to reverse drug resistance increases vincristine neurotoxicity. Am J Hematol 1992; 40:158–159.
39. Tobe SW, Siu LL, Jamal SA, Skorecki KL, Murphy GF, Warner E. Vinblastine and erythromycin: an unrecognized serious drug interaction. Cancer Chemother Pharmacol 1995; 35:188–190.
40. Thant M, Hawley RJ, Smith MT, et al. Possible enhancement of vincristine neuropathy by VP-16. Cancer 1982; 49:859–864.
41. Griffiths JD, Stark RJ, Ding JC, Cooper IA. Vincristine neurotoxicity enhanced in combination chemotherapy including both teniposide and vincristine. Cancer Treat Rep 1986; 70:519–521.
42. Jackson DV Jr, Wells HB, White DR, et al. Lack of potentiation of vincristine-induced neurotoxicity by VP-16-213. Am J Clin Oncol 1983; 6:327–330.
43. Richardson P, Hideshima T, Anderson K. Thalidomide: emerging role in cancer medicine. Annu Rev Med 2002; 53:629–657.

44. Figg WD, Dahut W, Duray P, et al. A randomized phase II trial of thalidomide, an angiogenesis inhibitor, in patients with angrogen-independent prostate cancer. Clin Cancer Res 2001; 7:1888–1893.

45. D'Amato RJ, Loughnan MS, Flynn E, Folkman J. Thalidomide is an inhibitor of angiogenesis. Proc Natl Acad Sci USA 1994; 91:4082–4085.

46. Gordon GB, Spielberg SP, Blake DA, Balasubramanian V. Thalidomide teratogenesis: evidence for a toxic arene oxide metabolite. Proc Natl Acad Sci USA 1981:78:2545–2548.

47. Braun AG, Harding FA, Weinreb SL. Teratogen metabolism: thalidomide activation is mediated by cytochrome *P*-450. Toxicol Appl Pharmacol 1986; 82:175–179.

48. Bauer KS, Dixon SC, Figg WD. Inhibition of angiogenesis by thalidomide requires metabolic activation, which is species-dependent. Biochem Pharmacol 1998; 55:1827–1834.

49. Braun AG, Weinreb SL. Teratogen metabolism: spontaneous decay products of thalidomide and thalidomide analogues are not bioactivated by liver microsomes. Teratogen Carcinogen Mutagen 1985; 5:149–158.

50. Eriksson T, Björkman S, Roth B, Björk H, Höglund P. Hydroxylated metabolites of thalidomide: formation in-vitro and in-vivo in man. J Pharmaceut Pharmacol 1998; 50:1409–1416.

51. Teo SK, Sabourin PJ, O'Brien K, Kook KA, Thomas SD. Metabolism of thalidomide in human microsomes, cloned human cytochrome P-450 isozymes, and Hansen's disease patients. J Biochem Toxicol 2000; 14:140–147.

52. Ando Y, Fuse E, Figg WD. Thalidomide metabolism by the CYP2C subfamily. Clin Cancer Res 2002; 8:1964–1973.

53. Ando Y, Price DK, Dahut WL, Cox MC, Reed E, Figg WD. Pharmacogenetic associations of *CYP2C19* genotype with in vivo metabolisms and pharmacological effects of thalidomide. Cancer Biol Ther 2002; 1:669–673.

54. Eiselt R, Domanski TL, Zibat A, et al. Identification and functional characterization of eight CYP3A4 protein variants. Pharmacogenetics 2001; 11:447–458.

55. Felix CA, Walker AH, Lange BJ, et al. Association of *CYP3A4* genotype with treatment-related leukemia. Proc Natl Acad Sci USA 1998; 95:13176–13181.

56. Ando Y, Tateishi T, Sekido Y, et al. Re: Modification of clinical presentation of prostate tumors by a novel genetic variant in CYP3A4. J Natl Cancer Inst 1999; 91:1587–1590.

57. Marre F, Sanderink GJ, de Sousa G, Gaillard C, Martinet M, Rahmani R. Hepatic biotransformation of docetaxel (Taxotere) *in vitro*: involvement of the CYP3A subfamily in humans. Cancer Res 1996; 56:1296–302.

58. Shou M, Martinet M, Korzekwa KR, Krausz KW, Gonzalez FJ, Gelboin HV. Role of human cytochrome P450 3A4 and 3A5 in the metabolism of taxotere and its derivatives: enzyme specificity, interindividual distribution and metabolic contribution in human liver. Pharmacogenetics 1998; 8:391–401.

59. Kamataki T, Yokoi T, Fujita K, Ando Y. Preclinical approach for identifying drug interactions. Cancer Chemother Pharmacol 1998; 42(Suppl):S50–S53.

60. Hirth J, Watkins PB, Strawderman M, Schott A, Bruno R, Baker LH. The effect of an individual's cytochrome CYP3A4 activity on docetaxel clearance. Clin Cancer Res 2000; 6:1255–1258.

61. Yamamoto N, Tamura T, Kamiya Y, Sekine I, Kunitoh H, Saijo N. Correlation between docetaxel clearance and estimated cytochrome P450 activity by urinary metabolite of exogenous cortisol. J Clin Oncol 2000; 18:2301–2308.

62. Fujitaka K, Oguri T, Isobe T, Fujiwara Y, Kohno N. Induction of cytochrome P450 3A4 by docetaxel in peripheral mononuclear cells and its expression in lung cancer. Cancer Chemoter Pharmacol 2001; 48:42–46.

63. Relling MV, Nemec J, Schuetz EG, Schuetz JD, Gonzalez FJ, Korzekwa KR. *O*-Demethylation of epipodophyllotoxins is catalyzed by human cytochrome P450 3A4. Mol Pharmacol 1994; 45:352–358.

64. Minami H, Shimokata K, Saka H, et al. Phase I clinical and pharmacokinetic study of a 14-day infusion of etoposide in patients with lung cancer. J Clin Oncol 1993; 11:1602–1608.

65. Hande KR, Krozely MG, Greco FA, Hainsworth JD, Johnson DH. Bioavailability of low-dose oral etoposide. J Clin Oncol 1993; 11:374–377.

66. Kobayashi K, Ratain MJ, Fleming GF, Vogelzang NJ, Cooper N, Sun BL. A phase I study of CYP3A4 modulation of oral (po) etoposide with ketoconazole (KCZ) in patients (pts) with advanced cancer (CA). Proc Am Soc Clin Oncol 1996; 15:471.

67. Miller AA, Herndon JE 2nd, Hollis DR, et al. Schedule dependency of 21-day oral versus 3-day intravenous etoposide in combination with intravenous cisplatin in extensive-stage small-cell lung

cancer: a randomized phase III study of the Cancer and Leukemia Group B. J Clin Oncol 1995; 13:1871–1879.

68. Malingré MM, Richel DJ, Beijnen JH, et al. Coadministration of cyclosporine strongly enhances the oral bioavailability of docetaxel. J Clin Oncol 2001; 19:1160–1166.

69. Chico I, Kang MH, Bergan R, et al. Phase I study of infusional paclitaxel in combination with the P-glycoprotein antagonist PSC 833. J Clin Oncol 2001; 19:832–842.

70. Kang MH, Figg WD, Ando Y, et al. The P-glycoprotein antagonist PSC 833 increases the plasma concentrations of 6α-hydroxypaclitaxel, a major metabolite of paclitaxel. Clin Cancer Res 2001; 7: 1610–1617.

71. Rahman A, Korzekwa KR, Grogan J, Gonzalez FJ, Harris JW. Selective biotransformation of taxol to 6α-hydroxytaxol by human cytochrome P450 2C8. Cancer Res 1994; 54:5543–5546.

72. Rodman JH, Murry DJ, Madden T, Santana VM. Pharmacokinetics of high doses of etoposide and the influence of anticonvulsants in pediatric cancer patients. Clin Pharmacol Ther 1992; 51:156.

73. Ando Y, Minami H, Saka H, Ando M, Sakai S, Shimokata K. Therapeutic drug monitoring of etoposide in a 14-day infusion for non-small cell lung cancer. Jpn J Cancer Res 1996; 87:200–205.

74. Ando Y, Minami H, Saka H, Ando M, Sakai S, Shimokata K. Therapeutic drug monitoring in 21-day oral etoposide treatment for lung cancer. Jpn J Cancer Res 1996; 87:856–861.

15 Polymorphisms in Genes of Drug Targets and Metabolism and in DNA Repair

Jan Stoehlmacher, MD, Syma Iqbal, MD, and Heinz-Josef Lenz, MD, FACP

CONTENTS

INTRODUCTION
MOLECULAR MARKERS IN CHEMOTHERAPY
SUMMARY AND CONCLUSIONS

1. INTRODUCTION

Although we have seen great improvements in both length and quality of life over the last decades, optimal treatment for major diseases such as neurological disorders, coronary artery disease, and cancer is not yet a reality. In the postgenomic era, new chemotherapeutic drugs are becoming more and more available, but the remaining challenge is the prospective identification of those patients who are most likely to benefit from a specific medication or drug combination.

It is a common phenomenon that drug response and host toxicity vary widely between patients. Interindividual differences in drug transport and metabolism, signaling, and cellular response pathways all contribute to the observed diversity of patients' reactions *(1)*.

The development of cancer is thought of as a process requiring the input of multiple genes and nongenetic factors *(2)*. Utilizing modern technology of high-throughput genomic analysis in conjunction with unique knowledge from the Human Genome Project dramatically improved our ability to identify new players of defined networks of genes that are involved in cell physiology and metabolism. Current techniques will speed up the evaluation process of newly identified genes in phamacogenetic studies, which have been shown to be very fruitful in the determination of drug activity and toxicity.

Genomic polymorphisms in genes of drug targets *(3,4)*, metabolizing enzymes *(5)*, and DNA repair enzymes *(6)* have been demonstrated to have important implications for drug efficacy. The discovery of significant associations between genomic variants and functionality of the gene product will contribute to providing tailored chemotherapy to cancer patients based on the molecular profile of the tumor.

Handbook of Anticancer Pharmacokinetics and Pharmacodynamics
Edited by: W. D. Figg and H. L. McLeod © Humana Press Inc., Totowa, NJ

2. MOLECULAR MARKERS IN CHEMOTHERAPY

Colorectal cancer was chosen as a model to describe the impact of genomic polymorphisms as a pharmacogenetic component to variability in drug activity.

Colorectal cancer is a very common disease with significant ethnic differences in incidence, causing more than 500,000 deaths per year worldwide *(7)*.

Crude measurement of tumor stage is still the most important, currently available marker of patient outcome. The relatively small number of chemotherapeutic drugs that is currently available for the treatment of this type of cancer (e.g., thymidylate synthase [TS] inhibitors such as capecitabine and 5-fluorouracil [5-FU], oxaliplatin, irinotecan) already demonstrates a high variability of response and toxicity. Furthermore, reports have already demonstrated that differences of expression of target genes within the tumor tissue have prognostic significance in colorectal cancer *(8)*.

The identification of powerful molecular predictive markers for these drugs might help to achieve the goal of giving the drug with minimal host toxicity and maximal tumor response at the right time. This chapter focuses on the predictive and the prognostic value of genomic polymorphisms in genes of metabolizing enzymes of 5-FU, CPT-11, and oxaliplatin, and DNA repair enzymes.

2.1. 5-FU Metabolizing Enzymes

2.1.1. THYMIDYLATE SYNTHASE

Fluoropyrimidines are widely used in the treatment of gastrointestinal cancers and the main mechanism of action is through the inhibition of TS. This enzyme catalyzes the intracellular conversion of deoxyuridylate to deoxythymidylate, which is the sole *de novo* source of thymidylate, an essential precursor for DNA synthesis *(9)*. The active metabolite of 5-FU, 5-fluorodeoxyuridylate (5-FdUMP), binds to TS and inhibits it by forming a stable ternary complex *(10)*. Thus, the therapeutic efficiency of action of fluoropyrimidines depends on the inhibition of TS.

It has consistently been reported that a low TS expression in the tumor is associated with an improved response to TS inhibitors and a superior overall survival in single and combination chemotherapy *(11–13)*.

TS gene expression is modulated by a polymorphism in the 5' regulatory region of the gene. The polymorphism consists of either two repeats *(2R)* or three repeats *(3R)* of a 28-basepair sequence, yielding greater TS gene expression and protein levels with the *3R* genotype *(14,15)*. It has been demonstrated that colorectal cancer patients with a double repeat genotype had a significantly lower TS gene expression in both the tumor and the normal tissue compared with the triple repeat genotype *(16)*. Direct correlation of the *TS* genotype that was determined from DNA of white blood cells or tumor tissue with clinical outcome to 5-FU in metastatic colorectal cancer revealed a better response rate and a survival benefit for patients possessing the *2R/2R* genotype *(16–18)*. Analyses by Pullarkat et al. further demonstrated that this *TS* polymorphism is also associated with host toxicity. The *3R/3R* genotype was found to be significantly associated with a lower rate of severe toxic side effects. High levels of TS gene expression, which are associated with the *3R/3R* genotype, are thought to mediate a protective effect on the normal tissue owing to a lower efficacy in TS inhibition. The resulting decreased cell death rate causes less tumor shrinkage (tumor cells), but also less toxic side effects in the normal tissue *(16)*. This information is important for clinicians, because a closer monitoring of patients receiving 5-FU, who are often outpatients, and a possible adjustment of the administered dose could be considered for *2R/2R* carriers.

Evidence also exists for a survival benefit for the *2R/2R* genotype in the adjuvant setting. Iacopetta et al. reported that patients who possess the *TS* double repeats showed significant gains in survival if adjuvant 5-FU chemotherapy was administered, but patients with the *3R/3R* genotype did not *(19)*. Furthermore, it has been demonstrated that this polymorphism within the *TS* gene, probably through its effect on TS expression levels, may be predictive for tumor down-staging in rectal cancer and useful to predict response to preoperative 5-FU-based chemoradiation *(20)*.

In addition, there is some evidence that the *TS* polymorphism in the 5' region of the *TS* gene has also predictive value for other TS inhibitors, such as capecitabine. Capecitabine is an oral prodrug of 5-FU; thus the target enzyme remains TS. A preliminary analysis revealed that patients possessing the *2R/2R* genotype were more likely to respond compared to carriers of the *2R/3R* or *3R/3R* genotype *(21)*.

Interestingly, it has been reported that a reasonable subgroup of patients who possess the *3R/3R* genotype respond well to chemotherapy with fluoropyrimidines, indicating that additional modifying factors may alter the association between TS expression and polymorphism in the 5' region of TS. One possible modifier could be another polymorphism in the *TS* gene, like the 6-basepair deletion of the 3' untranslated region *(22)*. Although the function of this variant is still unknown, it has been demonstrated in the past that alterations of the 3' UTR can significantly change the rate of transcription *(23,24)*.

The choice of the sample source may represent another parameter that needs to be taken into account when the true association between the polymorphism and expression is questioned. Loss of heterozygosity (LOH) of the short arm of chromosome 18, which contains the human *TS* locus, has been demonstrated in up to 40% of colorectal tumors. Therefore, some investigators argue that the resulting allelic imbalance in the tumor is not accurately reflected by the genotype analysis from white blood cells *(25)*. However, the reports available today suggest consistently that independent from the source of material (i.e., blood or tumor) the *2R/2R* genotype may be associated with a superior clinical outcome to 5-FU inhibitors.

Although different mechanisms have been postulated to explain how the difference in the TS promoter alters the TS level, without doubt the determination of this genomic variation provides significant information about TS functionality *(16,26)*. The predictive power of this polymorphism and the simplicity of its determination in a blood test render it a valuable part of any comprehensive analysis of TS function in addition to protein and gene expression analyses.

2.1.2. Dihydropyrimidine Dehydrogenase

The level of the target enzyme is not the only determinant of 5-FU efficacy and toxicity. The amount of chemotherapeutic drug that can be delivered to the cell is critical for the success of the treatment. Bioavailability of 5-FU mainly depends on the activity of dihydropyrimidine dehydrogenase (DPD), the rate-limiting enzyme in 5-FU catabolism *(27)*. Several reports demonstrated the importance of this key player in 5-FU metabolism by revealing the link between severe toxicity, including death, and deficiency of DPD activity in 5-FU-treated patients *(28–31)*. Retrospective analysis identified a common $G \rightarrow A$ mutation in the invariant GT splice donor site flanking exon 14 (IVS14+1G$\rightarrow$A) to cause dramatically diminished DPD activity levels *(31)*. Individuals homozygous for this mutation do not show any DPD activity *(30)*. Not surprisingly, a number of patients with severe toxic reactions to 5-FU treatment possessed a genotype associated with decreased DPD activity. Among more than 15 DPD allele variants that have been identified to be associated with decreases of the enzyme activity, the IVS14+1G$\rightarrow$A mutation appeared to be the most frequent one *(32)*. Recently, van Kuilenburg et al. reported a frequency of 0.91% for this mutation of the *DPD* gene among the Caucasian population *(33)*. A frequency of less than 1% may appear to be insignificant, if compared, for instance, to the frequency of the *TS* polymorphism, with 4–46% *(34)*. However, the consequences rising from a genomic change determine its importance. As very severe, even lethal toxicity to the widely used chemotherapeutic drug 5-FU is the consequence of this single base substitution, a genetic screening for its presence is clearly warranted before administration of the drug.

Several additional polymorphisms in genes that are involved in the 5-FU pathway such as ribonucleotide reductase M1, M2 (RRM1/RRM2), or dihydropyrimidinase (DPYS) have been identified, but their functional and clinical significance still remains unclear.

Another promising aspect rises from the related pathways of folate metabolism. The complex interactions of folate and fluoropyrimidine pathways suggest that alterations of the folate metabolism will also alter the therapeutic effectiveness and toxicity of administrated fluoropyrimidines. TS inhibitors such as 5-FU may induce acute folate depletion with possible severe toxic sequelae. Several genomic polymorphisms have been identified in genes of the folate cycle and should be investigated further in conjunction with polymorphisms of genes of the 5-FU pathway *(35)*.

2.2. Irinotecan Metabolizing Enzymes

The pathway of the prodrug irinotecan involves several proteins for drug activation and inactivation, drug efflux, and drug targeting. The functional significance of genomic variants in the corresponding genes has been identified for the *multidrug resistance (MDR)-1* gene (efflux pump) *(36)*, and the *uridine diphosphate glucosyltransferase 1* gene, *UGT1A1* (detoxification) *(37)*. The *MDR-1* gene encodes an integral membrane protein, P-glycoprotein, that regulates the energy-dependent efflux of several substances out of the cell. The transport of irinotecan out of the cell is also mediated by this membrane protein.

Hoffmeyer et al. showed that a C→T substitution in exon 26 of the *MDR-1* gene is associated with significantly decreased *MDR-1* expression in vivo *(36)*. Based on these data it can be speculated that less drug will finally reach the cell in individuals who show this C→T substitution. A possible consequence would be a decreased efficacy of the drug, represented by less tumor response. However, the significance of this polymorphism in the treatment with irinotecan still has to be elucidated.

After sequential activation of irinotecan to SN-38, the hepatic isoform 1A1 of UGT is primarily responsible for glucuronidation and thereby detoxification of the active drug metabolite. A common polymorphism of the *UGT1A1* gene, represented by an additional *TA* repeat in the *TATA* sequence of *UGT1A1* [(TA)7TAA] is associated with a significant decrease of SN-38 glucuronidation *(5,37)*. An increased bioavailability of active SN-38 would be the consequence for individuals possessing the seven *TA* repeats variant. The use of irinotecan is limited mainly by severe diarrhea and bone marrow suppression and dose adjustments are often necessary. Not surprisingly, recent data by Iyer et al. demonstrated that severe gastrointestinal toxicity and neutropenia were associated with the *(TA)7TAA* sequence of the *UGT1A1* gene in cancer patients who received intravenous infusion of irinotecan *(38)*.

Screening for this *TA* repeat polymorphism may select patients who are likely to experience severe toxicity on irinotecan administration. Alternative chemotherapy regimens might be considered for those individuals. Determination of the *UGT1A1* polymorphism becomes even more important if colorectal cancer patients are treated with combination chemotherapy of 5-FU and irinotecan. Administration of these drugs to a patient whose genomic profile reveals homozygosity for the *(TA)7TAA* variant of the *UGT1A1* gene and the

IVS14+1G→A mutation of the *DPD* gene may expose the patient to massive and even life-threatening toxicities.

2.3. DNA-Repair Enzymes

The transport of the drug into the cell, its metabolic fate, and the availability of the drug target have already been discussed as possible modifiers of tumor response and patient toxicity. The efficacy of those processes in terms of cell kill is finally related to the magnitude of DNA damage. Cell turnover is a physiological process of the human body, and therefore several mechanisms are in place to maintain a well-defined balance between damage and repair. Logically, disturbances of this balance might have significant implications for the effect of administrated chemotherapy. Several processes have been postulated to be important for this balance: (1) recognition of DNA damage, (2) mismatch repair, (3) translesional replication, and (4) excision repair.

The paradigm that reduced DNA repair capacity may be associated with increased efficacy of cytotoxic agents has been demonstrated in various studies *(6,11,39–42)*. Oxaliplatin is an increasingly used agent in the chemotherapy of colorectal cancers. The synergistic effects of the combination therapy of 5-FU/oxaliplatin has increased response rates up to 25% even in heavily pretreated relapsing patients *(43)*. Administration of this a 1,2-diamino-cyclohexane ring containing platinum compound results in the formation of bulky DNA adducts, the cause of its cytotoxic effect.

Proteins of the nucleotide excision repair pathway (NER) are thought to repair DNA damage caused by platinum agents *(43)*. The excision repair cross-complementing (*ERCC*) gene family prevents damage to DNA by nucleotide excision and repair. Modified nucleotides together with adjacent nucleotides are removed from the damaged strand during the first step (excision), followed by recovery of an intact strand through DNA polymerase activity (repair synthesis) *(44,45)*.

The *ERCC1* gene encodes a protein of 297 amino acids, which is considered to function in a complex with ERCC11, XPF, and ERCC4 *(44)*. Its role is critical in DNA damage recognition and DNA strand incision.

Previous studies have shown that increased *ERCC1* gene expression levels are associated with resistance to platinum-based chemotherapy in various cancers. For example, gastric cancer patients who received a combination of 5-FU and cisplatin with a low *ERCC1* gene expression in the tumor responded better to the chemotherapy compared to patients whose tumor showed a high *ERCC1* expression profile *(42)*. Very similarly, colorectal cancer patients possessing low *ERCC1* gene expression in the tumor demonstrated a superior survival after administration of second line chemotherapy of 5-FU/oxaliplatin *(11)*.

Yu et al. identified a common C→T transition in codon 118 of the *ERCC1* gene, which does not change the code for the amino acid asparagines *(46)*. Preliminary results from a retrospective clinical study in colorectal cancer identified a positive correlation between *ERCC1* mRNA expression and the number of T alleles (Table 1). Consistent with that observation, a survival benefit has been seen for colorectal cancer patients who received platinum-based chemotherapy and possessed a homozygous *C/C* genotype (Fig. 1) *(47)*.

It is difficult to explain how a genetic polymorphism leading to the same amino acid could affect clinical outcome to chemotherapy. Although the data seem to suggest an influence to gene expression, the mechanism for this is unclear. In fact, the polymorphism is not part of any known regulatory binding site. Another plausible explanation is that the polymorphism might be in linkage disequilibrium with another factor influencing survival to platinum-based chemotherapy within the same gene or a gene nearby, such as xeroderma pigmentosum group D gene (*XPD*) or X-ray cross-complementing gene 1 (*XRCC1*).

Table 1
Association Between *ERCC1* Polymorphism at Codon 118
and mRNA Expression Colorectal Tumor Tissue

	Patients	mRNA level[a]	95% CI[b]	p-Value[c]
Genotype				0.096
C/C	11	2.31	(1.47, 3.61)	
C/T	12	2.91	(1.89, 4.48)	
T/T	8	4.91	(2.90, 8.32)	
				0.041
Any C	23	2.60	(1.91, 3.54)	
T/T	8	4.91	(2.91, 8.28)	

[a] Geometric mean of mRNA expression.
[b] CI, Confidence interval.
[c] Based on least significant difference test.

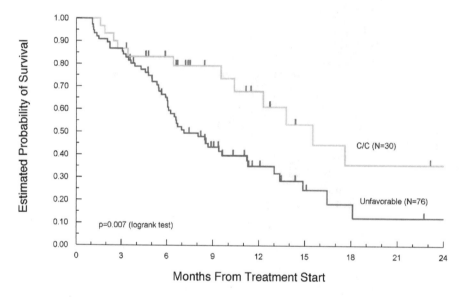

Fig. 1. Association of *ERCC1* polymorphism (exon 118) with survival of colorectal cancer patients treated with 5-FU/oxaliplatin chemotherapy.

In contrast, data from ovarian cancer cell lines indicated a 50% reduction of the codon usage and a reduced *ERCC1* mRNA level if the *T* allele is present *(48)*. However, the clinical data suggest that this *ERCC1* polymorphism may alter the efficacy of the *ERCC1* overall pathway. A change of the activity of this key enzyme in the NER would possibly have consequences for the removal of platinum-induced DNA adducts. Because the proteins of the NER have been identified as major determinants of DNA repair caused by platinum compounds, this polymorphism may become a powerful genomic predictor of response to platinum-based chemotherapy.

As mentioned earlier, the successful action of DNA repair requires participation of multiple proteins, and every player may modify the overall activity of the repair pathway. The xeroderma pigmentosum group D gene, also known as *ERCC2*, represents another protein of this critical pathway. Several common genomic polymorphisms have been identified for the *ERCC2* gene that might be associated with differential DNA repair capacity. A G→A change (codon 312) causes the amino acid change Asp→Asn whereas the A751C polymorphism causes the amino acid change Lys→Gln. A third single nucleotide polymorphism C156A is silent but it transforms a high usage codon into a low usage codon. However, studies yielded diverging results regarding their effects on the nucleotide excision repair *(49–51)*. This is especially true for the Lys751Gln polymorphism where the Lys variant was shown to be associated with decreased DNA repair in one study *(50)* while a much larger study reported the opposite *(49)*.

Recent clinical data indirectly confirmed the hypothesis that the Lys variant of XPD codon 751 is linked to a decreased activity of this DNA repair enzyme. Among 73 colorectal cancer patients treated with 5-FU/oxaliplatin chemotherapy those who possessed the Lys/Lys genotype survived 17.4 mo (median; 95% 7.9, 26.5) compared to only 3.3 mo (median; 95% CI 1.4, 6.5) in the Gln/Gln group *(21)*. Investigators posited that this amino acid change might have significant functional implications due to its proximity to the poly(A) signal, thereby affecting protein function *(51)*.

The examples of polymorphisms in genes of *ERCC1* and *ERCC2* impressively demonstrated that functional polymorphisms of DNA repair genes could result in significant alteration of the sensitive balance between damage and repair. Knowledge of an impaired capacity of this critical cellular function, determined by screening for polymorphism in those DNA repair genes might aid the clinicians' therapy decision.

The functional relevance of several polymorphisms in genes that are involved in other important pathways of the DNA repair process such as damage recognition (e.g., high mobility group protein 1 [HMG1]) or translesional replication (DNA polymerase eta [PolH]/DNA polymerase [PolB]) has been described. But their relevance to platinum toxicity and activity still has to be elucidated.

Impaired DNA repair function cannot be used as strict indicator for therapy success. First, other mechanisms such as increased drug detoxification may override and set off the suggested therapy benefit of reduced DNA repair capacity. Therefore several predictors should always be considered before a decision is made. Second, strong in vitro and in vivo evidence must confirm the linkage of a certain DNA-repair deficiency to a defined drug pathway.

Glutathione *S*-transferase P1 (GST-P1) represents another factor that should be considered in platinum-based treatment and is an example how the rate of drug detoxification determines clinical outcome.

GST-P1 belongs to a superfamily of dimeric phase II metabolic enzymes *(52)*. GST-P1 is the predominantly expressed GST subclass in colorectal epithelium and has been found to be highly overexpressed in human colorectal cancers *(53)*. In vitro studies revealed its direct participation in the detoxification of platinum compounds and identified GST-P1 as a mediator of both intrinsic and required resistance *(54,55)*. A single nucleotide substitution at position 313 (A→G) of the *GSTP1* gene, replacing isoleucine with valine, significantly diminishes the enzyme activity *(56)*.

Recent clinical data suggest that the GST-P1 Ile105Val polymorphism is associated in a dose-dependent fashion with superior survival of colorectal cancer patients receiving 5-FU/oxaliplatin chemotherapy. Patients with a *Val/Val* genotype survived more than three times longer (>24 mo) in median if compared to patients homozygous for the *Ile* allele (8 mo) *(57)*. Additional analysis by our group revealed the predictive value of this polymorphism.

Table 2
Summary of Clinically Significant Polymorphism
in Pathways of 5-FU, Irinotecan, and Oxaliplatin

Drug	Gene	Polymorphism	Clinical implication
5-FU	TS	28 bp repeat (5' region)	Response, toxicity, overall survival
5-FU	DPD	IVS14+1G→A (Exon 14)	Toxicity
CPT-11	UGT1A1	(TA)6/7TAA (TATA-Sequence)	Toxicity
Oxaliplatin	ERCC1	nt19007 C→G (Exon 118)	Overall survival
Oxaliplatin	GST-P1	ILE^{105}VAL (Exon 5)	Disease-free and overall survival
Oxaliplatin	XPD	Lys^{751}Gln (Exon 23)	Overall survival, response

Patients possessing the *Ile/Ile* GST-P1 genotype had an 86% increased relative risk of disease progression if compared to *Val/Val* carriers. Based on the biochemical evidence provided by other investigators, it is suggested that the low activity *Val*-containing GST-P1 variant leads to a prolonged length of stay of the platinum drug in the tissue, causing a more significant tumor shrinkage that finally leads to an improved overall survival of these patients compared to individuals possessing an *Ile* GST-P1 genotype.

GST-P1 polymorphism is an excellent example that demonstrates how molecular markers might provide additional guidance in therapy planning. Besides its detoxifying role in the platinum treatment, GST-P1 has also been characterized as activator of another cytotoxic drug, TLK286, whose efficacy in colorectal cancer is currently investigated in clinical trials *(58)*. Screening for this polymorphism in colorectal cancer patients might be helpful in the future to decide which of these drugs or whether a combination should be administered.

3. SUMMARY AND CONCLUSIONS

Screening of specific genes involved in drug metabolism, drug transport, and DNA repair in well-defined pathways of agents used in the treatment of colorectal cancer have already been identified. Clinical testing demonstrated the predictive value of some of these polymorphisms for tumor response, overall survival and toxicity in patients receiving currently available chemotherapy (TS inhibitors, platinum compounds, topoisomerase inhibitiors) (Table 2).

However, one of the remaining challenges in the future is to develop a comprehensive marker pattern for each drug or drug combination. For instance important information about the patient's risk to experience toxicity and to respond to anticipated 5-FU/CPT-11 chemotherapy could be derived from screening for polymorphisms in the following genes: *TS, DPD, UGT1A1,* and *MDR-1.*

Table 3
Combined Analysis of Association Between *XPD-751*, *ERCC1-19007*,
TS-3', and *GST-P1* Polymorphisms and Survival
After 5-FU/Oxaliplatin Chemotherapy for Disseminated Colorectal Cancer

Number of favorable genotypes [a]	No. of patients (N=102)	Median survival (95% CI)	p-Value [b]
LYS/LYS, C/C, VAL/VAL, +6BP/+6BP			<0.001
≥2	29	17.4 mo (9.4, 26.5)	
1	48	10.2 mo (6.8, 15.3)	
0	25	5.4 mo (4.3, 6.0)	

[a] Favorable genotypes of XPD-751 (LYS/LYS), ERCC1-19007 (C/C), GST-P1 (VAL/VAL), and TS-3' (+6BP/+6BP) polymorphisms.

[b] Based on logrank test.

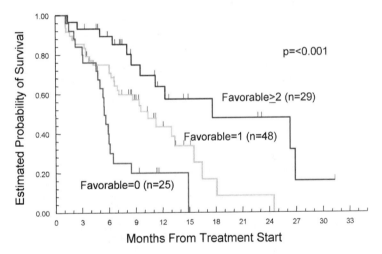

Fig. 2. Association between the number of favorable genotypes (*XPD751 = LYS/LYS*, *ERCC1 = C/C*, *GST-P1 = VAL/VAL*, *3'-TS = +6BP+6BP*) and survival of colorectal cancer patients treated with 5-FU/oxalipatin chemotherapy.

Lenz and colleagues demonstrated the power of a comprehensive analysis of genomic markers for clinical outcome in colorectal cancer patients receiving second line 5-FU/ oxaliplatin chemotherapy *(59)*. First, favorable genotypes (in terms of survival) of relevant polymorphisms of the following genes were identified: *TS* (3'-UTR), *XPD*, *ERCC2*, and *GST-P1*. Second, survival was re-analyzed according to the number of favorable genotypes. Table 3 summarizes the association between overall survival to 5-FU/oxaliplatin chemotherapy and number of favorable genotypes (see also Fig. 2).

This simple example of only four markers demonstrates, that combined analysis of molecular markers like functional genomic polymorphisms, may become powerful tools in tailoring chemotherapy.

Based on the presented data distinct marker pattern should include information about functional polymorphisms in genes of drug metabolism, drug transport and DNA repair. To discover true associations between genomic polymorphisms and clinical outcome (response and survival) to certain chemotherapies the genetic makeup of the tumor might be the most valuable sample source. However, if a patient's toxicity is questioned, a nontumor specimen is probably more relevant.

Clearly, functional genomic polymorphisms may, if the screening is applied in a prospective manner, help to eliminate unwanted effects in the patient in terms of chemotherapy resistance and toxicity. However, the limitation of genomic polymorphisms as molecular predictive or prognostic marker may arise from its *static* character. Expression profiles (gene and protein) might more accurately reflect the current situation in the tumor in second or third line chemotherapy. This is particularly true for genes of the metabolizing enzyme systems. For example up-regulation of TS after first-line TS-inhibitor therapy (e.g., 5-FU) might occur differently in different patients. This variability would not be detected by analysis of the genomic polymorphism of *TS*, but might be important if the second- or third-line chemotherapy regimen includes another drug of this group (e.g., capecitabine). This is especially true for tumor response. Instead the prediction of patient's toxicity based on a genomic polymorphism profile should show less variability if an agent from the same group is administrated more than once in the same patient.

Overall, the data suggest that knowledge of tumors' and hosts' genotypes might improve tailored chemotherapy in the future. The growing use of high-throughput techniques will rapidly identify additional important players of drug pathways and DNA repair and will speed up their clinical and pharmacological evaluation. The synthesis of the genetic profile of the tumor and the host, together with clinical–pathological criteria, will determine the chemotherapeutic treatment in the future.

REFERENCES

1. Evans WE, Relling MV. Pharmacogenomics: translating functional genomics into rational therapeutics. Science 1999; 286:487–491.
2. Guo SW, Lange K. Genetic mapping of complex traits: promises, problems, and prospects. Theor Popul Biol 2000; 57:1–11.
3. Lima JJ, Thomason DB, Mohamed MH, Eberle LV, Self TH, Johnson JA. Impact of genetic polymorphisms of the beta2-adrenergic receptor on albuterol bronchodilator pharmacodynamics. Clin Pharmacol Ther 1999; 65:519–525.
4. Gebhardt F, Zanker KS, Brandt B. Modulation of epidermal growth factor receptor gene transcription by a polymorphic dinucleotide repeat in intron 1. J Biol Chem 1999; 274:13,176–13,180.
5. Ando Y, Saka H, Ando M, et al. Polymorphisms of UDP-glucuronosyltransferase gene and irinotecan toxicity: a pharmacogenetic analysis. Cancer Res 2000; 60:6921–6926.
6. Park DJ, Stoehlmacher J, Zhang W, Tsao-Wei DD, Groshen S, Lenz HJ. A xeroderma pigmentosum group D gene polymorphism predicts clinical outcome to platinum-based chemotherapy in patients with advanced colorectal cancer. Cancer Res 2001; 61:8654–8658.
7. Greenlee RT, Murray T, Bolden S, Wingo PA. Cancer statistics, 2000. CA Cancer J Clin 2000; 50:7–33.
8. Aschele C, Lonardi S, Monfardini S. Thymidylate synthase expression as a predictor of clinical response to fluoropyrimidine-based chemotherapy in advanced colorectal cancer. Cancer Treat Rev 2002; 28:27–47.
9. Kundu NG, Heidelberger C. Cyclopenta(f)isoquinoline derivatives designed to bind specifically to native deoxyribonucleic acid. 3. Interaction of 6-carbamylmethyl-8-methyl-7H-cyclopenta(f)isoquinolin-3(2H)-one with deoxyribonucleic acids and polydeoxyribonucleotides. Biochem Biophys Res Commun 1974; 60:561–568.
10. Danenberg PV. Thymidylate synthetase—a target enzyme in cancer chemotherapy. Biochim Biophys Acta 1977; 473:73–92.

11. Shirota Y, Stoehlmacher J, Brabender J, et al. ERCC1 and thymidylate synthase mRNA levels predict survival for colorectal cancer patients receiving combination oxaliplatin and fluorouracil chemotherapy. J Clin Oncol 2001; 19:4298–4304.

12. Johnston PG, Lenz HJ, Leichman CG, et al. Thymidylate synthase gene and protein expression correlate and are associated with response to 5-fluorouracil in human colorectal and gastric tumors. Cancer Res 1995; 55:1407–1412.

13. Leichman L, Lenz HJ, Leichman CG, et al. Quantitation of intratumoral thymidylate synthase expression predicts for resistance to protracted infusion of 5-fluorouracil and weekly leucovorin in disseminated colorectal cancers: preliminary report from an ongoing trial. Eur J Cancer 1995; 31A:1306–1310.

14. Kawakami K, Omura K, Kanehira E, Watanabe Y. Polymorphic tandem repeats in the thymidylate synthase gene is associated with its protein expression in human gastrointestinal cancers. Anticancer Res 1999; 19:3249–3252.

15. Horie N, Aiba H, Oguro K, Hojo H, Takeishi K. Functional analysis and DNA polymorphism of the tandemly repeated sequences in the 5'-terminal regulatory region of the human gene for thymidylate synthase. Cell Struct Funct 1995; 20:191–197.

16. Pullarkat ST, Stoehlmacher J, Ghaderi V, et al. Thymidylate synthase gene polymorphism determines response and toxicity of 5-FU chemotherapy. Pharmacogenomics J 2001; 1:65–70.

17. Etienne MC, Chazal M, Laurent-Puig P, et al. Prognostic value of tumoral thymidylate synthase and p53 in metastatic colorectal cancer patients receiving fluorouracil-based chemotherapy: phenotypic and genotypic analyses. J Clin Oncol 2002; 20:2832–2843.

18. Marsh S, McKay JA, Cassidy J, McLeod HL. Polymorphism in the thymidylate synthase promoter enhancer region in colorectal cancer. Int J Oncol 2001; 19:383–386.

19. Iacopetta B, Grieu F, Joseph D, Elsaleh H. A polymorphism in the enhancer region of the thymidylate synthase promoter influences the survival of colorectal cancer patients treated with 5-fluorouracil. Br J Cancer 2001; 85:827–830.

20. Villafranca E, Okruzhnov Y, Dominguez MA, et al. Polymorphisms of the repeated sequences in the enhancer region of the thymidylate synthase gene promoter may predict downstaging after preoperative chemoradiation in rectal cancer. J Clin Oncol 2001; 19:1779–1786.

21. Park DJ, Stoehlmacher J, Zhang W, Tsao-Wei D, Groshen S, Lenz HJ. Thymidylate synthase gene polymorphism predicts response to capecitabine in advanced colorectal cancer. Int J Colorect Dis 2002; 17:46–49.

22. Ulrich CM, Bigler J, Velicer CM, Greene EA, Farin FM, Potter JD. Searching expressed sequence tag databases: discovery and confirmation of a common polymorphism in the thymidylate synthase gene. Cancer Epidemiol Biomark Prev 2000; 9:1381–1385.

23. Rajagopalan LE, Malter JS. Growth factor-mediated stabilization of amyloid precursor protein mRNA is mediated by a conserved 29-nucleotide sequence in the 3'-untranslated region. J Neurochem 2000; 74:52–59.

24. Gou Q, Liu CH, Ben-Av P, Hla T. Dissociation of basal turnover and cytokine-induced transcript stabilization of the human cyclooxygenase-2 mRNA by mutagenesis of the 3'-untranslated region. Biochem Biophys Res Commun 1998; 242:508–512.

25. Zinzindohoue F, Ferraz JM, Laurent-Puig P. Thymidylate synthase promoter polymorphism. J Clin Oncol 2001; 19:3442.

26. Kawakami K, Salonga D, Park JM, et al. Different lengths of a polymorphic repeat sequence in the thymidylate synthase gene affect translational efficiency but not its gene expression. Clin Cancer Res 2001; 7:4096–4101.

27. Heggie GD, Sommadossi JP, Cross DS, Huster WJ, Diasio RB. Clinical pharmacokinetics of 5-fluorouracil and its metabolites in plasma, urine, and bile. Cancer Res 1987; 47:2203–2206.

28. Milano G, Etienne MC. Potential importance of dihydropyrimidine dehydrogenase (DPD) in cancer chemotherapy. Pharmacogenetics 1994; 4:301–306.

29. Milano G, Etienne MC, Pierrefite V, Barberi-Heyob M, Deporte-Fety R, Renee N. Dihydropyrimidine dehydrogenase deficiency and fluorouracil-related toxicity. Br J Cancer 1999; 79:627–630.

30. Wei X, McLeod HL, McMurrough J, Gonzalez FJ, Fernandez-Salguero P. Molecular basis of the human dihydropyrimidine dehydrogenase deficiency and 5-fluorouracil toxicity. J Clin Invest 1996; 98:610–615.

31. Van Kuilenburg AB, Vreken P, Beex LV, et al. Heterozygosity for a point mutation in an invariant splice donor site of dihydropyrimidine dehydrogenase and severe 5-fluorouracil related toxicity. Eur J Cancer 1997; 33:2258–2264.

32. Van Kuilenburg AB, Vreken P, Abeling NG, et al. Genotype and phenotype in patients with dihydropyrimidine dehydrogenase deficiency. Hum Genet 1999; 104:1–9.
33. van Kuilenburg AB, Muller EW, Haasjes J, et al. Lethal outcome of a patient with a complete dihydropyrimidine dehydrogenase (DPD) deficiency after administration of 5-fluorouracil: frequency of the common IVS14+1G>A mutation causing DPD deficiency. Clin Cancer Res 2001; 7: 1149–1153.
34. Luo HR, Lu XM, Yao YG, et al. Length polymorphism of thymidylate synthase regulatory region in Chinese populations and evolution of the novel alleles. Biochem Genet 2002; 40:41–51.
35. Ulrich CM, Robien K, Sparks R. Pharmacogenetics and folate metabolism—a promising direction. Pharmacogenomics 2002; 3:299–313.
36. Hoffmeyer S, Burk O, von Richter O, et al. Functional polymorphisms of the human multidrug-resistance gene: multiple sequence variations and correlation of one allele with P-glycoprotein expression and activity in vivo. Proc Natl Acad Sci USA 2000; 97:3473–3478.
37. Iyer L, Hall D, Das S, et al. Phenotype–genotype correlation of in vitro SN-38 (active metabolite of irinotecan) and bilirubin glucuronidation in human liver tissue with UGT1A1 promoter polymorphism. Clin Pharmacol Ther 1999; 65:576–582.
38. Iyer L, Das S, Janisch L, et al. UGT1A1*28 polymorphism as a determinant of irinotecan disposition and toxicity. Pharmacogenomics J 2002; 2:43–47.
39. Bosken CH, Wei Q, Amos CI, Spitz MR. An analysis of DNA repair as a determinant of survival in patients with non-small-cell lung cancer. J Natl Cancer Inst 2002; 94:1091–1099.
40. Kartalou M, Essigmann JM. Mechanisms of resistance to cisplatin. Mutat Res 2001; 478:23–43.
41. Akiyama S, Chen ZS, Sumizawa T, Furukawa T. Resistance to cisplatin. Anticancer Drug Des 1999; 14:143–151.
42. Metzger R, Leichman CG, Danenberg KD, et al. ERCC1 mRNA levels complement thymidylate synthase mRNA levels in predicting response and survival for gastric cancer patients receiving combination cisplatin and fluorouracil chemotherapy. J Clin Oncol 1998; 16:309–316.
43. Bleiberg H. Role of chemotherapy for advanced colorectal cancer: new opportunities. Semin Oncol 1996; 23:42–50.
44. Hoeijmakers JH. Nucleotide excision repair. II: From yeast to mammals. Trends Genet 1993; 9:211–217.
45. Van Houten B. Nucleotide excision repair in Escherichia coli. Microbiol Rev 1990; 54:18–51.
46. Yu JJ, Mu C, Lee KB, et al. A nucleotide polymorphism in ERCC1 in human ovarian cancer cell lines and tumor tissues. Mutat Res 1997; 382:13–20.
47. Park D, Stoehlmacher J, Zhang W, et al. ERCC1 polymorphism is associated with different ERCC1 mRNA expression levels. Proc Am Assoc Cancer 2002, abstract 1591.
48. Yu JJ, Lee KB, Mu C, et al. Comparison of two human ovarian carcinoma cell lines (A2780/CP70 and MCAS) that are equally resistant to platinum, but differ at codon 118 of the ERCC1 gene. Int J Oncol 2000; 16:555–560.
49. Spitz MR, Wu X, Wang Y, et al. Modulation of nucleotide excision repair capacity by XPD polymorphisms in lung cancer patients. Cancer Res 2001; 61:1354–1357.
50. Lunn RM, Helzlsouer KJ, Parshad R, et al. XPD polymorphisms: effects on DNA repair proficiency. Carcinogenesis 2000; 21:551–555.
51. Dybdahl M, Vogel U, Frentz G, Wallin H, Nexo BA. Polymorphisms in the DNA repair gene XPD: correlations with risk and age at onset of basal cell carcinoma. Cancer Epidemiol Biomark Prev 1999; 8:77–81.
52. Nebert DW. Polymorphisms in drug-metabolizing enzymes: what is their clinical relevance and why do they exist? Am J Hum Genet 1997; 60:265–271.
53. Moscow JA, Fairchild CR, Madden MJ, et al. Expression of anionic glutathione-S-transferase and P-glycoprotein genes in human tissues and tumors. Cancer Res 1989; 49:1422–1428.
54. Goto S, Iida T, Cho S, Oka M, Kohno S, Kondo T. Overexpression of glutathione S-transferase pi enhances the adduct formation of cisplatin with glutathione in human cancer cells. Free Radic Res 1999; 31:549–558.
55. Ban N, Takahashi Y, Takayama T, et al. Transfection of glutathione S-transferase (GST)-pi antisense complementary DNA increases the sensitivity of a colon cancer cell line to adriamycin, cisplatin, melphalan, and etoposide. Cancer Res 1996; 56:3577–3582.
56. Watson MA, Stewart RK, Smith GB, Massey TE, Bell DA. Human glutathione S-transferase P1 polymorphisms: relationship to lung tissue enzyme activity and population frequency distribution. Carcinogenesis 1998; 19:275–280.

57. Stoehlmacher J, Park DJ, Zhang W, et al. Association between glutathione *S*-transferase P1, T1, and M1 genetic polymorphism and survival of patients with metastatic colorectal cancer. J Natl Cancer Inst 2002; 94:936–942.

58. Morgan AS, Sanderson PE, Borch RF, et al. Tumor efficacy and bone marrow-sparing properties of TER286, a cytotoxin activated by glutathione *S*-transferase. Cancer Res 1998; 58:2568–2575.

59. Lenz HJ, Park D, Zhang et al. A multivariate analysis of genetic markers for clinical response to 5-FU/ oxaliplatin chemotherapy in advanced colorectal cancer. Proc Am Soc Clin Oncol 2002, abstract 513.

16   Drug Interactions

Laurent P. Rivory

CONTENTS

1. INTRODUCTION

The setting of chemotherapy for cancer is rife with potential for significant drug interactions and this topic has been the subject of several excellent reviews *(1–4)*. Most patients receive multidrug combinations for their malignancy. Also, many of these patients are treated with intercurrent medication for co-morbidity or for cancer-related disorders (coagulopathy, infection, pain, seizures, etc.). The clinical significance of these potential drug interactions is also all the more relevant in cancer chemotherapy because the cytotoxic agents traditionally used do not have clear therapeutic windows. That is, the doses selected produce toxicity in a significant proportion of patients without necessarily providing benefit. Drug interactions causing an increased exposure of the patient to the cytotoxic agent may produce more severe side effects, whereas those causing a decreased exposure may jeopardize tumor control. Unfortunately, both the good and bad effects of chemotherapy are unpredictable, and the influence of drug interactions in either eventuality is almost impossible to detect in individual patients. These, however, may be borne out in large-scale studies, or when combined with pharmacokinetic data (for example, see refs. *5,6*). Therefore, most drug interactions in cancer chemotherapy may go undetected unless some *a priori* knowledge alerts the clinician or oncology pharmacist to their likelihood.

When we think of drug–drug interactions, we usually think about classical interactions with the cytochrome P450 enzymes, as these have been well recognized and characterized over the last few decades. Certainly, this mechanism remains at the forefront of clinically significant drug–drug interactions. However, the pathways involved in the classical ADME of drug disposition (absorption, distribution, metabolism, and elimination) are all candidates for drug interactions. In particular, our understanding of transporters and their role in the systemic disposition of anticancer drugs has evolved exponentially over the last few years.

Handbook of Anticancer Pharmacokinetics and Pharmacodynamics
Edited by: W. D. Figg and H. L. McLeod © Humana Press Inc., Totowa, NJ

They are now recognized as a major locus of drug–drug interaction *(7)*. Also, the routes of metabolism of importance for the elimination of anticancer drugs are almost as diverse as their mechanisms of action, and some unexpected drug interactions have arisen as a result.

The aim of this chapter is to review some of the potential mechanisms of drug–drug interactions and to illustrate these with published data. The focus here is to examine the possible loci of drug interactions that should be considered in the setting of drug development rather than an exhaustive listing of all the known interactions. In addition, the possibility of exploiting drug–drug interactions to improve cancer chemotherapy is raised.

2. THE LOCI FOR DRUG INTERACTIONS: PROCESS BY PROCESS

As mentioned briefly in the previous section, any of the traditional processes implicated in drug pharmacokinetics (i.e., ADME) is a potential locus for drug–drug interactions.

2.1. Drug Absorption

Drug interactions can occur at the site of absorption by a multitude of mechanisms. Although oral chemotherapy has traditionally been limited in the past, many of the newer agents are being developed with the possibility of oral administration. Part of this challenge has arisen following demonstration that some of the newer "targeted" therapies are likely to require protracted exposure to ensure maximal benefit. Repeated intravenous administration in this context is impractical and there has been a push toward orally bioavailable drugs.

2.1.1. GASTRIC TRANSIT TIME AND ENVIRONMENT

For oral drugs, interactions leading to significant pharmacokinetic changes may arise as a result of changes in the gastric emptying time *(8)*. Food is the most widely accepted factor for increasing gastric transit time, but a number of drug-related factors may have similarly important roles. Drugs may affect directly the rate of gastric emptying with most slowing this process, although some, such as metoclopramide, actually speed it up *(9)*. Many cancer drugs produce transient nausea and vomiting. Nausea produces a slowing down of gastric emptying and may influence the rate and extent of absorption of oral chemotherapy. Many of the anticancer drugs given orally to date display wide variability in their absorption (e.g., mercaptopurine *[10]*), which would possibly mask these subtle effects. Small-intestinal transit time is also likely to be an important factor *(11)*. Certainly, the advent of rationally developed oral chemotherapy may, in the future, require specific consideration of these factors *(12,13)*.

Drug interactions during absorption may also follow from alterations in the gastrointestinal environment. For example, the camptothecins are unstable at physiological pH and drugs affecting intragastric pH could be of concern for the administration of these agents by the oral route. This was the basis for a study of oral topotecan with and without ranitidine *(14)*. Conversely, temozolomide is unstable at low pH and ranitidine was examined for an effect on drug absorption *(15)*. In neither case was there any significant effect. In some cases, the instability of drugs at acidic pH has led to the direct incorporation of inhibitors of gastric acid production into oral bioavailability studies *(16)*. Antacids may also be worthy of investigation from this point of view *(17)*.

Other nonspecific interactions that may modulate drug absorption can arise from the coadministration of binding drugs such as cholestyramine. Some parenteral formulations have surfactants to solubilize hydrophobic drugs in aqueous solutions. Although it is attractive to use intravenous formulations to investigate the oral route of administration of these drugs by simply administering these, the nonspecific effects of these agents may significantly modify the absorption of the compound of interest. In the case of paclitaxel, coadministration with its intravenous formulation surfactant, Cremophor EL, was shown to decrease greatly paclitaxel bioavailability whereas polysorbate 80 (Tween 80) had the opposite effect *(18)*.

2.1.2. DRUG METABOLISM

During their absorption from the gastrointestinal tract, drugs run the gauntlet of gut mucosal and hepatic drug metabolism, the so-called "first-pass effect." As reviewed elsewhere in this book, a multitude of pathways are implicated in the metabolism of anticancer drugs. One of the first drug interactions observed in oncology was that which occurs between 6-mercaptopurine and allopurinol *(4)*. An important metabolic pathway for the catabolism of 6-mercaptopurine is mediated by xanthine oxidase, which is inhibited by allopurinol. In the study by Zimm et al., administration of allopurinol increased peak concentrations and the area under the concentration–time curve (AUC) of 6-mercaptopurine by fivefold, but only when 6-mercapoturine was administered orally *(19)*. Methotrexate is another, albeit weaker, known inhibitor of xanthine oxidase *(20)*.

Inhibition of gut wall and hepatic metabolism may well be a requisite for appreciable absorption of some drugs from oral formulations. For example, the bioavailability of oral 5-fluorouracil (5-FU), which is of the order of 20–30 % *(21)*, is limited by intestinal and hepatic dihydropyrimidine dehydrogenase (DPD), the major catabolic pathway for 5-FU *(22)*. Novel oral formulations of fluoropyrimides often contain a DPD inhibitor to minimize this loss of drug to improve bioavailability. In the case of UFT, uracil is added in a 4:1 molar ratio as a competitive inhibitor of DPD with the 5-FU prodrug tegafur *(23)*. With the DPD inhibitor ethyniluracil, the bioavailability of orally administered 5-FU approaches 100% *(24)*. These are examples of how drug interactions can be exploited to improve the pharmacokinetic properties of important drugs.

Another major class of drug metabolizing enzymes present in the mucosa and liver is the cytochrome P450 (CYP450) superfamily. Again, these enzymes have been reviewed elsewhere in this book. In general, drug–drug interactions occurring at the CYP450 locus have been documented mostly in the context of parenterally administered cytotoxic drugs and these are discussed later.

2.1.3. DRUG TRANSPORT

There has been a revolution in the pharmacology of drug interactions following the demonstration that several of the ABC transporters, including P-glycoprotein, line the gastrointestinal lumen. Aside from the context of multidrug resistance, there has been the realization that these transporters, in facilitating basal to apical fluxes of drugs, are able to reduce greatly drug absorption following oral administration *(25)*. This mechanism is now being extensively manipulated in the experimental setting to try and achieve oral chemotherapy of drugs previously considered too poorly absorbed *(26)*. The taxanes are avid substrates of P-glycoprotein and particularly suitable for testing the concept of modulation of this transporter on drug bioavailability *(25)*. Cyclosporin A and its nonimmunosuppressive analog PSC833 were some of the first blockers of P-glycoprotein to be tested for this modulation, demonstrating impressive improvements in paclitaxel bioavailability in mice *(27,28)*. Results in clinical trials of 60 mg/m^2 of oral paclitaxel combined with 15 mg/kg of oral cyclosporin also showed large increases in oral bioavailability of paclitaxel *(29)*. The bioavailability of the combination was approx 30%, which may, however, have been underestimated because of the nonlinearity of paclitaxel kinetics *(29)*. Nevertheless, targeting relevant concentrations (i.e., those achieved by intravenous administration) may prove difficult although possible *(30)*. Other P-glycoprotein modulators (e.g., GF120918) are being investigated in this setting *(31,32)*.

In the same vein, topotecan is a substrate of both P-glycoprotein and the half-transporter breast-cancer-related protein (BCRP) and both these transporters are expressed in the gut mucosa *(33)*. The P-glycoprotein modulator GF120918 is also a potent modulator of BCRP and caused a further increase in topotecan bioavailability in the mouse as a result of blocking this second transporter *(33)*.

2.2. Drug Distribution

2.2.1. TRANSPORTERS

Aside from controlling the transfer of drugs across the gastrointestinal mucosa, the same transporters also control the distribution of drugs into other compartments (e.g., central nervous system, placenta). Inhibition or induction of transporters may therefore have an impact on the distribution of anticancer drugs. An effect of drug distribution would be detectable either from an effect on the volume of distribution of the drug or its pharmacokinetics in a specific compartment (e.g., central nervous system [CNS], cerebrospinal fluid [CSF], etc.). In a study of PSC833, Advani et al. examined the effects of this P-glycoprotein blocker (5 mg/kg po four times per day for 3 d) on a regimen of doxorubicin and paclitaxel *(34)*. Importantly, this was a crossover study and, although the sequences were not randomized, this design enabled the effect of PSC833 to be observed in each individual. The presence of PSC833 led to a doubling of the terminal half-lives of both doxorubicin and paclitaxel. In the case of paclitaxel, the effect was due primarily to a trebling of the volume of distribution, indicating a substantial interaction with the distribution of this drug. In contrast, in the case of doxorubicin, the effect was attributable mostly to changes in total clearance. Specific compartments may well be targeted by such drug interactions. Indeed, there is the exciting possibility of improving drug distribution into the CNS by coadministration of blockers of P-glycoprotein and other transporters located at the blood–brain barrier *(25,35)*. Importantly, however, an increase in CNS toxicity may be a down side to such strategies *(36)*. Also, issues in relation to the concentrations required need clarification *(25)*. There are conflicting data in animal models on the potential of cyclosporin A to modulate brain uptake of drugs *(37–39)* and this may reflect subtle differences in the probe drugs and their schedules of administration. However, this is a clear area of concern for potential drug–drug interactions.

2.2.2. PROTEIN BINDING

In theory, the competition by two drugs for a plasma binding protein can lead to an increase in the free concentration of the displaced drug. This, however, depends largely on the physicochemical and pharmacokinetic properties of the drug in question. In most cases, the displaced drug distributes rapidly into tissue compartments and/or is eliminated more rapidly with no net effect on free plasma concentrations. If the tissue compartment contains the tumor or organs of toxicity, then there may be a clinical effect of this displacement. These are, however, relatively rare but may need to be considered for drugs with very high plasma binding and small volumes of distribution. Cyclosporin A has been reported as being able to cause an increase in the unbound fraction of teniposide and increase the myelosuppressant effect of the latter *(40)*. In such cases, however, it is difficult to discern whether the effect is exclusively pharmacokinetic. Methotrexate is a drug suspected of being the subject of many drug–drug interactions, some of which may possibly be mediated in part through protein-binding alterations *(41)*. However, the data on this mechanism are relatively sparse, although a significant effect was shown with trimethoprim–sulfamethoxazole in pediatric leukemia patients *(42)* with the free fraction of methotrexate rising from 37% to 52 % in the presence of the antibiotic. The significance of this modest change is not evident. Other compounds can produce similar effects and these include the salicylates, other nonsteroidal anitiinflammatory drugs (NSAIDs), sulfonamides, phenytoin, tetracycline, chloramphenicol, and *p*-aminobenzoic acid (PABA).

2.2.3. DIRECT INTERACTIONS

Thiol protective agents (e.g., amifostine) provide nucleophiles able to react directly with platinum drugs *(43)*. This could potentially alter the distribution and activity of these drugs. However, studies looking at possible pharmacokinetic interactions have so far not revealed clinically significant interactions with either cisplatin or carboplatin *(44,45)* or other drugs for that matter *(46,47)*.

2.2.4. NONSPECIFIC EFFECTS

Several of the formulation vehicles are membrane-active compounds that may modify drug solubility and disposition. This was discussed briefly earlier in relation to the oral absorption of drugs. Similar effects may be relevant with regard to peripheral distribution of drugs. In fact some of these can be significant and the cause of apparent drug–drug interactions. This is covered in more detail in Subheading 4.

2.3. Drug Metabolism

Arguably, the most clinically significant drug–drug interactions in medical oncology are caused by interference at this locus. Several specific and nonspecific mechanisms are possible. Although it is beyond the scope of this chapter to explore all the possible enzymatic interactions, it is worth differentiating between some of the major mechanisms.

2.3.1. COMPETITIVE INHIBITION

Competitive inhibition is the dominant mechanism when two drugs compete for the same metabolic enzyme and a reduction of the metabolism of one occurs due to competitive displacement by the other. Erythromycin and cyclosporin A, for example, are competitive inhibitors of cytochrome P450 3A *(48)*. A feature of many substrate inhibitors of CYP3A, however, is their ability to form a reversible nitrosoalkane intermediate, which forms a tight complex with the CYP3A heme. Although reversible in theory, this complex is almost impossible to dissociate under physiological conditions. This is true for many of the compounds that undergo *N*-dealkylation reactions such as the macrolide antibiotics (erythromycin, troleandomycin, clarithromycin), some local anesthetics (e.g., lidocaine), diltiazem, fluoxetine, and tamoxifen *(49)*. The complex typically requires significant preincubation with NADPH and enzyme to form and so may not be detected on a casual screen, in which preincubations with drug are the exception rather than the norm. As a result, the screen may detect only the immediate competitive component and greatly underestimate the possible interaction in vivo. Indeed, this form of complex may explain why some drug interactions with drugs such as erythromycin are much more extensive (see Fig. 1) than predicted from inhibition constants estimated from competitive inhibition experiments *(50)*. Long-term treatment with such drugs depletes the affected CYP until an equilibrium of CYP synthesis and deactivation occurs *(51)*.

The most potent inhibitors of CYP3A activity are the azole antifungals and some of the HIV protease inhibitors (ritonavir, indinavir, etc.). Although the latter may be problematic in the setting of HIV-related malignancy, interactions with azole antifungals are much more likely in the routine setting where they are sometimes used in antifungal prophylaxis. This may lead to severe, occasionally fatal interactions *(52)*. The clearance of cyclophosphamide in children receiving fluconazole is reduced by almost 50% relative to controls, and in vitro experiments were in support of a role of decreased CYP metabolism in this interaction *(53)*.

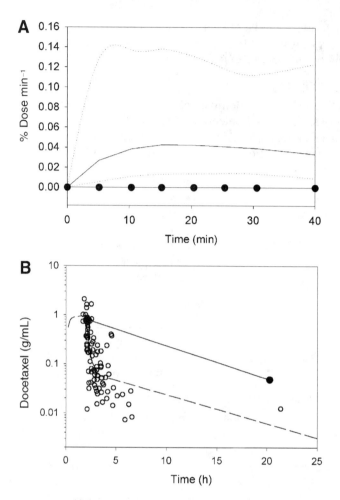

Fig. 1. (**A**) The results of the [^{14}C]erythomycin breath test performed on 54 cancer patients prior to treatment with single-agent docetaxel. The *solid* and *dotted lines* represent the mean and 95% confidence intervals, respectively, for the evolution of breath radioactivity as part of this test. In general, subjects with early appearing radioactive have greater cytochrome P450 3A activity *(162)*. The results from a subject who was receiving intercurrent clarithromycin for a chest infection at the time of treatment are shown as a *solid line* and *symbols*. The lack of measurable radioactivity in this individual suggests substantial impairment of drug metabolism as a result of a drug–drug interaction. (**B**) Sparse docetaxel plasma concentration data for the same individuals as in (**A**). The patient with impaired CYP3A drug metabolism is identified again with *solid symbols* and *line*. Identification of outliers in such data "clouds" may lead to the detection of unsuspected drug–drug interactions.

The azole antifungals are also inhibitors of CYP2C8, albeit at higher concentrations *(54)*. Paclitaxel is metabolized more avidly by this isoform *(55)* and an interaction with high-dose ketoconazole was thought possible on the basis of in vitro studies *(56)*. However, acute administration of ketoconazole after paclitaxel or 200 mg orally 3 h prior to paclitaxel had no pharmacokinetic consequences *(57)*. Whether this implies safety of paclitaxel with steady-state ketoconazole administration cannot necessarily be implied.

Other drugs metabolized by CYP3A include topotecan, irinotecan *(58,59)*, paclitaxel *(55)*, and docetaxel *(60)*. With irinotecan, the importance of this pathway was recently made clear in a study of ketoconazole pretreatment. Administration of 200 mg of ketoconazole 1 h prior to and 23 h after the infusion of irinotecan did not impact on the clearance of irinotecan. However, it significantly shifted the metabolic profile away from CYP3A deactivation toward carboxylesterase-mediated activation *(61)*. The apparent metabolic ratio for CYP3A was decreased approx 10-fold. Therefore, this interaction could provide a significant safety risk to patients receiving this combination.

Ketoconazole and the other azole antifungals are also inhibitors of P-glycoprotein *(62)* (but possibly not substrates *[63]*) and Kehrer et al. considered this as a potential factor in the drug interaction with irinotecan. Drug–drug interactions with azole antifungals may therefore be mediated at least partially through modulation of P-glycoprotein transport. For example, as mentioned previously, vinblastine does not readily penetrate into the CNS largely because of P-glycoprotein function, and mdr1a/1b knockout mice are at greater risk of neurotoxicity following administration of this agent *(64)*. The clinical interaction between itraconazole and vincristine *(65,66)* therefore may be due to modulation of CNS distribution of vincristine by P-glycoprotein. Fluconazole, in contrast, is a poor inhibitor of P-glycoprotein and given that doxorubicin is not appreciably metabolized by CYP450, a clinical interaction would not be predicted. This appears to be the case, at least in nonhuman primates *(67)*.

Conversely, many of the investigated inhibitors of P-glycoprotein are inhibitors of CYP3A4, and this may contribute to drug–drug interactions *(27)*. This includes some of the later generation inhibitors such as PSC833 *(68)*.

The metabolism of thiotepa, which is at least partially mediated by CYP enzymes *(69)*, has been shown to interfere with that of cyclophosphamide. Significant reductions in the C_{max} and AUC of the active 4-hydroxycyclophosphamide metabolite were observed when thiotepa was administered 1 h prior to cyclophosphamide *(70)*. Recently, it has been demonstrated that thiotepa is a potent, selective inhibitor of CYP 2B6, one of the key pathways in oxazaphosphorine metabolism *(71)*. One of the issues with investigating drug–drug interactions involving the oxazaphosphorines is the fact that their metabolism is extremely complex, with some pathways responsible for both activation and deactivation reactions. Carmustine, which inhibits human aldehyde dehydrogenase 1, causes a reduction in the deactivation of the aldocyclophosphamide intermediate *(72)*.

2.3.2. SUICIDE INHIBITION

Occasionally, the inhibiting drug is transformed into a highly reactive species by the action of the enzyme, and the two react to form a covalent complex. This type of inhibition is potentially more significant than competitive inhibition because the extent and duration of enzyme inactivation can both be extensive. In Japan, an interaction between an antiviral nucleoside, sorivudine, and 5-FU was suspected as being responsible for a series of 18 deaths *(73)*. An investigation into the metabolism of sorivudine found that the drug was hydrolyzed into 5-(2-bromovinyl)uracil by intestinal bacteria *(74)*. The latter is a potent suicide inhibitor of DPD, the major catabolic pathway of 5-FU. Blockage of DPD effectively transforms these patients to a DPD-deficient phenotype *(75)* with possible lethal consequences. Ironically, 5-(2-bromovinyl)uracil was a well-recognized inhibitor of DPD and had previously been shown to be of benefit when combined with reduced doses of 5-FU in animal models *(76)*. Indeed, tumoral overexpression of DPD is a recognized mechanism of resistance to fluoropyrimidines, and other suicide inhibitors of DPD have been developed clinically to reduce both the systemic and intratumoural metabolism of 5-FU *(77)*.

Although suicide inhibition is an attractive mechanism to exploit in cancer chemotherapy (e.g., exemestane and aromatase *[78]*), the situation with sorivudine exemplifies that drugs that produce suicide inhibition of key catabolic enzymes can have serious consequences unless they are administered for the specific purpose. Preclinical screening of compounds for their potential to inhibit DPD has become commonplace (79,80).

Several 17α-ethinyl-substituted steroids such as gestodene and ethinylestradiol are suicide inhibitors of CYP3A and this would suggest potentially multiple drug–drug interactions. However, clinical studies looking for such effects with, for example, ethinylestradiol, have not been in support of a major effect under therapeutically relevant conditions (81).

2.3.3. ENZYME ALKYLATION

Alkylating agents have the potential to interact with most cellular and extracellular macromolecules including enzymes and transporters. For example, the active product of cyclophosphamide, 4-hydroxyphosphoramide, and an eventual byproduct of its metabolism, acrolein, are able to react with cytochrome P450 enzymes (82). This can be blocked by the addition of thiol protective agents, suggesting a reaction with CYP sulfydryl groups. However, it is unclear what the clinical consequences of this are, if there are indeed any. Likewise, aquated platinum species can react with CYP enzymes leading to inactivation, but although these interactions can be demonstrated in vitro, pharmacokinetic interactions of this nature appear to be minor in vivo, as demonstrated with etoposide (83). Nevertheless, the demonstration that JM216, another recently developed platinum analog, also inhibits multiple CYP enzymes (84), indicates that some care should be taken with this class of drugs. Interaction of platinum compounds may extend to other enzyme systems, and, indeed, the clearance of 5-FU is reduced approx 25% by coadministration of oxaliplatin. The effect, however, does not appear to be mediated via an inhibition of DPD (85).

2.3.4. REDUCED EXPRESSION

Enzyme activity also relates to the expression of the protein and drugs able to modify the expression of the enzyme in question will also potentially lead to drug–drug interactions.

2.3.4.1. Cytotoxic Drugs

Exposure of cells to cytotoxic agents may lead to differential expression of metabolic enzymes. In a rat model, Yoshisue et al. demonstrated that oral administration of 5-FU reduced the activity of several drug-metabolizing enzymes (phases I and II). The loss of activity was apparently mediated by a reduction of these proteins within the cells and displayed little specificity (86). The effect was more marked in enterocytes than hepatocytes, suggesting that interactions might be more pronounced for orally administered drugs. Certainly, some drug interactions involving fluoropyrimidines have been reported, but these have so far been limited to a handful of substrates, implying greater selectivity of this effect in human subjects. In particular, clinically significant interactions between fluoropyrimidines and substrates of CYP2C9 such as phenytoin and (S)warfarin have been reported (87–89).

In male rats, the mRNA expression of the sexually dimorphic CYP isoform 2C11 can be repressed by treatment with cisplatin whereas the expression of "female" cytochrome p450s is increased (90). Similar observations have been made by the same laboratory using cyclophosphamide (91). The mechanism and clinical relevance of these observations are both unclear and only serve to highlight the species differences that may cloud the investigation of drug–drug interactions in animal models.

2.3.4.2. Biological Agents

Cytokines are able to down-regulate the expression of many cytochrome P450 enzymes, and this may explain the apparent link between inflammatory diseases and decreased metabolic drug clearance observed in several disease states *(92)* including cancer *(93)*. Exogenous cytokines can have the same effect and the administration of interferon-α to patients was associated with a significant 37% decrease in cyclophosphamide clearance *(94)*. This was consistent with a reduction in metabolic activation, because the AUC of the activated metabolite 4-hydroxycyclophosphamide was correspondingly reduced by 45%. Similar data demonstrating a reduction in 5-FU clearance when administered with interferon-α have been reported *(95)*, but this effect has varied between studies, possibly reflecting differences in schedules and doses *(96–98)*.

2.3.5. ENZYME INDUCTION

Cytochrome P450s in general are inducible enzymes. In the case of CYP3A4, it is well recognized that glucocorticoids (dexamethasone), barbiturates, rifampicin, and several anticonvulsant agents (phenytoin, carbamazepine) are able to up-regulate enzyme activity transcriptionally *(99)*. Indeed, drug interactions resulting from increased CYP3A-mediated metabolism following the administration of anticonvulsants and steroids are among the most commonly encountered and problematic drug–drug interactions in medical oncology *(5)*. Among the CYP3A substrates that have been demonstrated as being affected are the *Vinca* alkaloids *(100)*, cyclophosphamide *(6)*, irinotecan *(101)*, etoposide, and teniposide *(102)*. In the study of Baker et al., *(102)* the range of teniposide clearance in six children on anticonvulsants was 21–54 mL/min per m^2 (22 courses) as compared to 7–17 mL/min per m^2 in a control group matched for age and sex. The clearance of topotecan has also been shown to increase by approx 50% when phenytoin is coadministered with concomitant increases in the AUC of the CYP3A metabolite *N*-desmethyltopotecan *(103)*. Steroids have been reported to induce the metabolism and/or clearance of other drugs, including paclitaxel *(104,105)*.

Many of these inducers also induce other CYP450 isoforms, including members of the CYP2C superfamily *(106)*.

The oxazaphosphorines ifosfamide and cyclophosphamide display autoinduction of metabolism with unregulated expression of several enzymes in vitro *(107)*. However, this is a complex effect and its role in drug interactions is not well established. It is complicated by the fact that cyclophosphamide metabolites can also inactivate CYPs, as discussed previously.

A confounding factor for the interpretation of drug–drug interactions with drugs such as the anticonvulsants, steroids, and other CYP-inducing drugs (e.g., rifampin and phenobarbital) is that these compounds can coordinately up-regulate P-glycoprotein and other transporters. Hence, even drugs that are not extensively metabolized by the cytochrome P450 system may have altered pharmacokinetics, presumably through an effect on transporter-mediated excretion *(108)*.

2.4. Excretion

Drug interactions leading to modified drug excretion generally relate to interference with transporter function. Specifically, drug transporters in the proximal tubule of the kidney and the bile canaliculi are most likely involved. A major problem is identifying the tissue and transporter most at play in any observed drug–drug interaction. For example, cyclosporin A is an inhibitor of not only CYP3A but also of the transporters MRP-2 and P-glycoprotein. In addition to the effects on drug distribution discussed previously, cyclosporin also modulates both the renal and nonrenal clearance of several drugs including etoposide *(109)*.

2.4.1. RENAL EXCRETION

Many drugs undergo active tubular secretion in the kidney, and there is the potential for drug interactions at that locus. The interaction between methotrexate and probenecid is one of the best known examples *(110)*. Several transporters of the organic anion transporter (OAT) family are present in the tubular epithelium of the kidney and their inhibition by probenecid, various antibiotics, and NSAIDs is the likely mechanism *(111–114)*. These interactions are indeed now being determined at the molecular level, which was not possible until relatively recently. This type of interaction may be important for other antifolate analogues with significant tubular secretion, although there is a paucity of data on this subject.

Alterations in tubular secretion may also be modified through less direct effects. For example, Beorlegui et al. reported an apparent interaction between omeprazole and methotrexate *(115)*. They argued that inhibition of the tubular proton pump by omeprazole caused a reduction in methotrexate secretion because of the requirement for protons by the latter.

2.4.2. BILIARY EXCRETION

Biliary excretion is a major route of excretion of many anticancer drugs *(116,117)*. As mentioned previously, several transporters are present at the canalicular membrane including P-glycoprotein, MRP1, MRP-2 (cMOAT), and MRP-3. The development and discovery of drugs that act on these transporters has recently enabled the elucidation and exploitation of drug interactions at this locus.

2.4.2.1. Inhibition of Biliary Excretion

There are no documented cases of drug interactions specifically involving biliary excretion of anticancer drugs. Mostly, the problem is that measurement of biliary excretion is not routinely possible. Therefore, some of the pharmacokinetic interactions that have been reported might be attributable to this locus *(118)*, but confirmatory evidence is not available. Preclinical experiments using perfused rat liver preparations have shown that inhibitors of P-glycoprotein may reduce biliary excretion of compounds known to be excreted such as doxorubicin *(119,120)*. Using a similar model, Smit et al. demonstrated the potential for interactions between *Vinca* alkaloids and doxorubicin *(120)*.

2.4.2.2. Induction of Biliary Excretion

Transporters, as with metabolic enzymes, can be involved in drug–drug interactions as a result of induction of activity. It is increasingly recognized that the induction of transporters such as P-glycoprotein can be caused by agents that overlap substantially with those capable of inducing CYP3A *(121)*. As a result, some interactions with anticonvulsants may actually be the results of up-regulation of important transporters. This is a possible mechanism for the interaction between methotrexate and anticonvulsants *(108)*.

3. PREDICTING INTERACTIONS

The prediction and evaluation of significant drug–drug interactions has in many instances been a rather piecemeal process. However, significant inroads in our understanding of the loci of these interactions have been made in vitro through to in vivo *(50)* and there are now instances of systematic screening for these interactions during drug development *(122)*.

3.1. Historical Data

In assessing likely interactions for a new drug, it is enormously useful if the compound has metabolism and excretion similar to those of previously characterized analogs. In the absence of such information, the usual sequential processes of in vitro and preclinical studies need to be carried out. One of the major problems is the manner in which these experiments have been performed often varies significantly from study to study and the data often reported are in different formats. There is therefore a real need for consistent experimental design and reporting in such studies *(123)*. In the absence of such a platform, however, other groups have assembled electronic databases, which at least should enable some qualitative predictions of potential drug–drug interactions *(124)*. A drug–drug interaction locus identified in vitro will be relevant only if this pathway represents a major route of elimination for the candidate drug *(125)*. This is one of the major issues that databases such as the one proposed by Bonnabry et al. are trying to address *(124)*.

3.2. Predicted from In Vitro Experiments

The advantage of being able readily to obtain drug metabolism enzymes from recombinant sources (insect cells, human lymphoblastoid cells, yeast, bacteria) has greatly facilitated the task of establishing the important routes of metabolism likely to be encountered when administered to patients. Similarly, these systems can also be used to search for potential drug interactions. Rapid throughput systems have been developed that use specific fluorogenic substrates to facilitate the large-scale and thorough screening required *(126,127)*. The much larger potential problem is that relating to drug transporters. Here, the best systems are likely to be panels of stably transfected cells expressing each known transporter, starting probably with P-glycoprotein, BCRP, and MRP-1 and MRP-2. Alternatively, cells mimicking the relevant in vivo system may be used to test simultaneously the effects of expression of transporters and metabolic enzymes *(128)*. A specific problem with the in vitro testing of drug interactions with alkylating anticancer drugs relates to the fact that these have complex pharmacology featuring multiple, often unstable species. Comprehensive studies of metabolic interactions with such drugs are difficult to perform and to interpret *(53,70–72,82,91,107,129,130)*.

3.3. In Silico

Ultimately, the structure–activity relationships for each enzyme/transporter may become sufficiently documented by the use of large databases to enable direct *in silico* predictions of the metabolic and transporter properties of new drugs. These in turn would enable extrapolation of likely in vivo disposition, pharmacogenetics, and possible drug interactions. The use of such predictive models and their validation has been reviewed recently *(131)*.

As mentioned previously, predictions are complicated by the overlap between transporters and metabolism. The interaction of etoposide with cyclosporin reported by Bisogno et al. *(132)* could, on the basis of other observations discussed above, be the result of interaction with metabolism, biliary and intestinal secretion, and protein binding. Likewise cimetidine, which is often used as a relatively nonselective CYP450 inhibitor, is also an inhibitor of OAT in the kidney. Hence the mechanism for the drug interaction reported between cimetidine and epirubicin is also difficult to identify *(133)*. Ultimately, therefore, classical in vitro and in vivo approaches for the investigation of drug interactions are required.

3.4. Preclinical Studies

Animal models may enable certain drug–drug interactions to be examined in a more physiologically meaningful fashion *(134)*. However, some major interspecies differences exist with respect to the metabolism and excretion of drugs. For example, rats are relatively deficient in the aldo–keto reductases that metabolize anthracyclines to their corresponding C-13 alcohols *(135)*. The cytochrome P450 enzymes also often differ markedly between species, not only in terms of their substrate affinities and reaction products *(136,137)* but also in their susceptibility to inducers and inhibitors *(138)*. The regulation of CYP450 is also highly species dependent. For example, induction of CYP3A by rifampicin is pronounced in humans and rabbits but not in rats *(139)*. Hence, investigations of drug interactions require the use of the most representative animal or in vitro system to ensure relevance.

3.5. Clinical Studies

Many of the clinical drug interactions reported have been detected on the basis on comparisons of relatively small patient groups. In most cases, data are compared to historical or case-matched groups. Even less reliable are isolated case reports that report suspected drug interactions on the basis of abnormal drug disposition. Because of the large interindividual differences in metabolism and disposition, many of these studies are underpowered and biased. Ideally, clinical studies should be performed using a randomized crossover design as is normally used in trials to support of registration of compounds. FDA guidelines are available for the design of such trials (http://www.fda.gov/cder/guidance/2635fnl.htm). However, in medical oncology, many of the drugs are inherently unsafe. Usually drug–drug interactions are investigated because they pose a threat either to the safety or the efficacy of a compound and it becomes ethically difficult to propose such trials in patients who cannot really afford either. One alternative is to incorporate extensive population pharmacokinetics as part of Phase II and III trials of anticancer drugs. This then enables the identification of patients with unusual pharmacokinetic data and the identification of possible interactions *(140,141)*.

One of the down sides of this approach is that studies may require a very large number of subjects (several hundred) unless the interacting drug is very commonly used in the intended setting (e.g., anticonvulsants in CNS malignancy).

The drug candidates most worthy of further study for possible interactions are obviously those that are likely to be coadministered and for which there is some support from *in silico*, in vitro, preclinical, or clinical data. Other factors to be considered include the doses of the agents, their dosing regimen (single or multiple doses), and the timing of the administration (A before B, A after B, or A + B). The latter is particularly important when the drug interaction is modulated through alteration of gene expression. For example, a study on the effects of rifampicin on drug clearance would require several days of rifampicin treatment prior to administration of the test drug to ensure maximal induction of the relevant enzyme system.

4. WHEN THE PROBLEM IS NOT THE DRUG

In some instances, apparently classical drug–drug interactions have subsequently been shown to have little to do with the drugs involved. Consideration of these alternate mechanisms should be part of the investigation of drug–drug interactions.

4.1. Vehicle Effects

Many drugs are not sufficiently soluble to be administered in purely aqueous solvents. Instead a formulation component is frequently a surfactant (e.g., Cremophor EL, sorbitol, Tween, etc.). These compounds should not be dismissed as inactive and inconsequential. For example, Cremophor EL has some membrane effects and has been investigated for its ability to reverse P-glycoprotein-mediated multidrug resistance *(142)*. It also modulates differentially the toxicity of cisplatin to marrow and tumor cells *(143,144)*. Cremophor EL has been shown to modulate the distribution and elimination of doxorubicin in both preclinical and clinical studies *(142,145,146)*. In the study of Millward et al., 11 patients were randomized to receive either 50 mg/m^2 of doxorubicin alone or in combination with 30 mL/m^2 of Cremophor EL. They were then crossed over to the alternative regimen.

Cremophor significantly reduced the clearance of doxorubicin by approx 20%. The metabolite doxorubicinol was present in higher concentrations after Cremophor EL administration, resulting in an almost doubling of its AUC. Cremophor EL is also the likely major component of the interaction between Taxol® and anthracyclines. When Taxol® (paclitaxel formulated in Cremophor EL) is administered immediately prior to a doxorubicin infusion or as an infusion prior to bolus doxorubicin, the clearance of doxorubicin is reduced by 20–30% and concentrations of doxorubicinol are again greatly increased *(118,147,148)*. The latter suggests a possible reduction in the biliary clearance of the metabolite or a redistribution phenomenon secondary to the membrane effects of the Cremophor EL. Indeed, even when paclitaxel is administered 24 h after doxorubicin, sudden rebound profiles of doxorubicinol are observed *(148)*. The effects of Cremophor EL on the hepatic disposition of paclitaxel itself also appear to be due to nonspecific effects on distribution rather than direct effects on biliary excretion *(149)*.

Polysorbate 80 (also known as Tween 80) is used in the current formulation of docetaxel and etoposide. The coadministration of polysorbate 80 by itself or in the etoposide formulation had up to a twofold effect on doxorubicin AUC, mainly through increased early tissue distribution *(150)*. The effect of etoposide on methotrexate pharmacokinetics reported by Paal et al. may also be due to the nonspecific effects of the Tween 80 present in etoposide *(151)*. Indeed, the rebound profile of plasma methotrexate that occurred a few hours following etoposide is qualitatively similar to the rebound of doxorubicinol concentrations when paclitaxel is administered in Cremophor EL *(148)*.

4.2. Effects of Dose Form

Several drugs are now marketed in liposomal formulations (doxorubicin, daunorubicin, amphotericin B). Theoretically, drugs can self-load into preformed liposomes in the circulation, and this was first demonstrated in a mouse model *(152)*. When combination therapy includes a liposomal agent, the fact that many anticancer drugs are amphiphilic compounds that can interact with membranes suggests that drug–liposome interactions could take place. By binding to liposomes, it is possible that the release of the encapsulated drug would be modified and this has indeed been demonstrated in vitro *(153)*. In vivo, however, this appears less likely and the predominant effect appears to be the uptake of the free drug into the circulating liposomes. In the study of Waterhouse et al., mice administered idarubicin and liposomal vincristine had a 3.6-fold increase in circulating concentrations of idarubicin 15 min later.

4.3. Effects of Treatment Regimens

Apart from aspects of formulation composition, specific treatment regimens require additional procedures to ensure adequate safety. For example, fluid loading is usually undertaken prior to cisplatin or methotrexate to ensure adequate renal function. Therefore, administration of another drug also cleared by the kidneys with either cisplatin or methotrexate might possibly result in altered disposition relative to drug alone. Some data are in support of such an effect. For example, Hudes et al. reported an increase in the renal clearance of trimetrexate when administered with cisplatin *(154)*. Paradoxically, the urinary recovery of pemitrexed was reduced and its total clearance increased when administered with cisplatin *(155)*. It is expected that effects of volume loading on renal clearance would be most pronounced in patients with some degree of renal dysfunction. For example, Kaye et al. *(156)* found greatly increased methotrexate clearance when coadministered with cisplatin and forced diuresis only in a patient with renal clearance < 60 mL/min.

Administration of premedication agents for nausea/vomiting and hypersensitivity reactions may also be implicated. For example, interaction studies of a drug regimen with or without cisplatin might reasonably introduce not only the cisplatin but also antiemetics in the regimen. Ondansetron, for example, has been suggested to cause a slight decrease in the clearance of cyclophosphamide in high-dose regimens *(157)* as compared to historical controls. Other studies have also noticed similar modest effects on both cyclophosphamide and cisplatin elimination by ondansetron *(158)*, again when compared to historical controls.

Similarly, the requirement for steroid prophylaxis for hypersensitivity reactions with docetaxel has been suggested to be the mechanism behind the interaction between ifosfamide and docetaxel *(159)*.

5. WHEN THE CYTOTOXIC AGENT IS NOT THE VICTIM

Because cytotoxic agents are potentially dangerous drugs we are actually more concerned about the effects of concomitant therapy on the cytotoxic drug rather than the reverse. However, many drugs that are used for the intercurrent treatment of the patient may also suffer from small therapeutic windows. As discussed above, there have been reports of perturbed coagulation parameters in patients on warfarin receiving capecitabine. Similarly, blood concentrations of phenytoin are increased under similar circumstances. The effect is unlikely to be mediated by an acute interaction, given that capecitabine does not inhibit the cytochrome involved in the metabolism of warfarin. However, as mentioned previously, it appears that oral fluoropyrimidines can affect the expression and activity of cytochrome P450s.

6. CAN WE EXPLOIT DRUG INTERACTIONS?
6.1. Oral Delivery of Drugs

Drug interactions, as shown in the relevant sections above can have both detrimental and beneficial effects in chemotherapy. In particular, the inhibition of gastrointestinal transporters and enzymes greatly improves the bioavailability of oral drugs and enables oral delivery of some drugs that could previously not be administered orally. Poor bioavailability is usually associated with highly variable systemic concentrations and an additional possible benefit could be a reduction in intra- and interpatient variability in pharmacokinetics, although this is unlikely to be reduced to less than that encountered with parenteral administration. An example of successful exploitation of this strategy is the development of orally administered fluoropyrimidines that incorporate an inhibitor of DPD *(23)*.

Many transport and enzyme modulators are currently being investigated in the setting of oral chemotherapy, although analogues that are specifically not substrates for these pathways provide an alternative route of development. For example, several taxanes that are not P-glycoprotein substrates are currently being evaluated for oral chemotherapy.

6.2. Systemic Administration

As previously discussed for the DPD inhibitors, administration of an inhibitor may greatly reduce intratumoral metabolism that in some cases may act as a significant mechanism of resistance in vivo. The second possible advantage of the suicide inhibitors of DPD (e.g., ethinyluracil) is that when coadministered, the elimination of 5-FU is no longer mostly via DPD catabolism but by renal excretion. The latter pathway is inherently less variable and more predictable than DPD, thereby potentially facilitating the dose individualization of treatment *(24)*, although this has not been exploited in Phase III trials of the combination *(160)*.

Other DPD inhibitors have been developed in combination with oral prodrugs of 5-FU. These combination products include S-1 and UFT. S-1 also contains potassium oxonate as an inhibitor of thymidine kinase, and this assists in reducing activation of the 5-FU in the gastrointestinal mucosa.

The reduction in fluoropyrimidine dose that is made possible with DPD inhibitors underscores another way in which drug interactions can be exploited. In the early years of cyclosporin A use, the interaction between diltiazem was characterized and exploited to enable substantial cost savings. However, interactions based on reversible mechanisms are very difficult to predict because of constantly varying profiles on the target and inhibitor drug. In oncology, because of the limited safety of many of these agents, introduction of an additional variable into the chemotherapy regimen may become counterproductive, and such strategies are used only in the experimental setting. Such interactions also need to be proven from the aspect of activity, and the substantial costs of the additional Phase III trials probably outweigh the savings. Ironically, cyclosporin has now been proposed as a modulator of several agents to improve their pharmacokinetic and pharmacodynamic properties.

7. FUTURE DIRECTIONS

From a drug development aspect, the most exciting proposition is that accumulated knowledge about current drugs and their metabolism will enable some *in silico* prediction of likely mechanism of clearance and the potential drug interactions that might arise. This could greatly assist the rational refinement of drug leads and reduce the expense of development.

The possibility of using well-characterized drug–drug interactions to enable oral therapy may prove obvious potential advantages, but this has not yet been developed into the routine clinical setting.

Finally, genomic advances are likely to advance greatly our understanding of drug–drug interactions, particularly as they relate to instances in which drug metabolism is induced. For example, cytochrome P450 3A expression is extremely sensitive to control from interactions of nuclear receptors with the RXR. Some of the nuclear factors involved (CAR, PXR, and PPAR) have recently been shown to be subject to functional polymorphic variation *(161)*. The elucidation of genotype/phenotype associations may help ultimately enable prediction of drug–drug interactions in individual subjects.

REFERENCES

1. Balis FM. Pharmacokinetic drug interactions of commonly used anticancer drugs. Clin Pharmacokinet 1986; 11:223–235.
2. Loadman PM, Bibby MC. Pharmacokinetic drug interactions with anticancer drugs. Clin Pharmacokinet 1994; 26:486–500.
3. van Meerten E, Verweij J, Schellens JH. Antineoplastic agents. Drug interactions of clinical significance. Drug Safety 1995; 12:168–182.
4. McLeod HL. Clinically relevant drug–drug interactions in oncology. Br J Clin Pharmacol 1998; 45:539–544.
5. Relling MV, Pui CH, Sandlund JT, et al. Adverse effect of anticonvulsants on efficacy of chemotherapy for acute lymphoblastic leukaemia. Lancet 2000; 356:285–290.
6. Yule SM, Boddy AV, Cole M, et al. Cyclophosphamide metabolism in children. Cancer Res 1995; 55:803–809.
7. Yu DK. The contribution of P-glycoprotein to pharmacokinetic drug–drug interactions. J Clin Pharmacol 1999; 39:1203–1211.
8. Reigner B, Verweij J, Dirix L, et al. Effect of food on the pharmacokinetics of capecitabine and its metabolites following oral administration in cancer patients. Clin Cancer Res 1998; 4:941–948.
9. Nimmo W. Drugs, diseases and altered gastric emptying. In: Gibaldi M, Prescott, L (eds). Handbook of Clinical Pharmacokinetics. New York, NY: ADIS Health Science Press, 1983.

10. Riccardi R, Balis FM, Ferrara P, Lasorella A, Poplack DG, Mastrangelo R. Influence of food intake on bioavailability of oral 6-mercaptopurine in children with acute lymphoblastic leukemia. Pediatr Hematol Oncol 1986; 3:319–324.

11. Pearson AD, Craft AW, Eastham EJ, et al. Small intestinal transit time affects methotrexate absorption in children with acute lymphoblastic leukemia. Cancer Chemother Pharmacol 1985; 14:211–215.

12. Swaisland H, Laight A, Stafford L, et al. Pharmacokinetics and tolerability of the orally active selective epidermal growth factor receptor tyrosine kinase inhibitor ZD1839 in healthy volunteers. Clin Pharmacokinet 2001; 40:297–306.

13. Hughes AN, Rafi I, Griffin MJ, et al. Phase I studies with the nonclassical antifolate nolatrexed dihydrochloride (AG337, THYMITAQ) administered orally for 5 days. Clin Cancer Res 1999; 5: 111–118.

14. Akhtar S, Beckman RA, Mould DR, Doyle E, Fields SZ, Wright J. Pretreatment with ranitidine does not reduce the bioavailability of orally administered topotecan. Cancer Chemother Pharmacol 2000; 46:204–210.

15. Beale P, Judson I, Moore S, et al. Effect of gastric pH on the relative oral bioavailability and pharmacokinetics of temozolomide. Cancer Chemother Pharmacol 1999; 44:389–394.

16. Saven A, Cheung WK, Smith I, et al. Pharmacokinetic study of oral and bolus intravenous 2-chlorodeoxyadenosine in patients with malignancy. J Clin Oncol 1996; 14:978–983.

17. Reigner B, Clive S, Cassidy J, et al. Influence of the antacid Maalox on the pharmacokinetics of capecitabine in cancer patients. Cancer Chemother Pharmacol 1999; 43:309–315.

18. Malingre MM, Schellens JH, Van Tellingen O, et al. The co-solvent Cremophor EL limits absorption of orally administered paclitaxel in cancer patients. Br J Cancer 2001; 85:1472–1477.

19. Zimm S, Collins JM, O'Neill D, Chabner BA, Poplack DG. Inhibition of first-pass metabolism in cancer chemotherapy: interaction of 6-mercaptopurine and allopurinol. Clin Pharmacol Ther 1983; 34: 810–817.

20. Balis FM, Holcenberg JS, Zimm S, et al. The effect of methotrexate on the bioavailability of oral 6-mercaptopurine. Clin Pharmacol Ther 1987; 41:384–387.

21. Phillips TA, Howell A, Grieve RJ, Welling PG. Pharmacokinetics of oral and intravenous fluorouracil in humans. J Pharmaceut Sci 1980; 69:1428–1431.

22. DiAsio R. Clinical implications of dihydropyrimidine dehydrogenase on 5-FU pharmacology. Oncology 2001; 15:21–26.

23. Jones R, Twelves C. Oral uracil-tegafur: an alternative to intravenous 5-fluorouracil? Exp Opin Pharmacother 2001; 2:1495–1505.

24. Baker SD, Khor SP, Adjei AA, et al. Pharmacokinetic, oral bioavailability, and safety study of fluorouracil in patients treated with 776C85, an inactivator of dihydropyrimidine dehydrogenase. J Clin Oncol 1996; 14:3085–3096.

25. Ayrton A, Morgan P. Role of transport proteins in drug absorption, distribution and excretion. Xenobiotica 2001; 31:469–497.

26. Schellens JH, Malingre MM, Kruijtzer CM, et al. Modulation of oral bioavailability of anticancer drugs: from mouse to man. Eur J Pharmaceut Sci 2000; 12:103–110.

27. van Asperen J, van Tellingen O, van der Valk MA, Rozenhart M, Beijnen JH. Enhanced oral absorption and decreased elimination of paclitaxel in mice cotreated with cyclosporin A. Clin Cancer Res 1998; 4:2293–2297.

28. van Asperen J, van Tellingen O, Sparreboom A, et al. Enhanced oral bioavailability of paclitaxel in mice treated with the P-glycoprotein blocker SDZ PSC 833. Br J Cancer 1997; 76:1181–1183.

29. Meerum Terwogt JM, Malingre MM, Beijnen JH, et al. Coadministration of oral cyclosporin A enables oral therapy with paclitaxel. Clin Cancer Res 1999; 5:3379–3384.

30. Britten CD, Baker SD, Denis LJ, et al. Oral paclitaxel and concurrent cyclosporin A: targeting clinically relevant systemic exposure to paclitaxel. Clin Cancer Res 2000; 6:3459–3468.

31. Bardelmeijer HA, Beijnen JH, Brouwer KR, et al. Increased oral bioavailability of paclitaxel by GF120918 in mice through selective modulation of P-glycoprotein. Clin Cancer Res 2000; 6:4416–4421.

32. Malingre MM, Beijnen JH, Rosing H, et al. Co-administration of GF120918 significantly increases the systemic exposure to oral paclitaxel in cancer patients. Br J Cancer 2001; 84:42–47.

33. Jonker JW. Role of breast cancer resistance protein in the bioavailability and fetal penetration of topotecan. J Natl Cancer Inst 2000; 92:1651–1656.

34. Advani R, Fischer G, Lum B, et al. A phase I trial of doxorubicin, paclitaxel and valspodar (PSC 833), a modulator of multidrug resistance. Clin Cancer Res 2001; 7:1221–1229.

35. Bart J, Groen HJ, Hendrikse NH, van der Graaf WT, Vaalburg W, de Vries EG. The blood–brain barrier and oncology: new insights into function and modulation. Cancer Treat Rev 2000; 26:449–462.

36. Schinkel AH, Wagenaar E, Mol C, Deemter L. P-glycoprotein in the blood–brain barrier of mice influences the brain penetration and pharmacological activity of many drugs. J Clin Invest 1996; 97: 2517–2524.

37. Hendrikse NH, Schinkel AH, de Vries EG, et al. Complete in vivo reversal of p-glycoprotein pump function in the blood–brain barrier visualized with positron emission tomography. Br J Pharmacol 1998; 124:1413–1418.

38. Hendrikse NH, de Vries EG, Eriks-Fluks L, et al. A new in vivo method to study P-glycoprotein transport in tumors and the blood–brain barrier. Cancer Res 1999; 59:2411–2416.

39. Warren KE, Patel MC, McCully CM, Montuenga LM, Balis FM. Effect of P-glycoprotein modulation with cyclosporin A on cerebrospinal fluid penetration of doxorubicin in non-human primates. Cancer Chemother Pharmacol 2000; 45:207–212.

40. Toffoli G, Aita P, Sorio R, et al. Effect of cyclosporin A on protein binding of teniposide in cancer patients. Anticancer Drugs 1999; 10:511–518.

41. Long KS, Frenia ML. Methotrexate and nonsteroidal antiinflammatory drug interactions. Ann Pharmacother 1992; 26:234–237.

42. Ferrazzini G, Klein J, Sulh H, Chung D, Griesbrecht E, Koren G. Interaction between trimethoprim–sulfamethoxazole and methotrexate in children with leukemia. J Pediatr 1990; 117:823–826.

43. Treskes M, Holwerda U, Klein I, Pinedo HM, van der Vijgh WJ. The chemical reactivity of the modulating agent WR2721 (ethiofos) and its main metabolites with the antitumor agents cisplatin and carboplatin. Biochem Pharmacol 1991; 42:2125–2130.

44. Korst AE, van der Sterre ML, Eeltink CM, Fichtinger-Schepman AM, Vermorken JB, van der Vijgh WJ. Pharmacokinetics of carboplatin with and without amifostine in patients with solid tumors. Clin Cancer Res 1997; 3:697–703.

45. Korst AE, van der Sterre ML, Gall HE, Fichtinger-Schepman AM, Vermorken JB, van der Vijgh WJ. Influence of amifostine on the pharmacokinetics of cisplatin in cancer patients. Clin Cancer Res 1998; 4:331–336.

46. Czejka M, Schueller J, Eder I, et al. Clinical pharmacokinetics and metabolism of paclitaxel after polychemotherapy with the cytoprotective agent amifostine. Anticancer Res 2000; 20:3871–3877.

47. Martens-Lobenhoffer J, Fuhlroth J, Ridwelski K. Influence of the administration of amifostine on the pharmacokinetics of 5-fluorouracil in patients with metastatic colorectal carcinoma. Int J Clin Pharmacol Ther 2000; 38:41–44.

48. Thummel KE, Wilkinson GR. In vitro and in vivo drug interactions involving human CYP3A. Annu Rev Pharmacol Toxicol 1998; 38:389–430.

49. Jones DR, Gorski JC, Hamman MA, Mayhew BS, Rider S, Hall SD. Diltiazem inhibition of cytochrome P-450 3A activity is due to metabolite intermediate complex formation. J Pharmacol Exp Ther 1999; 290:1116–1125.

50. Weaver RJ. Assessment of drug–drug interactions: concepts and approaches. Xenobiotica 2001; 31:499–538.

51. Mayhew BS, Jones DR, Hall SD. An in vitro model for predicting in vivo inhibition of cytochrome P450 3A4 by metabolic intermediate complex formation. Drug Metab Dispos 2000; 28: 1031–1037.

52. Bosque E. Possible drug interaction between itraconazole and vinorelbine tartrate leading to death after one dose of chemotherapy. Ann Intern Med 2001; 134:427.

53. Yule S, Walker D, Cole M, et al. The effect of fluconazole on cyclophosphamide metabolism in children. Drug Metab Dispos 1999; 27:417–421.

54. Ong CE, Coulter S, Birkett DJ, Bhasker CR, Miners JO. The xenobiotic inhibitor profile of cytochrome P4502C8. Br J Clin Pharmacol 2000; 50:573–580.

55. Rahman A, Korzekwa KR, Grogan J, Gonzalez FJ, Harris JW. Selective biotransformation of taxol to 6 alpha-hydroxytaxol by human cytochrome P450 2C8. Cancer Res 1994; 54:5543–5546.

56. Jamis-Dow CA, Klecker RW, Katki AG, Collins JM. Metabolism of taxol by human and rat liver in vitro: a screen for drug interactions and interspecies differences. Cancer Chemother Pharmacol 1995; 36:107–114.

57. Jamis-Dow CA, Pearl ML, Watkins PB, Blake DS, Klecker RW, Collins JM. Predicting drug interactions in vivo from experiments in vitro. Human studies with paclitaxel and ketoconazole. Am J Clin Oncol 1997; 20:592–599.

58. Haaz MC, Rivory L, Riche C, Vernillet L, Robert J. Metabolism of irinotecan (CPT-11) by human hepatic microsomes: participation of cytochrome P-450 3A and drug interactions. Cancer Res 1998; 58:468–472.

59. Dodds HM, Haaz MC, Riou JF, Robert J, Rivory LP. Identification of a new metabolite of CPT-11 (irinotecan): pharmacological properties and activation to SN-38. J Pharmacol Exp Ther 1998; 286: 578–583.

60. Marre F, Sanderink GJ, de Sousa G, Gaillard C, Martinet M, Rahmani R. Hepatic biotransformation of docetaxel (Taxotere) in vitro: involvement of the CYP3A subfamily in humans. Cancer Res 1996; 56:1296–1302.

61. Kehrer D, Mathijssen R, Verweij J, de Bruijn P, Sparreboom A. Modulation of irinotecan metabolism by ketoconazole. J Clin Oncol 2002; 20:3122–3129.

62. Siegsmund MJ, Cardarelli C, Aksentijevich I, Sugimoto Y, Pastan I, Gottesman MM. Ketoconazole effectively reverses multidrug resistance in highly resistant KB cells. J Urol 1994; 151:485–491.

63. Kim RB, Wandel C, Leake B, et al. Interrelationship between substrates and inhibitors of human CYP3A and P-glycoprotein. Pharmaceut Res 1999; 16:408–414.

64. Schinkel AH, Smit JJ, van Tellingen O, et al. Disruption of the mouse mdr1a P-glycoprotein gene leads to a deficiency in the blood-brain barrier and to increased sensitivity to drugs. Cell 1994; 77:491–502.

65. Bohme A, Ganser A, Hoelzer D. Aggravation of vincristine-induced neurotoxicity by itraconazole in the treatment of adult ALL. Ann Hematol 1995; 71:311–312.

66. Gillies J, Hung KA, Fitzsimons E, Soutar R. Severe vincristine toxicity in combination with itraconazole. Clin Lab Haematol 1998; 20:123–124.

67. Warren KE, McCully CM, Walsh TJ, Balis FM. Effect of fluconazole on the pharmacokinetics of doxorubicin in nonhuman primates. Antimicrob Agents Chemother 2000; 44:1100–1101.

68. Fischer V, Rodriguez-Gascon A, Heitz F, et al. The multidrug resistance modulator valspodar (PSC 833) is metabolized by human cytochrome P450 3A. Implications for drug–drug interactions and pharmacological activity of the main metabolite. Drug Metab Dispos 1998; 26:802–811.

69. Ng SF, Waxman DJ. *N,N',N''*-triethylenethiophosphoramide (thio-TEPA) oxygenation by constitutive hepatic P450 enzymes and modulation of drug metabolism and clearance in vivo by P450-inducing agents. Cancer Res 1991; 51:2340–2345.

70. Huitema AD, Kerbusch T, Tibben MM, Rodenhuis S, Beijnen JH. Reduction of cyclophosphamide bioactivation by thioTEPA: critical sequence-dependency in high-dose chemotherapy regimens. Cancer Chemother Pharmacol 2000; 46:119–127.

71. Rae J, Soukhova N, Flockhart D, Desta Z. Triethylenethiophosphoramide is a specific inhibitor of cytochrome P450 2B6: implications for cyclophosphamide metabolism. Drug Metab Dispos 2002; 30: 525–530.

72. Ren S, Slatterly J. Inhibition of carboxyethylphosphoramide mustard formation from 4-hydroxy-cyclophosphamide by carmustine. AAPS Pharmaceut Sci 1999; 1:E14.

73. Okuda H, Ogura K, Kato A, Takubo H, Watabe T. A possible mechanism of eighteen patient deaths caused by interactions of sorivudine, a new antiviral drug, with oral 5-fluorouracil prodrugs. J Pharmacol Exp Ther 1998; 287:791–799.

74. Nakayama H, Kinouchi T, Kataoka K, Akimoto S, Matsuda Y, Ohnishi Y. Intestinal anaerobic bacteria hydrolyse sorivudine, producing the high blood concentration of 5-(E)-(2-bromovinyl)uracil that increases the level and toxicity of 5-fluorouracil. Pharmacogenetics 1997; 7:35–43.

75. Yan J, Tyring SK, McCrary MM, et al. The effect of sorivudine on dihydropyrimidine dehydrogenase activity in patients with acute herpes zoster. Clin Pharmacol Ther 1997; 61:563–573.

76. Desgranges C, Razaka G, De Clercq E, et al. Effect of (E)-5-(2-bromovinyl)uracil on the catabolism and antitumor activity of 5-fluorouracil in rats and leukemic mice. Cancer Res 1986; 46: 1094–1101.

77. Ahmed FY, Johnston SJ, Cassidy J, et al. Eniluracil treatment completely inactivates dihydropyrimidine dehydrogenase in colorectal tumors. J Clin Oncol 1999; 17:2439–2445.

78. Evans TR, Di Salle E, Ornati G, et al. Phase I and endocrine study of exemestane (FCE 24304), a new aromatase inhibitor, in postmenopausal women. Cancer Res 1992; 52:5933–5939.

79. Yamazaki S, Hayashi M, Toth LN, Ozawa N. Lack of interaction between bropirimine and 5-fluorouracil on human dihydropyrimidine dehydrogenase. Xenobiotica 2001; 31:25–31.

80. Watanabe M, Tateishi T, Takezawa N, et al. Effects of PR-350, a newly developed radiosensitizer, on dihydropyrimidine dehydrogenase activity and 5-fluorouracil pharmacokinetics. Cancer Chemother Pharmacol 2001; 47:250–254.

81. Belle D, Callaghan J, Gorski J, et al. The effects of an oral contraceptive containing ethinyloestradiol and norgestrel on CYP3A activity. Br J Clin Pharmacol 2002; 53:67–74.

82. Gurtoo HL, Marinello A, Struck R, Paul B, Dahms R. Studies on the mechanism of denaturation of cytochrome P-450 by cyclophosphamide and its metabolites. J Biol Chem 1981; 256:11,691–11,701.

83. Thomas H, Porter D, Bartelink I, et al. Randomized cross-over clinical trial to study potential pharmacokinetic interactions between cisplatin or carboplatin and etoposide. Br J Clin Pharmacol 2002; 53: 83–91.

84. Ando Y, Shimizu T, Nakamura K, et al. Potent and non-specific inhibition of cytochrome P450 by JM216, a new oral platinum agent. Br J Cancer 1998; 78:1170–1174.

85. Boisdron-Celle M, Craipeau C, Brienza S, et al. Influence of oxaliplatin on 5-fluorouracil plasma clearance and clinical consequences. Cancer Chemother Pharmacol 2002; 49:235–243.

86. Yoshisue K, Nagayama S, Shindo T, Kawaguchi Y. Effects of 5-fluorouracil on the drug-metabolizing enzymes of the small intestine and the consequent drug interaction with nifedipine in rats. J Pharmacol Exp Ther 2001; 297:1166–1175.

87. Kolesar J, Johnson C, Freeberg B, Berlin J, Schiller J. Warfarin-5-FU interaction: a series of consecutive case series. Pharmacotherapy 1999; 19:1445–1449.

88. Reigner B, Blesch K, Weidekamm E. Clinical pharmacokinetics of capecitabine. Clin Pharmacokinet 2001; 40:85–104.

89. Gilbar P, Brodribb T. Phenytoin and fluorouracil interaction. Ann Pharmacother 2001; 35:1367–1370.

90. LeBlanc GA, Sundseth SS, Weber GF, Waxman DJ. Platinum anticancer drugs modulate P-450 mRNA levels and differentially alter hepatic drug and steroid hormone metabolism in male and female rats. Cancer Res 1992; 52:540–547.

91. Chang TK, Waxman DJ. Cyclophosphamide modulates rat hepatic cytochrome P450 2C11 and steroid 5 alpha-reductase activity and messenger RNA levels through the combined action of acrolein and phosphoramide mustard. Cancer Res 1993; 53:2490–2497.

92. Morgan ET. Regulation of cytochrome p450 by inflammatory mediators: why and how? Drug Metab Dispos 2001; 29:207–212.

93. Rivory LP, Slaviero K, Clarke J. Hepatic cytochrome P450 3A drug metabolism is reduced in cancer patients who have an acute-phase response. Br J Cancer 2002; 87:277–280.

94. Hassan M, Nilsson C, Olsson H, Lundin J, Osterborg A. The influence of interferon-alpha on the pharmacokinetics of cyclophosphamide and its 4-hydroxy metabolite in patients with multiple myeloma. Eur J Haematol 1999; 63:163–170.

95. Danhauser LL, Freimann JH, Jr, Gilchrist TL, et al. Phase I and plasma pharmacokinetic study of infusional fluorouracil combined with recombinant interferon alfa-2b in patients with advanced cancer. J Clin Oncol 1993; 11:751–761.

96. Grem JL, McAtee N, Murphy RF, et al. A pilot study of gamma-1b-interferon in combination with fluorouracil, leucovorin, and alpha-2a-interferon. Clin Cancer Res 1997; 3:1125–1134.

97. Yee LK, Allegra CJ, Steinberg SM, Grem JL. Decreased catabolism of fluorouracil in peripheral blood mononuclear cells during combination therapy with fluorouracil, leucovorin, and interferon alpha-2a. J Natl Cancer Inst 1992; 84:1820–1825.

98. Kim J, Zhi J, Satoh H, et al. Pharmacokinetics of recombinant human interferon-alpha 2a combined with 5-fluorouracil in patients with advanced colorectal carcinoma. Anticancer Drugs 1998; 9:689–696.

99. Guengerich FP. Cytochrome P-450 3A4: regulation and role in drug metabolism. Annu Rev Pharmacol Toxicol 1999; 39:1–17.

100. Villikka K, Kivisto KT, Maenpaa H, Joensuu H, Neuvonen PJ. Cytochrome P450-inducing antiepileptics increase the clearance of vincristine in patients with brain tumors. Clin Pharmacol Ther 1999; 66:589–593.

101. Friedman HS, Petros WP, Friedman AH, et al. Irinotecan therapy in adults with recurrent or progressive malignant glioma. J Clin Oncol 1999; 17:1516–1525.

102. Baker DK, Relling MV, Pui CH, Christensen ML, Evans WE, Rodman JH. Increased teniposide clearance with concomitant anticonvulsant therapy. J Clin Oncol 1992; 10:311–315.

103. Zamboni WC, Gajjar AJ, Heideman RL, et al. Phenytoin alters the disposition of topotecan and N-desmethyl topotecan in a patient with medulloblastoma. Clin Cancer Res 1998; 4:783–789.

104. Anderson CD, Wang J, Kumar GN, McMillan JM, Walle UK, Walle T. Dexamethasone induction of taxol metabolism in the rat. Drug Metab Dispos 1995; 23:1286–1290.

105. Monsarrat B, Chatelut E, Royer I, et al. Modification of paclitaxel metabolism in a cancer patient by induction of cytochrome P450 3A4. Drug Metab Dispos 1998; 26:229–233.

106. Gerbal-Chaloin S, Pascussi JM, Pichard-Garcia L, et al. Induction of CYP2C genes in human hepato-cytes in primary culture. Drug Metab Dispos 2001; 29:242–251.
107. Chang TK, Yu L, Maurel P, Waxman DJ. Enhanced cyclophosphamide and ifosfamide activation in primary human hepatocyte cultures: response to cytochrome P-450 inducers and autoinduction by oxazaphosphorines. Cancer Res 1997; 57:1946–1954.
108. Riva M, Landonio G, Defanti CA, Siena S. The effect of anticonvulsant drugs on blood levels of methotrexate. J Neurooncol 2000; 48:249–250.
109. Lum BL, Kaubisch S, Yahanda AM, et al. Alteration of etoposide pharmacokinetics and pharmaco-dynamics by cyclosporine in a phase I trial to modulate multidrug resistance. J Clin Oncol 1992; 10: 1635–1642.
110. Aherne GW, Piall E, Marks V, Mould G, White WF. Prolongation and enhancement of serum meth-otrexate concentrations by probenecid. Br Med J 1978; 1:1097–1099.
111. Uwai Y, Saito H, Inui K. Interaction between methotrexate and nonsteroidal anti-inflammatory drugs in organic anion transporter. Eur J Pharmacol 2000; 409:31–36.
112. Ronchera CL, Hernandez T, Peris JE, et al. Pharmacokinetic interaction between high-dose methotr-exate and amoxicillin. Ther Drug Monit 1993; 15:375–379.
113. Blum R, Seymour JF, Toner G. Significant impairment of high-dose methotrexate clearance following vancomycin administration in the absence of overt renal impairment. Ann Oncol 2002; 13:327–330.
114. Dalle JH, Auvrignon A, Vassal G, Leverger G. Interaction between methotrexate and ciprofloxacin. J Pediatr Hematol Oncol 2002; 24:321–322.
115. Beorlegui B, Aldaz A, Ortega A, Aquerreta I, Sierrasesumega L, Giraldez J. Potential interaction between methotrexate and omeprazole. Ann Pharmacother 2000; 34:1024–1027.
116. Koren G, Beatty K, Seto A, Einarson TR, Lishner M. The effects of impaired liver function on the elimination of antineoplastic agents. Ann Pharmacother 1992; 26:363–371.
117. Donelli MG, Zucchetti M, Munzone E, D'Incalci M, Crosignani A. Pharmacokinetics of anticancer agents in patients with impaired liver function. Eur J Cancer 1998; 34:33–46.
118. Gianni L, Vigano L, Locatelli A, et al. Human pharmacokinetic characterization and in vitro study of the interaction between doxorubicin and paclitaxel in patients with breast cancer. J Clin Oncol 1997; 15:1906–1915.
119. Booth CL, Brouwer KR, Brouwer KL. Effect of multidrug resistance modulators on the hepatobiliary disposition of doxorubicin in the isolated perfused rat liver. Cancer Res 1998; 58:3641–3648.
120. Smit JW, Duin E, Steen H, Oosting R, Roggeveld J, Meijer DK. Interactions between P-glycoprotein substrates and other cationic drugs at the hepatic excretory level. Br J Pharmacol 1998; 123:361–370.
121. Schuetz EG, Beck WT, Schuetz JD. Modulators and substrates of P-glycoprotein and cytochrome P4503A coordinately up-regulate these proteins in human colon carcinoma cells. Mol Pharmacol 1996; 49:311–318.
122. Fuhr U, Weiss M, Kroemer HK, et al. Systematic screening for pharmacokinetic interactions during drug development. Int J Clin Pharmacol Ther 1996; 34:139–151.
123. Rodrigues AD, Winchell GA, Dobrinska MR. Use of in vitro drug metabolism data to evaluate meta-bolic drug–drug interactions in man: the need for quantitative databases. J Clin Pharmacol 2001; 41: 368–373.
124. Bonnabry P, Sievering J, Leemann T, Dayer P. Quantitative drug interactions prediction system (Q-DIPS): a dynamic computer-based method to assist in the choice of clinically relevant in vivo studies. Clin Pharmacokinet 2001; 40:631–640.
125. Rodrigues AD. Integrated cytochrome P450 reaction phenotyping: attempting to bridge the gap between cDNA-expressed cytochromes P450 and native human liver microsomes. Biochem Pharmacol 1999; 57:465–480.
126. Crespi CL, Stresser DM. Fluorometric screening for metabolism-based drug–drug interactions. J Pharmacol Toxicol Methods 2000; 44:325–331.
127. Stresser DM, Blanchard AP, Turner SD, et al. Substrate-dependent modulation of CYP3A4 catalytic activity: analysis of 27 test compounds with four fluorometric substrates. Drug Metab Dispos 2000; 28:1440–1448.
128. Crespi CL, Fox L, Stocker P, Hu M, Steimel DT. Analysis of drug transport and metabolism in cell monolayer systems that have been modified by cytochrome P4503A4 cDNA-expression. Eur J Phar-maceut Sci 2000; 12:63–68.
129. Baumhakel M, Kasel D, Rao-Schymanski RA, et al. Screening for inhibitory effects of antineoplastic agents on CYP3A4 in human liver microsomes. Int J Clin Pharmacol Ther 2001; 39:517–528.

130. Yule SM, Walker D, Cole M, et al. The effect of fluconazole on cyclophosphamide metabolism in children. Drug Metab Dispos 1999; 27:417–421.

131. Rodrigues AD, Lin JH. Screening of drug candidates for their drug–drug interaction potential. Curr Opin Chem Biol 2001; 5:396–401.

132. Bisogno G, Cowie F, Boddy A, Thomas HD, Dick G, Pinkerton CR. High-dose cyclosporin with etoposide—toxicity and pharmacokinetic interaction in children with solid tumours. Br J Cancer 1998; 77:2304–2309.

133. Murray LS, Jodrell DI, Morrison JG, et al. The effect of cimetidine on the pharmacokinetics of epirubicin in patients with advanced breast cancer: preliminary evidence of a potentially common drug interaction. Clin Oncol 1998; 10:35–38.

134. Kamataki T, Yokoi T, Fujita K, Ando Y. Preclinical approach for identifying drug interactions. Cancer Chemother Pharmacol 1998; 42(Suppl):S50–S53.

135. Lovless H, Arena E, Felsted RL, Bachur NR. Comparative mammalian metabolism of adriamycin and daunorubicin. Cancer Res 1978; 38:593–598.

136. Guengerich FP. Comparisons of catalytic selectivity of cytochrome P450 subfamily enzymes from different species. Chem Biol Interact 1997; 106:161–182.

137. Turesky RJ, Constable A, Fay LB, Guengerich FP. Interspecies differences in metabolism of heterocyclic aromatic amines by rat and human P450 1A2. Cancer Lett 1999; 143:109–112.

138. Boobis AR, Sesardic D, Murray BP, et al. Species variation in the response of the cytochrome P-450-dependent monooxygenase system to inducers and inhibitors. Xenobiotica 1990; 20:1139–1161.

139. Waxman DJ. P450 gene induction by structurally diverse xenochemicals: central role of nuclear receptors CAR, PXR, and PPAR. Arch Biochem Biophys 1999; 369:11–23.

140. Grasela TH, Jr, Antal EJ, Ereshefsky L, Wells BG, Evans RL, Smith RB. An evaluation of population pharmacokinetics in therapeutic trials. Part II. Detection of a drug–drug interaction. Clin Pharmacol Ther 1987; 42:433–441.

141. Bauer LA, Horn JR, Pettit H. Mixed-effect modeling for detection and evaluation of drug interactions: digoxin-quinidine and digoxin–verapamil combinations. Ther Drug Monit 1996; 18:46–52.

142. Millward MJ, Webster LK, Rischin D, et al. Phase I trial of Cremophor EL with bolus doxorubicin. Clin Cancer Res 1998; 4:2321–2329.

143. Badary OA, Abdel-Naim AB, Khalifa AE, Hamada FM. Differential alteration of cisplatin cytotoxicity and myelotoxicity by the paclitaxel vehicle cremophor EL. Naunyn Schmiedebergs Arch Pharmacol 2000; 361:339–344.

144. de Vos AI, Nooter K, Verweij J, et al. Differential modulation of cisplatin accumulation in leukocytes and tumor cell lines by the paclitaxel vehicle Cremophor EL. Ann Oncol 1997; 8:1145–1150.

145. Badary OA, Al-Shabanah OA, Al-Gharably NM, Elmazar MM. Effect of Cremophor EL on the pharmacokinetics, antitumor activity and toxicity of doxorubicin in mice. Anticancer Drugs 1998; 9: 809–815.

146. Webster LK, Cosson EJ, Stokes KH, Millward MJ. Effect of the paclitaxel vehicle, Cremophor EL, on the pharmacokinetics of doxorubicin and doxorubicinol in mice. Br J Cancer 1996; 73:522–524.

147. Holmes FA, Madden T, Newman RA, et al. Sequence-dependent alteration of doxorubicin pharmacokinetics by paclitaxel in a Phase I study of paclitaxel and doxorubicin in patients with metastatic breast cancer. J Clin Oncol 1996; 14:2713–2721.

148. Moreira A, Lobato R, Morais J, et al. Influence of the interval between the administration of doxorubicin and paclitaxel on the pharmacokinetics of these drugs in patients with locally advanced breast cancer. Cancer Chemother Pharmacol 2001; 48:333–337.

149. Ellis AG, Webster LK. Inhibition of paclitaxel elimination in the isolated perfused rat liver by Cremophor EL. Cancer Chemother Pharmacol 1999; 43:13–18.

150. Cummings J, Forrest GJ, Cunningham D, Gilchrist NL, Soukop M. Influence of polysorbate 80 (Tween 80) and etoposide (VP-16-213) on the pharmacokinetics and urinary excretion of adriamycin and its metabolites in cancer patients. Cancer Chemother Pharmacol 1986; 17:80–84.

151. Paal K, Horvath J, Csaki C, Ferencz T, Schuler D, Borsi JD. Effect of etoposide on the pharmacokinetics of methotrexate in vivo. Anticancer Drugs 1998; 9:765–772.

152. Mayer LD, Reamer J, Bally MB. Intravenous pretreatment with empty pH gradient liposomes alters the pharmacokinetics and toxicity of doxorubicin through in vivo active drug encapsulation. J Pharmaceut Sci 1999; 88:96–102.

153. Waterhouse DN, Dos Santos N, Mayer LD, Bally MB. Drug-drug interactions arising from the use of liposomal vincristine in combination with other anticancer drugs. Pharmaceut Res 2001; 18:1331–1335.

154. Hudes GR, LaCreta F, Walczak J, et al. Pharmacokinetic study of trimetrexate in combination with cisplatin. Cancer Res 1991; 51:3080–3087.
155. Thodtmann R, Depenbrock H, Dumez H, et al. Clinical and pharmacokinetic phase I study of multitargeted antifolate (LY231514) in combination with cisplatin. J Clin Oncol 1999; 17:3009–3016.
156. Kaye SB, McWhinnie D, Hart A, et al. The treatment of advanced bladder cancer with methotrexate and cis-platinum—a pharmacokinetic study. Eur J Cancer Clin Oncol 1984; 20:249–252.
157. Gilbert CJ, Petros WP, Vredenburgh J, et al. Pharmacokinetic interaction between ondansetron and cyclophosphamide during high-dose chemotherapy for breast cancer. Cancer Chemother Pharmacol 1998; 42:497–503.
158. Cagnoni PJ, Matthes S, Day T, Bearman SI, Shpall EJ, Jones RB. Modification of the pharmacokinetics of high-dose cyclophosphamide and cisplatin by antiemetics. Bone Marrow Transplant 1999; 24:1–4.
159. Schrijvers D, Pronk L, Highley M, et al. Pharmacokinetics of ifosfamide are changed by combination with docetaxel: results of a phase I pharmacologic study. Am J Clin Oncol 2000; 23:358–363.
160. Schilsky RL, Levin J, West WH, et al. Randomized, open-label, phase III study of a 28-day oral regimen of eniluracil plus fluorouracil versus intravenous fluorouracil plus leucovorin as first-line therapy in patients with metastatic/advanced colorectal cancer. J Clin Oncol 2002; 20:1519–1526.
161. Hustert E, Zibat A, Presecan-Siedel E, et al. Natural protein variants of pregnane X receptor with altered transactivation activity toward CYP3A4. Drug Metab Disp 2001; 29:1454–1459.
162. Rivory LP, Slaviero KA, Hoskins JM, Clarke SJ. The erythromycin breath test for the prediction of drug clearance. Clin Pharmacokinet 2001; 40:151–158.

17 ABC Transporters
Involvement in Multidrug Resistance and Drug Disposition

Susan E. Bates, MD and Tito Fojo, MD

1. INTRODUCTION

Drug resistance can occur at several levels and is ultimately the cause of treatment failure in oncology. Cellular resistance has been the most widely studied, although host factors and host–tumor interactions may also play critical roles. Cellular resistance mediated by a reduced accumulation of chemotherapy can be due to the expression of drug transporters in tumor cells. The ATP-binding cassette (ABC) transporters, the largest transporter family, are found in a wide range of normal tissues and transport a wide range of substrates important in normal physiology. The normal tissue function of these transporters may be protection from toxic compounds such as xenobiotics. Because chemotherapeutic drugs have been found to be substrates for several of these transporters, some are referred to as multidrug transporters. This chapter reviews the role of these multidrug transporters in oncology and in normal tissues.

2. MECHANISMS OF DRUG RESISTANCE

2.1. Cellular Mechanisms of Drug Resistance

Multiple cellular mechanisms of drug resistance have been described, and a schematic for these is shown in Fig. 1. These can be classified as those that (1) affect drug accumulation through reduced uptake or enhanced efflux; (2) impact drug metabolism as a result of decreased activation or increased inactivation; (3) alter the molecular target either by reduc-

Handbook of Anticancer Pharmacokinetics and Pharmacodynamics
Edited by: W. D. Figg and H. L. McLeod © Humana Press Inc., Totowa, NJ

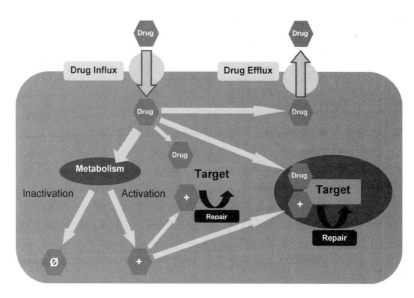

Fig. 1. Schematic showing levels of cellular mechanisms of drug resistance: reduced accumulation through reduced drug influx or increased drug efflux; altered drug metabolism including both decreased activation and increased inactivation; altered drug target through mutation or changed expression level; altered repair through enhanced damage repair pathways or enhanced survival pathways. Most cellular mechanisms of drug resistance can be classified according to this schema.

ing expression or altering affinity; (4) increase repair of drug-induced damage; and (5) support cell survival following drug exposure, allowing time for repair and /or adjustments to be made. Anticancer agents may be subject to one or all of these mechanisms of resistance. Doxorubicin is an illustrative example: (1) drug accumulation may be reduced by the multidrug resistance 1 (MDR1)/P-glycoprotein (P-gp) multidrug transporter; (2) glucuronidation may inactivate the drug once inside the cell; (3) its molecular target, topoisomerase IIα, may be reduced to levels that impair drug activity, or may be rendered insensitive by an acquired mutation; and (4) p53-mediated G1 arrest or bcl2 overexpression may promote cell survival by inhibiting apoptosis. Recognizing that a focus on one mechanism of resistance may be misleading, most investigators have found that defining any one component of resistance is sufficiently daunting to warrant no greater range of investigation.

2.2. ABC Transporters

ABC transporters are the largest transporter family. Comprised of similar structures, a functional ABC transporter is thought to contain two transmembrane and two ATP-binding domains (1). The latter bind and hydrolyze ATP, and the derived energy is used for transport of the substrate across the cell membrane. The ATP binding domains are highly conserved across the ABC superfamily, and characteristic sequences known as the Walker A, Walker B, and C signature regions are critical for ATP binding and hydrolysis. Conservation of these regions is such that ABC transporters can be identified by homology searches in genetic databases. With completion of the sequencing of the human genome, it appears that there are 48 human ABC transporters. Using clustering tools, ABC genes can be grouped into seven subfamilies, designated *ABCA* through *ABCG*. To date, this classification based on homology appears to allow only modest predictions about function. Table 1 *(1–4)* lists the seven ABC subfamilies and known members of each, with currently understood functions.

Table 1
Human ABC Transporters

HUGO name[a]	Common name	Disease associated with absence or mutation	Function
ABCA1	ABC1	Tangier disease	Cholesterol efflux onto HDL
ABCA2	ABC2		
ABCA3	ABC3, ABCC		
ABCA4	ABCR	Stargardt disease, retinitis pigmentosum, cone-rod dystrophy	N-Retinylidiene-PE efflux
ABCA5			
ABCA6			
ABCA7			
ABCA8			
ABCA9			
ABCA10			
ABCA12			
ABCA13			
ABCB1	MDR1	Xenobiotic protection	
ABCB2	TAP1	Immune deficiency	Peptide transport
ABCB3	TAP2	Immune deficiency	Peptide transport
ABCB4	MDR2, MDR3	Progressive familial intrahepatic cholestasis type 3	Phosphatidylcholine transport
ABCB5			
ABCB6	MTABC3		
ABCB7	ABC7	X-linked sideroblastic anemia and ataxia	
ABCB8	MABC1		
ABCB9			
ABCB10	MTABC2		
ABCB11	SPgp, BSEP	Progressive familial intrahepatic cholestasis type 2	Bile salts
ABCC1	MRP1		Xenobiotic protection
ABCC2	MRP2, CMOAT	Dubin–Johnson syndrome	Bilirubin-glucuronide
ABCC3	MRP3		
ABCC4	MRP4		
ABCC5	MRP5		
ABCC6	MRP6	Pseudoxanthoma elasticum	
CFTR	CFTR	Cystic fibrosis	Choride ion channel
ABCC8	SUR	Familial hyperinsulinemic hypoglycemia of infancy	Regulation of insulin secretion
ABCC9	SUR2		
ABCC10	MRP7		
ABCC11	MRP8		
ABCC12	MRP9		
ABCD1	ALD	X-linked adrenoleukodystrophy	Regulation of VLCFA transport
ABCD2	ALDL1, ALDR		
ABCD3	PXMP1, PMP70		
ABCD4	PMP69, P70R		
ABCE1	OABP, RNS4I		
ABCF1	ABC50		
ABCF2			
ABCF3			
ABCG1	ABC8, White		
ABCG2	MXR, ABCP, BCRP		Xenobiotic protection
ABCG4	White2		
ABCG5	White3	Sitosterolemia	Plant sterols
ABCG8		Sitosterolemia	Plant sterols

VLCFA, Very long chain fatty acids.

[a]Adapted from Dean et al. *(1,4)*, Gottesman et al. *(2)*, and Klein et al. *(3)*.

Table 2
Chemotherapy Substrate Specificities of ABC Transporters

HUGO name[a]	ABCA2	ABCB1	ABCB4	ABCB11	ABCC1	ABCC2	ABCC3	ABCC4	ABCC5	ABCC6	ABCC10	ABCC11	ABCC12	ABCG2
Common name	ABC2	MDR1	MDR2 MDR3	SPgp BSEP	MRP1	MRP2 cMOAT	MRP3	MRP4	MRP5	MRP6	MRP7	MRP8	MRP9	BCRP MXR ABCP
Adriamycin		+			+	+								
Paclitaxel		+	+	+										
Vinblastine		+												
Vincristine		+			+	+								
Etoposide		+			+	+	+							
Cisplatin						+								
Organic Anions					+	+	+	+	+	+				
Methotrexate					+	+	+	+	+	+				
17β-E2G					+	+	+	+		+				
6-Mercaptopurine								+	+					
6-Thioguanine								+	+					
Topotecan		+												+
SN-38						+								+
Mitoxantrone		+												+
Estramustine	+													

17β-E2G, 17β-Estradiol glucuronide; SN38, active metabolite of irinotecan.
[a]Adapted from Gottesman et al. (2), Borst et al. (5), and Kruh et al. (6). MRP 7–9 not yet characterized.

270

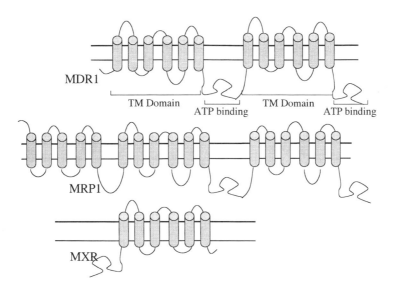

Fig. 2. Schematic drawing of three ABC transporters involved in drug resistance. ABC transporters are organized into domains: the ATP-binding domain includes the Walker A and B regions together with the C signature region, which is unique to the ABC transporter superfamily. The transmembrane (TM) domains are comprised typically of six transmembrane segments. A fully functional transporter is classically considered to include two transmembrane domains and two ATP binding domains. MRP1 also contains the five-segment TMD_0 region, 5' to the MDR1-like core. TMD_0 is thought to confer the anionic transport capacity of MRP1. ABCG2 is a half-size ABC transporter, and is thought to dimerize in order to function. Note the reverse orientation, with the ATP binding domain 5' to the transmembrane segments. It is not known what significance this orientation has.

2.3. Multidrug Transporters

Although 48 ABC transporters have been definitely identified, a more limited number are thought to transport anticancer compounds and to have a potential role in multidrug resistance (Table 2) *(2,5,6)*. These include Pgp, MRP1–5, bile salt exporter protein (BSEP) (sPgp), ABCA2, and ABCG2. Their investigation has the ultimate goal of developing clinical therapies that evade or inhibit transporter-mediated resistance.

3. P-GLYCOPROTEIN

3.1. Background

The most intensively studied multidrug transporter is Pgp, the product of the *MDR1* gene. Pgp has the characteristic "full transporter" structure with two ATP binding domains and two transmembrane domains each comprised of six transmembrane segments that confer substrate specificity (Fig. 2). Pgp is known to transport commonly used cancer chemotherapeutic agents including anthracyclines such as daunorubicin and doxorubicin, taxanes, vinca alkaloids, and podophyllotoxins (Table 2). However, work with the National Cancer Institute (NCI) drug screen suggested there were hundreds, if not thousands, of Pgp substrates *(7)*. This is perhaps not surprising given the presumed role of Pgp in normal physiology: protection of normal tissues and the organism as a whole from exposure to xenobiotics.

Table 3
Pgp Substrates and Inhibitors in Clinical Use or Development in Oncology

	Pgp Inhibitors		
Pgp substrates	First-generation agents	Second-generation agents	Third-generation agents
Doxuribicin	Verapamil	R-Verapamil	GF120918
Daunorubicin	Quinidine	PSC833	R101933
Epirubicin	Quinine	Dexniguldipine	XR9576
Paclitaxel	Amiodarone	VX710	LY335979
Taxotere	Nifedipine		OC144-093
Pgp substrates	Cyclosporine A		
Vincristine			
Vinblastine			
VP-16			
Mitoxantrone			
Bisantrene			
Homoharringtonine			
Actinomycin D			

3.2. The Physiologic Role of Pgp

A protective role for Pgp has received support from several sources. First, the substrate profile encompasses a wide array of structurally unrelated natural products, or xenobiotics, naturally occurring toxins. This broad substrate profile would be expected for a protein designed to perform a protective function. Second, the distribution of Pgp suggests a protective role. High levels of Pgp expression are found in the gastrointestinal tract, the kidney, and the liver, three organs involved in the elimination of toxins from the body. High levels are also found in the adrenal cortex, where Pgp is thought to protect the adrenal cell membrane from the toxic effects of glucocorticoids. High levels are also found in the capillary endothelium of the brain and the testis, where Pgp is thought to have a role in the blood–brain and blood–testis barriers (8–10). Finally, high levels are also found on the apical surface of the epithelial cells of the choroid plexus, suggesting Pgp may prevent movement of compounds out of the cerebrospinal fluid (CSF) (11). Third, knockout studies in mice support a protective role for Pgp. Early studies showed that mice have two mdr1 genes, designated mdr1a and mdr1b. When mice lacking both of these murine homologs were initially bred, neither survival to adulthood nor reproduction was affected, suggesting no critical function for Pgp. However, death occurred unexpectedly when these mice were exposed to the neurotoxic pesticide ivermectin, which is routinely used to protect mice from mite infestation (12). Pharmacokinetic studies demonstrated an 87-fold increase in ivermectin levels in the brain with a 3.3-fold increase in plasma levels in the knockout mouse. This study confirmed the suspicion that the main role of Pgp was protection of the organism from toxic compounds. As shown in Table 3, further studies in knockout mice have shown altered blood and brain accumulation of numerous compounds, including vinblastine, colchicine, dexamethasone, cortisone, quinidine, morphine, and digoxin (13,15–24).

These studies in mice lacking the MDR1 homologs have provided pharmacokinetic information not otherwise attainable in humans. The experiments cannot be replicated in humans, and the extent to which the findings in the murine model can be extrapolated to humans remains unclear. For example, drug accumulation in the brain of mdr-deficient mice is 35-, 29-, 22-, and 17-fold higher for digoxin, quinidine, vinblastine, and cyclosporin A, respectively. If these differences were predictive of alterations occurring in patients treated with Pgp inhibitors, it is surprising that Pgp antagonists have not induced some symptoms in patients receiving concurrent Pgp substrates. Yet, apart from a reversible ataxia observed with the Pgp antagonists PSC 833 and tamoxifen, central nervous system (CNS) toxicities have not been observed in clinical trials with Pgp inhibitors.

In accordance with a protective role for Pgp, several studies have shown that Pgp limits the absorption of its substrates from the gastrointestinal tract, presumably by pumping them back into the intestinal lumen. Support for this observation includes studies with Pgp inhibitors administered either orally or intravenously (discussed in more detail below) that have shown increased bioavailability of orally administered Pgp substrates by coadministration of a Pgp inhibitor. For example, oral absorption of paclitaxel was increased eightfold when administered concurrently with cyclosporin A *(25)*. Similarly, oral bioavailability of paclitaxel, calculated at 30% ± 15% when the drug was administered alone, was increased to 50% in patients when administered in combination with GF120918 *(26)*. In animal models, similar increases have also been reported for paclitaxel in combination with PSC 833, OC144-093, and MS-209 *(27–29)*. Thus, independent of the efficacy of Pgp inhibitors to alter drug resistance in cancer cells, a role in modulating the oral bioavailability of anticancer agent would be an important contribution to the treatment of cancer patients. Anticancer agents available as oral formulations are widely accepted by patients, and in many cases a preferable alternative to parenteral administration

3.3. Pgp in Multidrug Resistance

The role of Pgp in conferring multidrug resistance has been addressed in numerous preclinical and clinical studies. Pgp expression has been found in numerous tumor types, with high levels of expression reported in renal, gastrointestinal, adrenocortical, hepatocellular, and pancreatic cancer *(30)*. Lower levels that increase with treatment have been observed in breast cancer, ovarian cancer, leukemia, lymphoma, lung cancer, and sarcoma *(31)*. The most consistent data have been reported in acute myelogenous leukemia (AML), where expression is observed in 30–50% of newly diagnosed cases. Pgp expression has been detected either using antibodies or by performing functional studies to examine daunorubicin accumulation. However, unlike the results in AML, the level of expression reported in the literature for many tumors can vary enormously. For example, a meta-analysis concluded that 40% of breast cancers express Pgp but the studies included in the analysis reported expression levels ranging from 0 to 80% *(32)*. To be sure, the patient population studied may explain some of the variability as evidenced by a report examining Pgp expression in breast cancer pre- and post-therapy *(33)*. In this study, Pgp expression was documented in 11% of pretherapy and 30% of posttreatment samples, suggesting a role for Pgp in the development of drug resistance in breast cancer.

3.4. First-Generation Pgp Inhibitors

With the description by Tsuruo in 1981 of the ability of verapamil to inhibit Pgp-mediated drug efflux, the reversal of drug resistance became a tantalizing possibility *(34)*; and verapamil became the beginning of a series of inhibitors to be tested in patients (Table 4). The identification of verapamil was all the more provocative because it was a compound already in clinical use. It meant that clinical trials could be launched without the need to perform time-consuming trials establishing the safety of a Pgp inhibitor. Soon thereafter, additional agents were identified as inhibitors of Pgp-mediated efflux, and like verapamil, these were already available for use in clinical trials. These first-generation agents were rapidly tested as inhibitors of Pgp in numerous clinical trials, but the outcome of these studies was disappointing and inconclusive. A common problem encountered was clinical toxicity of the inhibitor as investigators attempted to achieve serum concentrations comparable to those used in the in vitro model systems. For example, because of the occurrence of hypoten-

Table 4
Increased Drug Levels in MDR-Deficient ($mdr1a^{-/-}$ or $1a/1b^{-/-}$) Mice

Drug	T	Deleted	Plasma	Liver	Kidney	Lung	Testis	Brain	Reference
Ivermectin	4.0 h	$1a^{-/-}$	3.3	3.8	3.0	4.0	n.a.	87.0	(12)
Cyclosporin A	4.0 h	$1a^{-/-}$	1.4	1.2	1.0	1.2	2.6	17.0	(13)
Digoxin	4.0 h	$1a^{-/-}$	1.9	2.0	1.9	2.2	2.8	35.3	(13)
Morphine	4.0 h	$1a^{-/-}$	1.1	1.1	0.8	1.1	0.7	1.7	(13)
	4.0 h	$1a^{-/-}$	1.2	n.a.	n.a.	n.a.	n.a.	2.6	(14)
Dexamethasone	4.0 h	$1a^{-/-}$	1.0	1.1	1.2	0.8	1.2	2.5	(13)
	1.0 h	$1a^{-/-}$	1.2	1.1	n.a.	n.a.	n.a.	4.2	(15)
Vinblastine	4.0 h	$1a^{-/-}$	1.7	2.4	2.3	2.1	2.5	22.4	(16)
Loperamide	4.0 h	$1a^{-/-}$	2.0	3.1	1.5	1.7	3.8	13.5	(17)
Ondansetron	0.5 h	$1a^{-/-}$	1.0	0.9	0.9	1.1	1.9	4.0	(17)
Verapamil	1.0 h	$1a^{-/-}$	1.2	1.1	1.2	0.9	3.4	9.5	(18)
Doxorubicin	4.0 h	$1a^{-/-}$	0.9	4.5	1.0	1.0	n.a.	2.8	(19)
Quinidine	4.0 h	$1a^{-/-}$	3.7	4.3	2.5	2.7	n.a.	29.2	(20)
Nelfinavir	2.0 h	$1a^{-/-}$	1.1	n.a.	n.a.	n.a.	4.1	27.9	(21)
Corticosterone	1.0 h	$1a^{-/-}$	0.9	1.0	n.a.	n.a.	1.1	1.3	(22)
Cortisol	1.0 h	$1a^{-/-}$	1.0	1.0	n.a.	n.a.	1.1	3.9	(22)
Sparfloxacin	4.0 h	$1a^{-/-}$	0.97	n.a.	n.a.	n.a.	n.a.	3.2	(23)
Grepafloxacin	1.0 h	$1a/1b^{-/-}$	1.1	1.0	1.4	1.0	0.62	2.8	(24)

n.a., not available.

sion, management in the intensive care unit was required to achieve verapamil serum levels of 1 μM (35). However, these first generation trials did suggest that Pgp inhibitors could be safely administered with anticancer agents.

Recent studies allow a more accurate retrospective analysis of the results of these first-generation trials. Abraham et al. reported results of a trial in adrenocortical cancer using the first-generation inhibitor mitotane (36). Rhodamine efflux from circulating CD56+ cells expressing high levels of Pgp, an established surrogate used in clinical trails, failed to demonstrate inhibition of Pgp in patients with steady-state mitotane levels exceeding 10 μg/mL, a level that could readily block Pgp in vitro. Similarly, Cisternino could not demonstrate increased brain uptake of vinblastine in mice following brain perfusion with 1–2 μM verapamil, although vinblastine accumulation was increased 2.7-fold in $mdr1a^{-/-}$ mice and threefold in PSC 833- or GF120918-treated mice (37). Admittedly, this last assay may have been relatively insensitive, as a previous study had demonstrated that following intravenous administration, the level of vinblastine accumulation in the brain of $mdr1a^{-/-}$ mice is 22-fold that in normal mice (Table 3) (16). However, these and other studies suggest first generation antagonists were at best only able to marginally inhibit Pgp in vivo.

3.5. Second-Generation Pgp Inhibitors

A group of second-generation antagonists were then developed with the hope of achieving increased potency to inhibit Pgp. One of these, PSC 833, an analog of cyclosporine, was widely tested in Phase I clinical trials but required reductions of the dosage of the anticancer agents to avoid excessive toxicity. For some anticancer agents, a reduction of as much as 66% in dosage was needed to avoid toxicity when PSC 833 was coadministered. Dose reductions required in a series of clinical trials with PSC 833 are summarized in Table 5 (38–61). VX710, another second-generation agent, was also found to reduce the clearance of anticancer agents, requiring a dose reduction of 54% for paclitaxel.

Table 5
Clinical Trials with Second- and Third-Generation Pgp Inhibitors

	n	Drug regimen	% Dose reduction required for Pgp substrate drugs[a]	Author/year	Reference
PSC 833 Phase I trials	34	Etoposide (75 mg/m²)	25	Boote1996	(38)
	38	Doxorubicin (35 mg/m²)[b]	30	Giaccone 1997	(39)
	31	Doxorubicin (40 mg/m²)[b]	20	Minami 2001	(40)
	16	Paclitaxel, 3 h (122.5 mg/m²)[b]	30	Fracasso 2000	(41)
	41	Paclitaxel, 96 h (17.5 mg/m²/d)	50	Chico 2001	(42)
	79	Vinblastine, 120 h (0.6 mg/m²/d)	50–66	Bates 2001	[43]
	22	Vincristine (0.3 mg)/doxorubicin (6.75 mg/m²)/dexamethasone	25/25	Sonneveld 1996	(44)
	58	Paclitaxel (67.5–81 mg/m²)/carboplatin	50–60	Patnaik 2000	(45)
	33	Doxorubicin (20 mg/m²)/paclitaxel (90 mg/m²)	42/40	Advani 2001	(46)
	58	Paclitaxel, 3 h (70 mg/m²)[b]	60	Fracasso 2001	(47)
	33	Doxorubicin (35 mg/m²)/cisplatin	30	Baekelandt 2001	(48)
	10	Mitoxantrone (2.5 mg/m²)/etoposide (170 mg/m²)	66/66	Kornblau 1997	(49)
	37	Mitoxantrone (4 mg/m²)/etoposide (40 mg/m²)/Ara-C	44/58	Advani 1999	(50)
	66	Daunorubicin (40 mg/m²)/etoposide (60 mg/m²)/Ara-C	33/45	Lee 1999	(51)
	30	Mitoxantrone (6 mg/m²)/etoposide (60 mg/m²)	40/40	Chauncey 2000	(52)
	43	Daunorubicin/Ara-C	None	Dorr 2001	(53)
	23	Mitoxantrone/VP-16/Ara-C	25/62.5	Visani 2001	(54)
Phase III trials	762	Paclitaxel (80 mg/m²)/carboplatin/PSC 833	54	Joly 2002	(55)
		Paclitaxel (175 mg/m²)/carboplatin			
	59	Daunorubicin/VP-16/Ara-C/PSC 833	33/40	Baer 2002	(52)
	61	Daunorubicin/VP-16/Ara-C			
VX-710 Phase I trials	25	Paclitaxel, 3 h (60–80 mg/m²)[b]	54–66	Rowinsky 1998	(57)
	25	Doxorubicin (45 mg/m²)[b]	10	Peck 2001	(58)
Phase II trials	37	Paclitaxel, 3 h (80 mg/m²)[b]	54	Toppmeyer 2002	(59)
	29	Doxorubicin (60 mg/m²)	none	Bramwell 2002	(60)
	50	Paclitaxel, 3 h (80 mg/m²)[b]	54	Seiden 2002	(61)

Drugs separated by the slash mark, /, correspond to dose reductions separated by slash mark for the Pgp substrate drugs only.

[a] Dose reduction at the MTD in the presence of the Pgp inhibitor, compared to MTD in the absence of the Pgp inhibitor.

[b] Dose reductions relative to doxorubicin, based on 50 mg/m² q 3 wk as standard dose; and for paclitaxel, 175 mg/m² as standard dose.

The mechanism underlying this reduction in drug clearance is likely multifactorial, but has been primarily attributed to interactions with cytochrome P450. For example, in vitro studies have shown that PSC 833 is an inhibitor of cytochrome 3A4. Although an assessment of the contribution of Pgp inhibition to the pharmacokinetic effect that necessitated dose reductions has to be inferred, many investigators believe Pgp inhibition was not a critical contributor. Support for this conclusion includes data from murine knockouts showing at most a twofold increase in plasma concentrations of vinblastine and from studies with third-generation inhibitors that do not interact with P450 and have a much reduced impact on the clearance of the anticancer agents tested. A third mechanism underlying the reduction in drug clearance seen with PSC 833 may have been a decrease in biliary clearance. Drug clearance is determined in part by biliary flow, which in turn is influenced by the transport of bile salts through the ABC transporter BSEP (bile salt exporter protein) (62,63). Initially termed "sister of Pgp" owing to its high homology with Pgp, BSEP is a member of the ABCB subfamily and has been shown to transport taurocholate along with other bile salts (64). Cyclosporine A and PSC 833 have been shown to inhibit taurocholate transport, and in animal models PSC833 has been shown to reduce bile flow (65,66). Thus, it is likely that bile flow was impacted in patients receiving PSC 833, and this in turn may have impacted drug clearance. Certainly, bilirubin elevations were commonly seen with PSC 833 administration.

In animal studies, the delay in drug clearance resulted in both an increase in peak concentrations and a prolonged half-life. It was hoped that in patients the reduction in anticancer drug doses in combination with the inhibitor would result in AUCs for the anticancer agent under study that were comparable to those archieved without the inhibitor. Initially this appeared to be true. However, significant interpatient variation was observed, most likely due to differences in P450 expression. This would not be surprising given the variability demonstrated using indices of P450 activity, such as the erythromycin breath test and midazolam clearance (67). For example, as much as a 10-fold variation in midazolam pharmacokinetics ascribed to differences in P450 has been reported, and this could account for the interpatient variability in the impact of PSC 833 on drug clearance (68). In our study combining PSC 833 with paclitaxel, this interpatient variability was striking. The calculated mean AUCs for paclitaxel were comparable with and without PSC 833. However, if individual changes in AUCs were examined at the maximum tolerated dose of the combination, it became evident that reduction in anticancer drug dose resulted in striking interpatient variability. One third of patients had no major change in AUC, one third of patients had a reduction in AUC, and one third of patients had a marked increase in AUC. This finding echoed that of Dorr et al., who reported a trial combining PSC 833 with daunomycin and Ara-C for AML. According to these authors, had dose reductions been incorporated into the trial design, one third of patients would have been undertreated (53).

Concurrent with and most likely related to the problematic dose reductions summarized in Table 5 were the poor response rates in the reported trials (39–61). Although no one expected high response rates in these Phase I trials, it was hoped that some evidence of drug resistance reversal would be observed with these second-generation agents. If first generation agents failed because toxicity prevented the administration of doses sufficient to overcome drug resistance, this was certainly not the problem for PSC 833 or VX-710. Both compounds were shown to overcome Pgp in patients using surrogate studies that were developed to reflect Pgp inhibition. Yet, response rates in the Phase I studies were no better than expected for the given drugs and disease types studied. Several of the AML trials were performed in newly diagnosed, high-risk or elderly patients, and complete response rates seldom exceeded 50%.

Despite these disappointing results, several reports suggest this strategy should be explored further. Randomized studies, which offer the most rigorous test of Pgp inhibition, have in several cases suggested a survival advantage for patients receiving the inhibitor. Long-term results of a recently published trial in AML suggest an overall survival advantage when cyclosporine A is added to a standard daunorubicin and ara-C regimen *(69)*. In this trial, there was no difference in complete response rates (33% vs 39% for the combination), but a statistically significant difference in resistant disease (47% vs 31%), 2-yr relapse-free survival (9% vs 34%), and overall survival (12% vs 22%). One interpretation of the unchanged complete response rate is that the majority of cells at the initiation of treatment are drug sensitive. Thus, instead of increasing the initial response rate, Pgp inhibition may be more effective in preventing the survival and eventual emergence of resistant clones that will ultimately impact response duration. Although the result of this trial is promising, it must be recognized that it used cyclosporine A as the Pgp inhibitor, a compound that is not without its own separate activities. Therefore, final conclusions regarding this trial await its confirmation with one or more of the highly specific third-generation Pgp antagonists.

Two additional reports describing randomized trials with PSC 833 are available, one in abstract form. In the first of these, PSC 833 plus paclitaxel and carboplatin showed no improvement over paclitaxel and carboplatin alone in ovarian cancer *(55)*. However, the paclitaxel dose was reduced from 175 mg/m^2 to 80 mg/m^2, a 54% dose reduction. Because the low overall prevalence of Pgp in ovarian cancer also may have undermined the results, it could be argued that a subset of patients with this disease may yet benefit from addition of a Pgp inhibitor. The second randomized trial, in AML, closed early because of toxicity in the PSC 833 arm. However, subset analysis suggested a potential benefit with the combination in patients whose leukemic cells displayed PSC 833-inhibitable drug efflux, consistent with the presence of Pgp.

3.6. Third-Generation Pgp Inhibitors

Third-generation agents have entered clinical trials. These agents are thought to have little impact on drug clearance, have no significant P450 interactions, and should require minimal or no reductions in the dose of the anticancer agent. Structures for four third-generation agents currently in clinical development are shown in Figure 3. Animal studies showed no effect on drug clearance when OC144-093 was administered concurrently with paclitaxel *(70)*. R101933 was shown to have no effect on docetaxel plasma levels in patients *(71)*. Dose reductions were not required for XR9576 in combination with doxorubicin, paclitaxel, and vinorelbine, although conservative doses were selected for the trials: 50 mg/m^2 of doxorubicin, 135 mg/m^2 of paclitaxel, and 20–22.5 mg/m^2 vinorelbine (unpublished observations). XR9576 has been shown to be effective in preventing the efflux of ^{99m}Tc-sestamibi from Pgp-bearing tumors and tissues, as shown in Fig. 4, and discussed further below. A single 150-mg dose inhibits efflux from CD56$^+$ circulating cells for 48–72 h without readministration. Lacking significant toxicities, this agent will be of value in combination with Pgp substrates in clinical trials testing Pgp inhibition.

3.7. Surrogate Endpoints

One major accomplishment derived from the conduct of the second-generation Pgp inhibitor trials was the development of surrogate studies to confirm inhibition of Pgp in patients. Two surrogate assays were developed: (1) the CD56$^+$ rhodamine assay and (2) the ^{99m}Tc-sestamibi scan. The rhodamine efflux assay takes advantage of the expression of Pgp in circulating CD56$^+$ mononuclear cells. These cells have naturally high levels of

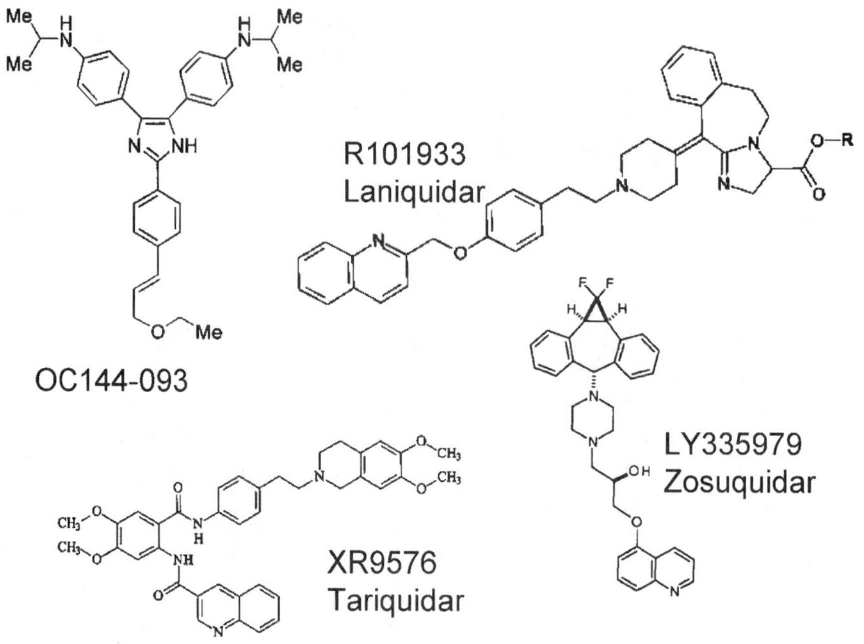

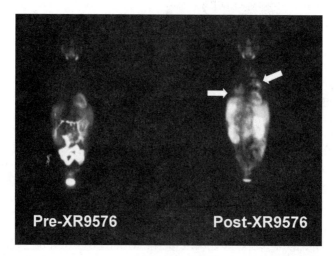

R101933
Laniquidar

OC144-093

XR9576
Tariquidar

LY335979
Zosuquidar

Fig. 3. Structures of newer Pgp inhibitors.

Pre-XR9576   Post-XR9576

Fig. 4. ^{99m}Tc-Sestamibi imaging of Pgp inhibition. The cardiac imaging agent Sestamibi has been shown to be a Pgp substrate and has been used to indicate Pgp inhibition. In this figure, images were obtained before (left) and after (right) administration of the Pgp inhibitor tariquidar (XR9576) to a patient with adrenocortical cancer enrolled on a clinical trial combining tariquidar with vinorelbine. In the image on the left, Sestamibi accumulation is observed in the gastrointestinal tract and in the bladder following excretion from the liver and kidney. In the image on the right, Sestamibi accumulation is observed in pulmonary metastases (arrows), in metastases in the retroperitoneum, in the liver, and in the kidneys. The retention in normal tissues indicates that Sestamibi can be used as a marker of Pgp inhibition, while retention in tumor tissue indicates that Sestamibi can be used as a diagnostic assay for Pgp function.

Pgp and rapidly efflux rhodamine, a fluorescent Pgp substrate, when a 1-h accumulation period in rhodamine is followed by a 30-min efflux period without rhodamine. The fluorescence of rhodamine in the $CD56^+$ cells can be detected by flow cytometry. When administered to patients, the second-generation inhibitor PSC 833 revealed excellent inhibition of efflux from $CD56^+$ cells (72,73). The second strategy used to confirm Pgp inhibition was ^{99m}Tc-sestamibi imaging. Shown by Pinwica-Worms et al. to be a Pgp substrate, ^{99m}Tc-sestamibi has long been used in cardiac imaging (74), and was thus easily adapted to imaging tumors and tissues for Pgp inhibition. As shown in Fig. 4, the liver and kidneys are not well visualized in scans obtained prior to the administration of the Pgp inhibitor. However, following the administration of XR9576, a third-generation inhibitor administered to the patient in this image, both the liver and the kidney retain ^{99m}Tc-sestamibi. This confirms the inhibition of Pgp in these normal tissues.

4. THE MRP FAMILY OF DRUG TRANSPORTERS

4.1. Background

As already noted, several explanations have been advanced for the failure of clinical trials attempting to modulate Pgp. For the first-generation agents, insufficient concentrations or potency of the inhibitor can explain the failure. For the second-generation agents, pharmacokinetic interactions required lowering of the anticancer drug dose, most likely compromising efficacy in a subset of patients. Apart from these concerns, the presence of other resistance mechanisms, particularly other drug transporters, may have confounded results of clinical trials. As noted above, only a select number of ABC transporters are thought to transport drugs and most have a far more narrow substrate profile than Pgp. Among these, the MRP or ABCC transporter subfamily contains nine putative drug transporters.

The first member of the ABCC subfamily to be cloned was the multidrug resistance protein, MRP1. Cloned by Cole et al. in 1992, MRP1 was found to have an additional five transmembrane segments in a single domain at the amino terminus of the protein (the TMD_0 domain) (75) (Fig. 2). Since the original description of MRP1, 12 members of the ABCC subfamily have been described, of which nine have been labeled as MRPs because of their homology to MRP1. All MRP transporters that have been characterized appear to be organic anion transporters of varying specificity (Table 2). MRPs 1, 2, 3, 6, and 7 contain the TMD_0 domain, while MRPs 4, 5, 8, and 9 lack this feature, suggesting the TMD_0 domain is not critical for transport (5). However, the adjacent linker region is essential and is present in all of the MRPs (76,77). MRPs 1–3 have been shown to transport glutathione and glucuronide conjugates, sulfates, and other organic anions. MRP2, or multispecific organic anion transporter (cMOAT), was originally identified as an organic anion transporter and transports bilirubin glucuronide from the liver. MRP4 and MRP5 have been shown to transport cyclic nucleotides including cAMP and cGMP, as well as nucleoside analogs (78–81). Interestingly, glutathione depletion was recently reported to reduce the export of cAMP in MRP4-expressing cells (82). MRP6 has also been confirmed as a glutathione conjugate transporter.

4.2. Subcellular Localization and Substrate Specificity

The substrate specificity as well as localization within the body varies for the different members of the MRP family. MRP1 is ubiquitously expressed at low levels in most normal tissues. It routes to the basolateral surface of epithelial cells, including the choroid plexus epithelium, where it may be involved in the transport of substrates from the CSF into the bloodstream (11). Thus, when etoposide was instilled into the CSF a 10-fold increase in accumulation occurred in $mdr1a/1b^{-/-}/mrp1^{-/-}$ (triple knockout) mice, relative to that observed in $mdr1a/1b^{-/-}$ mice (83). In the liver, MRP 2 is found on the apical surface of the hepatocyte, transporting substrates into the biliary cannaliculi, while MRP3 is found on the basolateral surface, presumably there to pump substrates back into the bloodstream should biliary flow be interrupted (84). Like MRP1 and MRP3, MRP6 demonstrates a basolateral localization (85), while MRP4 demonstrates apical localization similar to MRP2 (86).

The substrate profile for the MRPs with regard to anticancer agents is less straightforward than that for Pgp. Currently understood substrate profiles for the MRP family members are shown in Table 2. It has been shown that in addition to the transport of glutathione conjugates, MRP1 is able to cotransport vincristine and adriamycin together with glutathione, without conjugation (6). This may also be true for etoposide. Methotrexate, which has been determined to be a substrate for MRP1, is also transported by MRP2, MRP3, and MRP4 (6,87). Because methotrexate is an organic anion, transport does not require conjugation or cotransport with glutathione. In contrast, the polyglutamylated forms of methotrexate are not transported by the MRPs. MRP3 has been shown to confer resistance primarily to etoposide, and to favor glucuronides over glutathione conjugates (88). MRP4 and MRP5 have been shown to confer resistance to the nucleoside analogs 6-mercaptopurine and 6-thioguanine (79,81). Similarly, 9-(2-phosphonylmethoxyethyl)-adenine (PMEA), an antiretroviral nucleoside agent, is an MRP4 substrate (78). With overexpression of MRP4, both the cytotoxicity and antiviral activity of PMEA are reduced.

4.3. Physiologic Role of MRP Family Members

Like Pgp, MRP1 is thought to protect the organism from xenobiotics. This idea is reinforced by in vitro studies using fibroblasts from knockout mice. When fibroblasts from mice lacking the orthologs for both Pgp and MRP were studied, increased in vitro sensitivity was observed compared to the Pgp knockout alone: for paclitaxel (22- vs 16-fold), vincristine (28- vs 2.4-fold), doxorubicin (7.1- vs 4.7-fold), and etoposide (7.0- vs 1.0-fold) was observed (89). These results suggest that there is redundancy in the protection of normal tissues from xenobiotics, and that the drug transporters contribute substantively to intrinsic drug resistance. Knockout mice in which Mrp alone had been deleted exhibited increased sensitivity to etoposide in the oropharynx (90), but little difference in most drug pharmacokinetic profiles. MRP2 or cMOAT is responsible for the efflux of bilirubin glucuronide from the liver. Mutations that result in a nonfunctional MRP2 are the basis of the Dubin–Johnson disorder, characterized by failure to transport bilirubin into the bile. Mutations in patients with pseudoxanthoma elasticum render MRP6 unable to transport the glutathione conjugates leukotriene and NEM-GS (91).

5. ABCG2: A MITOXANTRONE TRANSPORTER

Cloned by three independent labs, ABCG2 was originally named BCRP for breast cancer resistance protein, ABCP for ABC transporter in placenta, and MXR for mitoxantrone-resistance gene (92–94). Unlike other multidrug transporters, ABCG2 is a "half-transporter," comprised of six transmembrane segments in one TM domain and a single ATP binding site at the amino terminus (Fig. 2). Although conclusive proof is lacking, ABCG2 is thought to dimerize to generate a fully functional ABC transporter. Nonreducing conditions and studies using crosslinking agents show high molecular weight forms suggesting that more than two proteins may be involved in the dimerization (95,96). Immunofluorescence localization (97) studies have localized ABCG2 to the plasma membrane of drug resistant selected cell lines (95).

ABCG2 is expressed in the placenta, the small and large intestine, the liver, and the endothelium of CNS tissues, suggesting that like Pgp the role of ABCG2 in normal human physiology may be protection of the organism from exposure to environmental xenobiotics. In the placenta, ABCG2 is found at high levels in the syncytiotrophoblast, suggesting a role in the excretion of toxins from the fetal circulation, or transport of substrates in from the maternal circulation (98). Consistent with this, increased fetal penetration of topotecan was demonstrated following treatment with an inhibitor of ABCG2 efflux, supporting a role for ABCG2 in protecting the fetus from toxins (99). Evidence for a protective role in the gastrointestinal tract includes studies showing that in mice lacking the Pgp homologs oral administration of GF120918, an ABCG2 inhibitor, increased the absorption of orally administered topotecan, an ABCG2 substrate (99). This provides support for the hypothesis that ABCG2 may be involved in the control of drug absorption from the gastrointestinal tract. If so, inhibition of ABCG2, like Pgp, may be exploitable in the development of oral agents for anticancer therapy. Because there is some overlap in substrate specificity, inhibitors such as GF1201918 that block both Pgp and ABCG2 may be desirable candidates for this purpose (98). Finally, recent studies have also shown that the "side population" of stem cells found in bone marrow, skeletal muscle, and neural cells have ABCG2-mediated Hoechst 33342 dye efflux (100). The side population had been previously defined by its ability to efflux Hoechst dye. However, mice lacking the *ABCG2* gene mature normally and reproduce, despite the absence of this Hoechst 33342-defined side population of stem cells (101). Furthermore, mice lacking ABCG2 have normal steady-state hematopoiesis, although marrow cells are more sensitive to the toxic effects of mitoxantrone. The normal hematopoiesis suggests stem cell maturation can occur in the absence of ABCG2.

Overexpression of ABCG2 confers resistance to mitoxantrone, topotecan, and irinotecan, mediated by reduced drug accumulation (102–106). Studies have also demonstrated that in some but not all cell lines, ABCG2 overexpression results in resistance to the anthracyclines doxorubicin, daunorubicin, and epirubicin, as well as resistance to rhodamine and VP-16. This discrepancy was resolved by the recognition that two cell lines had mutations at amino acid 482 (107). Arginine, the wild-type amino acid at 482, was replaced by a threonine in the breast-cancer-derived MCF-7 AdVp cell line (from which *BCRP* was originally cloned), and was substituted by a glycine in the colon-cancer-derived S1M180 cell line (from which *MXR* was originally cloned). This amino acid is predicted to lie at the entrance to the third transmembrane segment. An explanation of the mechanism underlying this alteration in substrate specificity remains to be elucidated. Interestingly, doxorubicin selection of murine fibroblasts obtained from mice deficient in Mdr1a, Mdr1b, and MRP led to the isolation of drug-resistant sublines containing mutations at the same site (108,109). Finally, a recent report shows that ABCG2 confers resistance to methotrexate (110), suggesting transport of a range of substrates including anionic compounds.

6. OTHER ABC TRANSPORTERS

At least two other ABC transporters with distinct roles in normal physiology have been shown to transport an anticancer agent (Fig. 5). These transporters provide a prototype or model for the concept that any transporter can be subverted for the purpose of protecting the cell from cytotoxic agents.

Returning to the ABCB subfamily of which Pgp is a member, ABCB11 has been shown to transport paclitaxel as well as its natural bile salt substrates. ABCB11 was originally termed "sister of Pgp (sPgp)" based on its homology with Pgp (111). The identification of ABCB11 mutations in liver tissue obtained from patients with progressive familial intrahepatic cholestasis, type II, led to the recognition that sPgp encoded the ATP-dependent BSEP

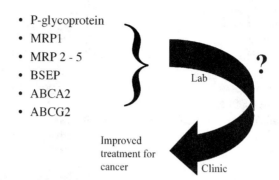

- P-glycoprotein
- MRP1
- MRP 2 - 5
- BSEP
- ABCA2
- ABCG2

Lab

?

Improved
treatment for
cancer

Clinic

Fig. 5. Cartoon listing ABC transporters with potential roles in clinical drug resistance. Although 48 ABC transporters have been described in the human genome, only the handful shown here have been shown to be capable of transporting anticancer agents. Among those shown to transport drugs, only Pgp, MRP1, and ABCG2 have been suggested as being clinically important. Although the ABC transporters represent potential molecular targets for anticancer drug development, no ABC transporter will be considered clinically important in oncology without translation of that discovery into improved treatment for cancer.

(112). Absence of ABCB11 leads to impaired bile salt transport and reduced bile with progressive liver damage. In vitro studies have demonstrated that the ability of BSEP/sPgp to confer resistance to paclitaxel can be reversed by CsA, PSC 833, or verapamil *(111)*.

Among ABCA subfamily members, ABCA2 was originally termed ABC2 when cloned from cells with high levels of estramustine resistance *(113)*. ABCA2 has a large 5' extracellular loop and a regulatory domain. It is expressed at high levels in the brain and as a member of the A subfamily is most likely involved in cholesterol transport *(1)*. However, following transfection ABCA2 colocalizes with fluorescently labeled estramustine and confers resistance to this drug *(114)*.

7. ABC TRANSPORTERS: AN EXPANDING LIST OF SUBSTRATES

Work with the NCI drug screen suggested that Pgp substrates number in the hundreds, if not thousands *(7)*. This is perhaps not surprising if one considers the important role of Pgp in protecting the organism from exposure to environmental toxins. Substrate profiles for the MRPs and for ABCG2 appear more restricted; however, this may reflect a less comprehensive inquiry. Recent reports have shown that MRP4 and MRP5 confer resistance to the nucleosides 6-MP and 6-TG, agents not previously considered substrates of ABC transporters, raising the possibility that transporters for other nucleoside analogs such as cytosine arabinoside will be identified. In addition to conferring resistance to mitoxantrone, topotecan, and irinotecan, wild-type ABCG2 has also been shown to confer resistance to flavopiridol *(115)*. Even the recently approved Bcr–abl kinase inhibitor Gleevec may be a substrate for Pgp *(116)*. Following this path to its conclusion, it could be argued that a drug transporter will likely be identified for every anticancer agent developed.

Furthermore, it is likely that ABC transporters will be important not only in oncology but also in other clinical disciplines. One has to think of ABC transporters as modulators of drug uptake, without limitation to anticancer agents. For example, the HIV-protease inhibitor nelfinavir is a substrate for Pgp. To the extent that Pgp is an important regulator of CNS uptake through the blood–brain barrier, nelfinavir may not achieve CNS levels sufficient for antiretroviral activity. The finding that another antiretroviral agent, PMEA, is a substrate for MRP4 and MRP 5 makes it important to identify the localization of that ABC transporter. Because MRP4 and MRP5 have been identified in circulating mononuclear cells, this has direct implications for human immunodeficiency virus (HIV) resistance to PMEA.

Finally, as suggested above, there may be a role for Pgp inhibition in the modulation of absorption of orally administered Pgp substrates. This could result in the ability to administer agents orally that otherwise must be given parenterally. Alternatively, it may be found that interpatient variability in drug absorption can be reduced by coadministration of a Pgp inhibitor. Similar considerations may also apply to other transporters, including ABCG2.

8. CONCLUSIONS

The role of ABC transporters in multidrug resistance, in oncology, in pharmacology, and in medicine is still under investigation. The earliest studies with inhibitors of Pgp focused on reversal of drug resistance in oncology. These trials were limited by inferior antagonist potency and by the need to reduce the dose of the anticancer agent. Newer inhibitors of Pgp have been identified with reduced toxicity, greater potency, and minimal pharmacokinetic interaction. Surrogate studies have confirmed that these inhibitors are able to inhibit Pgp in vivo, setting the stage for studies that will provide a definitive answer to the question of whether drug resistance modulation by Pgp inhibition can be beneficial. The expanding list of ABC transporters has identified additional potential mediators of drug resistance. Strategies for characterizing the expression of these transporters in cancer samples and identifying agents for inhibiting efflux mediated by them will be a necessary prelude to testing in the clinic. Established agents, newer agents, and agents in development are likely to be substrates for drug efflux by one or more than one ABC transporter, which could potentially limit their therapeutic benefit. If this hypothesis is correct then, despite the long and winding road these studies have followed, efforts to develop inhibitors of ABC transporters may soon be rewarded.

REFERENCES

1. Dean M, Hamon Y, Chimini G. The human ATP-binding cassette (ABC) transporter superfamily. J Lipid Res 2001; 42:1007–1017.
2. Gottesman MM, Fojo T, Bates SE. Multidrug resistance in cancer: role of ATP-dependent transporters. Nat Rev Cancer 2002; 2:48–58.
3. Klein I, Sarkadi B, Varadi A. An inventory of the human ABC proteins. Biochim Biophys Acta 1999; 1461:237–262.
4. Dean M, Rzhetsky A, Allikmets R. The human ATP-binding cassette (ABC) transporter superfamily. Genome Res 2001; 11:1156–1166.
5. Borst P, Evers R, Kool M, Wijnholds J. A family of drug transporters: the multidrug resistance-associated proteins. J Natl Cancer Inst 2000; 92:1295–1302.
6. Kruh GD, Zeng H, Rea PA, et al. MRP subfamily transporters and resistance to anticancer agents. J Bioenerg Biomembr 2001; 33:493–501.
7. Lee JS, Paull K, Alvarez M, et al. Rhodamine efflux patterns predict P-glycoprotein substrates in the National Cancer Institute Drug Screen. Mol Pharmacol 1994; 46:627–638.
8. Schinkel AH. P-Glycoprotein, a gatekeeper in the blood–brain barrier. Adv Drug Deliv Rev 1999; 36: 179–194.
9. Thiebaut F, Tsuruo T, Hamada H, Gotesman MM, Pastan I, Willingham MC. Immunohistochemical localization in normal tissues of different epitopes in the multidrug transport protein P170: evidence for localization in brain capillaries and cross reactivity of one antibody with muscle protein. J Histochem Cytochem 1989; 37:159–164.
10. Bart J, Groen HJ, van der Graaf WT, et al. An oncological view on the blood–testis barrier. Lancet Oncol 2002; 3:357–363.

11. Rao VV, Dahlheimer JL, Bardgett ME, et al. Choroid plexus epithelial expression of MDR1 P glyco-protein and multidrug resistance-associated protein contribute to the blood–cerebrospinal-fluid drug–permeability barrier. Proc Natl Acad Sci USA 1999; 96:3900–3905.

12. Schinkel AH, Smit JJ, van Tellingen O, et al. Disruption of mouse mdr-1a p-glycoprotein gene leads to a deficiency in the blood-brain barrier and to increased sensitivity to drugs. Cell 1994; 77:491–502.

13. Schinkel AH, Wagenaar E, van Deemter L, Mol CA, Borst P. Absence of the mdr1a P-Glycoprotein in mice affects tissue distribution and pharmacokinetics of dexamethasone, digoxin, and cyclosporin A. J Clin Invest 1995; 96:1698–1705.

14. Xie R, Hammarlund-Udenaes M, de Boer AG, de Lange EC. The role of P-glycoprotein in blood–brain barrier transport of morphine: transcortical microdialysis studies in *mdr1a (–/–)* and *mdr1a (+/+)* mice. Br J Pharmacol 1999; 128:563–568.

15. Meijer OC, de Lange EC, Breimer DD, de Boer AG, Workel JO, de Kloet ER. Penetration of dexamethasone into brain glucocorticoid targets is enhanced in mdr1A P-glycoprotein knockout mice. Endocrinology 1998; 139:1789–1793.

16. van Asperen J, Schinkel AH, Beijnen JH, Nooijen WJ, Borst P, van Tellingen O. Altered pharmaco-kinetics of vinblastine in Mdr1a P-glycoprotein-deficient Mice. J Natl Cancer Inst 1996; 88:994–999.

17. Schinkel AH, Wagenaar E, Mol CA, van Deemter L. P-Glycoprotein in the blood–brain barrier of mice influences the brain penetration and pharmacological activity of many drugs. J Clin Invest 1996; 97:2517–2524.

18. Hendrikse NH, Schinkel AH, de Vries EG, et al. Complete in vivo reversal of P-glycoprotein pump function in the blood-brain barrier visualized with positron emission tomography. Br J Pharmacol 1998; 124:1413–1418.

19. van Asperen J, van Tellingen O, Tijssen F, Schinkel AH, Beijnen JH. Increased accumulation of doxorubicin and doxorubicinol in cardiac tissue of mice lacking mdr1a P-glycoprotein. Br J Cancer 1999; 79:108–113.

20. Fromm MF, Kim RB, Stein CM, Wilkinson GR, Roden DM. Inhibition of P-glycoprotein-mediated drug transport: a unifying mechanism to explain the interaction between digoxin and quinidine. Circulation 1999; 99:552–557.

21. Choo EF, Leake B, Wandel C, et al. Pharmacological inhibition of P-glycoprotein transport enhances the distribution of HIV-1 protease inhibitors into brain and testes. Drug Metab Dispos 2000; 28:655–660.

22. Karssen AM, Meijer OC, van der Sandt IC, et al. Multidrug resistance P-glycoprotein hampers the access of cortisol but not of corticosterone to mouse and human brain. Endocrinology 2001; 142:2686–2694.

23. de Lange EC, Marchand S, et al. In vitro and in vivo investigations on fluoroquinolones; effects of the P-glycoprotein efflux transporter on brain distribution of sparfloxacin. Eur J Pharm Sci 2000; 12:85–93.

24. Yamaguchi H, Yano I, Saito H, Inui K. Pharmacokinetic role of P-glycoprotein in oral bioavailability and intestinal secretion of grepafloxacin in vivo. J Pharmacol Exp Ther 2002; 300:1063–1069.

25. Meerum Terwogt JM, Malingre MM, Beijnen JH, et al. Coadministration of oral cyclosporin A enables oral therapy with paclitaxel. Clin Cancer Res 1999; 5:3379–3384.

26. Malingre MM, Beijnen JH, Rosing H, et al. Co-administration of GF120918 significantly increases the systemic exposure to oral paclitaxel in cancer patients. Br J Cancer 2001; 84:42–47.

27. van Asperen J, van Tellingen O, Sparreboom A, Schinkel AH, Borst P, Nooijen WJ, et al. Enhanced oral bioavailability of paclitaxel in mice treated with the P- glycoprotein blocker SDZ PSC 833. Br J Cancer 1997; 76:1181–1183.

28. Guns ES, Denyssevych T, Dixon R, Bally MB, Mayer L. Drug interaction studies between paclitaxel (Taxol) and OC144-093—a new modulator of MDR in cancer chemotherapy. Eur J Drug Metab Phar-macokinet 2002; 27:119–126.

29. Kimura Y, Aoki J, Kohno M, Ooka H, Tsuruo T, Nakanishi O. P-Glycoprotein inhibition by the multidrug resistance-reversing agent MS-209 enhances bioavailability and antitumor efficacy of orally administered paclitaxel. Cancer Chemother Pharmacol 2002; 49:322–328.

30. Fojo AT, Ueda K, Slamon DJ, Poplack DG, Gottesman MM, Pastan I. Expression of a multidrug resistance gene in human tumors and tissues. Proc Natl Acad Sci USA 1987; 84:265–269.

31. Bates SE. Solving the problems of multidrug resistance: ABC transporters in clinical oncology. In: Holland IB, Cole SPC, Kuchler K, Higgins CF (eds). ABC Proteins: From Bacteria to Man. London, UK: Elsevier Science, 2002, pp. 359–391.

32. Trock BJ, Leonessa F, Clarke R. Multidrug resistance in breast cancer: a meta-analysis of MDR1/gp170 expression and its possible functional significance. J Natl Cancer Inst 1997; 89:917–931.

33. Mechetner E, Kyshtoobayeva A, Zonis S, et al. Levels of multidrug resistance (MDR1) P-glycoprotein expression by human breast cancer correlate with in vitro resistance to taxol and doxorubicin. Clin Cancer Res 1998; 4:389–398.

34. Tsuruo T, Iida H, Tsukagoshi S, et al. Overcoming of vincristine resistance in P388 leukemia in vivo and in vitro through enhancing cytotoxicity of vincristine and vinblastine by verapamil. Cancer Res 1981; 41:1967–1972.

35. Ozols RF, Cunnion RE, Klecker RW, et al. Verapamil and adriamycin in the treatment of drug-resistant ovarian cancer patients. J Clin Oncol 1987; 5:641–647.

36. Abraham J, Bakke S, Rutt A, et al. A phase II trial of combination chemotherapy and surgical resection for the treatment of metastatic adrenocortical carcinoma: continuous infusion doxorubicin, vincristine, and etoposide with daily mitotane as a P-glycoprotein antagonist. Cancer 2002; 94:2333–2343.

37. Cisternino S, Rousselle C, Dagenais C, Scherrmann JM. Screening of multidrug-resistance sensitive drugs by in situ brain perfusion in P-glycoprotein-deficient mice. Pharm Res 2001; 18:183–190.

38. Boote DJ, Dennis IF, Twentyman PR, et al. Phase I study of etoposide with SDZ PSC 833 as a modulator of multidrug resistance in patients with cancer. J Clin Oncol 1996; 14:610–618.

39. Giaccone G, Linn SC, Welink J, et al. A dose-finding and pharmacokinetic study of reversal of multidrug resistance with SDZ PSC 833 in combination with doxorubicin in patients with solid tumors. Clin Cancer Res 1997; 3:2005–2015.

40. Minami H, Ohtsu T, Fujii H, et al. Phase I study of intravenous PSC-833 and doxorubicin: reversal of multidrug resistance. Jpn J Cancer Res 2001; 92:220–230.

41. Fracasso PM, Westerveldt P, Fears CA, et al. Phase I study of paclitaxel in combination with a multidrug resistance modulator, PSC 833 (Valspodar), in refractory malignancies. J Clin Oncol 2000; 18:1124.

42. Chico I, Kang MH, Bergan R, et al. Phase I study of infusional paclitaxel in combination with the P-glycoprotein antagonist PSC 833. J Clin Oncol 2001; 19:832–842.

43. Bates S, Kang M, Meadows B, et al. A Phase I study of infusional vinblastine in combination with the P-glycoprotein antagonist PSC 833 (valspodar). Cancer 2001; 92:1577–1590.

44. Sonneveld P, Marie J-P, Huisman C, et al. Reversal of multidrug resistance by SDZ PSC 833, combined with VAD (vincristine, doxorubicin, dexamethasone) in refractory multiple myeloma. A Phase I study. Leukemia 1996; 10:1741–1750.

45. Patnaik A, Warner E, Michael M, et al. Phase I dose-finding and pharmacokinetic study of paclitaxel and carboplatin with oral valspodar in patients with advanced solid tumors. J Clin Oncol 2000; 18:3677–3689.

46. Advani R, Fisher GA, Lum BL, et al. A phase I trial of doxorubicin, paclitaxel, and valspodar (PSC 833), a modulator of multidrug resistance. Clin Cancer Res 2001; 7:1221–1229.

47. Fracasso PM, Brady MF, Moore DH, et al. Phase II study of paclitaxel and valspodar (PSC 833) in refractory ovarian carcinoma: a gynecologic oncology group study. J Clin Oncol 2001; 19:2975–2982.

48. Baekelandt M, Lehne G, Trope CG, et al. Phase I/II trial of the multidrug-resistance modulator valspodar combined with cisplatin and doxorubicin in refractory ovarian cancer. J Clin Oncol 2001; 19:2983–2993.

49. Kornblau SM, Estey E, Madden T, et al. Phase I study of mitoxantrone plus etoposide with multidrug blockade by SDZ PSC-833 in relapsed or refractory acute myelogenous leukemia. J Clin Oncol 1997; 15:1796–1802.

50. Advani R, Visani G, Milligan D, et al. Treatment of poor prognosis AML patients using PSC833 (valspodar) plus mitoxantrone, etoposide, and cytarabine (PSC-MEC). In: Kaspers G, Pieters R (eds). Drug Resistance in Leukemia and Lymphoma III. New York, NY: Kluwer Academic/Plenum, 1999, pp. 47–56.

51. Lee EJ, George SL, Caligiuri M, et al. Parallel Phase I studies of daunorubicin given with cytarabine and etoposide with or without the multidrug resistance modulator PSC-833 in previously untreated patients 60 years of age or older with acute myeloid leukemia: results of cancer and leukemia group B study 9420. J Clin Oncol 1999; 17:2831–2839.

52. Chauncey TR, Rankin C, Anderson JE, et al. A Phase I study of induction chemotherapy for older patients with newly diagnosed acute myeloid leukemia (AML) using mitoxantrone, etoposide, and the MDR modulator PSC 833: a Southwest Oncology Group study 9617. Leuk Res 2000; 24:567–574.

53. Dorr R, Karanes C, Spier C, et al. Phase I/II study of the P-glycoprotein modulator PSC 833 in patients with acute myeloid leukemia. J Clin Oncol 2001; 19:1589–1599.

54. Visani G, Milligan D, Leoni F, et al. Combined action of PSC 833 (Valspodar), a novel MDR reversing agent, with mitoxantrone, etoposide and cytarabine in poor-prognosis acute myeloid leukemia. Leukemia 2001; 15:764–771.

55. Joly F, Joly F, Mangioni C, et al. A Phase 3 study of PSC 833 in combination with paclitaxel and carboplatin (PC-PSC) versus paclitaxel and carboplatin (PC) alone in patients with stage IV or suboptimally debulked stage III epithelial ovarian cancer or primary cancer of the peritoneum. Proc Am Soc Clin Oncol 2002; abstract 809.

56. Baer MR, George SL, Dodge RK, et al. Phase 3 study of the multidrug resistance modulator PSC-833 in previously untreated patients 60 years of age and older with acute myeloid leukemia: Cancer and Leukemia Group B Study 9720. Blood 2002; 100:1224–1232.

57. Rowinsky EK, Smith L, Wang YM, et al. Phase I and pharmacokinetic study of paclitaxel in combination with biricodar, a novel agent that reverses multidrug resistance conferred by overexpression of both MDR1 and MRP. J Clin Oncol 1998; 16:2964–2976.

58. Peck RA, Hewett J, Harding MW, et al. Phase I and pharmacokinetic study of the novel MDR1 and MRP1 inhibitor biricodar administered alone and in combination with doxorubicin. J Clin Oncol 2001; 19:3130–3141.

59. Toppmeyer D, Seidman AD, Pollak M, et al. Safety and efficacy of the multidrug resistance inhibitor Incel (biricodar; VX-710) in combination with paclitaxel for advanced breast cancer refractory to paclitaxel. Clin Cancer Res 2002; 8:670–678.

60. Bramwell VH, Morris D, Ernst DS, et al. Safety and efficacy of the multidrug-resistance inhibitor biricodar (VX-710) with concurrent doxorubicin in patients with anthracycline-resistant advanced soft tissue sarcoma. Clin Cancer Res 2002; 8:383–393.

61. Seiden MV, Swenerton KD, Matulonis U, et al. A Phase II study of the MDR inhibitor biricodar (INCEL, VX-710) and paclitaxel in women with advanced ovarian cancer refractory to paclitaxel therapy. Gynecol Oncol 2002; 86:302–310.

62. Rollins DE, Klaassen CD. Biliary excretion of drugs in man. Clin Pharmacokinet 1979; 4:368–379.

63. Kullak-Ublick GA, Stieger B, Hagenbuch B, Meier PJ. Hepatic transport of bile salts. Semin Liver Dis 2000; 20:273–292.

64. Gerloff T, Stieger B, Hagenbuch B, et al. The sister of P-glycoprotein represents the canalicular bile salt export pump of mammalian liver. J Biol Chem 1998; 273:10,046–10,050.

65. Bohme M, Muller M, Leier I, Jedlitschky G, Keppler D. Cholestasis caused by inhibition of the adenosine triphosphate-dependent bile salt transport in rat liver. Gastroenterology 1994; 107:255–265.

66. Song S, Suzuki H, Kawai R, Tanaka C, Akasaka I, Sugiyama Y. Dose-dependent effects of PSC 833 on its tissue distribution and on the biliary excretion of endogenous substrates in rats. Drug Metab Dispos 1998; 26:1128–1133.

67. Danielson PB. The cytochrome p450 superfamily: biochemistry, evolution and drug metabolism in humans. Curr Drug Metab 2002; 3:561–597.

68. Gorski JC, Hall SD, Jones DR, VandenBranden M, Wrighton SA. Regioselective biotransformation of midazolam by members of the human cytochrome P450 3A (CYP3A) subfamily. Biochem Pharmacol 1994; 47:1643–1653.

69. List AF, Kopecky KJ, Willman CL, et al. Benefit of cyclosporine modulation of drug resistance in patients with poor-risk acute myeloid leukemia: a Southwest Oncology Group study. Blood 2001; 98: 3212–3220.

70. Newman MJ, Rodarte JC, Benbatoul KD, et al. Discovery and characterization of OC144-093, a novel inhibitor of P-glycoprotein-mediated multidrug resistance. Cancer Res 2000; 60:2964–2972.

71. van Zuylen L, Sparreboom A, van der Gaast A, et al. The orally administered P-glycoprotein inhibitor R101933 does not alter the plasma pharmacokinetics of docetaxel. Clin Cancer Res 2000; 6: 1365–1371.

72. Witherspoon SM, Emerson DL, Kerr BM, Lloyd TL, Dalton WS, Wissel PS. Flow cytometric assay of modulation of P-glycoprotein function in whole blood by the multidrug resistance inhibitor GG918. Clin Cancer Res 1996; 2:7–12.

73. Robey R, Bakke S, Stein W, et al. Efflux of rhodamine from CD56+ cells as a surrogate marker for reversal of P-glycoprotein-mediated drug efflux by PSC 833. Blood 1999; 93:306–314.

74. Piwnica-Worms D, Chiu ML, Budding M, Kronaauge JF, Kramer RA, Croop JM. Functional imaging of multidrug-resistant P-glycoprotein with an organotechnetium complex. Cancer Res 1993; 53: 977–984.

75. Cole SPC, Bhardwaj G, Gerlach JH, et al. Overexpression of a transporter gene in a multidrug-resistant human lung cancer cell line. Science 1992; 258:1650–1654.

76. Bakos E, Evers R, Szakacs G, Tusnady GE, Welker E, Szabo K, et al. Functional multidrug resistance protein (MRP1) lacking the N-terminal transmembrane domain. J Biol Chem 1998; 273:32,167–32,175.

77. Tammur J, Prades C, Arnould I, et al. Two new genes from the human ATP-binding cassette transporter superfamily, ABCC11 and ABCC12, tandemly duplicated on chromosome 16q12. Gene 2001; 273: 89–96.

78. Schuetz JD, Connelly MC, Sun D, et al. MRP4: A previously unidentified factor in resistance to nucleoside-based antiviral drugs. Nat Med 1999; 5:1048–1051.

79. Wijnholds J, Mol CA, van Deemter L, et al. Multidrug-resistance protein 5 is a multispecific organic anion transporter able to transport nucleotide analogs. Proc Natl Acad Sci USA 2000; 97:7476–7481.

80. Jedlitschky G, Burchell B, Keppler D. The multidrug resistance protein 5 functions as an ATP-dependent export pump for cyclic nucleotides. J Biol Chem 2000; 275:30,069–30,074.

81. Chen ZS, Lee K, Kruh GD. Transport of cyclic nucleotides and estradiol 17-beta-D-glucuronide by multidrug resistance protein 4: resistance to 6-mercaptopurine and 6-thioguanine. J Biol Chem 2001; 276:33,747–33,754.

82. Lai L, Tan TM. Role of glutathione in the multidrug resistance protein 4 (MRP4/ABCC4)-mediated efflux of cAMP and resistance to purine analogues. Biochem J 2002; 361:497–503.

83. Wijnholds J, deLange EC, Scheffer GL, et al. Multidrug resistance protein 1 protects the choroid plexus epithelium and contributes to the blood–cerebrospinal fluid barrier. J Clin Invest 2000; 105:279–285.

84. Konig J, Rost D, Cui Y, Keppler D. Characterization of the human multidrug resistance protein isoform MRP3 localized to the basolateral hepatocyte membrane. Hepatology 1999; 29:1156–1163.

85. Scheffer GL, Hu X, Pijnenborg AC, Wijnholds J, Bergen AA, Scheper RJ. MRP6 (ABCC6) detection in normal human tissues and tumors. Lab Invest 2002; 82:515–518.

86. van Aubel RA, Smeets PH, Peters JG, Bindels RJ, Russel FG. The MRP4/ABCC4 gene encodes a novel apical organic anion transporter in human kidney proximal tubules: putative efflux pump for urinary cAMP and cGMP. J Am Soc Nephrol 2002; 13:595–603.

87. Chen ZS, Lee K, Walther S, et al. Analysis of methotrexate and folate transport by multidrug resistance protein 4 (ABCC4): MRP4 is a component of the methotrexate efflux system. Cancer Res 2002; 62: 3144–3150.

88. Zelcer N, Saeki T, Reid G, Beijnen JH, Borst P. Characterization of drug transport by the human multidrug resistance protein 3 (ABCC3). J Biol Chem 2001; 276:46400–46407.

89. Allen JD, Brinkhuis RF, van Deemter L, Wijnholds J, Schinkel AH. Extensive contribution of the multidrug transporters P-glycoprotein and Mrp1 to basal drug resistance. Cancer Res 2000; 60:5761–5766.

90. Lorico A, Rappa G, Finch RA, Yang D, Flavell RA, Sartorelli AC. Disruption of the murine MRP (multidrug resistance protein) gene leads to increased sensitivity to etoposide (VP-16) and increased levels of glutathione. Cancer Res 1997; 57:5238–5242.

91. Ilias A, Urban Z, Seidl TL, et al. Loss of ATP-dependent transport activity in pseudoxanthoma elasticum-associated mutants of human ABCC6 (MRP6). J Biol Chem 2002; 277:16,860–16,867.

92. Miyake K, Mickley L, Litman T, et al. Molecular cloning of cDNAs which are highly overexpressed in mitoxantrone-resistant cells: demonstration of homology to ABC transport genes. Cancer Res 1999; 59:8–13.

93. Doyle LA, Yang W, Abruzzo LV, et al. A multidrug resistance transporter from human MCF-7 breast cancer cells. Proc Natl Acad Sci USA 1998; 95:15,665–15,670.

94. Allikmets R, Schriml LM, Hutchinson A, Romano-Spica V, Dean M. A human placenta-specific ATP-binding cassette gene (ABCP) on chromosome 4q22 that is involved in multidrug resistance. Cancer Res 1998; 58:5337–5339.

95. Litman T, Jensen U, Hansen A, et al. Use of peptide antibodies to probe for the mitoxantrone resistance-associated protein MXR/BCRP/ABCP/ABCG2. Biochim Biophys Acta 2002; 1565:6–16.

96. Kage K, Tsukahara S, Sugiyama T, et al. Dominant-negative inhibition of breast cancer resistance protein as drug efflux pump through the inhibition of S–S dependent homodimerization. Int J Cancer 2002; 97:626–630.

97. Rocchi E, Khodjakov A, Volk EL, et al. The product of the ABC half-transporter gene ABCG2 (BCRP/MXR/ABCP) is expressed in the plasma membrane. Biochem Biophys Res Commun 2000; 271:42–46.

98. Maliepaard M, Scheffer GL, Faneyte IF, et al. Subcellular localization and distribution of the breast cancer resistance protein transporter in normal human tissues. Cancer Res 2001; 61:3458–3464.

99. Jonker JW, Smit JW, Brinkhuis RF, et al. Role of breast cancer resistance protein in the bioavailability and fetal penetration of topotecan. J Natl Cancer Inst 2000; 92:1651–1656.

100. Zhou S, Schuetz JD, Bunting KD, et al. The ABC transporter Bcrp1/ABCG2 is expressed in a wide variety of stem cells and is a molecular determinant of the side-population phenotype. Nat Med 2001; 7:1028–1034.

101. Zhou S, Morris JJ, Barnes Y, Lan L, Schuetz JD, Sorrentino BP. Bcrp1 gene expression is required for normal numbers of side population stem cells in mice, and confers relative protection to mitoxantrone in hematopoietic cells in vivo. Proc Natl Acad Sci USA 2002; 99:12,339–12,344.

102. Litman T, Brangi M, Hudson E, et al. The multidrug-resistant phenotype associated with overexpression of the new ABC half-transporter, MXR (ABCG2). J Cell Sci 2000; 113:2011–2021.

103. Brangi M, Litman T, Ciotti M, et al. Camptothecin resistance: role of the ATP-binding cassette (ABC), mitoxantrone-resistance half-transporter (MXR), and potential for glucuronidation in MXR-expressing cells. Cancer Res 1999; 59:5938–5946.

104. Ross DD, Yang W, Abruzzo LV, et al. Atypical multidrug resistance: breast cancer resistance protein messenger RNA expression in mitoxantrone-selected cell lines. J Natl Cancer Inst 1999; 91:429–433.

105. Maliepaard M, van Gastelen MA, de Jong LA, Pluim D, van Waardenburg RC, Ruevekamp-Helmers MC, et al. Overexpression of the BCRP/MXR/ABCP gene in a topotecan-selected ovarian tumor cell line. Cancer Res 1999; 59:4559–4563.

106. Kawabata S, Oka M, Shiozawa K, et al. Breast cancer resistance protein directly confers SN-38 resistance of lung cancer cells. Biochem Biophys Res Commun 2001; 280:1216–1223.

107. Honjo Y, Hrycyna CA, Yan QW, Medina-Perez WY, Robey RW, van de Laar A, et al. Acquired mutations in the *MXR/BCRP/ABCP* gene alter substrate specificity in *MXR/BCRP/ABCP*-overexpressing cells. Cancer Res 2001; 61:6635–6639.

108. Allen JD, Brinkhuis RF, Wijnholds J, Schinkel AH. The mouse *Bcrp1/Mxr/Abcp* gene: amplification and overexpression in cell lines selected for resistance to topotecan, mitoxantrone, or doxorubicin. Cancer Res 1999; 59:4237–4241.

109. Allen JD, Jackson SC, Schinkel AH. A mutation hot spot in the bcrp1 (abcg2) multidrug transporter in mouse cell lines selected for doxorubicin resistance. Cancer Res 2002; 62:2294–2299.

110. Volk EL, Farley KM, Wu Y, Li F, Robey RW, Schneider E. Overexpression of wild-type breast cancer resistance protein mediates methotrexate resistance. Cancer Res 2002; 62:5035–5040.

111. Childs S, Yeh RL, Hui D, Ling V. Taxol resistance mediated by transfection of the liver-specific sister gene of P-glycoprotein. Cancer Res 1998; 58:4160–4167.

112. Strautnieks SS, Bull LN, Knisely AS, et al. A gene encoding a liver-specific ABC transporter is mutated in progressive familial intrahepatic cholestasis. Nat Genet 1998; 20:233–238.

113. Laing NM, Belinsky MG, Kruh GD, et al. Amplification of the ATP-binding cassette 2 transporter gene is functionally linked with enhanced efflux of estramustine in ovarian carcinoma cells. Cancer Res 1998; 58:1332–1337.

114. Vulevic B, Chen Z, Boyd JT, et al. Cloning and characterization of human adenosine 5'-triphosphate-binding cassette, sub-family A, transporter 2 (ABCA2). Cancer Res 2001; 61:3339–3347.

115. Robey RW, Medina-Perez WY, Nishiyama K, et al. Overexpression of the ATP-binding cassette half-transporter, ABCG2 (MXR/BCRP/ABCP1), in flavopiridol-resistant human breast cancer cells. Clin Cancer Res 2001; 7:145–152.

116. Mahon FX, Deininger MW, Schultheis B, Chabrol J, Reiffers J, Goldman JM, et al. Selection and characterization of BCR-ABL positive cell lines with differential sensitivity to the tyrosine kinase inhibitor STI571: diverse mechanisms of resistance. Blood 2000; 96:1070–1079.

18 Intrathecal Chemotherapy

Jeff Stone, MD and Susan M. Blaney, MD

1. INTRODUCTION

The central nervous system (CNS) is an increasingly recognized site of tumor recurrence. Tumor spread to the CNS, manifest as either neoplastic meningitis or intraparenchymal metastases, is in part due to the pharmacologic sanctuary created by the blood–brain (BBB) and blood–cerebrospinal fluid (CSF) barriers. As a result, tumor cells within the CNS are protected from the cytotoxic effects of systemically administered chemotherapy. Leukemias and lymphomas remain the most common cancers with a predilection for leptomeningeal spread. However, there are many solid tumors that may also disseminate within the CNS including breast and small-cell lung cancer *(1–3)*; primary CNS tumors such as medulloblastoma and glioma *(4,5)*; and childhood tumors such as neuroblastoma, retinoblastoma, and rhabdomyosarcoma *(6–9)*.

Strategies to treat metastatic CNS disease include intrathecal (IT) chemotherapy, radiation therapy, and high-dose systemic chemotherapy. These therapeutic strategies have been used successfully for the prevention and treatment of CNS leukemia. In fact, IT chemotherapy is currently incorporated into all front-line leukemia treatment protocols, and is the primary therapeutic modality for the prevention of leptomeningeal dissemination. Unfortunately, for most patients with neoplastic meningitis from underlying solid tumors or for patients with recurrent/refractory CNS leukemias, there is no effective therapy. Ongoing challenges to the successful treatment of these high-risk patients include the limited spectrum of antineoplastic agents that are currently available for IT administration as well as the lack of effective IT combination chemotherapy regimens.

The primary focus of this chapter is to describe the role of IT therapy in the treatment and/ or prevention of neoplastic meningitis, including a brief review of the limitations of systemi-

Handbook of Anticancer Pharmacokinetics and Pharmacodynamics
Edited by: W. D. Figg and H. L. McLeod © Humana Press Inc., Totowa, NJ

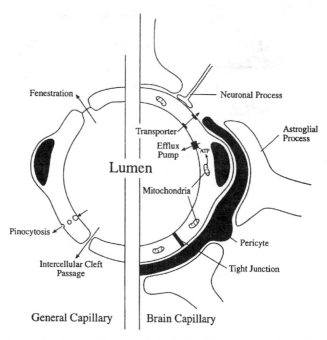

Fig. 1. Differences between brain capillary endothelial cells and endothelial cells in other organs. Brain capillary endothelial cells have tight intercellular junctions and lack fenestrations and pinocytic vesicles. The cytoplasm of the brain capillary endothelial cells are rich in mitochondria that supply energy to the various transport systems for passage of nutrients into the brain and to pump out potentially toxic compounds. Processes from astrocytes, pericytes, and neurons are closely associated with brain capillaries and trophically influence the specialized functions of brain capillary endothelial cells. (From ref. *16*, with permission.)

cally administered chemotherapy in the treatment of neoplastic meningitis, an overview of important pharmacologic principles that are relevant to intrathecal administration of anti-cancer agents, and a review of the pharmacokinetics and toxicities of the most commonly administered intrathecal agents. In addition, we provide an overview of new agents for IT administration that are in early stages of preclinical or clinical evaluation.

2. IT CHEMOTHERAPY

2.1. Rationale

The BBB and the blood–CSF barrier are natural membrane barriers that, among other physiologic functions, regulate drug delivery and egress from the central nervous system *(10,11)*. The BBB, located at the level of the CNS endothelial cell, and the blood–CSF barrier, located in the epithelium of the tiny organs surrounding the ventricles (e.g., choroid plexus, median eminence, area postrema), effectively limit the CNS penetration of toxic substances, including most hydrophilic anticancer agents, from the bloodstream (Fig. 1) *(10)*. Drug egress from the CSF generally occurs via passive diffusion. However, in contrast to non-CNS endothelial cells, there are metabolic enzymes and transporters (e.g., P-glyco-protein [Pgp], multidrug-resistance associated proteins [MRPs], and organic acid transporters [OATs]), in the blood–brain and blood–CSF barriers that play an important role in the clearance or egress of specific drugs from the CSF *(12–16)*.

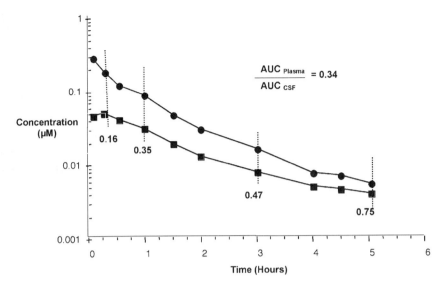

Fig. 2. Plasma (●) and CSF (■) concentration of topotecan in nonhuman primates after an intravenous dose. Ratios of CSF to plasma concentrations at individual time points are shown on the graph for the 0.25-h, 1-h, 3-h, and 5-h samples. The CSF/plasma ratios range from 0.16 to 0.75, and the ratio increases over time because of the difference in the shapes of the plasma and CSF concentration vs time curves. The ratio of drug exposure (AUC) in CSF to plasma is 0.34. Ratios obtained from single-timepoint measurements at later timepoints overestimate the drug exposure in CSF relative to exposure in plasma. (From ref. *88*, with permission.)

CSF drug exposure is often used as a surrogate for drug exposure in the brain interstitial space *(16)*. Since the cytotoxic activity of many anticancer agents is best correlated with exposure, an estimate of CSF drug exposure following systemic drug administration provides insight into whether or not an agent has potential utility in the treatment or prevention of CNS disease. CSF drug exposure is most accurately determined by comparing the ratio of steady-state concentrations in plasma and CSF or the ratio of the area under the plasma and CSF concentration–time curves (AUC_{CSF}/AUC_{plasma}) (Fig. 2). CSF exposure data are frequently derived from preclinical models, as it is neither practical nor feasible to routinely obtain serial CSF and plasma drug levels after systemic administration in humans. As demonstrated in Table 1, the CSF exposure for the most commonly used anticancer agents is <10% of the plasma exposure. As a result of this limited exposure, other approaches, such as high-dose chemotherapy and IT drug delivery, were developed to circumvent the blood–brain and blood–CSF barriers.

2.2. Systemic Chemotherapy

The primary advantages of systemic therapy compared with IT chemotherapy are that it is technically easier to administer and that it provides more uniform drug distribution throughout the neuraxis. In addition, there is the potential for prolonged CNS drug exposure after protracted infusions, which is of critical importance for cell-cycle specific cytotoxic agents. The primary disadvantage of systemic chemotherapy is that there is limited penetration of most hydrophilic agents into the CSF. Therefore, to attain cytotoxic levels of drug in the CSF after systemic dosing, very high doses of drug may be required.

Table 1
Central Nervous System Penetration
of Commonly Used Anticancer Drugs

Agent	CSF/Plasma ratio (%)
Alkylating agents	
Cyclophosphamide	
Total drug	50
Active metabolite	15
Ifosfamide	
Total drug	30
Active metabolite	15
Thiotepa	>95
Carmustine	>90
Cisplatin	
Free platinum	40
Total platinum	<5
Carboplatin	
Free platinum	30
Total platinum	<5
Antimetabolites	
Methotrexate	3
6-Mercaptopurine	25
Cytarabine	15
5-Fluorouracil	
Bolus	50
Infusion	15
Gemcitabine	7
Antitumor antibiotics	
Anthracyclines	ND
Dactinomycin	ND
Plant alkaloids	
Vinca alkaloids	5
Epipodophyllotoxins	<5
Topoisomerase I inhibitors (85,86)	
Topotecan	32
Irinotecan	
CPT-11 lactone	14
SN-38 lactone	<8
Miscellaneous	
Prednisolone	<10
Dexamethasone	15
l-Asparaginase	ND[a]

For most antineoplastic agents the total CSF drug exposure following administration of a systemic dose is <10% of the systemic exposure (87).
ND, Not detectable in CSF.
[a]Although drug is ND in CSF, CSF L-asparagine is depleted by systemic administration of L-asparaginase.

Although a high-dose strategy has been employed effectively with methotrexate, an agent for which calcium leucovorin provides adequate rescue from systemic toxicities *(17)*, this approach is generally not feasible because specific rescue agents or treatment strategies are not available for most antineoplastic agents. As a result, systemic toxicities, specifically the potential for severe or life-threatening myelosuppression, preclude the widespread use of high-dose chemotherapy without stem cell rescue.

2.3. Intrathecal Drug Delivery

IT chemotherapy is usually administered via lumbar puncture or via an indwelling ventricular access device (e.g., Ommaya reservoir). The primary advantage of intrathecally administered therapy is that it facilitates direct delivery of drug to the principal target tumor site, that is, the CSF and leptomeninges, using a relatively small drug dose. This is possible because the CSF volume of distribution is relatively small compared to the plasma volume of distribution (150 cm^3 vs 3500 cm^3). Therefore, high CSF drug exposure can be achieved using a relatively small drug dose, which minimizes the potential for systemic toxicity. In addition, because CSF drug clearance is often slower than systemic clearance, there is the potential for more prolonged drug exposure at the target site following bolus intrathecal drug administration *(18)*.

Although there are pharmacokinetic advantages associated with IT drug delivery, there are also disadvantages. Intralumbar drug administration may be associated with pain or suboptimal delivery to the subarachnoid space, owing to leakage or inadvertent injection into the subdural or epidural space *(19)*. In addition, there is heterogeneous drug distribution throughout the neuraxis after IT dosing due to the cephalo–caudad flow of CSF. As a result, after intralumbar dosing some agents may undergo metabolic inactivation or clearance via active transport or bulk flow prior to reaching the ventricles and cerebral convexities *(20–22)*. Finally, there is limited drug penetration (2–3 mm) from the CSF into the surrounding tissue, thereby limiting potential efficacy in patients with bulky leptomeningeal disease *(23)*. This is of particular concern for solid tumor metastases that may frequently include isolated or disseminated nodular tumor deposits, ranging in size from millimeters to centimeters, within the subarachnoid space or on the cranial or spinal nerve roots *(24)*.

Lumbar puncture is the most common method of IT drug delivery. Children with leukemia routinely receive intralumbar methotrexate, either as a single agent or in combination with cytarabine and hydrocortisone, in addition to their frontline systemic chemotherapy. Although lumbar punctures may cause local pain or discomfort, the procedure is generally well tolerated with the use of local anesthesia. In infants and very young children, the potential for pain and discomfort is reduced further by the use of either conscious or general sedation. Some investigators have attempted to use indwelling lumbar access devices to minimize procedural pain and to ensure drug delivery to the subarachnoid space. However, there is limited oncologic experience with intralumbar access devices. Such devices have inherent risks including bleeding and infection plus additional risks such as catheter breakage or leakage *(25)*. These devices are not recommended for routine IT drug administration for patients receiving preventative IT therapy.

Many of the limitations associated with intralumbar drug delivery can be overcome by the use of an intraventricular access device such as an Ommaya reservoir (Fig. 3). Ommaya reservoirs are frequently used in adults with leptomeningeal cancer because of technical difficulties in performing repeated lumbar punctures in patients with spinal stenosis. Ommaya reservoirs are also routinely used in children with nonleukemic neoplastic meningitis or refractory CNS leukemia. An obvious advantage to an Ommaya reservoir is that

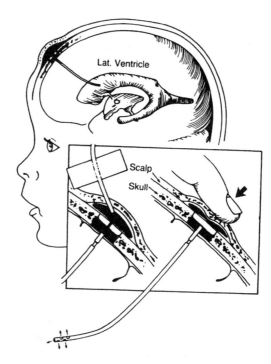

Fig. 3. Diagram of an intraventricular drug delivery system consisting of a subcutaneously implanted Ommaya reservoir attached to a catheter, the tip of which sits in the lateral ventricle. (Reprinted with permission from ref. *89.*)

it facilitates reliable drug delivery to the subarachnoid space. In addition, Ommaya reservoir injections are more convenient and less painful than intralumbar injections. In fact, the relative ease of intra-Ommaya drug delivery facilitates more effective, less toxic dosing schedules (*see* below). Finally, CSF drug distribution throughout the neuraxis is theoretically faster and more uniform after intraventricular injection, as CSF flow is not against gravity *(26).* The obvious disadvantage of an Ommaya reservoir is that it requires a neurosurgical procedure for placement. There is also the associated inherent risk of infection.

The classic example of an IT dosing approach facilitated by the placement of an Ommaya reservoir is the "concentration times time" ("$C \times T$") dosing schedule which involves administration of relatively small but frequent consecutive doses (daily × 3) of methotrexate or cytarabine (Fig. 4). The goal of "$C \times T$" dosing is to maximize efficacy, by attaining drug levels above a cytotoxic threshold level for a prolonged period of time, while minimizing toxicity, by avoiding high peak concentration–associated neurotoxicity (Fig. 5) *(27,28).* Several studies of the "$C \times T$" approach have suggested improved therapeutic results for intraventricular vs intralumbar chemotherapy in patients with recurrent CNS leukemia or lymphoma *(29,30).* The "$C \times T$" regimen was found to be as efficacious as the standard regimen and was associated with less neurotoxicity in a study of 19 patients with meningeal leukemia who were randomized to receive 12 mg/m^2 of intrathecal methotrexate twice weekly vs "$C \times T$" methotrexate (1 mg every 12 h for six doses) *(29).* In another study, the complete response duration following "$C \times T$" dosing was 15 mo for 14 of 15 patients (93%) with refractory meningeal leukemia or lymphoma *(30).*

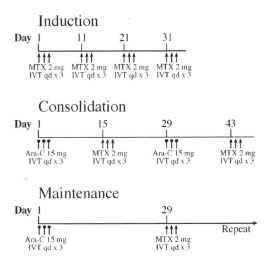

Fig. 4. Schematic diagram of the concentration × time ("$C \times T$") regimen for methotrexate and cytarabine. MTX, Methotrexate; Ara-C, cytarabine; IVT, intraventricular, qd, daily. *Note*: Doses are for patients > 3 yr of age. (Reprinted with permission from ref. *30*.)

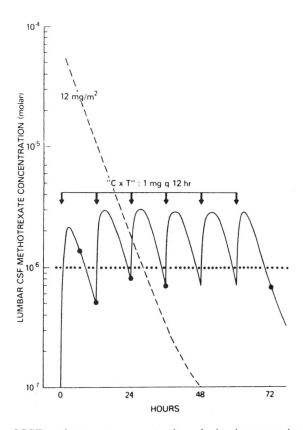

Fig. 5. Comparison of CSF methotrexate concentrations during intraventricular "$C \times T$" therapy (*solid line*) and after intraventricular injection of a single 12-mg/m² dose. *Horizontal dotted line*, approximation of the therapeutically effected methotrexate concentration. (Reprinted with permission from ref. *29*.)

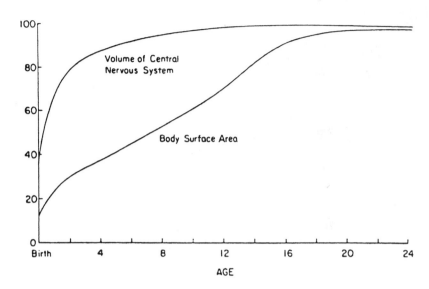

Fig. 6. Relationship between body surface area and CNS volume as a function of age. The CSF volume increases at a more rapid rate than BSA, reaching adult volume by 3 yr of age. (Reprinted with permission from ref. *33*.)

3. FACTORS AFFECTING DRUG EXPOSURE AND DISTRIBUTION AFTER IT ADMINISTRATION

Other unique considerations to IT drug administration that greatly affect CSF drug exposure and distribution include: relative changes in CSF volume of distribution with age; alterations in drug distribution due to alterations in CSF flow that directly or indirectly result from the underlying disease process; and alterations in drug distribution based on site of administration, that is, intraventricular or intralumbar; as well as on patient position following drug administration

3.1. Age-Based Dosing Recommendations for IT Agents

Whereas most systemically administered anticancer agents are dosed based on body surface area (BSA) or weight, dosing for IT anticancer agents is based on patient age *(31–33)*. This is because the CSF volume of infants and young children increases at a proportionally greater rate than BSA (Fig. 6). As a result, the CSF volume of infants and children is large relative to their BSA. In fact, by 3 yr of age the CSF volumes of adults and children are essentially the same. Thus, dosing practices based on age rather than BSA avoid "underdosing" infants and avoid "overdosing" adolescents and adults. As a result, age-based dosing recommendations for the commonly used IT agents are standard (Table 2). The direct advantages of age-based dosing for IT agents in children with CNS leukemia included less neurotoxicity, less variability in drug concentrations, and a reduction in the incidence of CNS relapse *(31–33)*.

3.2. Alterations in IT Drug Distribution

Unobstructed physiologic CSF flow and normal rates of CSF production and resorption are required for optimal drug distribution following IT administration. Nonuniform drug

Table 2
Dosage Regimens for Intralumbar Methotrexate
and Cytarabine Based on Patient Age

Patient age (yr)	Methotrexate dose (mg)	Cytarabine dose (mg)
<1	6	12
1	8	16
>2	10	20
≥3–9	12	24
≥10	15[a]	30

[a] Some investigators do not exceed methotrexate doses of 12 mg for patients ≥3 yr of age.

distribution throughout the neuraxis may compromise efficacy, as a result of inadequate drug exposure, or may increase the risk of local or delayed toxicities, owing to increased local drug exposure. Even in the absence of bulky leptomeningeal or parenchymal CNS disease, patients with neoplastic meningitis may have significant alterations in obstruction to normal CSF flow (34–36). Neuroimaging modalities, such as computed tomography (CT) or magnetic resonance imaging (MRI), are less sensitive in evaluating alterations in or obstruction to CSF flow than radionuclide CSF flow studies. Therefore, strong consideration should be given to obtaining a radionuclide CSF flow study, such as 111-DTPA or ^{99m}Tc-DTPA scan, prior to the initiation of IT chemotherapy, especially in patients with nonhematologic neoplastic meningitis. In some circumstances, focal CSF flow abnormalities can be readily restored through the use of local radiation to relieve the obstruction (35). IT chemotherapy should not be administered to patients with significant abnormalities in or obstruction to CSF flow.

3.3. Patient Position After IT Drug Administration

Patient position after IT drug administration may also have a major impact on CSF drug distribution, especially after intralumbar drug dosing. This has been confirmed in nonhuman primates that were maintained in either an upright or prone position for 1 h after intralumbar methotrexate dosing. Peak ventricular methotrexate concentrations and ventricular drug exposure were up to 10-fold greater in animals that remained prone. In addition, there was less variability in ventricular methotrexate levels when the animals were prone (37).

4. PHARMACOLOGY OF STANDARD ANTICANCER
AGENTS FOR IT ADMINISTRATION

4.1. Methotrexate

4.1.1. INTRALUMBAR METHOTREXATE

Intralumbar methotrexate is the most commonly used drug for IT administration. Interval administration of IT methotrexate for presymptomatic treatment of leptomeningeal leukemia, a standard component of front-line protocols for acute lymphocytic leukemias (ALL) and many lymphomas, has been instrumental in significantly decreasing the risk of CNS relapse in these settings (38,39). IT methotrexate is also effective in inducing CNS remissions in patients with overt CNS leukemia (40–42) and is commonly used for palliative treatment in the treatment of solid tumor neoplastic meningitis *(43)*. Nevertheless, the utility of methotrexate for most solid tumors is limited or has not been demonstrated due to its restricted spectrum of antitumor activity.

The initial detailed pharmacokinetic studies of methotrexate were performed prior to the development and routine implementation of age-based dosing guidelines. These studies revealed that after an intralumbar dose of 12 mg/m^2, CSF methotrexate elimination is biphasic with terminal half-lives of 4.5 and 14 h *(44)*. Average methotrexate levels in lumbar CSF exceed 10 μM at 6 h and fall to 0.1 μM by 48 h, while ventricular CSF levels averaged only 10% of simultaneous lumbar levels *(26,44)*. Drug elimination occurs primarily via bulk CSF resorption, although a nonspecific transport mechanism exists *(45)*.

As was previously discussed, intraventricular methotrexate administration may overcome many of the limitations associated with intralumbar dosing. Pharmacokinetic studies following an intraventricular methotrexate dose of 6.25 mg/m^2 reveal that peak ventricular methotrexate concentrations exceed 200 μM and remain above 0.2 μM for 48 h. In addition, there is good distribution throughout the neuraxis; lumbar CSF methotrexate is detected within 1 h and lumbar CSF levels exceed ventricular levels within 4 h after intraventricular dosing *(26)*.

4.1.2. TOXICITIES OF IT METHOTREXATE

The neurological toxicities associated with IT methotrexate can be characterized as acute, subacute, or delayed *(46)*. Acute toxicities are not uncommon and occur within several hours to a few days after drug administration. Commonly observed toxicities include headache, stiff neck, back pain, vomiting, fever, and lethargy. These adverse events may occur in isolation or may be associated with a CSF pleocytosis, indicative of a chemical arachnoiditis *(47)*. Subacute toxicities, occurring days to weeks after administration are relatively uncommon and are not always reversible. Subacute toxicities include paraplegia, myelopathy, or encephalopathy, with concomitant symptoms of weakness, ataxia, cranial nerve palsies, seizures, depression of mental status, or coma *(27,47)*. Leukoencephalopathy, a chronic progressive, demyelinating process, is a late neurotoxicity that may occur months to years after treatment. Leukoencephalopathy has most commonly been observed patients who received IT methotrexate combined with craniospinal irradiation *(28,47,48)*.

Plasma drug exposure after IT methotrexate is approx 100 times less than CSF exposure *(44)*. However, plasma levels of methotrexate exceed 0.01 μM for twice as long as following a systemic equivalent dose. Nonetheless, systemic toxicity is minimal, demonstrating one of the advantages of regional chemotherapy.

An unfortunate, albeit rare, event is the occurrence of an accidental overdose of IT methotrexate. This has most often occurred when a patient inadvertently receives the dose of methotrexate that was intended for intravenous administration. If untreated, the resultant overdose causes overwhelming acute neurotoxicity with subsequent severe morbidity or death. Treatment for such an overdose should include immediate CSF drainage, ventriculolumbar perfusion, and administration of systemic leucovorin and steroids *(49)*. In addition, carboxypeptidase-G2, a more specific antidote that converts methotrexate to an inactive metabolite, has recently been developed by Adamson and Widemann. Evaluation of carboxypeptidase-G2 in a preclinical nonhuman primate model demonstrated that after a methotrexate overdose of 50 mg (equivalent to 500 mg in humans), carboxypeptidase-G2 successfully reduced CSF methotrexate concentrations 400-fold within 5 min of administration *(49)*. Widemann et al. recently confirmed these observations in six patients who received accidental intrathecal methotrexate overdoses (median dose 482 mg). CSF methotrexate concentrations decreased in all but one patient by >95% following carboxypeptidase administration. Furthermore, all patients recovered completely with the exception of impaired short-term memory in one *(50)*. This potentially life-saving antidote is available to all Children's Oncology Group institutions in the United States. It should be available for immediate use in pharmacies of any hospital that routinely administers IT methotrexate.

4.2. Cytosine Arabinoside

Cytosine arabinoside (cytarabine, or ara-C) is the second most commonly used intrathecal agent. Similar to methotrexate, cytarabine is primarily used in the treatment and prevention of leptomeningeal leukemias and lymphomas. The disposition of cytarabine in the CSF after IT dosing is very different than plasma disposition after intravenous dosing owing to relative differences in cytidine deaminase levels between these two sites. Cytidine deaminase, a ubiquitous enzyme in the liver and blood, rapidly converts systemically administered cytarabine to an inactive metabolite, ara-U *(51,52)*. However, cytidine deaminase levels in human CSF are markedly lower than plasma levels. As a result, there is minimal conversion of cytarabine to ara-U following IT dosing *(52–54)*. Thus, there is a marked reduction in cytarabine clearance after IT vs systemic dosing. Cytarabine clearance after IT dosing is essentially that of CSF bulk flow, that is, 0.4 mL/min *(54)*, vs plasma clearance after intravenous dosing which approximates 1000–3600 mL/min/m^2 *(55)*. Thus, there is a tremendous pharmacokinetic advantage for IT cytarabine administration.

As with methotrexate, the duration of neoplastic cell exposure to cytotoxic concentrations of cytarabine is an important determinant of response. After intraventricular administration of a 30-mg cytarabine dose, elimination from CSF is biphasic with terminal half-lives of 1 and 3.4 h *(54)*. Peak CSF concentrations are > 2 mM and exceed 1 μM for more than 24 h. Plasma concentrations after a dose of IT cytarabine are undetectable.

In a simulated schedule of ara-C administered using a "$C \times T$" dosing approach, 30 mg daily for 3 d, cytotoxic concentrations were achieved for more than 72 h compared with approx 24 h after a single larger dose of 70 mg *(54)*. Thus, a "$C \times T$" approach is the preferred approach for attaining sustained CSF levels when the standard cytarabine formulation is utilized. Another alternative is use of a sustained-release cytarabine formulation, DTC101, that has recently been approved for use in the treatment of lymphomatous meningitis (discussed below).

4.2.1. TOXICITIES

The most common toxicity of cytarabine after IT administration is chemical arachnoiditis *(47)*. Less commonly, seizures, paraplegia, peripheral neuropathy, and encephalopathy have been reported *(47,56–58)*. Leukoencephalopathy has been reported with combined IT therapy and radiation *(59)*.

4.3. DTC101

DTC101 (DepoCyt™), a sustained-release formulation of cytarabine for intrathecal administration, was specifically developed to maximize the therapeutic efficacy of this S-phase-specific agent *(60)*. Pharmacokinetic studies after a single dose of DTC101 demonstrate that this novel formulation improves drug distribution throughout the neuraxis. Within 6 h of intraventricular delivery, lumbar CSF concentrations are equivalent to ventricular concentrations. In addition, DTC101 increases the terminal CSF half-life, vs that of standard cytarabine, by approx 40-fold (3.4–141 h) *(61)*. Thus, an obvious advantage of DTC101 is that it can be administered less frequently than standard cytarabine.

Randomized multicenter trials comparing DTC101 vs methotrexate in adults with lymphomatous meningitis demonstrated that there was a trend to improvement in neurologic progression and median survival in the DTC101 arm (62). Likewise, in adults with neoplastic meningitis due to solid tumors, there was a trend toward increased time to neurological progression in the DTC101-treated patients (62).

Studies in children demonstrate that despite equivalent CSF volumes, pediatric patients ≥ 3 yr of age appear to tolerate a somewhat lower dose of DTC101 than adults. The recommended treatment dose for adults is 50 mg while in the Phase I pediatric study the maximum tolerated dose (MTD) was 35 mg (63). At higher doses, children experience protracted headaches. Despite the lower dosage recommendation, DTC101 appears to be an active agent in children with refractory leptomeningeal leukemia with seven of nine patients experiencing an objective response. Pharmacokinetic studies at the pediatric recommended Phase II dose of 35 mg demonstrated that 8 d after DTC101 administration, four of five patients still had free cytarabine CSF levels ≥ 0.4 µM.

The primary disadvantage of DTC101 vs standard cytarabine is the toxicity profile. DTC101 must be given with concomitant oral dexamethasone for approx 5 d to prevent chemical meningitis. Otherwise, the toxicity profile of intrathecal DTC101 plus dexamethasone is very similar to that of the standard cytarabine formulation. Acute toxicities include fever, headache, back pain, nausea, and encephalopathy (61).

4.4. Thiotepa

Thiotepa is a lipid-soluble alkylating agent that has been administered by the IT route to children and adults with neoplastic meningitis. Thiotepa is rapidly converted to an active metabolite, TEPA, after intravenous administration; and both thiotepa and TEPA readily and extensively penetrate into the CSF after systemic dosing. In contrast, after IT administration there is no intra-CSF conversion to TEPA, and CSF clearance exceeds bulk flow by almost ninefold (64). Therefore, there is not a pharmacokinetic advantage for this lipophilic agent after regional drug administration.

Clinical studies of IT thiotepa have failed to provide compelling evidence for its use. In a randomized prospective study evaluating IT methotrexate vs IT thiotepa in adults with neoplastic meningitis, the overall toxicity and efficacy of these agents were essentially identical and overall quite dismal. The median survival for the methotrexate group was 15.9 wk vs 14.1 wk for the thiotepa group (65). Likewise, in a retrospective study of 15 children with neoplastic meningitis who received IT thiotepa in combination with other therapy the median survival was only 15.1 wk (66).

5. NEW AGENTS FOR IT ADMINISTRATION

The limited number and spectrum of antineoplastic agents that significantly penetrate the blood–brain and blood–CSF barriers and the paucity of agents that are available for IT administration impose significant limitations on the development of strategies to successfully prevent or treat solid tumor neoplastic meningitis or refractory CNS leukemia. Combination chemotherapy regimens are an integral component of successful treatment regimens for many systemic cancers. However, similar strategies cannot be employed for neoplastic meningitis because, with the exception of IT, combination regimens are not available. Therefore, we must identify additional agents suitable for IT administration or agents with favorable toxicity profiles and high CSF/plasma exposure ratios. We have used a nonhuman primate model to identify several candidate agents for IT administration. In this section we summarize the current status of ongoing clinical trials with these novel agents that hold promise for future widespread study.

5.1. Mafosfamide

Cyclophosphamide is a widely used alkylating agent that has a broad spectrum of antitumor activity against many pediatric and adult cancers. However, cyclophosphamide requires oxidation by hepatic microsomal enzymes to express activity and thus is not a candidate for IT or other regional therapeutic approaches. Mafosfamide is a cyclophosphamide derivative that does not require hepatic activation for tumoricidal effect. The spectrums of antitumor activity for mafosfamide and cyclophosphamide are essentially identical. Thus, mafosfamide was deemed an excellent candidate for further study.

Preclinical in vitro studies, using a representative panel of tumor cell lines with a predilection for leptomeningeal spread, were performed to define an optimal cytotoxic exposure. Preclinical studies in a nonhuman primate demonstrated the feasibility of this dosing approach and provided data for a safe starting dose *(67)*. A Phase I study of IT mafosfamide as a single agent is ongoing. Initial results demonstrate that headache and pain during or shortly after drug administration are dose limiting at the 6.5-mg dose level. Unfortunately, pharmacokinetic studies at this dose level showed there was not adequate drug exposure throughout the neuraxis for optimal cytotoxicity *(68)*. Therefore, strategies to facilitate dosage escalation, including decreasing the dose rate of administration and prophylactic treatment with analgesics, have been employed. Patients are currently being enrolled at the 12-mg dose level with a plan to continue dose escalations until, in the absence of neurotoxicity, exposure is deemed to be adequate in both the ventricular and lumbar CSF.

IT mafosfamide has also been incorporated into a Pediatric Brain Tumor Consortium front-line treatment protocol for infants and young children (< 3 yr of age) with embryonal CNS tumors. The rationale for this front-line treatment approach is that infants and young children with primary CNS tumors frequently have leptomeningeal tumor involvement either at diagnosis or at time of tumor progression. In addition, they have a very poor overall prognosis *(69)*. Therefore, we are evaluating the feasibility of a regional therapy approach using IT mafosfamide during the first 20 wk of systemic therapy, followed by conformal radiotherapy, and 20 more wk of systemic therapy. The ultimate goal of this approach is to improve leptomeningeal disease control and to minimize or eliminate the need for radiation therapy and its inherent morbidity.

5.2. Topotecan

Topotecan is a water-soluble topoisomerase I poison that has demonstrated objective antitumor activity against a variety of adult and pediatric malignancies including non-small-cell lung cancer, ovarian carcinoma, leukemias, and rhabdomyosarcomas. This spectrum of antitumor activity and lack of neurologic toxicity after systemic administration led to a series of preclinical studies that demonstrated the feasibility of IT drug delivery. A Phase I study of IT topotecan was recently completed. Arachnoiditis characterized by fever, nausea, vomiting, and headache with or without back pain was the dose-limiting toxicity in two of four patients enrolled at the 0.7-mg dose level. The MTD was subsequently defined as 0.4 mg. Six of the 23 evaluable patients had evidence of benefit manifested as prolonged disease stabilization or response *(70)*. A pediatric Phase II trial of IT toptecan was subsequently initiated by the Children's Oncology Group. The primary study endpoints of this ongoing study are response rate in patients with CNS leukemia in second or greater relapse and response rate and progression-free survival in children with leptomeningeal medulloblastoma.

5.3. Busulfan

Busulfan is a dimethanesulfonyloxyalkane that functions as a cell-cycle nonspecific alkylating agent. Clinical busulfan use is generally restricted to preparative regimens for bone marrow transplant owing to profound systemic toxicities, including severe myelosuppression and pulmonary fibrosis. Historically, regional busulfan administration was limited by its poor solubility in aqueous solutions *(71)*. However, a microcrystalline formulation of busulfan with greatly enhanced aqueous solubility, Spartaject busulfan, was recently developed. This formulation was specifically developed for IT administration based on preclinical studies demonstrating antitumor activity against medulloblastoma cell lines and xenografts. Subsequent studies in a nude rat model of neoplastic meningitis demonstrated antitumor activity, although toxicity studies suggested that there may be a very narrow therapeutic window *(71)*. Phase I studies to evaluate the safety and feasibility and to identify a dose of intrathecal busulfan for subsequent evaluation of efficacy are currently in progress *(72)*.

5.4. Gemcitabine

Gemcitabine (2', 2'-difluorodeoxycytidine or dFdC), a deoxycytidine analog, has a broad spectrum of clinical antitumor activity against a variety of tumors with potential for leptomeningeal spread *(73–77)*. Similar to cytarabine, gemcitabine is rapidly deaminated to an inactive metabolite following intravenous administration, thereby limiting CSF gemcitabine exposure *(78)*. Studies in the nonhuman primate model were thus performed to evaluate the feasibility and toxicity of IT administration of gemcitabine *(79)*. After a 5-mg IT gemcitabine dose (equivalent to 50 mg in humans), CSF drug exposure (measured by AUC) was eight times that in plasma after a 400-fold higher intravenous dose *(79)*. A Phase I study of IT gemcitabine for neoplastic meningitis has recently been initiated.

6. CONCLUSION

Significant advances in the treatment and prevention of CNS leukemias and lymphomas have been a direct result of a better understanding of CNS pharmacology and the development of effective therapeutic strategies to circumvent the limitations imposed by the blood–brain and blood–CSF barriers. Unfortunately, the treatment and prevention of leptomeningeal metastases from solid tumors and the treatment of recurrent CNS leukemia remain unsatisfactory. Further advancements in the treatment of this devastating disease require continued preclinical and clinical research efforts to identify new agents and combination regimens for IT administration and to evaluate new treatment strategies such as IT delivery of monoclonal antibodies or immunotherapies *(80–84)*. Furthermore, correlative clinical pharmacology studies to maximize efficacy and minimize toxicity are of paramount importance in ensuring that optimal dosing strategies are developed.

REFERENCES

1. Nugent J, Bunn PJ, Matthews M, et al. CNS metastases in small cell bronchogenic carcinoma: increasing frequency and changing pattern with lengthening survival. Cancer 1979; 44:1885–1883.
2. Rosen S, Aisner J, Makuch R, et al. Carcinomatous leptomeningitis in small cell lung cancer: a clinicopathologic review of the National Cancer Institute experience. Medicine 1982; 61:45–53.
3. Yap H, Yap B, Tashima C, DiStefano A, Blumenschein G. Meningeal carcinomatosis in breast cancer. Cancer 1978; 42:283–286.
4. Chintagumpala M, Berg SL, Blaney S. Treatment controversies in medulloblastoma. Curr Opin Oncol 2001; 13:154–159.
5. Whelan H, Sung J, Mastri A. Diffuse leptomeningeal gliomatosis: report of three cases. Clin Neuropathol 1987; 6:164–168.
6. Meli F, Boccaleri C, Manzitti J, Lylyk P. Meningeal dissemination of retinoblastoma: CT findings in with patients. Am J Neuroradiol 1990; 11:983–986.
7. Blatt J, Fitz C, Mirro J, Jr. Recognition of central nervous system metastases in children with metastatic primary extracranial neuroblastoma. Pediatr Hematol Oncol 1997; 14:233–241.

8. Shaw PJ, Eden T. Neuroblastoma with intracranial involvement: an ENSG study. Med Pediatr Oncol 1992; 20:149–155.

9. Kline R, Oseas R, Jolley S, et al. Leptomeningeal metastasis from a paraspinal rhabdomyosarcoma with a del(13)t(1:13)(q23,q32) in a 14-month-old boy. Cancer Genet Cytogenet 1997; 15:97–101.

10. Pardridge W, Oldendorf W, Cancilla P, et al. Blood–brain barrier: interface between internal medicine and the brain. Ann Intern Med 1986; 105:82–95.

11. Betz A. An overview of the multiple functions of the blood-brain barrier. NIDA Res Monogr 1992; 120:5–72.

12. Rao VV, Dahlheimer JL, Bardgett ME, et al. Choroid plexus epithelial expression of MDR1 P glyco-protein and multidrug resistance-associated protein contribute to the blood-cerebrospinal-fluid drug-permeability barrier. Proc Natl Acad Sci USA 1999; 96:3900–3905.

13. Schinkel A. P-glycoprotein, a gatekeeper in the blood-brain barrier. Adv Drug Deliv Rev 1999; 36:179–194.

14. Angeletti RH, Novikoff PM, Juvvadi SR, Fritschy JM, Meier PJ, Wolkoff AW. The choroid plexus epithelium is the site of the organic anion transport protein in the brain. Proc Natl Acad Sci USA 1997; 94:283–286.

15. Wijnholds J, deLange EC, Scheffer GL, et al. Multidrug resistance protein 1 protects the choroid plexus epithelium and contributes to the blood–cerebrospinal fluid barrier. J Clin Invest 2000; 105: 279–285.

16. Patel M, Blaney S, Balis F. Pharmacokinetics of drug delivery to the central nervous system. In: Grochow L, Ames M (eds). A Clinician's Guide to Chemotherapy Pharmacokinetics and Pharmaco-dynamics. Baltimore, MD: Williams & Wilkins, 1998, pp. 67–90.

17. Balis F, Savitch J, Bleyer B, Reaman G, Poplack D. Remission induction of meningeal leukemia with high-dose intravenous methotrexate. J Clin Oncol 1985; 11:74–86.

18. Poplack D, Bleyer W, Horowitz M. Pharmacology of antineoplastic agents in cerebrospinal fluid. In: Wood JH (ed). Neurobiology of Cerebrospinal Fluid, Vol. II. New York, NY: Plenum Press, 1980, pp. 561–568.

19. Larson S, Schall G, DiChiro G. The influence of previous lumbar puncture and pneumoencephalog-raphy on the incidence of unsuccessful radioisotope cisternography. J Nucl Med 1971; 12:555–557.

20. Di Chiro G, Hammock MK, Bleyer WA. Spinal descent of cerebrospinal fluid in man. Neurology 1976; 26:1–8.

21. Rieselbach RE, Di Chiro G, Freireich EJ, Rall DP. Subarachnoid distribution of drugs after lumbar injection. N Engl J Med 1962; 267:1273–1278.

22. Haaxma-Reiche H, Piers DA, Beekhuis H. Normal cerebrospinal fluid dynamics: a study with intra-ventricular injection of 111-In-DTPA in leukemia and lymphoma without meningeal involvement. Arch Neurol 1989; 46:997–999.

23. Blasberg R, Patlak C, Fernstermacher J. Intrathecal chemotherapy. Brain tissue profiles after ventriculo-cisternal perfusion. J Pharmacol Exp Ther 1975; 195:73–83.

24. Sagar S. Carcinomatous meningitis: it does not have to be a death sentence. Oncology 2002; 237–243.

25. Penn R, York M, Paice J. Catheter systems for intrathecal drug delivery. J Neurosurg 1995; 83:215–217.

26. Shapiro W, Young D, Mehta M. Methotrexate: distribution in cerebrospinal fluid after intravenous, ventricular and lumbar injections. N Engl J Med 1975; 293:161–166.

27. Bleyer W, Drake J, Chabner B. Neurotoxicity and elevated cerebrospinal fluid methotrexate concen-tration in meningeal leukemia. N Engl J Med 1973; 289:770–773.

28. Price R, Jamieson P. The central nervous system in childhood leukemia. II. Subacute leukoencepha-lopathy. Cancer 1975; 35:306–318.

29. Bleyer W, Poplack D, Simon R, et al. 'Concentration × time' methotrexate via a subcutaneous reser-voir: a less toxic regimen for intraventricular chemotherapy of central nervous system neoplasms. Blood 1978; 51:835–842.

30. Moser AM, Adamson PC, Gillespie AJ, Poplack DG, Balis FM. Intraventricular concentration times time (C × T) methotrexate and cytarabine for patients with recurrent meningeal leukemia and lym-phoma. Cancer 1999; 85:511–516.

31. Bleyer W, Savitch J, Holcenberg J. An improved regimen for intrathecal chemotherapy. Clin Pharmacol Ther 1976; 19:103.

32. Bleyer W. Clinical pharmacology of intrathecal methotrexate. II. An improved dosage regimen derived from age-related pharmacokinetics. Cancer Treat Rep 1977; 61:1419–1425.

33. Bleyer W, Coccia P, Sather H, et al. Reduction in central nervous system leukemia with a pharmacokinetically derived intrathecal methotrexate dosage regimen. J Clin Oncol 1983; 1:317–325.

34. Chamberlain MC. Leptomeningeal metastasis: a comparison of gadolinium-enhanced MR and contrast-enhanced CT of the brain. Neurology 1990; 40:435–447.
35. Glantz M, Hall W, Cole B, et al. Diagnosis, management, and survival of patients with leptomeningeal cancer based on cerebrospinal fluid-flow status. Cancer 1995; 75:2919–2931.
36. Grossman S, Trump D, Chen D, Thompson G, Camargo E. Cerebrospinal fluid flow abnormalities in patients with neoplastic meningitis: an evaluation using [111]Indium-DTPA ventriculography. Am J Med 1982; 73:641–647.
37. Blaney S, Poplack D, Godwin K, McCully C, Murphy R, Balis F. The effect of body position on ventricular cerebrospinal fluid methotrexate concentration following intralumbar administration. J Clin Oncol 1995; 13:177–179.
38. Pullen J, Boyett J, Shuster J, et al. Extended triple intrathecal chemotherapy trial for prevention of CNS relapse in good-risk and poor-risk patients with B-progenitor acute lymphoblastic leukemia: a Pediatric Oncology Group study. J Clin Oncol 1993; 11:839–849.
39. Tubergen D, Gilchrist G, O'Brien R, et al. Prevention of CNS disease in intermediate-risk acute lymphoblastic leukemia: comparison of cranial radiation and intrathecal methotrexate and the importance of systemic therapy: a Children's Cancer Group report. J Clin Oncol 1993; 11:520–526.
40. Kumar P, Kun L, Hustu H, et al. Survival outcome following isolated central nervous sytem relapse treated with additional chemotherapy and craniospinal irradiation in childhood acute lymphoblastic leukemia. Int J Radiat Oncol Biol Phys 1995; 31:477–483.
41. Kun L, Camitta B, Mulhern R, et al. Treatment of meningeal relapse in childhood acute lymphoblastic leukemia. I. Results of craniospinal irradiation. J Clin Oncol 1984; 2:359–364.
42. Ribiero R, Rivera G, Hudson M, et al. An intensive re-treatment protocol for children with an isolated CNS relapse of acute lymphoblastic leukemia. J Clin Oncol 1995; 13:333–338.
43. Grossman SA, Spence A. NCCN clinic practice guidelines for carcinomatous/lymphomatous meningitis. Oncology 1999; 13:144–152.
44. Bleyer W, Poplack D. Clinical studies on the central-nervous-system pharmacology of methotrexate. In: Pinedo H (ed). Clinical Pharmacology of Antineoplastic Drugs. Amsterdam: Elsevier/North-Holland Biomedica, 1978, pp. 115–131.
45. Bode U, McGrath I, Bleyer W, Poplack D, Glaubiger D. Active transport of methotrexate from cerebrospinal fluid in humans. Cancer Res 1980; 40:2184–2187.
46. Bleyer W. Neurologic sequelae of methotrexate and ionizing radiation: a new classification. Cancer Treat Rep 1981; 65:89–98.
47. Kaplan R, Wiernik P. Neurotoxicity of antineoplastic drugs. Semin Oncol 1982; 9:103–130.
48. Price R. Therapy related central nervous system disease in children with acute lymphocytic leukemia. In: Mastrangelo R, Poplack D, Riccardi R (eds). Central Nervous System Leukemia. Boston, MA: Martinus Nijhoff, 1983, pp. 71–81.
49. Adamson P, Balis F, McCully C, et al. Rescue of experimental intrathecal methotrexate overdose with carboxypeptidase-G$_2$. J Clin Oncol 1991; 9:670–674.
50. Widemann B, Balis F, Shalabi A, et al. Carboxypeptidase-G2 (CPDG2) treatment of accidental intrathecal (IT) methotrexate (MTX) overdose. Proc Am Soc Clin Oncol 2002; 21:123a.
51. Camiener G, Smith C. Studies of the enzymatic deamination of cytosine arabinoside. I. Enzyme distribution and species specificity. Biochem Pharmacol 1965; 14:1405–1416.
52. Ho D, Frei E. Clinical pharmacology of 1-β-D-arabinofuranosyl cytosine. Clin Pharmacol Ther 1971; 12:944–954.
53. Przuntek H, Breithaupt H. Cytarabine: distribution in ventricular cerebrospinal fluid after lumbar injection. J Neurol 1981; 226:73–76.
54. Zimm S, Collins J, Miser J, Chatterji D, Poplack D. Cytosine arabinoside cerebrospinal fluid kinetics. Clin Pharmacol Ther 1984; 35:826–830.
55. Berry B, Erlichman C. Clinical pharmacology of anticancer agents. In: Schilsky R, Milano G, Ratain M (eds). Principles of Antineoplastic Drug Development and Pharmacology. New York, NY: Marcel Dekker, 1996, pp. 75–122.
56. Russell JA, Powles RL. Neuropathy due to cytosine arabinoside. Br Med J 1974; 14:652–653.
57. Wolff L, Zighelboim J, Gale R. Paraplegia following intrathecal cytosine arabinoside. Cancer 1979; 43:83–88.
58. Eden O, Goldie W, Wood T, Etcubanas E. Seizures following intrathecal cytosine arabinoside in young children with acute lymphocytic leukemia. Cancer 1978; 42:53–58.
59. Baker W, Royer G, Weiss R. Cytarabine and neurologic toxicity. J Clin Oncol 1992; 9:679–693.

60. Kim S, Khatibi S, Howell S, McCully C, Balis F, Poplack D. Prolongation of drug exposure in cerebrospinal fluid by encapsulation into DepoFoam. Cancer Res 1993; 53:1596–1598.
61. Kim S, Chatelut E, Kim J, et al. Extended CSF cytarabine exposure following intrathecal administration of DTC 101. J Clin Oncol 1993; 11:2186–2193.
62. Glantz MJ, Jaeckle KA, Chamberlain MC, et al. A randomized controlled trial comparing intrathecal sustained-release cytarabine (DepoCyt) to intrathecal methotrexate in patients with neoplastic meningitis from solid tumors. Clin Cancer Res 1999; 5:3394–3402.
63. Bomgaars L, Geyer J, Franklin J, et al. A Phase I study of intrathecal liposomal cytarabine (DepoCytTM) in pediatric patients with advanced meningeal malignancies. Proc Am Soc Clin Oncol 2002; 21:109a.
64. Strong J, Collins J, Lester C, Poplack D. Pharmacokinetics of intraventricular and intravenous N,N',N''-triethylenethiophosphoramide (thiotepa) in Rhesus monkeys and humans. Cancer Res 1986; 46:6101–6104.
65. Grossman S, Finkelstein D, Ruckdeschel J, Trump D, Moynihan T, Ettinger D. Randomized prospective comparison of intraventricular methotrexate and thiotepa in patients with previously untreated neoplastic meningitis. Eastern Cooperative Oncology Group. J Clin Oncol 1993; 11:561–569.
66. Fisher P, Kadan-Lottick N, Korones D. Intrathecal thiotepa: reappraisal of an established therapy. J Pediatr Hematol Oncol 2002; 24:274–278.
67. Blaney S, Balis F, Murphy R, Arndt C, Gillespie A, Poplack D. A Phase 1 study of intrathecal mafosfamide (MF) in patients with refractory meningeal malignances. Proceedings of American Society of Clinical Oncology. 1992; 11:113, abstract 274.
68. Blaney S, Balis F, Murphy R, Arndt C, Gillespie A, Poplack D. A Phase I study of intrathecal mafosfamide in patients with refractory meningeal malignancies. Proc Am Soc Clin Oncol 1992; 11:113.
69. Blaney S, Boyett J, Friedman H, et al. Phase I trial of intrathecal mafosfamide in infants with embryonal CNS tumors: a Pediatric Brain Tumor Consortium Study, International Symposium on Pediatric Neuro-Oncology, London, England, 2002.
70. Blaney S, Heideman R, Berg S, et al. Phase I clinical trial of intrathecal topotecan in patients with neoplastic meningitis. J Clin Oncol 2003; 21:143–147.
71. Archer GE, Sampson JH, McLendon RE, et al. Intrathecal busulfan treatment of human neoplastic meningitis in athymic nude rats. J Neuro-Oncol 1999; 44:233–241.
72. Quinn JA, Glantz M, Petros W, et al. Phase I trial of intrathecal Spartaject busulfan for patients with neoplastic meningitis. Proc Am Soc Clin Oncol 2002; 21:80a.
73. Hui YF, Reitz J. Gemcitabine: a cytidine analog active against solid tumors. Am J Hlth Syst Pharm 1997; 54:162–170.
74. Storniolo AM, Enas NH, Brown CA, Voi M, Rothenberg ML, Schilsky R. An investigational new drug treatment program for patients with gemcitabine: results for over 3000 patients with pancreatic carcinoma. Cancer 1999; 85:1261–1268.
75. Luftner D, Flath B, Akrivakis C, Grunewald R, Mergenthaler HG, Possinger K. Gemcitabine for palliative treatment in metastatic breast cancer. J Cancer Res Clin Oncol 1998; 124:527–531.
76. Postmus PE, Schramel FMNH, Smit EF. Evaluation of new drugs in small cell lung cancer: the activity of gemcitabine. Semin Oncol 1998; 25:79–82.
77. Vogelzang NJ, Stadler WM. Gemcitabine and other new chemotherapeutic agents for the treatment of metastatic bladder cancer. Urology 1999; 53:243–250.
78. Kerr JZ, Berg SL, Egorin MJ, et al. Pharmacokinetics of intravenous (IV) gemcitabine (DFDC) in nonhuman primates (NHP). Proc Am Assoc Cancer Res 2000; 41:706, abstract 4488A.
79. Egorin MJ, Zuhowski EG, McCully CM, et al. Pharmacokinetics of intrathecal (I.T.) gemcitabine (DFDC) in non-human primates (NHP). Proc Am Assoc Cancer Res 2000; 41:490, abstract 3128.
80. Papanastassiou V, Pizer B, Chandler C, Zananiri T, Kemshead J, Hopkins K. Pharmacokinetics and dose estimates following intrathecal administration of ^{131}I-monoclonal antibodies for the treatment of central nervous system malignancies. Int J Radiat Oncol Biol Phys 1995; 31:541–552.
81. Brown MT, Coleman RE, Friedman AH, et al. Intrathecal ^{131}I-labeled antitenascin monoclonal antibody 81C6 treatment of patients with leptomeningeal neoplasms or primary brain tumor resection cavities with subarachnoid communication: Phase 1 trial results. Clin Cancer Res 1996; 2:963–972.
82. Pastan I, Archer C, McLendon R, et al. Intrathecal administration of single-chain immunotoxin, LMB-7 [B3(Fv)-PE38], produces cures of carcinomatous meningitis in a rat model. Proc Natl Acad Sci USA 1995; 92:2765–2769.

83. Gunther R, Chelstrom L, Tuel-Ahlgren L, Simon J, Myers D, Uckun F. Biotherapy for xenografted human central nervous system leukemia in mice with severe combined immunodeficiency using B43 (Anti-CD19)-pokeweed antiviral protein immunotoxin. Blood 1995; 85:2537–2545.
84. Puri RK, Hoon DS, Leland P, et al. Preclinical development of a recombinant toxin containing circularly permuted interleukin 4 and truncated *Pseudomonas* exotoxin for therapy of malignant astrocytoma. Cancer Res 1996; 56:5631–5637.
85. Blaney S, Cole D, Godwin D, Sung C, Poplack D, Balis F. Intrathecal administration of topotecan in nonhuman primates. Cancer Chemother Pharmacol 1995; 36:121–124.
86. Blaney S, Heideman R, Cole D, et al. A Phase I study of intrathecal topotecan. Proc Am Soc Cancer Res 1998; 39:2198.
87. Balis F, Poplack D. Cancer Chemotherapy. In: Nathan DG, Oski FA (eds). Hematology of Infancy and Childhood, 4th Edit. Philadelphia, PA: WB Saunders, 1993, pp. 1207–1238.
88. Blaney S, Cole D, Balis F, Godwin K, Poplack D. Plasma and cerebrospinal fluid pharmacokinetic study of topotecan in nonhuman primates. Cancer Res 1993; 53:725–727.
89. Balis F, Poplack D. Central nervous system pharmacology of antileukemia drugs. Am J Pediatr Hematol Oncol 1989; 11:74–86.

19 Use of Microdialysis in Preclinical and Clinical Development of Anticancer Agents

William C. Zamboni, Pharm D

CONTENTS

INTRODUCTION
MICRODIALYSIS METHODOLOGY AND STUDY DESIGN
PRECLINICAL MICRODIALYSIS STUDIES IN TUMOR AND TISSUE
CLINICAL MICRODIALYSIS STUDIES
PHARMACODYNAMIC STUDIES USING MICRODIALYSIS
SUMMARY AND FUTURE DIRECTIONS

1. INTRODUCTION

1.1. Issues Related to Drug Delivery in Solid Tumors

Major advances have been made in the use of cancer chemotherapy *(1)*. However, most patients, especially those diagnosed with solid tumors, fail to respond to initial treatment or relapse after an initial response *(1)*. Thus, there is a need to identify factors associated with lack of response and to develop new treatment strategies that address those factors. The development of effective chemotherapeutic agents for the treatment of solid tumors depends, in part, on the ability of those agents to achieve cytotoxic drug concentrations or exposure within the tumor *(2,3)*.

It is currently unclear why within a patient with solid tumors there can be a reduction in the size of some tumors while other tumors can progress during or after treatment, even though the genetic composition of the tumors is similar *(4)*. Such variable antitumor responses within a single patient may be associated with inherent differences in tumor vascularity, capillary permeability, and/or tumor interstitial pressure that result in variable delivery of anticancer agents to different tumor sites *(2,3)*. However, studies evaluating the intratumoral concentration of anticancer agents and factors affecting tumor exposure in preclinical models and patients are rare *(3,5,6)*. In addition, preclinical models evaluating tumor exposure of anticancer agents and factors affecting tumor exposure may not reflect the disposition of chemotherapeutic agents in patients with solid tumors owing to differences in vascularity and lymphatic drainage *(2,3)*. Moreover, it is logistically difficult to perform the extensive studies required to evaluate the tumor disposition of anticancer agents and factors that determine the disposition in patients with solid tumors,

Handbook of Anticancer Pharmacokinetics and Pharmacodynamics
Edited by: W. D. Figg and H. L. McLeod © Humana Press Inc., Totowa, NJ

307

especially in tumors that are not easily accessible. Thus, there is an impending need to develop and implement techniques and methodologies to evaluate the disposition and exposure of anticancer agents within the tumor matrix.

The need to develop and readily gain information on the tumor disposition of agents may become more important with the increasing number of tumor targeting approaches, such as gene and antisense therapy, polyethylene glycol (PEG)-conjugated agents, and liposomal delivery *(7,8)*. In addition, methodology and study designs used to develop classic cytotoxic anticancer agents, such as platinum, taxane, and camptothecin analogs, may not be appropriate for the new generations of anticancer therapy, such as angiogenesis inhibitors, antiproliferative agents, and signal transduction inhibitors *(7,9)*. As these agents may not induce classic toxicities or any toxicities, it may be difficult to recommend a dose for future trials using the standard Phase I dose escalation methods and endpoints (i.e., maximum tolerable dose and dose-limiting toxicities). Alternatively, defining the dose for Phase II studies could be based on the dose that achieves exposures associated with pharmacologic modulation, optimal biological exposure, or cytotoxicity results from in vitro studies *(3,10)*. Historically, investigators have compared in vitro IC_{50} values with plasma concentrations in patients as a means to determine if sufficient exposure has been reached in clinical studies. However, the inherent tumor characteristics that influence tumor penetration and high intra- and intertumoral variability in tumor exposure makes this comparison highly unreliable *(2,3,11)*, especially when the ratio of tumor exposure to plasma exposure may be approx 0.2 to 0.5 *(3,12–15)*. Thus, comparing the in vitro exposures and plasma exposures in patients results in an overestimation of drug exposure in the tumor extracellular fluid (ECF), and thus the exposure required for an effect may be insufficient. The use of methodologies that measure the exposure of anticancer agents within the tumor may improve the level of information needed to make informed decisions during the drug development process.

1.2. Methods to Measure Drug Disposition in Tumors and Tissue

Until recently, drug uptake into tissues and tumors has been described indirectly based on modeling from plasma pharmacokinetics or measured directly from tissue biopsies. As stated above, modeling of tumor exposure based on plasma exposures without incorporation of factors representing tumor heterogenity is unreliable *(2,3,11)*. The use of tissue or tumor biopsies is associated with several problems. Obtaining serial biopsies is most often logistically impossible, highly invasive, and associated with patient discomfort *(3,16,17)*. Thus, biopsies are usually available only for a single time point or measurement. Measurements of drug concentrations from biopsies are obtained in tissue or tumor homogenates, where it may be difficult to control ex vivo catabolism and differentiate between various forms of the drug. Several new advanced techniques, such as magnetic resonance imaging (MRI), positron emission tomography (PET), and microdialysis, have been developed to quantify the concentrations of anticancer agents in vivo *(16–18)*. However, the use of MRI and PET is complicated by the lack of ability to differentiate between different forms and metabolites of a drug, availability, chemical synthesis of effective probes, and cost *(17,18)*. Microdialysis to evaluate the disposition of anticancer agents in tumors and surrounding tissue, on the other hand, is a methodology that has several advantages over other existing methods *(2,7,19,20)*.

1.3. Introduction and Advantages of Microdialysis

Microdialysis is an in vivo sampling technique used to study the pharmacokinetics and drug metabolism in the blood and ECF of various tissues *(19–21)*. The use of microdialysis methodology to evaluate the disposition of anticancer agents in tumors is relatively new *(3,5,6)*. Microdialysis has been used to evaluate the tumor disposition of 5-fluorouracil and

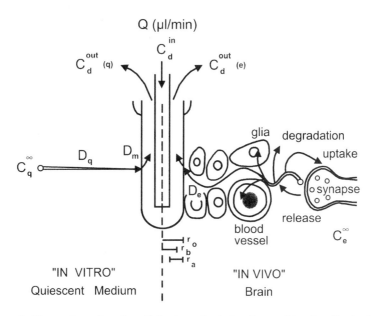

Fig. 1. Schematic illustration of a microdialysis probe in in vitro and in vivo (brain tissue) and the difference in diffusion paths.

carboplatin in patients with primary breast cancer lesions and melanoma, respectively *(5,6)*. These studies depict the clinical utility of microdialysis in evaluating the tumor disposition of anticancer agents in patients with accessible tumors. Microdialysis is based on the diffusion of non-protein-bound drugs from interstitial fluid across the semipermeable membrane of the microdialysis probe *(19–21)*. A schematic representation of a microdialysis probe in subcutaneous tissue or tumor is depicted in Fig. 1. Microdialysis provides a means to obtain samples from tumor ECF samples from which a concentration vs time profile can be determined within a single tumor *(3,5,6,20)*.

Microdialysis provides several advantages over autoradiographic studies of tumor biopsies as a method to evaluate anticancer drug concentrations in tumor tissue. With microdialysis techniques it is possible to obtain serial sampling of anticancer drugs from the ECF of a single tumor with minimal tissue damage or alteration of fluid balance *(3,19,20)*. The microdialysis probe can remain in peripheral or central nervous system (CNS) tissue for up to 72 h without complications, such as increased risk of infection, inflammation, or alteration in probe recovery. Samples can be immediately obtained and analyzed from a single probe that allows for the real time evaluation of physiologic, pharmacologic, and pharmacokinetic changes *(19,22–24)*. In addition, a single microdialysis probe can simultaneously sample several analytes of interest, thus allowing for the measurement of drug concentrations and pharmacologic endpoints that are required for pharmacodynamic studies. Furthermore, the drug concentration can be measured specifically rather than quantitating radioactivity, which may be nonspecific. Because of the pore cutoff size (20 kDa) of the semipermeable membrane, the use of microdialysis allows for the differentiation between liposomally encapsulated, conjugated drugs, protein-bound drugs, and active-unbound drug in the tumor ECF *(7,25)*. Using microdialysis techniques, serial sampling of the non-protein-bound, active form of anticancer agents can be obtained from a single sight in a brain tumor, peripheral tumor, or surrounding tissues. In addition, multiple microdialysis probes can be placed in a single tumor to evaluate intratumoral variabiltiy of the analyte of interest *(3,12)*. Thus, the data obtained with microdialysis techniques may more closely reflect the disposition of the active form of the drug within the tumor ECF *(12,19,26)*.

2. MICRODIALYSIS METHODOLOGY AND STUDY DESIGN

2.1. Microdialysis System and Setup

The principles of microdialysis sampling have been reviewed in detail previously *(20,21,26,27)*. In brief, a short length of hollow dialysis fiber is continuously perfused with a physiological solution. The presence of the analyte of interest in the ECF and its absence in the perfusate leads to a concentration gradient across the dialysis membrane. The analyte diffuses through the dialysis membrane, and is collected for analysis. This process is performed in vivo through the use of a microdialysis probe that is implanted into tissue and continuously perfused with a physiologic solution at a low flow rate (0.5–10 µL/min). After the probe is implanted into tumor tissue, substances are filtered by diffusion from the extracellular space through the semipermeable membrane into the perfusion medium, and carried via microtubing into the collection vials.

Commercially available microdialysis probes, microperfusion pumps, and microfraction collectors are available. The type of microdialysis probe used depends on the sight or tissues of interest (e.g., subcutaneous tumor or tissue, brain, or liver), size of the tumor, and the analyte of interest *(3,12)*. A microdialysis probe (CMA 20, Stockholm, Sweden) with a molecular cutoff of 20 kDa, membrane length of 4 mm, and outer diameter of 0.5 mm is the standard used for most pharmacokinetic studies of drugs in peripheral tissue and tumors *(3,5,6,12)*. The molecular weight cutoff (i.e., 20 kDa) of the semipermeable membrane of probe prevents albumin-bound drug from crossing the membrane. However, small plasma protein, such as α_1-acid-glycoprotein, can pass through the semipermeable membrane. Thus, depending on the protein binding characteristics of a drug, the recovery may not be limited to unbound drug. The microdialysis probe is perfused by a microperfusion pump and dialysate samples are collected by the microfraction collector. Ringer's solution (USP) is the standard perfusion solution because it is similar to the makeup of ECF. Alternatively, 0.9% NaCl (USP) can be used for tissue and CNS studies.

2.2. Microdialysis Methodology and Study Design

2.2.1. In Vitro Calibration

Only a fraction (i.e., 10–50%) of the analyte can cross the probe's semipermeable membrane and the percentage that crosses can vary between probes, drug type, and flow rate *(20,21,26,27)*. Thus, prior to in vivo studies it is standard to characterize the transfer rate, relative recovery, and the optimal flow rate of the drug and probe used in the studies. The recovery of drug across the membrane is concentration independent *(3,20,21,26,27)*. The objective is to use the lowest flow rate that achieves sufficient recovery of the analyte that can be detected by the analytical system. High flow rates should be avoided owing to the propensity to alter the fluid balance in the tumors. The flow rate and collection interval are then modified to attain the needed sample volume required by the analytical system.

In vitro calibration studies are performed by placing a microdialysis probe in a beaker that contains a clinically relevant concentration of the drug or analyte of interest. The probe is perfused at various flow rates (e.g., 0.5, 1, 2, 3, 8, and 16 µL/min) and dialysate samples are collected every 10–25 min based on the required sample volume for the assay.

The probe is allowed to reach equilibrium prior to sample collection at each flow rate. The time required to reach equilibrium is based on the flow rate and length of the microdialysis tubing. In vitro recovery is calculated as follows:

$$\text{In vitro recovery} = \frac{\text{Perfusate conc}_{out}}{\text{In vitro solution conc}} \tag{1}$$

2.2.2. Microdialysis In Vivo Study Design and Procedures

Microdialysis probes can be placed in any accessible tumor and tissue. However, areas of the tumor with pooled blood should be avoided to prevent false results. Probe placement can be confirmed by ultrasound or after tumor or tissue removal in animal studies. Dual-probe studies can also be performed to evaluate the intratumoral disposition of the analyte or drug.

After probe placement, a short period (i.e., 45–60 min) is allowed for probe and tumor ECF equilibration prior to the start of calibration (3,6,12,19). Although use of the microdialysis technique results in less tissue damage compared to other sampling methods (e.g., biopsy), insertion of the microdialysis probe into the tumor does induce some tissue damage and immune reactivity. Thus, samples collected immediately after probe insertion may not reflect basal tumor conditions because of acute tissue damage and changes in blood flow associated with probe insertion. Therefore, it is necessary to allow time for the probe and tumor ECF to equilibrate prior to the start of the probe calibration studies.

After probe placement, calibration and washout procedures are performed. Because of variability in recovery for various probes at various sights, the calibration procedure is performed to determine the extent of recovery for each probe at each site. The washout period is performed to remove any drug introduced into the ECF during retrocalibration. The length of the washout period is determined by concentration of drug introduced in the ECF during calibration and the $t_{1/2}$ of the drug in the ECF. After the washout period the drug is administered or the procedure is started, and the sample recovery procedure is performed.

2.2.3. In Vivo Calibration and Recovery

In vitro recovery may be substantially different from the in vivo (i.e., tumor ECF) recovery (19–21). In addition, recovery can vary between probes, drug type, flow rate, and tissue or tumor site. An in vivo microdialysis study is a dynamic process in which substances are continuously removed from the tumor ECF by diffusion into the probe. Consequently, the concentration of drug in the perfusate does not reach equilibrium with the tumor ECF. However, under constant conditions (i.e., perfusate flow rate) a steady-state percentage recovery, which represents a constant fraction of the ECF concentration, will be reached. Thus, the in vivo recovery value is determined for each probe in each tumor or tissue, and is specific for that single procedure. This provides the advantage of accounting for processes that affect recovery in tissues and tumors. The in vitro recovery values can be calculated by retrodialysis calibration, reference or marker compound, and point of zero net flux methods (20,21,27,28).

Retrodialysis calibration method can be used to estimate the steady-state percentage recovery (3,12–14,23,27,28). Retrodialysis quantification of in vivo recovery is based on the principle that the diffusion process across the microdialysis semipermeable membrane is equal in both directions. Therefore, the analyte of interest can be included in the perfusion medium and the disappearance from the perfusate into the tumor ECF is used as an estimation of in vivo recovery. In vivo recovery is calculated as follows (3,27):

$$\text{In vitro recovery} = \frac{\text{Perfusate conc}_{in} - \text{perfusate conc}_{out}}{\text{Perfusate conc}_{in}} \tag{2}$$

Thus, the estimated drug concentration in the tumor ECF is calculated as follows *(3,21,22)*:

$$\text{Estimated tumor ECF conc} = \frac{\text{Measured microdialysis sample}}{\text{In vitro recovery}} \tag{3}$$

One limitation of the retrodialysis method is the time required to perform the calibration studies (i.e., four to five samples over 1–1.5 h) and washout (three or four samples over approx 1 h). Alternatively, if the retrodialysis calibration studies could be performed at the same time as the samples are collected, the ratio of sample number to study duration could be increased. This can be performed by using a reference or marker compound that has the same recovery characteristics as the analyte of interest. This process occurs by placing the reference compound in the dialysis solution during sampling of the analyte of interest. The analyte of interest diffuses from the ECF into the probe at the same time, rate, and extent as the reference compound diffuses out of the probe and into the ECF. The in vivo recovery of the reference compound is determined using the standard retrodialysis procedure and calculations (Eq. 2). The in vivo recovery value for the reference compound is then used to calculate the estimated tumor concentration using Eq. (3).

The point of zero net flux is a calibration method that determines relative recovery of a drug or analyte by varying the concentrations of the drug included in the perfusate solution *(27–29)*. This procedure is performed by perfusing four or five varying concentrations of the drug into the microdialysis probe and measuring the concentration in the outflow dialysate. Plotting the difference between the inflow perfusate drug concentration and the outflow dialysate drug concentration as a function of the perfusate drug concentration results in a line with a slope that is equal to the relative recovery and an *x*-intercept that is equal to the steady-state tissue ECF concentration of the drug.

2.3. Online/Real-Time Analysis

A potential clinical implementation and advantage of microdialysis methodology is the real-time determination of drug concentration in tissue and tumors, measures of pharmacologic effect, and physiologic function *(19,22,23)*. The ability to link the microdialysis sampling system directly to an analytical system allows for the measurement of pharmacokinetic and pharmacodynamic endpoints within minutes of obtaining the sample. Thus, medical and pharmacologic interventions can be performed and modifications can be made immediately.

Leggas and colleagues developed a rapid and simultaneous system that measured the inactive carboxylate and active lactone forms of topotecan using an online microdialysis system linked to a microbore high-performance liquid chromatography system *(22)*. This system allowed for the continuous injection of small amounts of samples, the direct measure of both forms of the drug without loss of sensitivity, and the additional benefit of fast and automated analysis without the additional sample processing required for pharmacokinetic studies of camptothecin analogs *(30,31)*. This system is very versatile and can be used for other camptothecin analogs and anticancer agents *(32,33)*. The advantages of this system in pharmacokinetic studies of anticancer agents are the ability to measure the parent compound and metabolites within minutes without disrupting the fluid balance of the tissue, which is especially important in pharmacokinetic studies of drugs in the brain and cerebrospinal fluid (CSF).

Microdialysis techniques were initially developed to monitor changes in neurotransmitter levels in the brain of preclinical models *(34–37)*. The use of microdialysis to monitor dynamic changes in glucose and lactate concentrations in the cortex of freely moving rats has accelerated the move to human studies and produced interesting methodological adaptations and results *(36)*. A schematic diagram of an experimental setup using dual online microdialysis assay in rats is depicted in Fig. 2. The reduction of oxygen levels in the cage led to an immediate rise in lactate and glucose concentrations in the brain. These experiments reported the first temporal relationship between glucose and lactate changes during moderate hypoxia in unanesthetized animals *(36)*. However, the inability to have the analytical instruments that are required for the detection of specific neurotransmitters, such as lactate and glucose, at the bedside in clinical studies has complicated the need for real-time results. As the function of analytical instruments increase and their size decreases, the use of these systems in clinical practice will increase. Alternatively, delivering the microdialysis sample from the bedside to the analytical laboratory, as is done with other standard laboratory studies, can produce results in a relatively short period of time.

Tolias and colleagues used microdialysis to evaluate extracellular glutamate in the brains of children with severe head injuries *(38)*. A microdialysis probe was inserted next to an intracranial pressure bolt in the right frontal area of the brain. Dialysis samples were collected hourly and analyzed for glutamate, glutamine, and various structural amino acids. Clinical monitoring parameters were correlated with amino acid concentrations. A low glutamine to glutamate ratio was associated with increased morbidity. The authors concluded that glutamate metabolism may have a more significant role in the pathophysiology of pediatric head injury than had been recognized. As for the use of microdialysis to generate real-time results, the ability to obtain a sample over a relatively short period of time, send it to the clinical laboratory, and have the results sent back within hours may allow for modifications in the treatment of the patient.

3. PRECLINICAL MICRODIALYSIS STUDIES IN TUMOR AND TISSUE

3.1. Preclinical Studies of Tumor and Tissue Distribution

Studies comparing plasma and tumor ECF exposure associated with response in preclinical models have used microdialysis methodology *(3,14)*. Investigators reported a six-fold difference in dose and plasma exposure of topotecan associated with a complete response in mice bearing human neuroblastoma xenografts NB1691 (2.0 mg/kg and 290 ng/mL·h, respectively) as compared to NB1643 (0.36 mg/kg and 52 ng/mL·h, respectively) *(39)*. However, factors related to the difference in topotecan response in the two neuroblastoma xenograft lines were not identified. Moreover, macrotumor-related factors affecting sensitivity and the relationship between tumor ECF exposure to topotecan and antitumor activity in the xenograft model had not been established. As a result, the tumor ECF disposition of topotecan using microdialysis methodology was evaluated and the relationship between topotecan tumor ECF exposure and antitumor response in mice bearing the relatively resistant (NB1691) and sensitive (NB1643) human neuroblastoma xenografts was evaluated *(3)*.

The concentration vs time profiles of topotecan in plasma (top) and tumor ECF (bottom) in NB1643 (solid line) and NB1691 (dash line) human tumor xenografts are presented in Fig. 3. There was a 3.5-fold difference in tumor ECF exposure and penetration in NB1643 (25.6 ± 19.6 ng/mL·h and 0.15 ± 0.11, respectively) and NB1691 (7.3 ± 6.1 ng/mL·h and 0.04 ± 0.04, respectively) ($p < 0.05$), which was consistent with the difference in sensitivity of these xenografts based on dose and plasma exposure. These results suggest that topotecan tumor penetration may be one factor associated with neuroblastoma antitumor

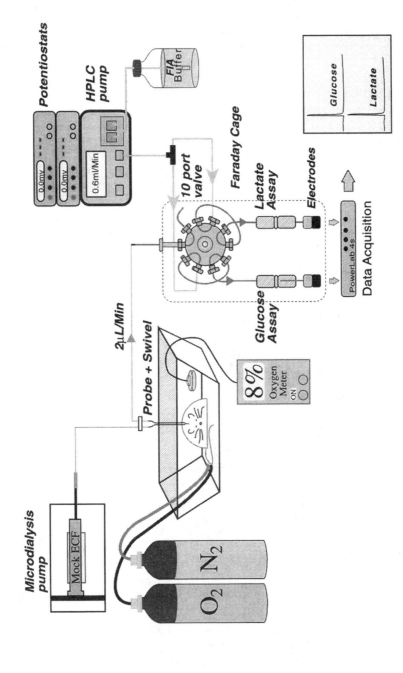

Fig. 2. Microdialysis probe in rat brain with online analytical system. Schematic diagram of the hypoxia experimental setup and dual online microdialysis assay. A 10-port injection valve is shown in the inject position.

314

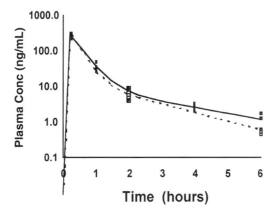

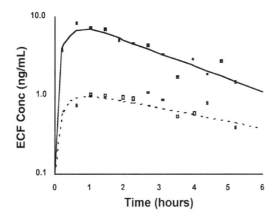

Fig. 3. Topotecan lactone concentration-time profiles in plasma and tumor ECF in resistant and sensitive neuroblastoma tumor xenografts. Representative topotecan plasma (**A**) and tumor ECF (**B**) concentration–time plots in mice bearing NB-1691 and NB-1643. Individual data points and best fit line of the data are represented for topotecan lactone plasma concentrations (**A**) in mice bearing NB-1643 (—, ●) and NB-1691 (---, ○) human neuroblastoma tumor xenografts. Individual data points and best fit line of the data are represented for topotecan lactone tumor ECF concentrations (**B**) in mice bearing NB-1643 (—, ■) and NB-1691 (---, □) human neuroblastoma tumor xenografts. The topotecan lactone tumor extracellular fluid $AUC_{0.5}$ for the representative NB-1643 (—, ■) and NB-1691 (---, □) tumor xenografts were 22.3 and 9.1 ng/mL-h, respectively.

response. Moreover, these data suggest inherent differences in tumor vascularity, capillary permeability, and/or tumor interstitial pressure between the sensitive and resistant neuroblastoma tumor xenografts. This was the first study reporting a relationship between the exposure of an anticancer agent in tumor ECF and antitumor response.

The significance of ECF as an important exposure for pharmacologic effect of anticancer agents and the inter- and intratumor variability was evaluated in preclinical studies of cisplatin using microdialysis *(12)*. The relationship between unbound platinum in tumor ECF, total platinum in tumor homogenates, and the formation of platinum–DNA (Pt-DNA) adducts were evaluated after administration of cisplatin in mice bearing B16 murine melanoma tumors. Intratumor variability in platinum disposition was evaluated by placing two

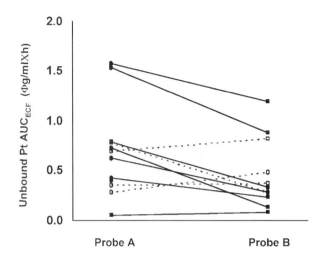

Fig. 4. Low intra- and high intertumoral disposition of cisplatin in murine melanoma tumors. Inter- and intratumoral variability in unbound platinum AUC_{ECF} in mice bearing B16 tumors and in mice bearing H23 xenografts after administration of at 10 mg/kg of cisplatin. In mice bearing B16 murine melanoma tumors, individual AUCs are represented by ●, and AUCs within the same tumor are connected by —. In mice bearing H23 human NSCLC xenografts, individual AUCs are represented by ○, and AUCs within the same tumor are connected by ---.

probes (A and B) in the same tumor. At the end of the 2-h sample period, tumor tissue was obtained at each probe site and analyzed for total platinum, and bifunctional intrastrand DNA adducts between platinum and two adjacent guanines (Pt-GG), and platinum and adenine and guanine (Pt-AG).

The concentration of unbound platinum in tumor ECF of B16 tumors was detectable from 12 min to 120 min after administration. In addition, the concentration vs time profile of unbound platinum in tumor ECF did not follow the plasma concentration vs time profile, suggesting that clearance of drug from tumor may be the primary factor affecting drug accumulation within a tumor. The median (range, % CV) area under the concentration vs time curve for ECF (AUC_{ECF}) and tumor penetration were 0.42 μg/mL·h (0.05–1.57, 78%) and 0.16 (0.02–0.62, 77%), respectively.

The relationship between unbound platinum AUC in tumor ECF from probe A and probe B is presented in Fig. 4. The median (range, % CV) AUC_{ECF} from probe A to probe B was 1.9 (1.3–5.5, 55%). The median (range, % CV) concentration of total platinum obtained at the end of the 2-h microdialysis procedure from probe A to probe B was 1.1 (1.0–2.0, 27%). Using an E_{max} model to describe the relationship between drug exposure and Pt-DNA adduct formation, there was a better correlation between unbound platinum AUC_{ECF} ($R^2 = 0.69$ and 0.63, respectively) and Pt-GG and Pt-AG compared to total platinum in tumor extracts ($R^2 = 0.29$ and 0.41, respectively). In addition, there was a poor correlation between unbound platinum AUC_{ECF} and total platinum in tumor extracts ($R^2 = 0.26$).

These results suggest there is relatively high inter- (approx a 30-fold range) and low intratumor (approx a fourfold range) variability in unbound and total platinum in B16 murine melanoma tumors, and a poor relationship between unbound and total platinum. In addition, these results suggest unbound platinum in tumor ECF is a better correlate of Pt-DNA adduct formation compared to total platinum measured in tumor extracts.

3.2. Evaluation of Angiogenesis Inhibitors

The angiogenic phenotype is associated with increased tumor neovascularization and hyperpermeability to drugs and other macromolecules *(40–42)*. Angiogenesis inhibitors could alter the increased tumor vascularization and permeability and have an untoward effect of decreasing tumor exposures of anticancer agents when coadministered with angiogenesis inhibitors. Thus, Ma and colleagues evaluated the tumor disposition of temozolomide administered alone and in combination with the angiogenesis inhibitor TNP-470 *(42)*. Temozolomide was administered alone and in combination with TNP-470 to nude rats bearing tumors that differentially expressed low or high vascular endothelial growth factor (VEGF). In both the subcutaneous and intracerebral tumors with high VEGF expression, TNP-470 treatment produced significant reductions in temozolomide tumor exposure and the ratio of tumor to plasma exposures. In conclusion, the pharmacodynamic effect of angiogenesis inhibitors on tumor angiogenesis can produce a reduction in tumor concentrations of coadministered anticancer agents. It is increasingly important to understand the pharmacokinetic impact of angiogeneis inhibitors when coadministered with anticancer agents and additional studies need to be performed to determine the optimal dosing schedules for combination regimens.

3.3. Evaluation of Liposomal Anticancer Agents

The theoretical advantages of encapsulated liposomal drugs are prolonged duration of exposure and selective delivery of entrapped drug to the site of action *(43–47)*. Major advances in the use of liposomes as vehicles delivering encapsulated pharmacologic agents and enzymes to sites of disease have occurred over the past 10 yr. Moreover, liposomal-encapsulated drugs, such as liposomal doxorubicin (Doxil®), are FDA-approved and have documented activity and decreased toxicity *(48,49)*. Studies evaluating the disposition and tumor penetration of liposomal and nonliposomal anticancer agents suggest liposomal agents extravasate selectively into solid tumors through the capillaries of tumor neovasculature *(47,50,51)*. However, the mechanisms by which liposomes enter tissue and tumors and release drug are not completely understood. In addition, the liposomes can be engineered to produce a complete spectrum of drug release rates that need to be evaluated in in vivo systems.

SPI-077 (ALZA Pharmaceuticals, Inc.) is cisplatin encapsulated in long-circulating STEALTH® liposome. The disposition of liposomal-cisplatin is dependent on the liposomal vehicle *(43,52,53)*. Once the cisplatin is released from the liposome, its disposition follows cisplatin pharmacology. SPI-077 has shown antitumor activity against a wide range of solid tumor xenografts, including murine colon tumors. In a study comparing SPI-077 and cisplatin tumor disposition in mice bearing murine colon tumors, the platinum exposure in tumors was several-fold higher and prolonged after SPI-077 as compared to cisplatin administration *(44)*. However, because the platinum exposure was measured in tumor extracts, it is unclear whether the platinum measured was encapsulated, protein-bound platinum, or unbound platinum. In addition, it is unclear whether the platinum exposure was intracellular or extracellular. Thus, it is currently unclear whether SPI-077 releases cisplatin into the tumor ECF, or penetrates into the cell as the liposome and then releases the cisplatin intracellularly.

Thus, the tumor disposition of platinum after administration of liposomal formulations of cisplatin (SPI-077) and nonliposomal cisplatin was evaluated using microdialysis in mice bearing B16 murine melanoma tumors *(25)*. Because of the pore cutoff size (20 kDa) of the semipermeable membrane of the microdialysis probe and the size of the liposome (100 nm), the microdialysis probe was able only to sample unbound platinum and allow the differentiation between liposomal-encapsulated cisplatin and cisplatin released into the tumor ECF.

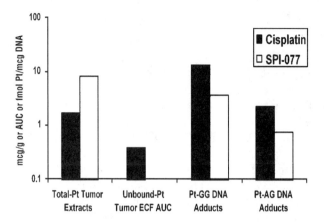

Fig. 5. Unbound platinum in tumor ECF, total platinum in tumor homogenates, and Pt-GG DNa adducts after administration of cisplatin and spi-077 in murine melanoma tumors.

After administration of cisplatin, the concentration of unbound platinum in tumor ECF was detectable from 12 min to 120 min after administration. However, there was no detectable unbound platinum in the tumor ECF after administration of SPI-077. The total platinum in tumor extracts, unbound platinum in tumor ECF as measured by AUC, and formation of Pt-GG DNA adducts after administration of cisplatin and SPI-077 are presented in Fig. 5 *(54)*. The results of this study suggest SPI-077 distributes into tumors, but releases significantly less platinum into tumor ECF, which results in lower formation of Pt-DNA adducts compared to cisplatin. This was the first study using microdialysis methodology to evaluate the tumor disposition of liposomally encapsulated anticancer agents.

3.4. Pharmacokinetic Brain Studies in Nonhuman Primates

Nonhuman primates are used as the standard model for the determination of drug penetration into the CNS *(10)*. These models primarily evaluate the exposure of drug in the CSF of the lateral, fourth ventricle, and lumbar space after intravenous administration. This may provide important information for the evaluation of cytotoxic exposures in the treatment of embryonal CNS tumors, such as medulloblastoma, leukemia, and bacterial or viral infections that have a high propensity to disseminate throughout the subarachnoid space. However, these exposures may be irrelevant for primary brain tumors that occur in the cerebral cortex *(10)*. This difference in clinically relevant exposure for primary brain tumors and tumors that spread throughout the subarachoid space is attributable to various components of the blood–brain barrier at each of these sights *(10,29)*. Thus, there is impending need to evaluate the penetration and exposure of anticancer agents in the cerebral cortex.

Fox and colleagues evaluated the exposure of zidovudine in brain ECF as measured by microdialysis in rhesus monkeys *(29)*. In vivo recovery was tissue dependent and was lower in brain than in blood or muscle. After intravenous administration, the steady-state concentrations of zidovudine in blood, temporalis muscle, and brain were $112 \pm 64 \mu M$, $105 \pm 51 \mu M$, and $14 \pm 10 \mu M$, respectively. The steady-state ultrafiltrate concentrations of zidovudine in serum and CSF were $81 \pm 40 \mu M$ and $14 \pm 8 \mu M$, respectively. The authors concluded that the CSF and brain ECF concentrations were comparable at steady state. Thus, zidovudine penetration in the brain ECF and CSF is limited to a similar extent, presumably by active transport, as in other species.

4. CLINICAL MICRODIALYSIS STUDIES

4.1. Clinical Microdialysis Studies in Tissue

In cancer treatment it is currently unclear if it is better to dose chemotherapeutic agents based on body surface area (i.e., mg/m^2), body weight (mg/kg), or fixed doses (i.e., mg). Several studies have shown that dosing anticancer agents based on body surface area does not reduce pharmacokinetic variability (55,56). Similarly, Hollenstein and colleagues investigated whether weight-adjusted ciprofloxacin dosing results in comparable concentrations of drug in tissue ECF in obese and lean subjects (57). Microdialysis was used to sample ECF concentrations of ciprofloxacin in the anterior aspect of the right thigh in age- and sex-matched obese (122 ± 23 kg) and lean (59 ± 9 kg) subjects after an intravenous dose of ciprofloxacin. The tissue penetration was significantly lower in obese patients (0.45 ± 0.27) as compared to lean patients (0.82 ± 0.36). The authors concluded that the penetration of drug into the ECF of muscle is impaired in obese patients. Therefore, antibiotic doses need not be adjusted for an increase in fat to water ratio, and weight-adjusted dosing based on actual body weight will yield adequate tissue levels of ciprofloxacin. Similar microdialysis studies evaluating the exposure of anticancer agents in tissue may help address the optimal method used to calculate doses of anticancer agents.

4.2. Clinical Microdialysis Studies in Tumors

Recently, microdialysis has been modified for use in human drug studies and has provided the opportunity to quantify drug concentrations in tissue and tumors (5,6,7,13). Microdialysis has been used to evaluate the ECF disposition of anticancer agents in patients with accessible solid tumors (5,6,7,13). The first study that demonstrated the utility of microdialysis in patients with solid tumors were studied by Blochl-Daum and colleagues. The disposition of carboplatin in blood and ECF of tumor and skin was studied in patients with cutaneous malignant melanoma metastases (6). Microdialysis probes were placed in cutaneous tumors and surrounding skin. The results indicated a rapid but incomplete equilibration between blood and the tumor compartment. Similar results were reported with subcutaneous tissue. The mean ± SD AUC of total (sum of unbound and bound) carboplatin in serum, tumor, and subcutaneous tissue were 1533 ± 189 µg/mL·min, 853 ± 172 µg/mL·min, and 506 ± 87 µg/mL·min, respectively. There was also significant interpatient variability in blood, tumor, and subcutaneous tissue. However, there was greater interpatient variability in tumor and skin exposure as compared to blood. These data suggest that in addition to systemic factors that control blood exposures, there are tumor- and tissue-related factors that add to the variability in the exposure at these sites.

Muller and colleagues evaluated the relationship between 5-fluorouracil (5-FU) exposure in tumor ECF and clinical response in patients with primary breast cancer (5). Microdialysis probes were placed into the primary tumor and periumbilical subcutaneous adipose layer in patients with breast cancer scheduled to receive neoadjuvant chemotherapy containing 5-FU. In addition, serial blood samples were obtained. The mean ± SD AUC of 5-FU in plasma, tumor, and subcutaneous tissue were 699 ± 75 µg/mL·min, 374 ± 62 µg/mL·min, and 401 ± 151 µg/mL·min, respectively. The pharmacokinetics of 5-FU were similar in tumor and adipose tissue. A high interstitial tumor exposure of 5-FU was associated with increased tumor response and there was no association between 5-FU exposure in adipose tissue or plasma and tumor response. The authors concluded that the exposure of 5-FU in tumor ECF may predict response in patients with breast cancer. Moreover, this information could be used to optimize dosing and administration schedules to increase the exposure of anticancer agents in tumors and thus improve response.

Muller and colleagues also evaluated the interstitial disposition of methotrexate in patients with primary breast cancer lesions *(13)*. Microdialysis probes were placed into the primary tumor and periumbilical subcutaneous adipose layer in patients with breast cancer receiving methotrexate as part of a three-drug regimen. The ratio of methotrexate AUC in tumor ECF to plasma was 0.60 ± 0.20. In addition, there was no correlation between methotrexate AUC in tumor ECF and plasma. Unlike in the previous study, the exposure of methotrexate in tumor ECF was not associated with response. The lack of a relationship between methotrexate exposure in tumor ECF and response may be associated with variability in transendothelial transfer of methotrexate. This study depicts the importance of not only the disposition of drug in tumor ECF, but also the intracellular exposure of anticancer agents as cytotoxic determinants of response.

5. PHARMACODYNAMIC STUDIES USING MICRODIALYSIS

5.1. Antibiotics

The ability of the microdialysis probe to recover any analyte that is small enough to pass through the semipermeable membrane makes it a useful technique for pharmacodyamic studies *(7,58)*. Microdialysis methodology has been used in clinical pharmacodynamic studies of antiinfective agents, diabetes, muscle physiology, and brian neurochemistry *(7,58–65)*. The specific advantage of microdialysis in the study of antiinfective agents is related to the ability of the probe to measure unbound, pharmacologically active drug in the ECF of tissue, which is the anatomically defined target site for most bacterial infections. In the study of antiinfective agents, microdialysis probes has been placed in subcutaneous tissues, brain, and lung *(7,58)*. Microdialysis studies have demonstrated that the concentrations of antiinfective agents in the ECF of subcutaneous tissue may be subinhibitory, whereas the concentrations in the serum may be sufficient for an antimicrobial effect. Thus, the use of tissue ECF or serum concentrations as an endpoint for determining the potential efficacy of antiinfective agents may have a significant impact on clinical decision making. Microdialysis also offers unique opportunities in pharmacokinetic and pharmacodynamic research and the potential to streamline the decision process on the drug development of antiinfective agents and also anticancer agents.

Delacher and colleagues evaluated a combined in vivo pharmacokinetic and in vitro pharmacodynamic approach to simulate the target site pharmacodynamics of antibiotics in humans *(59)*. This approach was based on the in vivo measurements of interstitial drug pharmacokinetics in tissue and a subsequent pharmacodynamic simulation of the drug concentration vs time profile in an in vitro setting. A schematic illustration of the general concept of the combined in vivo pharmacokinetic and in vitro pharmacodynamic approach is depicted in Fig. 6. Individual concentration vs time profiles of ciprofloxacin were measured in the interstitial space of patients following intravenous administration. Then different isolates of *Pseudomonas aeruginosa* were exposed in vitro to the interstitial ciprofloxacin concentration vs time profile obtained from the in vivo microdialysis experiments. Significant correlations were observed between pharmacokinetic and pharmacodynamic metrics. Moreover, the data were analyzed with an integrated pharmacokinetic–pharmacodynamic model, allowing for a much more detailed evaluation of the data than possible by strictly using minimum inhibitory concentrations. The results of these experiments showed that therapeutic success and failure in antiinfective therapy may be explained by pharmacokinetic variability at the target site, and therefore this in vivo pharmacokinetic and in vitro pharmacodynamic approach may provide valuable guidance for drug and dose selection for antiinfective agents. The use of pharmcokinetic drug exposure in the CSF of nonhuman

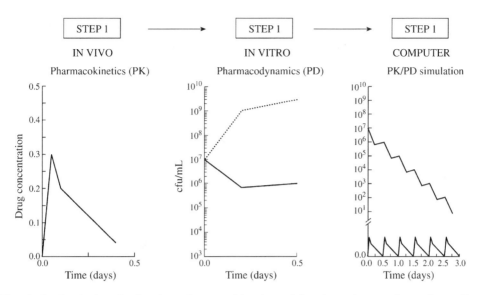

Fig. 6. Study design for in vivo pharmacokinetic and in vitro pharmcodynamic studies of antiinfective agents.

primates to guide in vitro cytotoxcity studies has been used in the development of topotecan for the treatment of medulloblastoma *(10)*. These procedures and study designs could be combined, along with microdialysis studies of anticancer agents in tumors, as described earlier, to provide information on drug and dose selection of anticancer agents as was performed for the antiinfective agents.

5.2. Brain Neurochemistry

The use of microdialysis probes in neuromonitoring is a new therapeutic opportunity for microdialysis systems *(63–65)*. The major value of microdialysis monitoring in severe head injury has been to demonstrate different brain pathophysiologic mechanisms in the living brain and to depict the time course of these changes. Interruption of substrate delivery is a major factor of vulnerability to ischemic damage to the brain in patients with severe head injury, stroke, or subarachnoid hemorrhage. Thus, continuous monitoring of substrate levels in the brain is required to optimize therapy for critically ill patients with brain injuries. Zauner and colleagues evaluated the delivery of oxygen via residual blood as an approach to protecting the brain during ischemia *(63)*. Therapy was evaluated by continuously measuring brain oxygen, brain CO_2, brain pH, and hourly glucose and lactate concentrations via a microdialysis system. As depicted in Fig. 7, there was an increase in brain tissue oxygen tension and a simultaneous decline in brain lactate during a stepwise increase in inspired oxygen. Although these new monitoring systems and methods are labor intensive and expensive, they can be readily applied in neurosurgical centers.

Disturbed ionic and neurotransmitter homeostasis are now recognized as the most important factor contributing to the development of secondary brain swelling after traumatic brain injury. Preclinical studies suggest that posttraumatic neuronal excitation by amino acids leads to an increase in extracellular potassium. Thus, Reinert and colleagues evaluated the relationship between extracellular potassium and high intracranial pressure after severe head

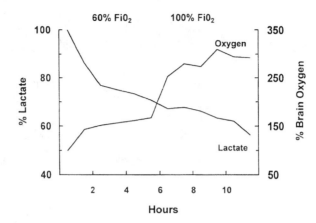

Fig. 7. Brain oxygenation tension and brain lactate concentrations during a stepwise increase in inspired oxygen.

injury *(64)*. An intracranial microdialysis procedure was used to monitor potassium, glutamate, and lactate concentrations in brain ECF. Dialysate potassium concentrations were increased for more than 3 h in approx 20% of patients. Moreover, a mean dialysate potassium > 2 m*M* throughout the entire monitoring period was associated with an intracranial pressure > 30 mmHg and fatal outcome, as were progressively rising concentrations of potassium in brain ECF. These studies show that microdialysis monitoring of physiologic and pharmacologic targets can be used to predict responses in patients.

The relationship between tissue oxygenation and excitatory amino acids in peritumoral edema has also been evaluated during glioma surgery *(65)*. Microdialysis was used to monitor glutamate and aspartate levels in peritumoral edema during resection of the tumor. Treatment with inspiratory oxygen led to an increase of tissue oxygenation and a decrease in glutamate and aspartate. Future microdialysis studies could evaluate the exposure of anticancer agents or pharmacologic markers of response in the ECF of a brain tumor after administration of a test dose of drug and prior to surgical resection. These studies could greatly enhance our knowledge of drug delivery and exposure in brain tumors.

6. SUMMARY AND FUTURE DIRECTIONS

Microdialysis has been used in the study of neurochemistry, muscle physiology, lipid metabolism, edema, diabetes, traumatic brain injury, antibiotics, and anticancer agents *(7,58,59,62,64,65)*. The possible uses of microdialysis in the pharmacokinetic and pharmacodynamic studies of anticancer agents are virtually endless. The use of microdialysis in the development of anticancer agents is based on preclinical and clinical results suggesting that tissue and tumor exposures do not equal plasma exposure, inter- and intratumoral exposure is highly variable, and the exposures of anticancer agents in CSF and CNS lobes are not identical. The advantages of microdialysis in the study of anticancer agents are sampling drug concentrations closer to the target site, as compared to plasma pharmacokinetic studies, obtaining serial samples from a single site within tissue and tumor, measurement of the active unbound forms of drugs, differentiation between various forms and metabolites of anticancer agents, and simultaneously obtaining samples for pharmacokinetic and pharmacodynamic studies *(3,7,58)*. The disadvantages of microdialysis are that it is invasive, requires in vivo calibration, and not all substances will cross the semipermeable membrane.

However, as compared to other sampling instruments and methods, these disadvantages are relatively minor.

The use of microdialysis in cancer-related studies will become more important as surrogate markers for response and toxicity are determined and new therapeutic agents are developed. The use of microdialysis can be especially important when evaluating the disposition of carrier-mediated agents (e.g., liposomes and PEG conjugates), gene therapy, antisense oligonucleotides, and angiogenesis inhibitors *(4,5,9,25)*. The disposition of carrier agents may be completely different than that of the parent compound and the release of drug systemically and in the tumor will be important in determining the antitumor effect and toxicity. The importance of microdialysis to address these issues is highlighted by the FDA's plan to inquire about methods to define and evaluate carrier systems. The pharmacokinetics and pharmacodynamics of gene therapy agents and antisense oligonucleotides may be drastically different than those of classical anticancer agents. In addition, owing to analytical assays and detection issues standard sampling strategies and processing may not be adequate for these agents. Thus, the use of methodology such as microdialysis that allows for rapid and accurate sampling and separation may become pivotal in the development of these agents. As the technology of microdialysis advances, the probe will be placed in more logistically difficult organs and tissues. Microdialysis probes can also be placed in blood vessels and obtain serial samples of unbound drug. These studies can be used to evaluate protein binding and reduce the need for repeated blood sampling and processing. Moreover, the ability to connect the mircrodialysis sampling instruments to online analytical equipment instruments allows for real-time analysis and may allow for the manipulation and modification of dosing regimens and strategies of anticancer agents.

REFERENCES

1. Grever MR, Chabner BA. Cancer drug development. In: DeVita VT, Hellman S, Rosenberg SA (eds). Cancer: Principles and Practice of Oncology, 5th Edit. Philadelphia, PA: Lippincott-Raven, 1997, p. 385.
2. Jain RK. Delivery of molecular medicine to solid tumors. Science 1996; 271:1079.
3. Zamboni WC, Houghton PJ, Hulstein JL, et al. Relationship between tumor extracellular fluid exposure to topotecan and response in human neuroblastoma xenografts and cell lines. Cancer Chemother Pharmacol 1999; 43:269–276.
4. Balch CM, Reintgen DS, Kirkwood JM, et al. Cutaneous melanoma. In: DeVita VT, Hellman S, Rosenberg SA (eds). Cancer: Principles and Practice of Oncology, 5th Edit. Philadelphia, PA: Lippincott-Raven, 1997, p. 1947.
5. Muller M, Mader RM, Steiner B, et al. 5-Fluorouracil kinetics in the interstitial tumor space: clinical response in breast cancer patients. Cancer Res 1997; 57:2598.
6. Blochl-Daum B, Muller M, Meisinger V, Eichler HG, Fassolt A, Pehamberger H. Measurement of extracellular fluid carboplatin kinetics in melanoma metastases with microdialysis. Br J Cancer 1996; 73:920.
7. Brunner M, Muller M. Microdialysis: an in vivo approach for measuring drug delivery in oncology. Eur J Clin Pharmacol 2002 ;58:227–234.
8. Zamboni WC, Gervais AC, Schellen JHM, et al. Disposition of platinum (Pt) in B16 murine melanoma tumors after administration of cisplatin & pegylated liposomal-cisplatin formulations (SPI-077 & SPI-077 B103). In: Proceedings of 11th NCI-EORTC-AACR Symposium on New Drugs in Cancer Therapy, November 2000: abstract 132.
9. Gelmon KA, Kisenhauer EA, Harris AL, Ratain MJ, Workman P. Anticancer agents targeting signaling molecules and cancer cell environment: challenges for drug development? J Natl Cancer Inst 1999; 91:1281–1287.
10. Zamboni WC, Gajjar AJ, Mandrell TD, et al. A four-hour topotecan infusion achieves cytotoxic exposure throughout the neuroaxis in the nonhuman primate model: implications for treatment of children with metastatic medulloblastoma. Clin Cancer Res 1998; 4:2537–2544.
11. Boucher Y, Jain RK. Microvascular pressure is the principal driving force for interstitial hypertension in solid tumors: implication for vascular collapse. Cancer Res 1992; 52:5110.

12. Zamboni WC, Gervias AC, Egorin MJ, et al. Inter- and intratumoral disposition of platinum in solid tumors after administration of cisplatin. Clin Cancer Res 2002; 8:2992–2999.
13. Muller M, Brunner M, Schmid R, et al. Interstitial methotrexate kinetics in primary breast cancer lesions. Cancer Res 1998; 58:2982–2985.
14. Ekstrom PO, Giercksky KE, Andersen A, Bruland OS, Slordal L. Intratumoral differences in methotrexate levels within human osteosarcoma xenografts studied by microdialysis. Life Sci 1997; 61:PL275–PL280.
15. Ekstrom PO, Andersen A, Warren DJ, Giercksky KE, Slordal L. Determination of extracellular methotrexate tissue levels by microdialysis in a rat model. Cancer Chemother Pharmacol 1996; 37:294–400.
16. Presant CA, Wolf W, Waluch V, et al. Association of intratumoral pharmacokinetics of fluorouracil with clinical response. Lancet 1994; 343:1184–1187.
17. Front D, Isreal O, Iosilevsky G, et al. Human lung tumors: SPECT quantitation of differences in Co-57 bleomycin uptake. Radiology 1987; 165:129–133.
18. Fishman AJ, Alpert NM, Babich JW, Rubin RH. The role of positron emission tomography in pharmacokinetic analysis. Drug Metab 1997; 29:923–956.
19. Muller M, Schmid R, Georgopoulos A, Buxbaum A, Wasicek C, Eichler HG. Application of microdialysis to clinical pharmacokinetics in humans. Clin Pharmacol Therapeut 1995; 57:371.
20. Johansen MJ, Newman RA, Madden T. The use of microdialysis in pharmacokinetics and pharmacodynamics. Pharmacotherapy 1997; 17:464.
21. Kehr J. A survey on quantitation microdialysis: theoretical models and practical limitations. J Neurosci Methods 1993; 48:251.
22. Leggas M, Welden J, Waters CM, Hanna SK, Stewart CF. Rapid and simulataneous determination of carboxylate and lactone forms of topotecan using microbore high performance liquid chromatography and online microdialysis sampling. J Pharmaceut Sci 2002, submitted.
23. Ettinger SN, Poellmann CC, Wisniewski NA, et al. Urea as a recovery marker for quantitative assessment of tumor interstitial solutes with microdialysis. Cancer Res 2001; 61:7964–7970.
24. Ekstrom PO, Andersen A, Saeter G, Giercksky KE, Slordal L. Continuous intratumoral microdialysis during high-dose methotrexate therapy in a patient with malignant fibrous histiocytoma of the femur; a case report. Cancer Chemother Pharmacol 1997; 39:267–272.
25. Thompson JF, Siebert GA, Anissimov YG, et al. Microdialysis and response during regional chemotherapy by isolated limb infusion of melphalan for limb malignancies. Br J Cancer 2001; 85:157–165.
26. Conley BA, Ramsland TS, Sentz DL, et al. Antitumor activity, distribution, and metabolism of 13-cis-retinoic acid as a single agent or in combination with tamoxifen in established human MCF-7 xenografts in mice. Cancer Chemother Pharmacol 1999; 43:183–197.
27. Bungay PM, Morrison PF, Dedrick RL. Steady-state theory for quantitative microdialysis of solutes and water in vivo and in vitro. Life Sci 1990; 46:105–119.
28. LeQuellec A, Dupin S, Genissel P, Saivin S, Marchand B, Houin G. Microdialysis probes calibration: gradient and tisue dependent changes in no net flux and reverse dialysis methods. J Pharmacol Toxicol Methods 1995; 33:11–16.
29. Fox E, Bungay PM, Bacher J, McGully CL, Dedrick RL, Balis FM. Zidovudine concentration in brain extracellular fluid measured by microdialysis: steady-state and transient results in rhesus monkey. J Pharmacol Exp Ther 2002; 361:1003–1011.
30. Zamboni WC, Bowman LC, Tan M, et al. Interpatient variability in bioavailability of the intravenous formulation of topotecan given orally to children with recurrent solid tumors. Cancer Chemother Pharmacol 1999; 43:454–460.
31. Furman WL, Stewart CF, Poquette CA, et al. Direct translation of protracted irinotecan schedule from a xenograft model to a phase I trial in children. J Clin Oncol 1999; 17:1815–1824.
32. Egorin MJ, Van Echo DA, Tipping SJ, et al. Pharmacokinetics and dosage reduction of cis-diammine (1, 1-cyclobutanedicarboxylato) platinum in patients with impaired renal function. Cancer Res 1984; 44:5432–5438.
33. Erkmen K, Egorin MJ, Reyno LM, Morgan R Jr, Doroshow JH. Effects of storage on the binding of carboplatin to plasma protein. Cancer Chemother Pharmacol 1995; 35:254–256.
34. Gerin C. Behavioral improvement and dopamine release in a Parkinsonian rat model. Neurosci Lett 2002; 330:5.
35. Mark GP, Finn DA. The relationship between hippocampal acetylcholine release and cholinergic convulsant sensitivity in withdrawal seizure-prone and withdrawal seizure-resistant selected mouse lines. Alchohol Clin Exp Res 2002; 26:1141–1152.

36. Jones DA, Ros J, Landolt H, Fillenz M, Boutelle MG. Dynamic changes in glucose and lactate in the cortex of the freely moving rat monitored using microdialysis. J Neurochem 2000; 75:1703–1708.

37. Zauner A, Doppenber E, Soukup J, Menzel M, Young HF, Bullock R. Extended neuromonitoring: new therapeutic opportunities? Neurol Res 1998; 20:S85–S90.

38. Tolias CM, Richards DA, Bowery NG, Sgouros S. Extracellular glutamate in the brains of children with severe head injuries: a pilot microdialysis study. Child Nerv System 2002; 18:368–374.

39. Zamboni WC, Stewart CF, Thompson J, et al. The relationship between topotecan systemic exposure and tumor response in human neuroblastoma xenografts. J Natl Can Inst 1998; 90:505–511.

40. Takamitsu O, Tjuvajev JG, Miyagawa T, et al. Tumor growth modulation by sense and antisense vascular endothelial growth factor gene expression: effects on angiogenesis, vascular permeability, blood volume, blood flow, fluorodeoxyglucose uptake, and proliferation of human melanoma intracerebral xenografts. Cancer Res 1998; 58:4185–4192.

41. Deviveni D, Klein-Szanto A, Gallo JM. Uptake of temozolomide in a rat glioma model in the presence and absence of the angiogenesis inhibitor TNP-470. Cancer Res 1996; 56:1983–1987.

42. Ma J, Pulfer S, Li S, Chu J, Reed K, Gallo JM. Pharmacodynamic-mediated reduction of temozolomide tumor concentrations by the angiogenesis inhibitor TNP-470. Cancer Res 2001; 61:5491–5498.

43. Harrington KJ, Lewanski CR, Northcote AD, et al. Phase I–II study of pegylated liposomal cisplatin (SPI-77) in patients with inoperable head and neck cancer. Ann Oncol 2001;493–496.

44. Newman MS, Colbern GT, Working PK, et al. Comparative pharmacokinetics, tissue distribution, and therapeutic effectiveness of cisplatin encapsulated in long-circulating, pegylated liposomes (SPI-077) in tumor bearing mice. Cancer Chemother Pharmacol 1999; 43:1–7.

45. Allen TM, Stuart DD. Liposomal pharmacokinetics. Classical, sterically-stabilized, cationic liposomes and immunoliposomes. In: Janoff AS (ed). Liposomes: Rational Design. New York, NY: Marcel Dekker, 1999, pp. 63–87.

46. Woodle MC, Lasic DD. Sterically stabilized liposomes. Biochem Biophys Acta 1992; 1113:171–199.

47. Harrington KJ, Rowlinson-Busza G, Synigos KN, et al. Biodistribution and pharmacokinetics of 111-In-DTPA-labeled pegylated liposomes in a human tumor xenograft model: implications for novel targeting strategies. Br J Cancer 2000; 83:232–238.

48. Muggia FM, Hainsworth JD, Jeffers S, et al. Phase II study of liposomal doxorubicin in refractory ovarian cancer: antitumor activity and toxicity modification by liposomal encapsulation. J Clin Oncol 1997; 15:987–993.

49. Stewart JSW, Jablonowski H, Goebel F-D, et al. Randomized comparative trial of pegylated liposomal doxorubicin versus bleomycin and vincristine in the treatment of AIDS-related Kaposi's sarcoma. International Doxorubicin Study Group. J Clin Oncol 1998; 16:683–691.

50. Harrington KJ, Monhammadtaghi S, Uster PS, et al. Effective targeting of solid tumors in patients with locally advanced cancers by radiolabeled pegylated liposomes. Clin Cancer Res 2001; 7:223–225.

51. Harrington KJ, Rowlinson-Busza G, Synigos KN, et al. Influence of tumor size on uptake of 111-In-DTPA-labeled pegylated liposomes in a human tumor xenograft model. Br J Cancer 2000; 83:684–688.

52. DeMario MD, Vogelzang NJ, Janisch L, et al. A Phase I study of liposome-formulated cisplatin (SPI-077) given every 3 weeks in patients with advanced cancer. Proc Am Soc Clin Oncol 1998; 17:883.

53. Veal GJ, Griffin MJ, Price E, et al. A Phase I study in paediatric patients to evaluate the safety and pharmacokinetics of SPI-77, a liposome encapsulated formulation of cisplatin. Br J Cancer 2001; 84: 1029–1035.

54. Pluim D, Maliepaard M, van Waardenburg RC, Beijnen JH, Schellens JHM. ^{32}P-postlabeling assay for the quantitation of the major platinum-DNA adducts. Analyt Biochem 1999; 274:30–38.

55. Baker SD, Verweij J, Rowinsky EK, et al. Role of body surface area in dosing of investigational anticancer agents in adults, 1991–2001. J Natl Cancer Inst 2002 Dec 18;94(24):1882–1888.

56. Kouno T, Katsumata N, Mukai H, et al. Standardization of the body surface area (BSA) formula to calculate the dose of anticancer agents in Japan. Jpn J Clin Oncol 2003 Jun;33(6):309–313.

57. Hollenstein UM, Brunner M, Schmid R, Muller M. Soft tissue concentrations of ciprofloxacin in obese and lean subjects following weight-adjusted dosing. Int J Obes 2001; 25:354–358.

58. Joukhadar C, Derendorf H, Muller M. Microdialysis: a novel tool for clinical studies of anticancer agents. Eur J Clin Pharmacol 2001; 57:211–219.

59. Delacher S, Derendorf H, Hollenstein U, et al. A combined in vivo pharmacokinetic and in vitro pharmacodynamic approach to simulate target site pharmacodynamics of antibiotics in humans. J Antimicrob Chemother 2000; 46:733–739.

60. Hickner RC. Applications of microdialysis in studies of exercise. Exerc Sport Sci Rev 2000; 28:117–222.

61. Hickner RC, Racette SB, Binder EF, Fisher JS, Kohrt WM. Suppression of whole body and regional lipolysis by insulin: effects of obesity and exercise. J Clin Endrocrinol Metab 1999; 84:3886–3895.
62. Hickner RC, Racette SB, Binder EF, Fisher JS, Kohrt WM. Effects of 10 days of endurance exercise training on the suppression of whole body and regional lipolysis by insulin. J Clin Endrocrinol Metab 2000; 85:1498–1504.
63. Zauner A, Doppenberg E, Soukup J, Menzel M, Young HF, Bullock R. Extended neuromonitoring: new therapeutic opportunities? Neurol Res 1998; 20:S85–S90.
64. Reinert M, Khaldi A, Zauner A, Doppenberg E, Choi S, Bullock R. High level of extracellular potassium and its correlates after severe head injury: relationship to high intracranial pressure. J Neurosurg 2000; 93:800–807.
65. Baunach S, Meixensberger J, Gerlach M, Lan J, Roosen K. Intraoperative microdialysis and tissue-pO2 measurement in human glioma. Acta Neurochir Suppl (Wein) 1998; 71:241–243.

20 Regional Therapy of Cancer Using Continuous Hyperthermic Peritoneal Perfusion or Vascular Isolation and Perfusion Techniques

H. Richard Alexander, MD, Maihgan A. Kavanagh, MD, Steven K. Libutti, MD, and James F. Pingpank, MD,

CONTENTS

INTRODUCTION
CONTINUOUS HYPERTHERMIC PERITONEAL PERFUSION
VASCULAR ISOLATION AND PERFUSION
SUMMARY

1. INTRODUCTION

Many individuals afflicted with solid organ malignancies suffer from recurrence of disease limited to a particular region or organ of the body that is not amenable to surgical resection. For these individuals systemic combination chemotherapy may offer palliative benefits and, except for ovarian carcinoma, is rarely curable. Moreover, the maximum doses of systemically administered chemotherapeutic agents are almost invariably limited by the occurrence of severe systemic toxicity. Regional cancer treatments are those that are directly delivered to a cancer-bearing organ or region of the body. The rationale for such therapies is to intensify treatment to the site of a progressively growing cancer while minimizing or potentially eliminating unnecessary systemic toxicity.

For many patients with peritoneal carcinomatosis secondary to gastrointestinal or ovarian carcinoma or mesothelioma, tumor progression in the peritoneum is the sole or life-limiting component of disease, and clinical evaluation of various forms of regional treatments for individuals afflicted with this condition have been long reported *(1–5)*. One such therapy is continuous hyperthermic peritoneal perfusion (CHPP), which is administered during a laparotomy at the time of maximum tumor debulking and is administered with a recirculating hyperthermic circuit throughout the peritoneal cavity using a perfusate containing one or more types of chemotherapy.

A second form of regional therapy that has been in clinical use for almost 50 yr is vascular isolation and perfusion of either the limb (ILP) or the liver (isolated hepatic perfusion or

Handbook of Anticancer Pharmacokinetics and Pharmacodynamics
Edited by: W. D. Figg and H. L. McLeod © Humana Press Inc., Totowa, NJ

Table 1
Consideration in Use of CHPP for Treatment of Carcinomatosis

Parameter	Favorable	Unfavorable
Patient	Opportunity to apply therapy early. CHPP can be done in conjunction with major procedures.	Most suitable patients are those with small-volume or microscopic disease.
Tumor	Peritoneal implants are surface malignancies: Do not invade peritoneal surface deeply.	Topically applied treatment may have variable tumor penetration.
Peritoneal cavity	Acts as a barrier: drug permeability should be less than plasma clearance; amenable to delivery of hyperthermia.	Complete and uniform distribution of perfusate is critical.
Chemotherapy	Much higher regional concentrations possible compared with systemic administration.	May have dose-limiting regional toxicity.
Hyperthermia	Neoplastic tissue is very sensitive to the lethal effects; synergizes with chemotherapy.	Difficult to heat tumors uniformly in vivo.

IHP). For individuals with in transit melanoma or high-grade unresectable sarcoma of the extremity, ILP with tumor necrosis factor (TNF) and melphalan has been in use as either a primary curative modality or as a limb salvage procedure (6–8). For individuals with unresectable malignancies confined to the liver, IHP has been used and shown to be associated with response rates of up to 75% (6,9,10). Vascular isolation and perfusion therapy is administered with an extracorporeal bypass circuit consisting of a heat exchanger, oxygenator, roller pump, and reservoir in which a saline-based perfusate containing packed red blood cells (PRBCs) and one or more therapeutic agents are administered directly through the vascular bed of the cancer-bearing region or organ of the body. The rationale, technique, pharmacokinetic advantage, and outcomes of CHPP and vascular isolation and perfusion (ILP and IHP) are the topics discussed in this chapter.

2. CONTINUOUS HYPERTHERMIC PERITONEAL PERFUSION

CHPP has been administered to patients with peritoneal carcinomatosis secondary to a variety of malignancies including gastrointestinal cancers, mesothelioma, and ovarian cancer. The treatment parameters, chemotherapeutics, degree of hyperthermia, and duration of treatment vary from one institution to another to some degree, but several overarching considerations of CHPP treatment apply (Table 1).

Patients with small-volume or completely resected peritoneal carcinomatosis appear to be the best candidates for CHPP. Peritoneal tumor implants must be exposed to sufficient doses of chemotherapeutic agents and hyperthermia at the center of the tumor to result in cell death. Because delivery of agents to tumor via CHPP is primarily by diffusion, tumor implants with a diameter > 6 mm are not likely to receive a tumoricidal dose (11–13). This was demonstrated by Dikhoff et al., who showed that cisplatin (CDDP) given intraperitoneally resulted in a fairly constant and high level of drug at a 3 mm depth into tumor, but CDDP concentrations decreased to 20% of tumor surface concentrations at a depth of 5 mm

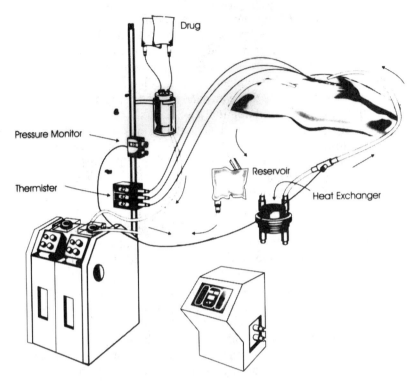

Fig. 1. Schema of the CHPP setup showing inflow and outflow cannulae positioned in the abdominal cavity and the perfusion circuit consisting of a roller pump heat exchanger and reservoir bag. Multiple temperature probes are placed within the peritoneal cavity to monitor adequate and uniform heating during treatment.

(11). Therefore, small implants such as those < 6 mm in diameter have the best theoretical likelihood of responding to intraperitoneal therapy.

A second potential limitation of intraperitoneal therapy is incomplete distribution of the therapeutic solution to all the serosal surfaces *(5,13)*. This has largely been overcome by using technical maneuvers during CHPP that physically promote distribution of the perfusate such as gentle agitation or manipulation of the abdominal contents during treatment *(3,14)*.

At laparotomy the peritoneal cavity is explored thoroughly and the nature and extent of the operative procedure are tailored based on the number, size, and location of peritoneal implants. In some circumstances when peritoneal disease is confined to a particular region of the abdomen, selective peritonectomy can be performed. Because tumors distributed in the peritoneal cavity are frequently limited to the serosa and not deeply infiltrative in nature, peritonectomy can be performed on the visceral and parietal peritoneum. Implants located on the serosa of the viscera can be excised or ablated with electrocautery. Some advocate a formal abdominal peritonectomy be performed to reduce the tumor burden as much as possible *(15)*. However, the extent of peritonectomy that is necessary to optimize the therapeutic effects of the subsequent CHPP and patient outcome has not been definitively established. When larger tumor masses are encountered segmental resection of stomach, small bowel, large bowel, or omentectomy with or without splenectomy may be indicated. Once adequate tumor debulking has been accomplished, inflow and outflow catheters are positioned at either end of the peritoneal cavity (Fig. 1). Typically the inflow catheters are placed at the upper portion of the abdominal cavity over the dome of the liver and left upper quadrant and the outflow catheters are placed in the pelvis. Several intra-peritoneal temperature probes are positioned to document uniform and sufficient heating of the peritoneal surfaces during treatment. The abdominal fascia is then temporarily closed and catheters are connected to a perfusion circuit consisting of a reservoir, roller pump, and heat exchanger (Fig. 1). Some have advocated using an open "coliseum" tech-nique in which the fascia of the abdominal cavity is suspended from a self-retaining retractor and a plastic seat is securely attached to the fascia *(14)*. A small slit is then made in the plastic cover to allow the surgeon's double-gloved hand access to the abdominal cavity for gentle manipulation of the perfusate. Because all the surfaces of the peritoneal cavity must be exposed to perfusate, great care is taken to lyse all intraperitoneal adhesions and ensure that the peritoneal surfaces are adequately exposed. For the closed CHPP technique, which is employed at the National Cancer Institute (NCI) and other institutions, the perfusion is initiated with saline that is heated until satisfactory perfusion parameters have been established and the peritoneal cavity has been adequately warmed *(3,4)*. The therapeutic agent is then administered into the reservoir bag and CHPP is continued for an additional 90 min.

Because the peritoneal cavity acts as a heat sink, flow rates of the perfusate should be high enough to achieve uniform and adequate intraperitoneal hyperthermia. In our expe-rience, this requires 1- to 1.5-L per minute flow rates through the peritoneal cavity. The patient should have a cooling blanket placed prior to the procedure and arms should be abducted on arm boards to allow both the cooling blanket and ice bags to be applied as necessary to maintain a core (esophageal) temperature of < 40°C. The therapeutic agent used at the NCI is CDDP at a dose of 250 mg/m^2, the maximum safe tolerated dose established in an initial Phase I study *(3,16)*. To minimize the likelihood of renal toxicity from systemically absorbed CDDP, sodium thiosulfate is administered systemically as described by Howell et al. *(17)* and urine output is increased using intravenous hydration and diuretics as necessary. Because CDDP is a large hydrophilic compound, it is less permeable across an intact peritoneal membrane than small lipophilic compounds. The estimated clearance across the peritoneal cavity during CHPP has been calculated to be approx 18 mm/min, which compares favorably to the absorbed plasma clearance of CDDP of 329 mm/min *(13)*.

2.1. Pharmacokinetics

The two most common agents used in CHPP are CDDP and mitomycin C. Both of these agents offer a pharmacological advantage when given via a perfusion in the peritoneal cavity. The pharmacokinetic advantage of cisplatin given to 27 patients via CHPP can be seen in Fig. 2. The concentration of CDDP in the perfusate over time, represented by the area under the curve of the concentration over time graph (AUC), was 3518 ± 1402 mg·min/mL compared with 287 ± 212 mg·min/mL in the plasma *(16)*. The ratio of perfu-sate to plasma CDDP concentrations at each time point ranged from 4.6 to 119, with a median of 14. The 14-fold greater perfusate concentration compared to systemic concen-tration illustrates the favorable regional pharmacokinetics achieved via CHPP. These data were supported further by Cho and co-workers, who analyzed pharmacokinetics of CDDP at doses between 100 and 450 mg/m^2 administered via CHPP in 56 patients *(18)*. They found that the percentage of total CDDP present in perfusate at the end of CHPP was about 28% of the total dose (Table 2).

TNF is an endogenously produced protein that has remarkable antitumor activity in murine models *(19)*. Its use as a systemic anticancer agent resulted in remarkable disappoint-

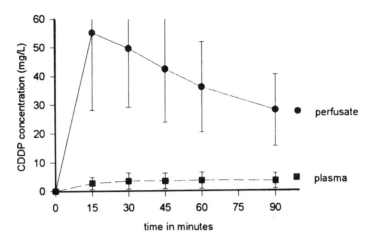

Fig. 2. Cisplatin concentrations in perfusate and plasma over time in 27 patients undergoing CHPP at a dose of 250 mg/m^2.

ment, as humans are exceedingly sensitive to the toxic side effects of the protein. In multiple Phase I and Phase II trials of intravenously administered TNF, significant toxicity, most commonly hypotension, was encountered at doses that were insufficient to produce any significant antitumor activity (20). However, regional administration of TNF has been surprisingly well tolerated, particularly when systemic levels of the protein can be largely reduced or eliminated. Several Phase I trials of recombinant TNF administered intraperitoneally as a dwell show that the protein was well tolerated at doses up to 350 μg/m^2 (21–23). Of note, concentrations of TNF in ascitic fluid were detectable up to 24 h after infusion and the estimated intraperitoneal half-life of the protein was between 8 and 12 h. No consistent serum levels of the protein could be detected in these trials. The reason for this is not entirely understood but may be related to the fact that the protein forms naturally occurring homotrimers that may limit systemic absorption from the peritoneal cavity. Resolution of malignant ascites was observed in a significant number of individuals, indicating that the protein may have exerted meaningful antitumor activity following this form of intracavitary administration (21,22).

Based on these data a Phase I trial of escalating dose TNF administrated with CDDP via CHPP was conducted at the NCI (16). In that trial 250 mg/m^2 of CDDP was administered with TNF at 0.1–0.3 mg/L of perfusate. At the first dose escalation of TNF (0.3 mg/L) severe dose-limiting nephrotoxicity was encountered and the maximum safe tolerated doses of CDDP and TNF given in combination were determined to be 250 mg/m^2 and 0.1 mg/L, respectively. The perfusate AUC for TNF was > 4000-fold higher than plasma AUC. Figure 3 shows the AUC of plasma CDDP with administration with various doses of TNF. Interestingly, there was a 1.6-fold higher plasma CDDP AUC in two patients treated at 0.3 mg/L of TNF compared to seven patients receiving 0.1 mg/L TNF and a 2.5-fold higher plasma CDDP AUC compared to the four patients who received no TNF at an equivalent dose of CDDP. Taken together, these data indicate that the dose-limiting renal toxicity observed with the combination therapy may have been related to some inflammatory changes secondary to TNF within the peritoneal cavity that promoted absorption of CDDP and resulted in higher systemic concentrations.

Table 2

Pharmacokinetic Parameters of CDDP Administered Intraperitoneally via CHPP over 90 Min

Dose (mg/m²)	No. of patients	C_{max}/plasma (mg/L)	C_{max}/perfusate (mg/L)	λ_2 h^{-1}	$t_{1/2\beta}$ (h)	AUC/plasma (mg·h/L)	AUC/perfusate (mg·h/L)	AUCpf/AUCpl
100	3	0.54 ± 0.21	14.2 ± 0.4	0.025 ± 0.002	27.4 ± 2.5	0.59 ± 0.32	25.4 ± 8.7	56.5 ± 45
150	3	1.38 ± 0.41	12.6 ± 5.5	0.027 ± 0.014	32.2 ± 28.9	1.42 ± 0.31	22.7 ± 3.4	16.7 ± 5.4
200	3	1.61 ± 0.25	41.3 ± 13.8	0.019 ± 0.014	50 ± 27.1	1.99 ± 0.043	85.4 ± 29.7	42 ± 6
250	19	3.86 ± 2.01	20.2 ± 15.3	0.023 ± 0.017	46.6 ± 35.2	4.42 ± 35.2	36.7 ± 30.9	10.1 ± 12.2
300	15	9.31 ± 7.79	40.9 ± 37.7	0.017 ± 0.007	47.2 ± 18.8	10.8 ± 8.46	75.3 ± 29.2	6.9 ± 3.2
350	9	12.7 ± 4.35	45.5 ± 21.4	0.011 ± 0.003	67 ± 17.4	13.6 ± 3.1	79.3 ± 29.2	6.9 ± 2.4
400	2	22.7 ± 5.82	41.4 ± 8.3	0.013 ± 0.004	55.9 ± 15.7	25 ± 8.7	145.6 ± 128	6.6 ± 6.8
Total	54			0.019 ± 0.012	48.9 ± 26.6			12.9 ±17.5
Median				0.015	46.9			7

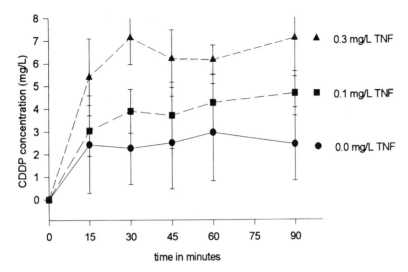

Fig. 3. Cisplatin perfusate concentrations over time in patients undergoing CHPP with increasing doses of TNF. The AUC of cisplatin was 2.5-fold higher in two patients treated with 0.3 mg/L of TNF compared to seven patients who received an equivalent dose of platinum alone.

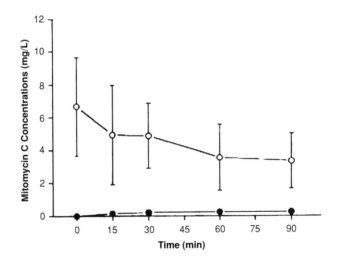

Fig. 4. Mitomycin C concentrations in perfusate (open circles) and plasma (filled circles) over time in patients undergoing CHPP at a dose of 10 mg/L.

Mitomycin C showed an advantage similar to CDDP when administered via CHPP (Fig. 4) *(24,25)*. Serial perfusate and plasma AUCs were determined for five patients with pancreatic or gastric cancer treated by laproscopic CHPP with both cisplatin and mitomycin C *(3)*. The AUC of MMC in perfusate was 389 ± 181 mg·min/mL compared to 18 ± 2 mg·min/mL in the plasma and represents a 22-fold higher dose in perfusate compared to serum. As would be expected, systemic toxicity is minimal, with no grade 3 or 4 toxicities.

2.2. Clinical Results with CHPP

The first reported CHPP, or the use of a recirculating infusion system to deliver hyperthermia and chemotherapy to the abdominal compartment, was performed in 1980 by Spratt et al. in a 35-yr-old male with pseudomyxoma peritoneii *(26)*. However, most of the early studies of this technique come from the Japanese experience using CHPP for prophylactic or therapeutic treatment after resection for gastric cancer. Koga et al. reported the first multiarm clinical trial of CHPP as prophylaxis against abdominal carcinomatosis in 60 patients with gastric cancer *(27)*. All patients underwent gastric resection with curative intent and were then randomized to receive no further treatment or CHPP with mitomycin C at 8–10 mg/L. Results from the subset analysis of 47 patients with serosal invasion by pathology showed a trend toward better survival at 3 yr in the CHPP treated group (83%) vs the standard therapy group (67%). In a similar trial, Fujimoto et al. selected 59 patients with gastric cancer to receive CHPP with perfusate containing mitomycin C at 10 mg/L vs no further treatment after resection *(28)*. At 1-yr follow-up, overall survival was significantly different at 80% for the CHPP-treated patients compared to 34% for the nonperfused controls. Moreover, in patients with peritoneal carcinomatosis, median posttreatment survival was 1 yr whereas the median survival for those who received CHPP had not been reached at the 3-yr follow-up. Hamazoe et al. treated 82 gastric cancer patients with gross serosal invasion but no peritoneal implants with either CHPP using mitomycin C or no further treatment after curative surgery *(29)*. The CHPP-treatment group had a trend toward lower incidence of peritoneal recurrence compared to the nonperfused control group ($p = 0.08$), but no statistically significant difference in survival at 5 yr (64% vs 53%). Fujimura et al. treated 31 patients with peritoneal carcinomatosis from gastric cancer using CHPP with 200 mg/m^2 of CDDP and 20 mg/m^2 of mitomycin C; subsequently, 12 patients underwent second-look laparotomy which showed four complete responses (CR) and one partial response (PR) with an overall response rate of 41% *(30)*. In patients with a CR or PR, overall survival at 2 yr was 50% compared with 0% of the nonresponders. Fujimura et al. followed this study with a three-arm randomized trial initially reported in 1994 comparing CHPP with CDDP/mitomycin C, continuous normothermia peritoneal perfusion (CNPP) with CDDP/mitomycin C vs surgery alone in 139 patients receiving curative surgery for T2–T4 gastric cancer *(31)*. The perfusate in CHPP-treatment group was heated to 42–43°C whereas that of the CNPP-treatment group remained at 37°C. Overall survival at 5 yr was 61% for CHPP, 43% for CNPP, and 42% for surgery alone.

More recent result of Phase II and I clinical trials of CHPP for a variety of tissue histologies other than gastric cancer have been reported. After treating 84 patients with peritoneal carcinomatosis from a variety of primary sites including colon ($n = 38$), appendix ($n = 22$), or stomach ($n = 19$) with CHPP using mitomycin C, Loggie et al. reported a median survival of 14.6, 31.1, and 10.1 mo, respectively *(32)*. The NCI reported the results of CHPP with CDDP on 18 patients with primary peritoneal mesothelioma. This cohort experienced a 26-mo progression-free survival and overall 2-yr survival of 80%, with nine out of ten patients having resolution of their ascites. In a Phase I trial of CHPP using carboplatin on six patients with residual epithelial ovarian cancer after standard debulking, Steller et al. reported five of six patients had no evidence of disease at a median follow-up of 15 mo *(33)*.

In summary, CHPP shows promise as a treatment option for peritoneal carcinomatosis for a wide variety of histologies. The administration of hyperthermia and chemotherapy to the peritoneal cavity, the minimal systemic absorption of these agents, and the resulting decrease in systemic toxicity make this an attractive treatment that certainly warrants further investigation.

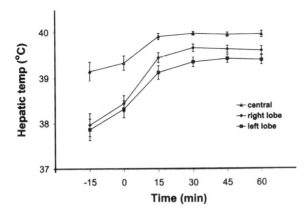

Fig. 5. Intrahepatic temperature levels during IHP showing prompt and uniform distribution of hyperthermia throughout the hepatic parenchyma during treatment.

3. VASCULAR ISOLATION AND PERFUSION

Vascular isolation and perfusion is a specialized operative procedure used to physically isolate blood flow to and from an organ or extremity to deliver chemotherapy, biological agents, and hyperthermia to a region of the body at doses higher than would otherwise be tolerated systemically (6). In general, the main artery and vein supplying blood to the region are prepared by dissecting and ligating all collateral vessels, cannulated, and connected to an extracorporeal bypass machine to circulate agents under hyperthermic conditions. In the liver, isolated hepatic perfusion (IHP) is performed for isolated unresectable hepatic metastases or primary hepatocellular carcinoma (34–38). In the extremity, isolated limb perfusion (ILP) has been utilized for metastatic extremity melanoma or unresectable high-grade sarcoma (7,8,39,40).

3.1. Isolated Hepatic Perfusion

There are both advantages and disadvantages to IHP when compared with other types of systemic and regional cancer therapies for unresectable cancers of the liver. IHP allows for the delivery of higher doses of agents directly to the liver than systemically tolerated, but, as a regional treatment, does not treat occult disease outside of the liver. Unlike surgical resection or regional ablative techniques such as radiofrequency ablation, cryotherapy, or ethanol injection, IHP can be used to treat large (>5 cm) deposits, bilobar disease, and potentially micrometastases (10). Although chemoembolization or infusion of chemotherapy into the hepatic artery through implantable pumps or percutaneous catheters can minimize systemic toxicity and treat the entire organ, these techniques still rely on the first-pass effect to remove the agent from the circulation (41–44). However, IHP allows for complete isolation of the vascular supply from the systemic circulation; therefore, the dose of therapeutic agent is limited only by the tissue tolerance of normal hepatic parenchyma (45). Also, at the end of the perfusion the circuit is flushed with normal saline to remove residual therapeutic agents from the hepatic vasculature and further decrease systemic exposure. IHP also effectively delivers potentially tumoricidal levels of hyperthermia uniformly to the liver (Fig. 5). However, IHP is a technically challenging procedure to perform and provides one relatively short exposure to the hyperthermia and chemotherapy, necessitating the use of a highly efficacious agent.

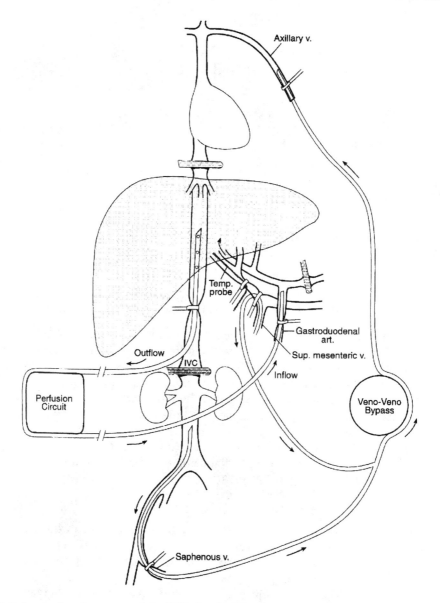

Fig. 6. Schema showing setup of the IHP circuit. The perfusion circuit inflow is via a catheter positioned in the gastroduodenal artery and outflow is via a catheter positioned in an isolated segment of retrohepatic inferior vena cava. A second veno–veno bypass machine is used to shunt inferior vena cava and portal blood flow back to the systemic circulation.

Figure 6 demonstrates the general layout of the IHP circuit. Initially, a right subcostal incision is made and the abdomen is explored to exclude extrahepatic metastases. Except for limited periportal lymphadenopathy which can be completely dissected, if no other extrahepatic disease is found then the incision is extended and the liver is mobilized. Complete dissection and identification of the arterial and venous structures are performed to ensure that all collateral flow from the hepatic to systemic system is controlled.

This involves mobilizing the retrohepatic inferior vena cava (IVC) and ligating the right adrenal vein, phrenic veins, and IVC tributaries to the retroperitoneum. The gallbladder is removed to prevent chemotherapy-induced postoperative cholecystitis. The porta hepatis is throughly dissected and all palpable lymphadenopathy is removed. The common hepatic artery, proper hepatic artery, and the gastroduodenal artery (GDA) are isolated. The GDA is cannulated for hepatic inflow. A catheter is advanced through a saphenous vein cut down into the IVC just below the renal veins and another in the portal vein. These two catheters are attached via veno–veno bypass pump to a catheter in the axillary vein shunting IVC and portal venous blood to the axillary vein (Fig. 6). The infrahepatic IVC is isolated and a catheter place in the retrohepatic IVC to collect the venous outflow from the perfusion. Probes are placed in the right and left lobes of the liver to monitor temperature.

The perfusion is performed with outflow from the retrohepatic IVC and inflow into the hepatic artery via the GDA. The perfusion circuit consists of a roller pump, membrane oxygenator, and heat exchanger. The temperature and pH of the perfusate are monitored. After completion of a 1-h perfusion, the liver is flushed via the GDA and the portal vein. The catheters are removed, the vasculature repaired, and the incision closed.

3.1.1. PHARMACOKINETICS

Despite the technical challenges of this procedure, the application of IHP for the delivery of therapy for liver metastases is particularly attractive because complete vascular isolation allows dose escalation and removes the need for drug elimination via the first pass effect. The most common agents used in IHP currently are TNF and melphalan and some centers have previously used 5-fluorouracil (5-FU), mitomycin C, or CDDP (10,35,36,46–49). In a Phase I trial of IHP at the NCI using TNF and melphalan with an alternating dose escalation design, hepatic venoocclusive disease occurred at a melphalan dose of 2 mg/kg body weight and dose-limiting coagulopathy was seen at 1.5 mg of TNF. The maximum safe tolerated doses are therefore 1.5 mg/kg of melphalan and 1 mg of TNF (34).

In the past, leakage of perfusate into the systemic circulation was monitored by using a radioactive tracer technique (50,51). However, the liver is an ideal organ for isolated perfusion, and in 50 patients undergoing IHP we detected a small leak in only two, both of which were easily corrected by adjusting vascular clamps (45). Enzyme-linked immunosorbent assay (ELISA) was used to measure TNF levels in the cohort of 50 patients from samples of serum and perfusate taken every 15 min during perfusion and are shown in Fig. 7. TNF levels in the perfusate rise within the first 15 min and stay consistently elevated throughout the length of the perfusion. However, serum TNF levels are undetectable at all time points, indicating no systemic leak.

Melphalan concentrations over time in perfusate are shown in Fig. 7. The decrease in melphalan concentration over time is presumably due to hydrolysis of drug under hyperthermic conditions, which has been demonstrated in mock perfusion (52) and no consistently measurable systemic levels could be identified.

3.1.2. CLINICAL RESULTS OF IHP

The first reported IHP on human subjects was performed by Ausman in 1961 at Roswell Park Cancer Institute in Buffalo, NY (53). Five patients received normothermic IHP with nitrogen mustard and although no response data were recorded, two of the five patients were long-term survivors, indicating some treatment response. No further studies were reported using this technique until 20 yr later (Table 3). In 1984, Aigner et al. used a 1-h hyperthermic IHP with 700–1100 mg of 5-FU to treat 32 patients (54). Although they did not report response data, median survival with IHP alone was only 8 mo and with IHP plus intraarterial

Table 3
Summary of Previous IHP Chemotherapy Trials

Chemotherapeutics and hyperthermia

Authors	n	Agents	Doses	Duration	Temperature (°C)	Results
Ausman 1961	5	Nitrogen mustard	0.2–0.4 mg/kg	N/A	37°	Two apparent long-term "survivors" no response data
Aigner 1984	32	5-FU	700–1100 mg	1 h	39.5°–40°	Median survival: 8 mo
Skibba 1986	8			4 h	42.0°–42.5°	5/6 responders
Schwemmle 1987	50	5-FU	300–1,250 mg	1 h	39.0°–39.5°	Median survival: 14 mo
		Mitomycin C ($n = 14$)	5–50 mg			CR: 9 (41%); PR: 28 (68%)
		Cisplatin ($n = 4$)	50 mg			PR: 20%
Hafström 1994	29	Melphalan	0.5 mg/kg	1 h	40.0°	5 survived 3 yr
		Cisplatin	0.5 mg/kg			
Marinelli 1996	9	Mitomycin	30 mg/m^2	1 h	37°	1 PR: 1 CR (28% RR)
van de Velde 1996	24	melphalan	0.54 mg/kg	1 h	37°	1 CR; 6 PR (41% RR)

Chemotherapeutics, TNF, and hyperthermia

Authors	n	Agents	Doses	Duration	Temperature (°C)	Results
De Vries 1998	8	Melphalan	1 mg/kg	1 h	>41°	Mortality 33%
		TNF				5/6 PR
	1	TNF alone	0.8 mg			
Hafström 1998	11	Melphalan	0.5 mg/kg	1 h	39°	Mortality 18%
		TNF	30–200 µg			Morbidity 45%
						3/11 PR
Oldhafer 1998	6	Melphalan	60–140 mg	1 h	40°–41°	Mortality 0%
		TNF	200–300 µg			1/6 CR, 2/6 PR
Alexander 1998	34	Melphalan	1.5 mg/kg	1 h	39.5°–40°	Mortality 3%
		TNF	1.0 mg			1 CR, 26 PR (75%)

PR, Partial response; CR, complete response; 5-FU, 5-fluorouacil; RR, response rate.

338

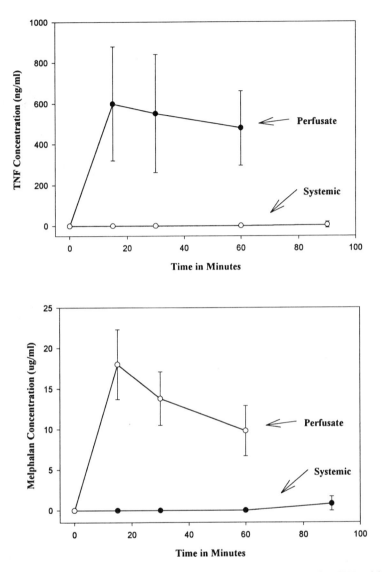

Fig. 7. TNF and melphalan concentrations over time in patients undergoing IHP with 1.5 mg/kg of melphalan and 1 mg of TNF. Of note, TNF concentrations stay largely stable during perfusion, indicating little degradation or tissue uptake of the protein. Melphalan concentrations decrease over time, consistent with hydrolysis of the drug under hyperthermic conditions and some tissue absorption. Systemic concentrations of TNF and melphalan were not reproducibly measurable.

chemotherapy it was only 12 mo. Treating six patients with a 4-h IHP with hyperthermia of 42.5°C alone, Skibba and Quebbeman demonstrated radiographic evidence of central tumor necrosis in five of six evaluable patients *(38,55)*. Schwemmle et al. treated 50 patients with 1-h IHP using moderate hyperthermia to 39.5°C and two chemotherapeutic regimens, 5-FU alone or 5-FU, mitomycin C, and CDDP *(56)*. They reported an overall response rate of 68% and complete response (CR) of 18% but used criteria such as decreased carcinoembryonic antigen (CEA) levels and nonstandard radiographic criteria to determine response.

There was a significant treatment and operative mortality of 10–25% in these early stud-ies. Most of these reports represented results of a single initial institutional experience with this technique in patients who frequently had very advanced conditions. Because the treat-ment risks are relatively high and the early results were equivocal, IHP has not been used except in a limited number of centers worldwide.

Within the last 10 yr, several European and United States clinical centers have reported their experiences with IHP. After treating 29 patients with melphalan and CDDP with a 1-h IHP at 40°C, Hafström reported a partial response (PR) rate of 20% and had five patients who survived 3 yr (50). Van de Velde and co-workers reported the results of 1-h normoth-ermic IHP using either mitomycin C or melphalan, with overall response rates of 28% and 41%, respectively (37). De Vries from the Netherlands treated eight patients with TNF and melphalan with a 1-h hyperthermic IHP and five of six patients experienced a PR (80%) but treatment had a 33% treatment-related mortality (57,58). Using melphalan and escalating doses of TNF in a 1-h hyperthermic IHP, Hafström et al. treated 11 patients, resulting in a 27% PR rate (3/11) but a high treatment mortality of 18% (36). Oldhafer and co-workers from Germany reported a 50% RR and no mortality from six patients treated with TNF and melphalan in a 1-h hyperthermic IHP (35). The largest series comes from the NCI where Alexander and colleagues treated 50 patients with 1-h hyperthermic IHP with melphalan and TNF with an overall response rate of 75% and mortality of 4% (10). Median duration of response was 9 mo, but some responses continued beyond 3 yr (Fig. 8).

In summary, IHP provides regional delivery of chemotherapeutic agents to the liver, but is technically challenging and has significant associated morbidity and mortality. Response rates are somewhat variable; current Phase III trials comparing hepatic arterial infusion (HAI) + IHP vs HAI alone in patients with colorectal cancer liver metastases may help to answer these continuing questions.

3.2. Isolated Limb Perfusion

ILP of the lower extremity is most commonly performed via the external iliac vessels and of the arm via the axillary vessels. However, the femoral, popliteal, or brachial vessels are also used in certain circumstances. With respect to lower extremity ILPs, the level of per-fusion should be based on the distribution of the disease and technical considerations such as patient body habitus or a history of prior surgery in the iliac or femoral region. The rate of inguinal nodal recurrence in melanoma patients who received femoral or iliac perfusion was comparable (25 vs 32%, respectively) indicating that perfusion through the more proxi-mal iliac vessels does not eradicate inguinal lymph node micrometastases (59).

Using a lower abdominal "transplant" incision, a retroperitoneal approach to the iliac vessels is made. The external iliac artery and vein are dissected distally and all venous tributaries and arterial branches arising proximal to, or under, the inguinal ligament are ligated and divided. Proximally the hypogastric vein is ligated in situ as it may contribute to increased systemic leak rates (50). The external iliac vessels are cannulated and a Steinmann pin is anchored into the anterior superior iliac spine and an Esmarch tourniquet is snugly wrapped at the root of the extremity. The heat exchanger and external warming blankets are used to maintain tissue temperatures in the range of 38.5–40.0°C.

The extracorporeal perfusion circuit is comprised of a roller pump, heat exchanger, and oxygenator. The circuit is typically primed with 700 mL of balanced salt solution, 1 U of packed red blood cells, and 1500 U of heparin. The resultant hematocrit of approx 25% provides adequate tissue oxygen tension, and perfusing at a higher hematocrit confers no additional benefit in preventing regional toxicity (60). Flow rates in the range of 50 mL/L of limb volume/min are desirable and adjusted depending on line pressure, reservoir volume, or the presence of systemic leak based on intraoperative monitoring.

Patient A

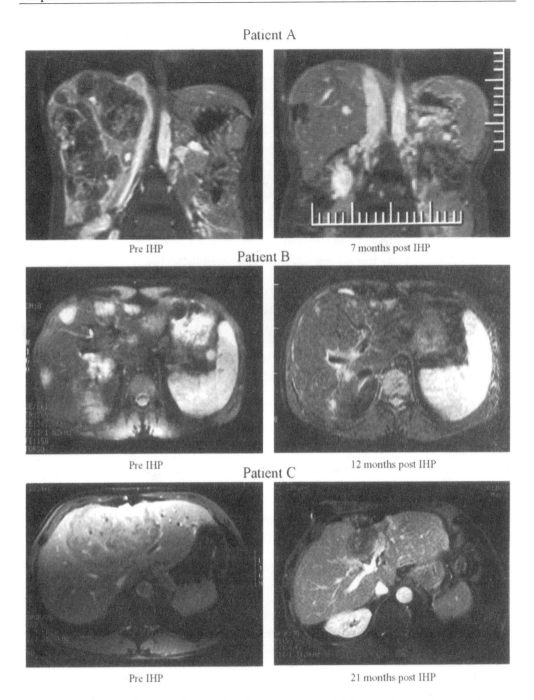

Patient B

Patient C

Fig. 8. Pretreatment (*left-sided panels*) and posttreatment (*right-sided panels*) magnetic resonance imaging studies of three patients undergoing IHP for colorectal cancer metastases. Patient A had large multiple bilobar metastases that responded significantly to a single 60-min IHP with TNF and melphalan. Patient B had multiple hepatic metastases as indicated by the bright signals in the hepatic parenchyma. Repeat imaging 12 mo after treatment showed a significant ongoing response. Patient C had a large centrally located hepatic metastasis from colorectal cancer treated by IHP using melphalan alone followed by HAI therapy with FUDR and leucovorin. He experienced a partial response in the liver for almost 2 yr.

Continuous intraoperative monitoring to assess perfusate leak into the systemic circulation is being used more routinely and is an important component of isolated perfusion therapy when one considers that perfusate doses of melphalan and tumor necrosis factor are at least 10-fold greater than maximally tolerated systemic doses. Careful monitoring of leak may reduce the severity of systemic complications and improve response rates in the limb *(50,61)*. Standard protocols using ^{131}I-radiolabeled albumin or ^{99m}Tc labeled red blood cells have been described for continuous intraoperative monitoring of leak during isolated limb perfusion *(51,62)*. A gamma detection camera is positioned over the precordium so the heart serves as a stable reservoir of blood to measure radioactivity leak. The detection system provides continuous assessment of leak rates and can discriminate a leak of < 1% *(62)*. Leak rates using this system have been shown to correlate with measured leak of TNF or melphalan from the perfusate and the development of systemic toxicity *(50,61)*.

3.2.1. Pharmacokinetics

The dose of melphalan that is typically administered in ILP is based on limb volume and 10–13 mg/L are associated with acceptable transient side effects but significant antitumor efficacy *(63)*. The disposition of melphalan in the perfusion circuit is influenced by several factors. First, there can be systemic leakage of the drug during limb perfusion and several investigators have shown that leak rates of > 5% occur in approx 10% of patients *(50)*. If there is systemic leakage, then several maneuvers can be performed to reverse or slow the efflux of melphalan into the systemic circulation such as altering the flow rate of the perfusion circuit *(64)*. Typically, isolated limb perfusion is performed for 30 min under hyperthermic conditions alone and then after tissue temperatures are approx 38.5°C melphalan is added slowly into the arterial line of the perfusion circuit over 5 min. The perfusion continues for an additional 60 min and then the perfusate is flushed from the extremity to remove residual melphalan prior to reestablishing the native blood flow to the extremity. We have analyzed melphalan concentrations in the perfusion circuit in 18 individuals undergoing lower extremity ILP with melphalan with or without 3–4 mg of TNF at the NCI. The data show that peak melphalan concentrations are observed immediately after the drug is administered and decrease progressively over the course of the perfusion (Fig. 9). It is also known that melphalan undergoes spontaneous hydrolysis under hyperthermic condition *(52)*, which may account for the decrease in concentrations in the perfusate observed over time.

Klasse and co-workers reported melphalan tissue concentrations for patients undergoing ILP for melanoma arising in the lower extremity. They found a direct correlation between increasing tumor concentrations of melphalan and the AUC of the drug in the perfusion circuit *(65)*. On the other hand, muscle concentrations were directly correlated with peak melphalan concentrations, suggesting that a lower peak level but a sustained higher AUC will be associated with better efficacy in minimal regional toxicity. As a consequence, several investigators administered the total dose of melphalan in the perfusion circuit as divided doses at time 0 and then at 30 min into the perfusion treatment. Concentrations of melphalan within tumor are likely due to the fact that melphalan is a phenylalanine derivative and is actively taken out by cells of melanocyte origin *(66)*. The concentration of TNF in the perfusion circuit, in contrast to melphalan concentrations, remain largely stable and indicate that there is very little degradation or absorption of the cytokine into tissues over the course of the treatment. It is known that patients who have leak of perfusate > 1% peak systemic concentrations of TNF occur within 4 h of treatment. The systemic exposure to low doses of TNF is associated with a variety of cardiovascular and metabolic alterations that have been well characterized but are easily managed with fluid hydration and close monitoring during the first 24 h after treatment *(67)*.

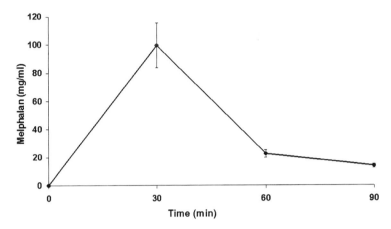

Fig. 9. Melphalan concentrations over time in patients undergoing a hyperthermic lower extremity ILP with 10 mg/L of limb volume of melphalan with ($n = 9$) or without ($n = 9$) TNF. Melphalan is added slowly to the perfusion circuit at 30 min of treatment and perfusion continues for an additional 60 min. Peak concentrations are therefore observed immediately after administration of melphalan.

3.2.2. Current Results with ILP for Extremity Melanoma or Sarcoma

In the initial report from Lièrard and Lejuenne, results from 29 patients treated with ILP using a combination of TNF, melphalan, and hyperthermia for in-transit melanoma or high-grade sarcoma of the extremity were presented *(68)*. The overall response rate in that initial trial was 100%, with 89% of patients having a complete response to treatment. In subsequent reports from various institutions, including a follow-up report from Lièrard and Lejuenne of a larger series of patients, the complete response rates were lower and ranged between 70% and 79% (Table 4) *(61,69,70)*. A prospective random assignment trial was initiated at the NCI and subsequently expanded to a multiinstitutional study but was closed prematurely in 1997 owing to a lack of available clinical grade TNF in the United States. The results of that trial showed no difference in overall or complete response rates between the groups *(71)*. It is also noteworthy that in several trials of ILP using melphalan alone, complete response rates between 56% and 82% have been reported *(72–75)*. A prospective random assignment trial comparing melphalan and TNF with melphalan alone administered via ILP for in-transit melanoma of the extremity was closed in Europe because of low accrual, suggesting a bias that for most patients with this histology, TNF does not substantially contribute to efficacy compared with melphalan alone.

ILP has been used for patients with unresectable high-grade extremity sarcoma for palliation, for potential cure in cases of multifocal disease, and as a neoadjuvant therapy to convert an unresectable lesion to a resectable one. Most data reported on ILP using chemotherapeutics alone indicate limited antitumor activity against this histology *(76,77)*. After the initial reports by Lièrard and Lejuenne using the combination of TNF, melphalan, and hyperthermia as a neoadjuvant treatment for high-grade unresectable sarcoma, a multi-institutional trial using this regimen for patients with condition was conducted in Europe and the results reported in two papers by Eggermont and co-workers *(8,79)*. In more than 219 patients, the overall clinical and pathologic response rate was > 80% and the limb salvage rate was 84%. Based on these results TNF is now licensed for administration via ILP for high-grade sarcoma in Europe, but no trials are currently being conducted in the United States.

Table 4
Selected Series of Isolated Limb Perfusion for Extremity Melanoma or Sarcoma

Author	Trial type	Agents	Assessable	Complete response(%)	Partial response(%)	Overall (%)
Lièñard	Phase II ILP Melanoma/sarcoma	Regimen A Mephalan, 10–13 mg/L TNF, 3–4 mg IFN, 0.2 mg	29	90	10	100
Lièñard	Phase III ILP Melanoma	Regimen A vs Melphalan, 10–13 mg/L TNF, 3–4 mg	31 33	78 69	22 22	100 91
Fraker	Phase III ILP Melanoma	Regimen A vs Melphalan, 10–13 mg/L	20 23	80 61	10 39	90 100
Eggermont	Phase II ILP Sarcoma	Melphalan, 10–13 mg/L TNF, 3–4 mg	186	29	53	82
Vaglini	Phase II ILP Melanoma	Melphalan, 10–13 mg/L TNF, 0.5–4.0 mg IFN, 0.2 mg	10	70		70
Hill	Phase I ILP Melanoma	Melphalan, 10–13 mg/L TNF, 0.125–0.5 mg IFN, 0.2 mg	7	100		100
Posner	Phase I/II ILP Melanoma	TNF, alone 1–4 mg	6	16	34	50[a]

ILP, Isolated limb perfusion; TNF, tumor necrosis factor.
[a]All responses short-lived (one 7-mo complete response, two 1-mo partial response).

4. SUMMARY

Regional delivery of hyperthermia and chemotherapy for patients with disease confined to the treatment field has shown promise as well as a decreasing treatment-related mortality. CHPP is being used to treat abdominal carcinomatosis for a wide variety of sources, with long-term results still pending. Vascular isolation techniques have become safer, and may present an option for the treatment of isolated liver, limb, lung, or renal disease. The pharmacokinetic advantage of these regional treatments has been well established, and continuing clinical evaluation will further define the best clinical applications of these therapies.

REFERENCES

1. Markman M. Principles of regional antineoplastic drug delivery. In: Markman M (ed). Regional Chemotherapy: Clinical Research and Practice. Totowa, NJ:Humana Press, 2000, pp. 1–4.
2. Dedrick RL. Theoretical and experimental bases of intraperitoneal chemotherapy. Semin Oncol 1985; XII:1–6.
3. Alexander HR, Bartlett DL, Libutti SK. National Cancer Institute experience with regional therapy for unresectable primary and metastatic cancer of the liver or peritoneal cavity. In: Markman M (ed). Current Clinical Oncology: Regional Chemotherapy: Clinical Research and Practice. Totowa, NJ: Humana Press, 1999, pp. 127–150.
4. Alexander HR, Buell JF, Fraker DL. Rationale and clinical status of continuous hyperthermic peritoneal perfusion (CHPP) for the treatment of peritoneal carcinomatosis. In: DeVita V, Hellman S, Rosenberg S (eds). Principles and Practices of Oncology Updates. Philadelphia, PA: JB Lippincott, 1995, pp. 1–9.
5. Sugarbaker PH. Intraperitoneal chemotherapy and cytoreductive surgery for the prevention and treatment of peritoneal carcinomatosis and sarcomatosis. Semin Surg Oncol 1998; 14:254–261.
6. Alexander HR Jr. Isolation perfusion. In: DeVita VT Jr, Hellman S, Rosenberg SA (eds). Cancer: Principles and Practice of Oncology. Philadelphia, PA: Lippincott Williams & Wilkins, 2001, pp. 769–776.
7. Alexander HR, Fraker DL, Bartlett DL. Isolated limb perfusion for malignant melanoma. Semin Surg Oncol 1996; 12:416–428.
8. Eggermont AMM, Koops HS, Klausner JM, et al. Isolated limb perfusion with tumor necrosis factor and melphalan for limb salvage in 186 patients with locally advanced soft tissue extremity sarcomas. Ann Surg 1996; 224:756–765.
9. Alexander HR, Bartlett DL, Libutti SK. Isolated hepatic perfusion: a potentially effective treatment for patients with metastatic or primary cancers confined to the liver. Cancer J Sci Am 1998; 4:2–11.
10. Alexander HR Jr, Bartlett DL, Libutti SK, Fraker DL, Moser T, Rosenberg SA. Isolated hepatic perfusion with tumor necrosis factor and melphalan for unresectable cancers confined to the liver. J Clin Oncol 1998; 16:1479–1489.
11. Dikhoff T, van der Heider J, Dubbelman R, ten Bokkel Huinink WW. Tissue concentration of platinum after intraperitoneal cisplatin administration in patients (PTS). Proc AACR 1985; 26:162.
12. Wientjes MG, Badalament RA, Au JL. Penetration of intravesical doxorubicin in human bladders. Cancer Chemother Pharmacol 1996; 37:539–546.
13. Dedrick RL, Flessner MF. Pharmacokinetic problems in peritoneal drug administration: tissue penetration and surface exposure. J Natl Cancer Inst 1997; 89:480–487.
14. Sugarbaker PH. Management of peritoneal-surface malignancy: the surgeon's role. Langenbecks Arch Surg 1999; 384:576–587.
15. Sugarbaker PH. Peritonectomy procedures. Ann Surg 1995; 221:29–42.
16. Bartlett DL, Buell JF, Libutti SK, et al. A Phase I trial of continuous hyperthermic peritoneal perfusion with tumor necrosis factor and cisplatin in the treatment of peritoneal carcinomatosis. Cancer 1998; 83: 1251–1261.
17. Howell SB, Pfeifle CG, Wung WE, et al. Intraperitoneal cisplatin with systemic thiosulfate protection. Ann Intern Med 1982; 97:845–851.
18. Cho H-K, Lush RM, Bartlett DL, et al. Pharmacokinetics of cisplatin administered by continuous hyperthermic peritoneal perfusion (CHPP) to patients with peritoneal carcinomatosis. J Clin Pharmacol 1999; 39:1–8.

19. Carswell EA, Old LJ, Kassel RL, Green S, Fiore N, Williamson B. An endotoxin-induced serum factor that causes necrosis of tumors. Proc Natl Acad Sci USA 1975; 72:3666–3670.
20. Alexander HR, Feldman AL. Tumor necrosis factor: basic principles and clinical application in systemic and regional cancer treatment. In: Rosenberg SA (ed). Biologic Therapy of Cancer. Philadelphia, PA: Lippincott, 2000, pp. 174–193.
21. Markman M, Reichman B, Ianotti N, et al. Phase I trial of recombinant tumor necrosis factor administered by the intraperitoneal route. Reg Cancer Treat 1989; 2:174–177.
22. Räth U, Kaufmann M, Schmid H, et al. Effect of intraperitoneal recombinant human tumour necrosis factor alpha on malignant ascites. Eur J Cancer 1991; 27:121–125.
23. Raeth U, Schmid H, Karck U, Kempeni J, Schlick E, Kaufmann M. Phase-II-trial of recombinant human tumor necrosis factora (rHuTNF) in patients with malignant ascites from ovarian carcinomas and non-ovarian tumors with intraperitoneal spread. Proc ASCO 1991; 10:187.
24. Gilly FN, Carry PY, Sayag AC, et al. Regional chemotherapy (with mitomycin C) and intra-operative hyperthermia for digestive cancers with peritoneal carcinomatosis. Hepato-Gastroenterol 1994; 41:124–129.
25. Fujimoto S, Shrestha RD, Kokubun M, et al. Pharmacokinetic analysis of mitomycin C for intraperitoneal hyperthermic perfusion in patients with far-advanced or recurrent gastric cancer. Reg Cancer Treat 1989; 2:198–202.
26. Spratt JS, Adcock RA, Muskovin M, Sherrill W, McKeown J. Clinical delivery system for intraperitoneal hyperthermic chemotherapy. Cancer Res 1980; 40:256–260.
27. Koga A, Watanabe K, Fukuyama T, Takiguchi S, Nakayama F. Diagnosis and operative indications for polypoid lesion of the gallbladder. Arch Surg 1988; 123:26–29.
28. Fujimoto S, Shrestha RD, Kokuban M, et al. Positive results of combined therapy of surgery and intraperitoneal hyperthermic perfusion for far-advanced gastric cancer. Ann Surg 1990; 212:592–596.
29. Hamazoe R, Maeta M, Kaibara N. Intraperitoneal thermochemotherapy for prevention of peritoneal recurrence of gastric cancer. Cancer 1994; 73:2048–2052.
30. Fujimura T, Yonemura Y, Fushida S, et al. Continuous hyperthermic peritoneal perfusion for the treatment of peritoneal dissemination in gastric cancers and subsequent second-look operation. Cancer 1990; 65:65–71.
31. Fujimura T, Yonemura Y, Muraoka K, et al. Continuous hyperthermic peritoneal perfusion for the prevention of peritoneal recurrence of gastric cancer: randomized controlled study. World J Surg 1994; 18:150–155.
32. Loggie BW, Fleming RA, Geisinger KR. Cytologic assessment before and after intraperitoneal hyperthermic chemotherapy for peritoneal carcinomatosis. Acta Cytologica 1996; 40:1154–1158.
33. Steller MA, Egorin MJ, Trimble EL, et al. A pilot phase I trial of continuous hyperthermic peritoneal perfusion with high-dose carboplatin as primary treatment of patients with small-volume residual ovarian cancer. Cancer Chemother Pharmacol 1999; 43:106–114.
34. Alexander HR, Bartlett DL, Libutti SK. Current status of isolated hepatic perfusion with or without tumor necrosis factor for the treatment of unresectable cancers confined to liver. Oncologist 2000; 5: 416–424.
35. Oldhafer KJ, Lang H, Frerker M, et al. First experience and technical aspects of isolated liver perfusion for extensive liver metastasis. Surgery 1998; 123:622–631.
36. Hafström L, Naredi P. Isolated hepatic perfusion with extracorporeal oxygenation using hyperthermia TNFa and melphalan: Swedish experience. Rec Results Cancer Res 1998; 147:120–126.
37. Marinelli A, de Brauw LM, Beerman H, et al. Isolated liver perfusion with mitomycin C in the treatment of colorectal cancer metastases confined to the liver. Jpn J Clin Oncol 1996; 26:341–350.
38. Skibba JL, Quebbeman EJ. Tumoricidal effects and patient survival after hyperthermic liver perfusion. Arch Surg 1986; 121:1266–1271.
39. Lejeune FJ, Lienard D, Eggermont A, et al. Administration of high-dose tumor necrosis factor alpha by isolation perfusion of the limbs. Rationale and results. J Infus Chemother 1995; 5:73–81.
40. Lienard D, Agermont AMM, Koops HS, et al. Isolated limb perfusion with tumour necrosis factor-α and melphalan with or without interferon-γ for the treatment of in-transit melanoma metastases: a multicentre randomized Phase II study. Melanoma Res 1999; 9:491–502.
41. Bartlett DL. Treatment of patients with hepatic metastases. Cancer J Sci Am 2000; 6(Suppl 2):S169–S176.
42. Alexander HR, Bartlett DL, Fraker DL, Libutti SK. Regional treatment strategies for unresectable primary or metastatic cancer confined to the liver. In: DeVita VT Jr, Hellman S, Rosenberg SA (eds). Cancer: Principles and Practice of Oncology. Philadelphia, PA: JB Lippincott, 1996, pp. 1–19.

43. Ridge JA, Sigurdson ER. Distribution of fluorodeoxyuridine uptake in the liver and colorectal hepatic metastases of human beings after arterial infusion. Surg Gynecol Obstet 1987; 164:318–323.
44. Venook AP. Update on hepatic intra-arterial chemotherapy. Oncology 1997; 11:947–970.
45. Libutti SK, Bartlett DL, Fraker DL, Alexander HR. Technique and results of hyperthermic isolated hepatic perfusion with tumor necrosis factor and melphalan for the treatment of unresectable hepatic malignancies. J Am Coll Surg 2000; 191:519–530.
46. Kuppen PJK, Jonges LE, Van de Velde CJH, et al. Liver and tumour tissue concentrations of TNF-α in cancer patients treated with TNF-α and melphalan by isolated liver perfusion. Br J Cancer 1997; 75: 1497–1500.
47. Vahrmeijer AL, Van Der Eb MM, Van Dierendonck JH, Kuppen PJ, van de Velde CJ. Delivery of anticancer drugs via isolated hepatic perfusion: a promising strategy in the treatment of irresectable liver metastases? Semin Surg Oncol 1998; 14:262–268.
48. Aigner KR, Walther H, Link KH. Isolated liver perfusion with MMC/5-FU—surgical technique, pharmacokinetics, clinical results. Contr Oncol 1988; 29:229–246.
49. Hafström LR, Holmberg SB, Naredi PLJ, et al. Isolated hyperthermic liver perfusion with chemotherapy for liver malignancy. Surg Oncol 1994; 3:103–108.
50. Klaase JM, Kroon BBR, van Geel AN, Eggermont AMM, Franklin HR. Systemic leakage during isolated limb perfusion for melanoma. Br J Surg 1993; 80:1124–1126.
51. Barker WC, Andrich MP, Alexander HR, Fraker DL. Continuous intraoperative external monitoring of perfusate leak using I-131 human serum albumin during isolated perfusion of the liver and limbs. Eur J Nucl Med 1995; 22:1242–1248.
52. Scott RN, Blackie R, Kerr DJ, et al. Melphalan concentration and distribution in the tissues of tumour-bearing limbs treated by isolated limb perfusion. Eur J Cancer 1992; 28:1811–1813.
53. Ausman RK. Development of a technic for isolated perfusion of the liver. NY State J Med 1961; 61:3393–3397.
54. Aigner KR, Walther H, Tonn JC, Link KH, Schoch P, Schwemmle K. Die isolierte leberperfusion bei fortgeschrittenen metastasen kolorektaler karzinome. Onkologie 1984; 7:13–21.
55. Skibba JL, Quebbeman EJ, Komorowski RA, Thorsen KM. Clinical results of hyperthermic liver perfusion for cancer in the liver. In: Aigner KR, Patt YZ, Link KH, Kreidler J (eds). Regional Cancer Treatment. Basel, Switzerland: Karger, 1988, pp. 222–228.
56. Schwemmle K, Link KH, Rieck B. Rationale and indications for perfusion in liver tumors: current data. World J Surg 1987; 11:534–540.
57. de Vries MR, Borel Rinkes IH, van de Velder CJH, et al. Isolated hepatic perfusion with tumor necrosis factor α and melphalan: experimental studies in pigs and Phase I data from humans. Rec Results in Cancer Res 1998; 147:107–119.
58. de Vries MR, Borel Rinkes IHM, Buurman WA, Wiggers Th. Soluble TNF-α receptor induction by isolated hepatic perfusion with TNF-α and melphalan. Eur Surg Res 1995; 27:108 abstract.
59. Klaase JM, Kroon BBR, van Geel AN, Eggermont AMM, Franklin HR, van Dongen JA. The role of regional isolated perfusion in the eradication of melanoma micrometastases in the inguinal nodes: a comparison between an iliac and femoral perfusion procedure. Mel Res 1992; 2:407–410.
60. Klaase JM, Kroon BBR, van Slooten GW, van Dongen JA. Comparison between the use of whole blood versus a diluted perfusate in regional isolated perfusion by continuous monitoring of transcutaneous oxygen tension: a pilot study. J Invest Surg 1994; 7:249–258.
61. Thom AK, Alexander HR, Andrich MP, Barker WC, Rosenberg SA, Fraker DL. Cytokine levels and systemic toxicity in patients undergoing isolated limb perfusion (ILP) with high-dose TNF, interferon-gamma and melphalan. J Clin Oncol 1995; 13:264–273.
62. Hoekstra HJ, Naujocks T, Schraffordt-Koops H, et al. Continuous leaking monitoring during hyperthermic isolated regional perfusion of the lower limb: techniques and results. Reg Cancer Treat 1992; 4:301–304.
63. Wieberdink J, Benckhuysen C, Braat RP, van Slooten EA, Olthuis GAA. Dosimetry in isolation perfusion of the limbs by assessment of perfused tissue volume and grading of toxic tissue reactions. Eur J Cancer Clin Oncol 1982; 18:905–910.
64. Sorkin P, Abu-Abid S, Lev D, et al. Systemic leakage and side effects of tumor necrosis factor alpha administered via isolated limb perfusion can be manipulated by flow rate adjustment. Arch Surg 1995; 130:1079–1084.
65. Klaase JM, Kroon BBR, Beijnen JH, van Slooten GW, van Dongen JA. Melphalan tissue concentrations in patients treated with regional isolated perfusion for melanoma of the lower limb. Br J Cancer 1994; 70:151–153.

66. Luck JM. Action of *p*-dichloroethyl amino-L-phenylalanine on Harding–Passey mouse melanoma. Science 1956; 123:984–985.
67. Fraker DL, Alexander HR, Andrich M, Rosenberg SA. Treatment of patients with melanoma of the extremity using hyperthermic isolated limb perfusion with melphalan, tumor necrosis factor, and interferon-gamma: results of a TNF dose escalation study. J Clin Oncol 1996; 14:479–489.
68. Lienard D, Ewalenko P, Delmotte JJ, Renard N, Lejeune FJ. High dose recombinant tumor necrosis factor alpha in combination with interferon gamma and melphalan in isolation perfusion of the limbs for melanoma and sarcoma. J Clin Oncol 1992; 10:52–60.
69. Lienard D, Lejeune F, Ewalenko I. In transit metastases of malignant melanoma treated by high dose rTNFa in combination with interferon-gamma and melphalan in isolation perfusion. World J Surg 1992; 16:234–240.
70. Vaglini M, Santinami M, Manzi R, et al. Treatment of in-transit metastases from cutaneous melanoma by isolation perfusion with tumour necrosis factor-alpha (TNF-α), melphalan and interferon-gamma (IFN-γ). Dose-finding experience at the National Cancer Institute of Milan. Melanoma Res 1994; 4:35–38.
71. Fraker DL. Limb perfusion with TNF: Current status of United States trials. Cambridge Symposia 1996; abstract 1, 13.
72. Minor DR, Allen RE, Alberts D, et al. A clinical and pharmacokinetic study of isolated limb perfusion with heat and melphalan for melanoma. Cancer 1985; 55:2638–2644.
73. Lejeune FJ, Deloof T, Ewalenko P, et al. Objective regression of unexcised melanoma in-transit metastases after hyperthermic isolation perfusion of the limbs with melphalan. Rec Results Cancer Res 1983; 86:268–276.
74. Skene AI, Bulman AS, Williams TR, et al. Hyperthermic isolated perfusion with melphalan in the treatment of advanced malignant melanoma of the lower limb. Br J Surg 1990; 77:765–767.
75. Klaase JM, Kroon BBR, van Geel AN, Eggermont AMM, Franklin HR, Hart AAM. Prognostic factors for tumor response and limb recurrence-free interval in patients with advanced melanoma of the limbs treated with regional isolated perfusion using melphalan. Surgery 1994; 115:39–45.
76. Klaase JM, Kroon BBR, Benckhuijsen C, van Geel AN, Albus-Lutter CE, Wieberdink J. Results of regional isolation perfusion with cytostatics in patients with soft tissue tumors of the extremities. Cancer 1989; 64:616–621.
77. di Filippo F, Calabro AM, Cavallari A, et al. The role of hyperthermic perfusion as a first step in the treatment of soft tissue sarcoma of the extremities. World J Surg 1988; 12:332–339.
78. Eggermont AMM, Koops HS, Liénard D, Kroon BBR, van Geel AN, Hoekstra HJ. Isolated limb perfusion with high dose tumor necrosis factor-α in combination with interferon-γ and melphalan for irresectable extremity soft tissue sarcomas: a multicenter trial. J Clin Oncol 1996; 14:2653–2665.

21 Isolated Lung Perfusion for the Treatment of Inoperable Pulmonary Malignancies

David S. Schrump, MD

1. INTRODUCTION

Primary and metastatic tumors involving the lungs cause considerable morbidity and mortality in cancer patients. Approximately 155,000 Americans will succumb to lung cancer in 2002 *(1)*. Many of these individuals will present with tumors that are confined to the chest, yet are unresectable owing to anatomic or physiologic limitations. Currently, median survival of patients with limited-stage small-cell or stage IIIA/B non-small-cell lung cancers treated with chemotherapy and/or radiation approximates 14 mo *(2)*. Whereas most of these individuals succumb to extrathoracic metastatic disease, a significant number develop life-threatening complications owing to uncontrolled growth of their primary tumors. Recalcitrant local disease following definitive induction therapy often precedes the development of systemic metastases in lung cancer patients.

Nearly one third of all patients dying from malignancies of nonthoracic origin suffer from pulmonary metastases. Many patients succumb to uncontrolled pulmonary metastases in the absence of other systemic disease; treatment of these individuals remains controversial *(3,4)*. A number of single-institution studies have demonstrated that resection alone may provide survival benefit in up to 40% of highly selected patients with pulmonary metastases *(5–7)*. A recent analysis of more than 5000 cases entered onto the International Registry of Pulmonary Metastases indicates that survival following pulmonary metastasectomy is contingent on histology, disease-free interval following resection of the primary malignancy, number of pulmonary nodules, and completeness of resection *(8)*. Overall, patients with metastatic melanomas do poorly despite complete resections (5-yr survival < 25%); in contrast, individuals with germ cell cancers fare much better following pulmonary metastasectomy, with 5-yr survivals of approx 60%. Patients with metastases from epithelial cancers have intermediate survivals. Collectively, these data indicate that whereas some

Handbook of Anticancer Pharmacokinetics and Pharmacodynamics
Edited by: W. D. Figg and H. L. McLeod © Humana Press Inc., Totowa, NJ

individuals with pulmonary metastases can be salvaged by resection alone, the majority of patients either present with or eventually develop multiple metastases that are inoperable. Recurrent disease following complete pulmonary metastasectomy is often attributable to outgrowth of micrometastases present at the time of initial resection.

Although efficacious for eradication of pulmonary metastases related to lymphoid or germ cell tumors, systemic chemotherapy has not proven to be beneficial for the treatment of pulmonary metastases secondary to epithelial or sarcomatous malignancies *(3,9)*. Frequently, systemic toxicities limit optimal dosing of chemotherapeutic agents in patients with these tumors. Conceivably, administration of cytotoxic agents by regional techniques may reduce tumor burden within the lungs while minimizing systemic toxicities in patients with pulmonary metastases. This chapter reviews recent developments pertaining to the regional perfusion of inoperable pulmonary malignancies.

2. ANATOMY OF THE PULMONARY SYSTEM

The high frequency of primary and metastatic cancers involving the lungs is attributable to the large surface area of respiratory epithelia at risk for malignant degeneration following carcinogen exposure, and the extensive capillary system that entraps circulating cancer cells within the pulmonary interstitium. The lungs are perfused by two circulatory systems *(10)*. The pulmonary artery (PA) normally delivers all of the output from the right ventricle; although deoxygenated, blood within the PA is sufficient to maintain viability of normal lung parenchyma. The bronchial arterial circulation, emanating from several branches off the descending aorta, provides additional nutrient support to the airway mucosa *(11)*. Primary lung cancers, as well as metastatic lesions, frequently derive significant, and at times preferential, nutrient support from the bronchial circulation *(12,13)*.

Inhalation or perfusion-related pulmonary injuries are manifested by desquamation of airway epithelia, alveolar protein accumulation, and edema with or without fibrosis within the interstitial space *(14,15)*. Depending on the severity of the insult, life-threatening, irreversible interstitial fibrosis may ensue, manifested either as acute respiratory failure, or more insidious, restrictive lung disease. The fragility of the pulmonary interstitium, and its limited potential for recovery following severe insults, must be considered when contemplating administration of cytotoxic agents to the lungs via isolated lung perfusion (ILuP) techniques.

3. ISOLATED LUNG PERFUSION

3.1. Nitrogen Mustard and Melphalan

Administration of cytotoxic agents by selective lung perfusion was first reported shortly after techniques for cardiopulmonary bypass had been established. In 1960, Pierpont and Blades *(16)* utilized a closed extracorporeal circuit to administer nitrogen mustard to dogs via antegrade (PA, inflow; PV, outflow) isolated lung perfusion techniques. Ten of 23 dogs receiving 0.4 mg/kg of nitrogen mustard via 15-min ILuP survived the procedure. No washout was used following the perfusion, and 3 of these 10 animals exhibited neutropenia. Histologic changes consistent with acute pneumonitis were evident in the perfused lungs. No dogs survived perfusion at higher doses. Subsequently, Jacobs et al. *(17)* administered escalating doses of nitrogen mustard to dogs via isolated lung perfusion techniques. In contrast to what was observed by Pierpont and Blades *(16)*, Jacobs et al. *(17)* noted that doses of nitrogen mustard up to 1.6 mg/kg were tolerated when this agent was administered by 30-min perfusion at flow rates that maintained normal physiologic pressures within the pulmonary arterial system. Creech et al. *(18)* described techniques for simultaneous bilateral lung perfusion in animals, and reported the results of bilateral ILuP in one lung cancer patient as part of a large study involving regional perfusion of a variety of malignancies involving limbs, pelvis, abdominal viscera, and lungs.

Although additional studies of isolated lung perfusion with nitrogen mustard were not pursued, a number of preclinical studies have been performed to determine the potential efficacy of the mustard derivative melphalan, for regional treatment of pulmonary metastases. Nawata et al. (19) evaluated the pharmacokinetics and antitumor activity of melphalan administered by ILuP techniques in a rodent sarcoma model. Rats received MCA-induced sarcoma cells via intrajugular vein injection, and 7 d later were randomized to receive 2 mg of melphalan intravenously, 1 mg of melphalan or ILuP with either 2 mg of melphalan (approx 7–8 mg/kg) administered over 20 min at a rate of 0.5 mL/min, or buffered hetastarch. Seven days following treatment, animals were euthanized and pulmonary nodules enumerated. Melphalan concentrations in pulmonary tissues following lung perfusion were 10-fold higher than those observed following systemic administration of a comparable melphalan dose. A 10-fold reduction in the number of pulmonary nodules was observed in melphalan-perfused lungs relative to lungs from animals receiving intravenous melphalan or hetastarch perfusions. Sixty-seven percent of animals receiving melphalan lung perfusions tolerated contralateral pneumonectomy, compared to 80% of animals receiving perfusions with hetastarch. No animals survived intravenous administration of melphalan.

Hendriks et al. (20) evaluated the efficacy of melphalan administered by ILuP in a rodent model of adenocarcinoma pulmonary metastases. Median survival of rats receiving unilateral melphalan lung perfusions was 81 ± 12 d compared to untreated animals with bilateral pulmonary metastases (18 ± 1 d) or unilateral metastases (28 ± 3 d), or animals treated with 0.5 mg of melphalan intravenously (37 ± 6 d). Collectively, these data suggest that when administered by ILuP techniques, melphalan may be efficacious for the treatment of sarcomatous or carcinomatous pulmonary metastases.

In another series of experiments, Ueda et al. (15) evaluated long-term pulmonary toxicity of melphalan in a rodent perfusion model. Rats underwent 20-min ILuP with 1 mg of melphalan, and were randomly euthanized at monthly intervals for 6 mo. In melphalan-treated lungs, perivascular as well as peribronchial edema with septal thickening and interstitial inflammation were observed 30 d following ILuP; all of these changes had resolved within 60 d of the perfusion. Transmission electron microscopy revealed minimal proliferation of type II pneumocytes in the perfused lung. Collectively, these experiments indicate that at a dose that mediates antitumor effects by ILuP, melphalan induces no long-term histologic sequellae in the rodent lung.

Melphalan is often administered in conjunction with tumor necrosis factor-α (TNF-α) during isolated limb perfusion (21). Hendriks et al. (22) evaluated the effects of melphalan and TNF-α administered by ILuP in a rodent model of pulmonary metastases secondary to colorectal carcinoma. Rats were injected intrajugularly with adenocarcinoma cells, and 7 d thereafter were randomized to undergo sham thoracotomy, or 25-min ILuP with either saline, melphalan, TNF, or melphalan/TNF; additional animals received melphalan intravenously; tumor nodules were enumerated 7 d later. In additional studies, animals underwent contralateral pneumonectomy on d 21, and were euthanized 5 d later. Consistent with data reported by Nawata et al. (19), Hendriks and colleagues (22) observed a 10-fold reduction in pulmonary metastases in animals receiving melphalan lung perfusions compared to control animals. The cytotoxic effects observed following ILuP with 1 mg of melphalan were comparable to those seen after ILuP with melphalan at 2 mg. TNF-α had no appreciable antitumor effects when administered alone, and did not appear to potentiate melphalan in this setting. Eighty percent of animals receiving melphalan (2.0 mg)/TNF (200 µg) lung perfusions tolerated contralateral pneumonectomy.

Table 1
Isolated Lung Perfusion Trials

Author	No. of patients	Agent	Dose	Technique	Duration	Mortality	Response
Johnston et al. (28)	6	Doxorubicin	1–10 mg	Closed circuit, antegrade perfusion	20 min	0	N/A
	2	Cisplatin	14–20 mg	Closed circuit, antegrade perfusion	20 min	1	N/A
Burt et al. (29)	8	Doxorubicin	40 mg/m^2 80 mg/m^2	Closed circuit, antegrade perfusion	20 min	0	N/A
Putnam et al. (30)	12	Doxorubicin	60 mg/m^2 75 mg/m^2	Single pass, antegrade infusion	20 min	1	1 MR 4 stable disease
Ratto et al. (33)	6	Cisplatin	200 mg/m^2	Closed circuit, antegrade perfusion	60 min	0	N/A
Schröder et al. (42)	4	Cisplatin	70 mg/m^2	Closed circuit, hyperthermic antegrade perfusion	20–30 min	0	N/A
Muller (43)	22	Cisplatin Mitomycin Navelbine	30 mg/m2 10 mg/m^2 25 mg/m^2	Torso perfusion	20 min × 2	0	1 CR, 12 PR
Pass et al. (50)	15	TNF-α IFN-α	0.3–0.6 mg 0.2 mg	Closed circuit, hyperthermic antegrade perfusion	90 min	0	0
Schrump et al. (unpublished)	8	Paclitaxel	100, 200, and 125 mg	Closed circuit, hyperthermic retrograde perfusion	90 min	0	4 stable disease

Collectively, these data indicate that melphalan can mediate antitumor effects without apparent long-term toxicities when administered by ILuP techniques in experimental model systems. The efficacy and toxicities of this mustard derivative in the treatment of slower growing pulmonary metastases in humans have not been defined as yet.

3.2. Doxorubicin

A series of animal experiments and clinical trials have been conducted to examine the toxicity and potential efficacy of doxorubicin administered by ILuP techniques. Minchin et al. (23) examined the pharmacokinetics of doxorubicin administered by 50-min ILuP in dogs using a closed, oxygenated, extracorporeal circuit; an in-line heat exchanger maintained a physiologic temperature of the perfusate that contained 1–80 mg of doxorubicin in 1 L of whole blood. Uptake of doxorubicin in the canine lung appeared uniform, time-dependent, and saturable. Maximal tissue to perfusate blood ratios were 10–15 at low doses of doxorubicin; however, with higher perfusate doses, doxorubicin tissue to blood ratios were < 2. Accumulation of doxorubicin in the canine lung appeared to occur via facilitated transport or tissue binding mechanisms. Doxorubicin was undetectable in the systemic circulation; a systemic to pulmonary circulation leak attributable to bronchial arterial blood flow approximated 10 mL/min.

In a series of rodent experiments, Minchin et al. (24) observed linear, nonsaturable uptake of doxorubicin in the rat lung following 20-min single-pass ILuP, and Weksler et al. (25) reported that uptake of doxorubicin in the normal rodent lung was 20–25 times higher following 20-min ILuP than that observed following systemic administration of a comparable dose of doxorubicin. In subsequent experiments, Weksler et al. (26) observed that rats undergoing single-pass ILuP with 1.6 mg of doxorubicin (320 µg/mL) over 10 min tolerated contralateral pneumonectomy 21 d later. In additional experiments, rats were injected intravenously with MCA-induced sarcoma cells 7 d prior to ILuP with either doxorubicin as described above, or with normal saline. Three weeks following the ILuP procedure, extensive tumor metastases were present bilaterally in all animals undergoing saline lung perfusions, and in nonperfused lungs of rats receiving doxorubicin ILuP; no tumor metastases were identified in lungs perfused with doxorubicin; histopathologic analysis revealed moderate interstitial fibrosis in doxorubicin perfused lungs.

Furrer et al. (27) evaluated the pharmacokinetics and immediate toxicities of doxorubicin (50 mg/m^2) administered either by 15-min single pass, or normothermic recirculating blood perfusion using similar flow rates (approx 100 mL/min), as well as intravenous systemic infusion in a porcine model. Doxorubicin lung tissue concentrations following single pass were comparable to those observed after recirculating blood perfusion (approx 18 µg/g of tissue vs 22 µg/g of tissue, respectively); in contrast, pulmonary doxorubicin levels were only 3.0 µg/g of tissue following intravenous drug administration. Wet to dry ratios were significantly lower following single pass compared to recirculating blood perfusions, suggesting that doxorubicin administered by single pass precipitated less acute perfusion-related edema than the same dose of doxorubicin delivered by recirculating blood perfusion techniques in large animals.

Several clinical studies have been performed to examine the toxicities and clinical efficacy of doxorubicin lung perfusions in patients with unresectable pulmonary malignancies (Table 1). Johnson et al. (28) treated six individuals with escalating doses of doxorubicin (1–10 µg/mL of perfusate in a closed extracorporeal circuit) via 20-min, normothermic ILuP. Three patients underwent unilateral lung perfusions, and three individuals had bilateral simultaneous lung perfusions. Flow rates were adjusted to maintain physiologic pulmonary arterial pressures. Following ILuP, residual perfusate was flushed from the lungs with either blood or low molecular weight dextran. Isolated lung perfusion circuits provided excellent separation of pulmonary and systemic circulations even under bilateral simultaneous perfusion conditions. Maximum doxorubicin levels in normal lung equaled or exceeded those observed in tumor tissues following lung perfusion *(23,28)*. In two individuals, doxorubicin was detected in mediastinal lymph nodes following lung perfusion, indicating transport of drug through the pulmonary interstitium to the regional lymphatics. One patient developed pneumonia that was fatal. No objective responses were noted in this pilot study in which maximum tolerated dose (MTD) was not determined.

In a more recent Phase I study, Burt et al. *(29)* utilized a closed, oxygenated, extracorporeal circuit to administer doxorubicin via ILuP to eight patients with unresectable sarcomatous metastases. Seven patients were treated at a dose of 40 mg/m^2, and one patient received 80 mg/m^2 doxorubicin via 20-min perfusion (300–500 mL/min) at ambient temperatures. Following ILuP, doxorubicin was flushed from the lungs with Hespan. Approximately 14% of the total dose of doxorubicin in perfusates was extracted by the lungs. Consistent with what was reported by Minchin et al. *(23)*, uptake of doxorubicin in tumors tended to be less than that observed in normal lung tissues (average drug concentration following ILuP with 40 mg/m^2 of doxorubicin were 11.1 µg/g of tissue for normal lung, and 8.7 µg/g of tissue for tumor nodules). A modified toxicity grading system was implemented by these investigators to assess pulmonary toxicity related specifically to drug exposure rather than the thoracotomy procedure itself. Six of the eight perfused patients experienced grade II pulmonary toxicity, defined as > 20% diminution in diffusion capacity for carbon monoxide (DLCO), or dyspnea at rest or with exertion. The single patient receiving 80 mg/m^2 of doxorubicin exhibited complete destruction of the perfused lung resulting in empyema and suppurative pericarditis requiring surgical intervention. Although none of the seven individuals perfused at a dose of 40 mg/m^2 experienced clinically significant pulmonary symptoms, postoperative pulmonary function tests revealed diminished forced expiratory volume in 1 s (FEV$_1$) as well as DLCO values indicative of subacute interstitial injury in these patients.

In a Phase I study, Putnam et al. *(30)* treated 12 sarcoma patients with doxorubicin administered via single-pass isolated lung perfusion. Eight patients received 200 mg/mL (approx 60 mg/m^2) and four patients received 250 mg/mL (approx 75 mg/m^2) doxorubicin in 1 L of crystalloid solution administered over 20 min. One patient experienced a major response, and four individuals exhibited stabilization of disease. Acute, pulmonary toxicity (interstitial pneumonitis) occurred in two individuals, both of whom were in the high-dose cohort; pneumonitis was fatal in one of these patients. Late pulmonary toxicity evidenced by diminution of ventilation and perfusion was observed in several patients in this study. Although extensive pharmacokinetic data have not been published, doxorubicin levels in normal tissues exceeded those in tumor nodules (median 592 µg/g of tissue [range 74–2750] vs 153 µg/g of tissue [range 12–1294], respectively). These observations, which were consistent with those reported by Minchin et al. *(23)* and Burt et al. *(29)*, may have accounted for the short- and long-term pulmonary toxicities observed following doxorubicin perfusions in this study.

3.3. Cisplatin

A series of laboratory experiments and clinical trials have been performed to evaluate the potential efficacy of cisplatin administered by ILuP techniques. Ratto et al. *(31)* reported that pulmonary tissue levels of cisplatin following bolus pulmonary artery infusion were not significantly higher than those observed following systemic administration of this cytotoxic agent. In subsequent experiments *(32)*, these investigators utilized a porcine model to evaluate the pharmacokinetics of cisplatin administered via 15-min infusion distal to a pulmonary artery tourniquet (stop-flow), 15-min infusion into a lung isolated by tourniquets on the ipsilateral pulmonary artery and pulmonary veins (stop-flow/occlusion), or by 4-h ILuP under normothermic conditions using a closed, oxygenated extracorporeal circuit. Pulmonary tissue cisplatin area under the concentration–time curve (AUC) values were approximately threefold higher in the stop-flow/occlusion animals compared to the stop-flow group ($11,538 \pm 4586 \, \mu g \cdot min^{-1} \cdot mL^{-1}$, vs $3658 \pm 824 \, \mu g \cdot min^{-1} \cdot mL^{-1}$, respectively). Interestingly, lung perfusions with 2.5 mg/kg of cisplatin did not increase pulmonary tissue AUC values relative to those observed following administration of the same dose by stop-flow/occlusion techniques; however, cisplatin AUCs in mediastinal lymph nodes were significantly higher following ILuP compared to stop-flow/occlusion, possibly owing to the duration of drug exposure in the perfusions. Drug uptake in lung tissues and mediastinal nodes following ILuP was dose dependent. Histopathologic analysis revealed no significant differences regarding acute toxicities in pulmonary tissues harvested 4 h after cisplatin administration by any technique.

In a more recent study, Ratto et al. *(33)* administered cisplatin (200 mg/m²) to six patients with sarcomatous pulmonary metastases via 60-min normothermic ILuP using a closed, oxygenated extracorporeal circuit. Two patients developed reversible interstitial pneumonitis, one of whom required mechanical ventilatory support. No systemic toxicities were observed. Cisplatin levels in normal lung and metastatic lesions were comparable, ranging between 60 and 70 μg/g tissue. In all likelihood, the low protein content of the perfusate (approx 1/7th that of normal serum) enhanced drug delivery during ILuP. Indices of interstitial injury (DLCO, pO_2, and pCO_2) assessed at 10, 30, and 90 d postoperatively were essentially unchanged from baseline values. Response to therapy was not evaluated in this trial.

Hyperthermia is known to increase cisplatin mediated cytotoxicity in cancer cells in vitro *(34,35)*, and is routinely utilized as a means to enhance delivery, uptake, and tumoricidal activity of cisplatin in clinical settings *(36–39)*. Previous studies by Rickaby et al. *(40)* and Cowen et al. *(41)* demonstrated tolerance of the canine lung to hyperthermia; when the temperature was < 44.4°C, 2-h hyperthermia had no effect on lung weight, vascular volume, extravascular water, serotonin uptake, perfusion pressure, or lung compliance. Recently, Schröder et al. *(42)* reported results of hyperthermic ILuP with cisplatin in four sarcoma patients. Following metastasectomy, patients underwent isolated lobar or unilateral whole lung perfusion with 70 mg/m² cisplatin administered at a temperature of 41°C for 20–30 min at a rate which maintained a mean pulmonary artery pressure less than baseline values (approx 300–500 mL/min). One individual underwent staged bilateral lung perfusions 1 1/2 mo apart. Maximal cisplatin concentrations at the completion of the perfusions approximated 98 μg/g of tissue. All patients experienced transient pulmonary toxicity manifested as noncardiogenic pulmonary edema and desquamation of perfused bronchial mucosa. The one patient who had undergone unilateral whole lung perfusion exhibited grade II pulmonary toxicity (> 20% decrease of FEV_1 and DLCO relative to baseline values) at 3 wk post-ILuP that gradually resolved over the next 9 wk. Two additional patients exhibited grade I pulmonary toxicity 3 wk following lung perfusion, and this toxicity was resolved in both patients within 6 wk following this procedure. One patient undergoing lobar perfusion experienced no clinically significant diminution in pulmonary function. Three of the four patients undergoing metastasectomy and perfusion were alive and free of disease with a median followup of 13 mo. Collectively, this limited clinical study demonstrated that hyperthermic lung perfusions with cisplatin are feasible in patients with pulmonary metastases, and that hyperthermia markedly enhances cisplatin uptake in the lung.

In a recent Phase I study, Muller et al. *(43)* evaluated the effects of combined regional and systemic chemotherapy for the treatment of inoperable non-small-cell lung cancer. Twenty-two chemo-naive patients underwent 20-min regional perfusion of the thorax with 10 mg/m² of mitomycin, 25 mg/m² of navelbine, and 30 mg/m² of cisplatin. Regional perfusion was accomplished by balloon catheter occlusion of the aorta above the celiac axis, and the inferior vena cava at the cavo–atrial junction as well as pneumatic tourniquets on the upper extremities. Three hundred micrograms of GM-CSF were administered intravenously during the perfusion, and thereafter patients received 250 mg/m² of 5-fluorouracil (5-FU) and 20 mg/m² of cisplatin via continuous intravenous infusion over 4 d. Two cycles of regional and systemic chemotherapy were administered 4 wk apart. The overall response rate was 59% (4.5% CR, 54.5% PR). Six additional patients exhibited minor responses. Nearly all patients responding to therapy experienced either improvement or stabilization of pulmonary function. No dose-limiting toxicities were observed during 45 cycles of therapy. Sixteen of 22 patients underwent surgery, 13 of whom had complete (RO) resections. Overall 1 yr survivals were 87% and 68% for patients with bulky IIIA and IIIB/IV disease, respectively. These data warrant further evaluation of the pharmacokinetics, toxicities, and efficacy of cisplatin administered alone or in conjunction with other cytotoxic agents via minimally invasive perfusion techniques for the treatment of pulmonary malignancies.

3.4. TNF-α

Although the macrophage derived cytokine TNF-α exhibits potent antitumor effects *(44,45)*, systemic administration of tumoricidal doses of recombinant TNF-α is not tolerated in cancer patients *(46,47)*. However, owing to the effects of TNF on tumor vasculature, this cytokine has been utilized with melphalan in hyperthermic isolated limb and liver perfusions resulting in complete response rates approximating 75% in melanoma and sarcoma patients *(21,48)*. Weksler et al. *(49)* evaluated the antitumor effects of TNF-α in a rodent perfusion model. Preliminary in vitro experiments revealed that 42 μg/mL of murine or human TNF-α inhibited in vitro proliferation of MCA-induced sarcoma cells by 20–40% relative to untreated cells. Tumor-bearing rats undergoing ILuP with 420 μg of TNF-α exhibited a five- to sevenfold reduction in the number of metastases in the perfused lung compared to the nonperfused lung. These data suggest that when administered by ILuP techniques, TNF-α can mediate significant antitumor effects without apparent systemic toxicity.

In a Phase I clinical trial, Pass et al. *(50)* treated 15 patients with pulmonary metastases from a variety of malignancies by 90-min hyperthermic ILuP using a closed, oxygenated extracorporeal circuit containing 0.2 mg of interferon-α, and escalating doses (0.3–0.6 mg) of TNF-α (approx 7 μg/mL in the highest cohort of patients). There were no operative deaths, and reduction of disease (not meeting criteria for partial response) was observed in three patients; TNF-α levels in pulmonary tissues were not ascertained in this study. One patient experienced reversible interstitial pneumonitis requiring mechanical ventilation. FEV_1 and DLCO, as well as ventilation and perfusion in the treated lung, were diminished 10–20% relative to baseline values 8 wk following ILuP, suggesting subclinical pulmonary toxicity following ILuP.

3.5. Paclitaxel

All of the animal and human lung perfusions described thus far have utilized antegrade (inflow via pulmonary artery, outflow via pulmonary vein) perfusion techniques that may not be optimal for drug delivery to pulmonary neoplasms which frequently derive their blood supply from the bronchial arteries *(12,13)*. The fact that chemotherapeutic agents adminis-tered by selective bronchial artery infusion can mediate significant regression of pulmonary ncoplasms *(51,52)*, attests to the relevance of this circulatory system regarding growth of pulmonary malignancies. By exploiting venous collaterals between the pulmonary and bron-chial arterial systems, retrograde perfusion (inflow via pulmonary vein; outflow via pulmo-nary artery) may enhance the efficiency of drug delivery to primary as well as metastatic tumors in the lung.

Recently, Schrump et al. *(53)* utilized a sheep model to evaluate the feasibility, phar-macokinetics, and immediate toxicities of paclitaxel administered via retrograde, hyper-thermic isolated lung perfusion techniques. Adult sheep underwent 90-min hyperthermic, retrograde ILuP using a closed, oxygenated, extracorporeal circuit with a 3-L perfusate containing crystalloid and packed red blood cells (pRBC) to a final hematocrit (Hct) of 10, and escalating doses of paclitaxel (2–800 mg). Paclitaxel levels in perfused tissues increased with escalating perfusate doses; drug levels in high-dose perfusates declined more slowly, suggesting that uptake of paclitaxel into pulmonary tissues was saturable. The average C_{max} (50 ng/mg) in lung tissues obtained when 200 mg of paclitaxel was utilized in the perfusion (78 μM paclitaxel) was approximately twofold higher than that observed following systemic infusion of the same dose of paclitaxel over 1 h; tissue AUCs under these conditions were relatively comparable. The plasma C_{max} and AUC following 1-h infusion of 200 mg of paclitaxel (approx 150 mg/m^2) in sheep were essentially com-parable to those reported by Maier-Lenz et al. *(54)* following 1-h infusion of 225 mg/m^2 of paclitaxel in cancer patients. When the dose of paclitaxel in the perfusate was increased to 800 mg (approx 325 μM), C_{max} of paclitaxel in perfused tissues was 86 ng/mL, and AUC was 165 ng-h/mg. Paclitaxel levels in the systemic circulation were undetectable at all perfusate doses during the ILuP; following restoration of circulation to the perfused lung (after washout), systemic levels were either undetectable or extremely low, indicating that retained drug was not rapidly released from the perfused lung into the systemic circulation. Histopathologic examination of lung tissues obtained 3 h following completion of the ILuP revealed no pulmonary hemorrhage, alveolar edema, or interstitial thickening. Sur-vival was not evaluated in these experiments, which were designed primarily to ascertain the pharmacokinetics of paclitaxel administered by retrograde, hyperthermic ILuP tech-niques that had not been described previously. The sheep model did not allow assessment of antitumor activity of paclitaxel administered in this manner.

Data from the above experiments provided the preclinical rationale for a Phase I study of hyperthermic, retrograde isolated lung perfusion in patients with unresectable pulmo-nary malignancies currently underway in the Thoracic Oncology Section, Surgery Branch, National Cancer Institute (Schrump, unpublished). The overall aims of this study include definition of the maximum tolerated dose and toxicities of paclitaxel administered in this manner. To date, ten lung perfusions (two left, eight right) have been performed in eight patients with refractory pulmonary metastases. Five of those perfusions were performed in the context of complete pulmonary metastasectomy. All patients received intravenous decadron, diphenhydryl, and cimetidine prior to ILuP. Inflow has been achieved by a single retrograde cardioplegia cannula placed into the isolated left atrial cuff, or by dual cannulation of the ipsilateral superior and inferior pulmonary veins. Outflow was estab-lished by cannulation of the ipsilateral main pulmonary artery. Flow rates have been adjusted to maintain a pressure of 14–16 mmHg within the pulmonary veins; under these conditions flow rates have ranged between 500 and 1000 mL/min. Temperature of the perfusate has been adjusted via in-line heat exchanger to maintain a temperature of 39.5–41°C in the lung, assessed by temperature probes placed into the upper and lower lobes.

Table 2
Paclitaxel Concentrations in Perfusate, Plasma, and Lung Tissues

Patient	Dose (mg)	C_{max} (mg/L)		Normal lung (ng/mg of tissue)		Tumor (ng/mg of tissue)	
		Perfusate	Plasma	90 min	120 min	90 min	120 mg
1	100	30	0.059	6.2	10.9	4.8	9.8
7	125	40	0.1	17.3	12.9	25.6	19.0
6	200	51	0.16	24.4	14.7	26.8	24.2

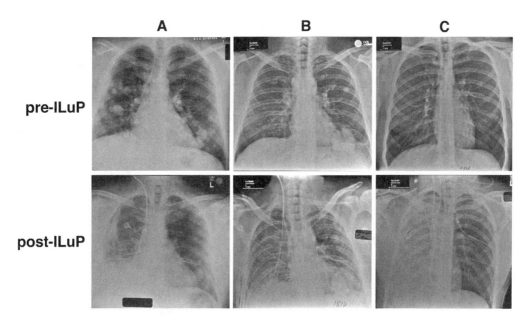

Fig. 1. Preoperative and 24-h postoperative chest X-ray films from three representative patients undergoing hyperthermic retrograde ILuP with 100 mg of paclitaxel (**A**), 125 mg of paclitaxel (**B**), or 200 mg of paclitaxel (**C**). Corresponding pharmacokinetic data for these patients are summarized in Table 2.

Prior to initiation of the perfusion the isolated lung is flushed with 1 L of Ringer's lactate containing 250 µg of prostaglandin E to dilute the pulmonary vasculature. Thereafter, the lung is perfused for 90 min with paclitaxel using a closed, oxygenated circuit containing a dilute blood perfusate (Hct = 10). Following completion of the paclitaxel perfusion, the lung is flushed with 2 L of Ringer's lactate prior to reestablishing normal blood flow to the isolated lung.

No dose-limiting toxicities were observed in three patients undergoing four perfusions with 100 mg of paclitaxel. However, significant pneumonitis requiring mechanical ventilation was observed in three patients perfused with 200 mg of paclitaxel. Although the pneumonitis was dramatically reversible in all three patients, the severity of the acute pulmonary injury warranted dose reduction. As such, three additional patients underwent four lung perfusions with 125 mg of paclitaxel; no pulmonary toxicity was observed in these individuals. Representative chest X-ray films and pharmacokinetic data for three individuals are depicted in Fig. 1 and Table 2. Uptake of paclitaxel in tumor tissue has equaled, if not exceeded, that in normal lung parenchyma. Although no objective responses have been observed, prolonged disease-free interval has been observed in four individuals who underwent ipsilateral metastasectomy at the time of ILuP; these individuals underwent contralateral metastasectomy shortly after ILuP, yet recurred in the nonperfused lung. These preliminary data suggest that eradication of micrometastases may have contributed to the apparent treatment effect in these individuals (Schrump, unpublished). Currently, patients are being accrued to this trial to further define the MTD and toxicities of paclitaxel delivered by hyperthermic, retrograde ILuP techniques, and to determine if other novel agents can be added to enhance the efficacy of this treatment regimen.

4. CONCLUSION

Only two of 61 patients undergoing invasive ILuP procedures in the aforementioned trials died as a result of perfusion (perioperative mortality = 3.3%); these data indicate that ILuP can be performed safely in properly selected individuals with resectable pulmonary neoplasms. Our experience (Schrump unpublished) as well as that of Schröder et al. *(42)* indicate that cisplatin and paclitaxel lung perfusions can be performed in the context of aggressive pulmonary metastasectomy (including lobar resections) without significant long-term sequellae.

At present, the major limitation of ILuP relates to the lack of specificity regarding uptake and cytotoxicity of drugs in normal lung parenchyma relative to tumor tissues; this phenomena has been well established for doxorubicin, and agents such as melphalan or TNF may have limited use in ILuP owing to their potential for inducing significant interstitial injury. Without question, continued efforts must focus on the identification of novel agents that mediate cytotoxicity preferentially in cancer cells. Furthermore, efforts should be undertaken to elucidate the pathophysiology of perfusion-related pneumonitis, and to identify agents that can ameliorate this lung injury. For instance, inhaled nitric oxide as well as the proteosome inhibitor gabexate mesilate can prevent reperfusion injury in transplanted lungs following warm ischemia *(55–57)*; conceivably, these agents may attenuate the pneumonitis observed following ILuP. In addition, a standardized system should be utilized for all future clinical trials to enable objective assessment of pulmonary toxicities following ILuP.

At present, ILuP appears most effective when performed in the context of pulmonary metastasectomy, and future trials at the NCI will directly compare resection with ILuP versus resection alone in patients with advanced pulmonary metastases. On the basis of preliminary results reported by Muller *(43)*, as well Osaki et al. *(52)*, efforts are underway to refine minimally invasive techniques for delivery of chemotherapeutic agents via torso perfusion or selective bronchial artery infusion. The rationale for regional cancer therapy is scientifically sound; although considerable work needs to be done to demonstrate efficacy, data thus far warrant further evaluation of ILuP for the treatment of inoperable pulmonary malignancies.

REFERENCES

1. American Cancer Society. Cancer facts and figures. 2002, 5–10.
2. Lee JD, Ginsberg RJ. The multimodality treatment of stage III A/B non-small cell lung cancer. The role of surgery, radiation, and hemotherapy. Hematol Oncol Clin North Am 1997; 11:279–301.
3. Putnam JB Jr. Metastatic cancer to the lung. In: DeVita VT Jr, Hellman S, Rosenberg SA (eds). Cancer, Principles & Practice of Oncology, 6th Edit. Philadelphia, PA: Lippincott, Williams & Wilkins, 2001, pp. 2670–2689.
4. Putnam JB Jr. New and evolving treatment methods for pulmonary metastases. Semin Thorac Cardiovasc Surg 2002; 14:49–56.
5. Putnam J, Roth JA, Wesley MN, Johnston MR, Rosenberg SA. Analysis of prognostic factors in patients undergoing resection of pulmonary metastases from soft tissue sarcomas. J Thorac Cardiovasc Surg 1984; 87:260–267.
6. McCormack PM, Burt ME, Bains MS, Martini N, Rusch VW, Ginsberg RJ. Lung resection for colorectal metastases—10-year results. Arch Surg 1992; 127:1403–1406.
7. Kavolius JP, Mastorakos DP, Pavlovich C, Russo P, Burt ME, Brady MS. Resection of metastatic renal cell carcinoma. J Clin Oncol 1998; 16:2261–2266.
8. Pastorino U, Buyse M, Friedel G, et al. Long-term results of lung metastasectomy: prognostic analyses based on 5206 cases. J Thorac Cardiovasc Surg 1997;113:37–47.
9. Spira AI, Ettinger DS. The use of chemotherapy in soft-tissue sarcomas. Oncologist 2002; 7:348–359.
10. Shields TW. Surgical anatomy of the lungs. In: Shields TW, Locicero III J, Ponn RB (eds). General Thoracic Surgery, 5th Edit. Philadelphia, PA: Lippincott, Williams & Wilkins, 2002, pp. 63–75.

11. Butler J. The Bronchial Circulation. 1992. New York, NY: Marcel Dekker.
12. Miller BJ, Rosenbarum A. The vascular supply to metastatic tumors of the lung. Surg Gynecol Obstet 1967; 125:1009–1012.
13. Neyazaki T, Ikeda M, Mitusi K, Kimura S, Suzuki M, Suzuki C. Angioarchitecture of pulmonary malignancics in humans. Cancer 1970; 26:1246–1255.
14. Flick MR. Pulmonary edema and acute lung injury. In: Murray JF, Nadel JA (eds). Respiratory Medicine, 2nd Edit. Philadelphia, PA: WB Saunders, 1994, pp. 1725–1777.
15. Ueda K, Sugi K, Li TS, Saeki K, Nawata S, Esato K. The long-term evaluation of pulmonary toxicity following isolated lung perfusion with melphalan in the rat. Anticancer Res 1999; 19:141–147.
16. Pierpont H, Blades B. Lung perfusion with chemotherapeutic agents. J Thorac Cardiovasc Surg 1960; 39:159–165.
17. Jacobs JK, Flexner JM, Scott HW Jr. Selective isolated perfusion of the right or left lung. J Thorac Cardiovasc Surg 1961; 42:546–552.
18. Creech O, Krementz E, Ryan RF, Winblad JN. Chemotherapy of cancer regional perfusion utilizing an extracorporeal circuit. Ann Surg 1958; 148:616–632.
19. Nawata S, Abecasis N, Ross HM, et al. Isolated lung perfusion with melphalan for the treatment of metastatic pulmonary sarcoma. J Thorac Cardiovasc Surg 1996; 112:1542–1547.
20. Hendriks JM, Van Schil PE, Van Oosterom, AA, Kuppen PJ, Van Marck E, Eyskens E. Isolated lung perfusion with melphalan prolongs survival in a rat model of metastatic pulmonary adenocarcinoma. Eur Surg Res 1999; 31:267–271.
21. Eggermont AM, Schraffordt KH, Klausner JM, et al. Isolation limb perfusion with tumor necrosis factor alpha and chemotherapy for advanced extremity soft tissue sarcomas. Semin Oncol 1997; 24:547–555.
22. Hendriks JM, Van Schil PE, De Boeck G, et al. Isolated lung perfusion with melphalan and tumor necrosis factor for metastatic pulmonary adenocarcinoma. Ann Thorac Surg 1998; 66:1719–1725.
23. Minchin RF, Johnston MR, Aiken MA, Boyd MR Pharmacokinetics of doxorubicin in isolated lung of dogs and humans perfused in vivo. J Pharmacol Exp Ther 1984; 229:193–198.
24. Minchin RF, Boyd MR. Uptake and metabolism of doxorubicin in isolated perfused rat lung. Biochem Pharmacol 1983; 32:2829–2832.
25. Weksler B, Ng B, Lenert JT, Burt ME. Isolated single-lung perfusion with doxorubicin is pharmacokinetically superior to intravenous injection. Ann Thorac Surg 1993; 56:209–214.
26. Weksler B, Lenert J, Ng B, Burt M. Isolated single lung perfusion with doxorubicin is effective in eradicating soft tissue sarcoma lung metastases in a rat model. J Thorac Cardiovasc Surg 1994; 107:50–54.
27. Furrer M, Lardinois D, Thormann W, et al. Isolated lung perfusion: single-pass system versus recirculating blood perfusion in pigs. Ann Thorac Surg 1998; 65:1420–1425.
28. Johnston MR, Minchen RF, Dawson CA. Lung perfusion with chemotherapy in patients with unresectable metastatic sarcoma to the lung or diffuse branchioloalveolar carcinoma. J Thorac Cardiovasc Surg 1995; 110:368–373.
29. Burt ME, Liu D, Abolhoda A, et al. Isolated lung perfusion for patients with unresectable metastases from sarcoma: a Phase I trial. Ann Thorac Surg 2000; 69:1542–1549.
30. Putnam JB, Madden T, Tran HT, Benjamin RS. Isolated single lung perfusion (ISLP) with Adriamycin® for unresectable sarcomatous metastases. Proc ASCO 1997; 16:500a.
31. Ratto GB, Esposito M, Vannozzi M, Fulco RA, Rovida S. Experimental models of regional chemotherapy via the pulmonary artery using cisplatin. Reg Cancer Treat 1990; 2:222–227.
32. Ratto GB, Esposito M, Leprini A, et al. In situ lung perfusion with cisplatin: an experimental study. Cancer 1993; 71:2962–2970.
33. Ratto GB, Toma S, Civalleri D, et al. Isolated lung perfusion with platinum in the treatment of pulmonary metastases from soft tissue sarcomas. J Thorac Cardiovasc Surg 1996; 112:614–622.
34. Hettinga JV, Konings AW, Kampinga HH. Reduction of cellular cisplatin resistance by hyperthermia—a review. Int J Hyperthermia 1997; 13:439–457.
35. Nakao K, Otsuki Y, Akao Y, et al. The synergistic effects of hyperthermia and anticancer drugs on induction of apoptosis. Med Electron Microsc 2000; 33:44–50.
36. Takahashi I, Emi Y, Hasuda S, Kakeji Y, Maehara Y, Sugimachi K. Clinical application of hyperthermia combined with anticancer drugs for the treatment of solid tumors. Surgery 2002; 131:S78–S84.
37. Cho HK, Lush RM, Bartlett DL, et al. Pharmacokinetics of cisplatin administered by continuous hyperthermic peritoneal perfusion (CHPP) to patients with peritoneal carcinomatosis. J Clin Pharmacol 1999; 39:394–401.

38. Eroglu A, Kocaoglu H, Demirci S, Akgul H. Isolated limb perfusion with cisplatin and doxorubicin for locally advanced soft tissue sarcoma of an extremity. Eur J Surg Oncol 2000; 26:213–221.
39. Yellin A, Simansky DA, Paley M, Refaely Y. Hyperthermic pleural perfusion with cisplatin: early clinical experience. Cancer 2001; 92:2197–2203.
40. Rickaby DA, Fehring JF, Johnston MR, Dawson CA. Tolerance of the isolated perfused lung to hyperthermia. J Thorac Cardiovasc Surg 1991; 101:732–739.
41. Cowen ME, Howard RB, Mulvin D, Dawson CA, Johnston MR. Lung tolerance to hyperthermia by in vivo perfusion. Eur J Cardiothorac Surg 1992; 6:167–172.
42. Schroder C, Fisher S, Pieck AC, et al. Technique and results of hyperthermic (41 degrees C) isolated lung perfusion with high-doses of cisplatin for the treatment of surgically relapsing or unresectable lung sarcoma metastasis. Eur J Cardiothorac Surg 2002; 22:41–46.
43. Muller H. Combined regional and systemic chemotherapy for advanced and inoperable non-small cell lung cancer. Eur J Surg Oncol 2002; 28:165–171.
44. Carswell EA, Old LF, Kassel RL. An endotoxin-induced serum factor that causes necrosis of tumors. Proc Natl Acad Sci USA 1975; 72:3666–3670.
45. Asher A, Mule JJ, Reichert CM, Shiloni E, Rosenberg SA. Studies on the anti-tumor efficacy of systemically administered recombinant tumor necrosis factor against several murine tumors in vivo. J Immunol 1987; 138:963–974.
46. Selby P, Hobbs S, Viner C, et al. Tumour necrosis factor in man: clinical and biological observations. Br J Cancer 1987; 56:803–808.
47. Spriggs DR, Sherman ML, Michie H, et al. Recombinant human tumor necrosis factor administered as a 24-hour intravenous infusion. A Phase I and pharmacologic study. J Natl Cancer Inst 1988; 80:1039–1044.
48. Alexander HR Jr, Bartlett DL, Libutti SK, Fraker DL, Moser T, Rosenberg SA. Isolated hepatic perfusion with tumor necrosis factor and melphalan for unresectable cancers confined to the liver. J Clin Oncol 1998; 16:1479–1489.
49. Weksler B, Blumberg D, Lenert JT, Ng B, Fong Y, Burt ME. Isolated single-lung perfusion with TNF-alpha in a rat sarcoma lung metastases model. Ann Thorac Surg 1994; 58:328–331.
50. Pass HI, Mew DJY, Kranda KC, Temeck BK, Donington JS, Rosenberg SA. Isolated lung perfusion with tumor necrosis factor for pulmonary metastases. Ann Thorac Surg 1996; 61:1609–1617.
51. Neyazaki T, Ikeda M, Seki Y, Egawa N, Suzuki C Bronchial artery infusion therapy for lung cancer. Cancer 1969; 24:912–922.
52. Osaki T, Hanagiri T, Nakanishi R, Yoshino I, Taga S, Yasumoto K. Bronchial arterial infusion is an effective therapeutic modality for centrally located early-stage lung cancer: results of a pilot study. Chest 1999; 115:1424–1428.
53. Schrump DS, Zhai S, Nguyen DM, et al. Pharmacokinetics of paclitaxel administered by hyperthermic retrograde isolated lung perfusion techniques. J Thorac Cardiovasc Surg 2002; 123:686–694.
54. Maier-Lenz H, Hauns B, Haering B, et al. Phase I study of paclitaxel administered as a 1-hour infusion: toxicity and pharmacokinetics. Semin Oncol 1997; 24:S19-16–S19-19.
55. Luh SP, Tsai CC, Shau WY, et al. Protective effects of inhaled nitric oxide and gabexate mesilate in lung reperfusion injury after transplantation from non-heart-beat donors. J Heart Lung Transplant 2002; 21:251–259.
56. Bacha EA, Sellak H, Murakami S, et al. Inhaled nitric oxide attenuates reperfusion injury in non-heartbeating-donor lung transplantation. Paris-Sud University Lung Transplantation Group. Transplantation 1997; 63:1380–1386.
57. Murakami K, Okajima K, Uchiba M, Okabe H, Takatsuki K. Gabexate mesilate, a synthetic protease inhibitor, attenuates endotoxin-induced pulmonary vascular injury by inhibiting tumor necrosis factor production by monocytes. Crit Care Med 1996; 24:1047–1053.

22 Pharmacokinetics of Isolated Lung Perfusion with Antitumor Agents

Suoping Zhai, *Pharm D*

CONTENTS

1. INTRODUCTION

1.1. Regional Chemotherapy and Pharmacokinetics

Regional chemotherapy provides a treatment approach designed to improve the selectivity of chemotherapy, by increasing drug concentrations at tumor sites and lowering systemic drug exposure. Isolated lung perfusion (ILP) provides an alternative to achieve high concentration of anticancer drugs in tumor tissue *(1,2)*. The main attractiveness of regional chemotherapy such as ILP is that high drug concentrations would target the tumor site, thus making the drug more efficacious. It is true that the therapy permits delivery of high drug levels over a relatively short period of time and this, in theory, results in considerably high tissue exposure. On the other hand, increased dose may not enhance the efficacy, but may induce toxicity when the maximum drug effect is reached. Therefore, it is important to keep in mind that regional drug therapy requires the knowledge of pharmacokinetics, such as the feasibility of reaching expected high concentrations in tumor tissue and the concentration–response relationship.

Evaluating the pharmacokinetics of anticancer agents via ILP is particularly important. It provides a quantitative perspective regarding the pharmacologic advantage of the anticancer drugs using ILP, and helps us to decide if clinical effort is necessary for a particular drug. Finally, pharmacodynamic factors must also be considered for the overall assessment of regional delivery.

Handbook of Anticancer Pharmacokinetics and Pharmacodynamics
Edited by: W. D. Figg and H. L. McLeod © Humana Press Inc., Totowa, NJ

1.2. Lung Anatomy and Physiology and Drug Pharmacokinetics

The lung is a complex and heterogeneous organ. There is considerable cellular heterogeneity, with approx 40 different cell types within the lung (3). Two classes of enzymes exist in the lungs that have direct implications for the disposition of drugs. The first class is the enzymes responsible for the active uptake of catecholamines and related drugs into the lung. These transport enzymes can be saturated and inhibited competitively. The other class is the enzymes that are required for drug metabolism in the lungs. The lung, generally, has low activities of many metabolic enzymes found in the liver. In humans, the enzyme activity in the lung varies from < 1% up to 34% of the liver enzyme activity for a range of drugs studied (4). Drug uptake into the lung is principally by diffusion, as well as active transportation. The lung has the smallest diffusion distances of all of the body organs; thus, the diffusion of drugs is very fast. The lung is also characterized by large surface areas in contact with blood and respiratory gases. The characteristics of lung anatomy and physiology have an influence on drug distribution and metabolism.

The evidence suggests that the kinetics of drugs in the lung is highly variable with respect to both drug distribution and metabolism. These can have a significant impact on pharmacokinetic studies. The lung kinetics of many drugs has not been extensively examined in animals and in humans. Regional chemotherapy using ILP provides an opportunity to evaluate the pharmacokinetic behavior of many drugs in the lung.

2. PRECLINICAL PHARMACOKINETIC STUDIES OF ILP WITH ANTICANCER AGENTS

Many animal studies have been performed using ILP with different anticancer agents. Different animal models of ILP have been developed in different laboratories. Pharmacokinetic advantages of ILP using different anticancer agents have been evaluated, together with the evaluation of pharmacodynamics.

2.1. Cisplatin

ILP with cisplatin was reported by several investigators. Li et al. evaluated ILP with cisplatin in a rat lung tumor model (5). The results demonstrated that a significantly higher platinum concentration in the tumor was observed in the ILP treated rats with 0.1 mg/mL of cisplatin than in the rats treated with a 1-mg intravenous injection (6.7 ± 1.6 vs 2.5 ± 0.6 µg/g of tissue [$p < 0.05$]). In accordance with the findings of Wang et al. (6), a lower cisplatin level was observed in the tumor nodule than in the lung tissue in the ILP rats, but almost the same levels were seen in the animals treated with intravenous cisplatin in this study. These results suggest that the pharmacokinetics for ILP and intravenous injection could be different. The study showed that ILP with cisplatin was pharmacokinetically superior to intravenous injection.

In another study, Li et al. investigated the pharmacokinetic differences of cisplatin in rat tumor and lung tissues after ILP, using different perfusion times and perfusate drug concentration (7). Isolated lungs were perfused over various times with perfusate cisplatin concentration of 25, 50, or 100 µg/mL. The total cisplatin concentration in the lung tissue increased significantly with perfusion time and increasing cisplatin perfusate concentration. The cisplatin concentrations in the lung tissue after a 60-min perfusion ranged from approx 4 to 21 µg/g of tissue. However, the total cisplatin concentrations in the perfused tumor tissues (tumor nodules developed were approx 4 mm in diameter) did not change significantly with the perfusion time or perfusate cisplatin concentration, ranging from 4.17 ± 0.82 to 4.95 ± 0.80 µg/g of tissue in all the perfusion groups (Table 1). It was also

Table 1
Cisplatin Concentration in Perfusate, Lung Tissue, and Tumor Tissue in Rats

Animals	Tumor	Route	Dose or initial conc.	Lung (μg/g)	Tumor (μg/g)	Reference
Rat	Sarcoma	ILP	0.1 mg/mL		6.67 (1.64)	5
		IV	1 mg		2.51 (0.60)	
Rat	Sarcoma	ILP	25 μg/mL	~ 4	4.76 (0.60)[a]	7
		ILP	50 μg/mL	~11	4.95 (0.80)[a]	
		ILP	100 μg/mL	~21	4.84 (0.74)[a]	
Rat	Sarcoma	ILP	25 μg/mL		5.08 (1.34)[a]	23
		ILP	50 μg/mL		4.93 (1.22)[a]	
		ILP	100 μg/mL		3.93 (1.19)[a]	

Data are presented as means and SD. ILP, Isolated lung perfusion; IV, intravenous infusion.
[a]Concentration at 60 min of ILP.

observed that the cisplatin concentration in tumor tissue was inversely related to the weight of tumor nodules after IPL with cisplatin. The results indicate that different pharmacokinetics in the tumor and lung tissues exist following ILP with cisplatin in the rat sarcoma model. Further studies are required to raise cisplatin concentration to the tumor tissue.

2.2. 2'-Deoxy-5-Fluorouridine

Port et al. studied the pharmacokinetics and effectiveness of ILP with 2'-deoxy-5-fluorouridine (FUDR) in a rat model (8). FUDR is well tolerated at 21 mg/mL at a rate of 0.5 mL/min for 20 min, which is above the rat lethal dose of intravenous bolus injection. The pharmacokinetics of FUDR via ILP was compared with intravenous administration. Isolated lung perfusion with FUDR at 21 mg/mL maximally elevated total lung FUDR and 5-fluorouracil (5-FU) levels (508.5 ± 96.4 μg/g) in comparison to the intravenous group (7.5 ± 4.1 μg/g). It is believed that the lung is an inefficient extractor of FUDR and is unable to catabolize FUDR beyond 5-FU. Less than 1% of FUDR extracted in this study supports the inefficient uptake by the lung. The pharmacokinetic advantage of high pulmonary FUDR levels, the lung's inefficient FUDR extraction, as well as the lung's inability to detoxify FUDR may be advantages for the treatment of pulmonary colorectal metastases with ILP.

2.3. Doxorubicin

Minchin and Boyd evaluated doxorubicin pharmacokinetics of ILP using an ex vivo rat model (9). The results demonstrated that doxorubicin concentration in the lung increased linearly with perfusion time and with increasing doxorubicin perfusate concentration. In another study, dog lungs were perfused with doxorubicin at concentrations ranging from 0.5 to 118.2 nmol/mL (0.27 to 64.1 μg/mL) (10). Doxorubicin uptake in the lung increased with time but was saturable at perfusate concentrations above 20 nmol/mL (10.9 μg/mL) after 50 min. Doxorubicin lung uptake ranged from 1.3 to 65.1 μg/g tissue (Table 2). Tumor levels of doxorubicin were always lower than in the pulmonary tissue surrounding the tumors. Random sampling of lung tissue from the upper, middle, and lower lobes showed that the drug was distributed uniformly throughout the tissue (10).

Table 2
Doxorubicin Concentration in Perfusate and Lung Tissue

Animals	Route	Dose or initial conc.	Perfusate (μg/mL)	Lung (μg/g)	Extraction (%)	Reference
Dog	ILP		0.27–64.1	1.3–65		10
Dog	ILP	1.95 μg/mL		3.9		11
	ILP	2.95 μg/mL		8.8 (1.2)		
	ILP	4.39 μg/mL		16.9 (1.7)		
	ILP	5.79 μg/mL		19.2 (0.8)		
	ILP	7.61 μg/mL		20.6 (4.5)		
Rat	ILP	80 μg/mL	72.1 (6.9)	107.8 (30.2)	38.3 (13.2)	12
	ILP	160 μg/mL	118.4 (12.1)	172.2 (64.4)	38.9 (15.2)	
	ILP	320 μg/mL	255.2 (12.8)	498.1 (180.6)	58.3 (13.1)	
	ILP	480 μg/mL	384.1 (46.2)	418.5 (69)	57 (9.8)	
	ILP	640 μg/mL	457.6 (32.5)	663.8 (350.2)	41.4 (9.3)	
	IV	5 mg/kg		19.9 (4.4)		
	IV	7 mg/kg		25.5 (1.5)		
Rat	ILP	80 μg/mL		170.5	5.5	13
	ILP	320 μg/mL		46.2	4.3	
Pig	ILP	50 mg/m^2		21.9		14
	IV	50 mg/m^2		3.0 (0.8)		

Numbers in parentheses are standard deviations. ILP, Isolated lung perfusion; IV, intravenous perfusion.

Baciewicz et al. studied the pharmacokinetics of ILP with doxorubicin in dog (11). Perfusate concentrations ranged from 1.95 μg/mL to 7.61 μg/mL and the lung concentration of doxorubicin ranged from 3.9 μg/g to 20.6 μg/g (Table 2). A plateau of doxorubicin concentration in lung tissue appeared to be reached at a perfusate concentration of 5.79 μg/mL. The observed plateau in tissue doxorubicin levels could be explained by the lung tissue uptake of doxorubicin, perhaps by means of a carrier-mediated mechanism. Another explanation of the plateau is that perfusate concentration of 7.6 μg/mL caused a significant histologic injury of the lung, and once the lung is injured, increased uptake might not be expected.

Weksler et al. evaluated doxorubicin pharmacokinetics of ILP and intravenous injection in rats (12). Lung doxorubicin concentrations after ILP were 107.8–663.8 μg/mL and were significantly higher than those after intravenous doxorubicin (19.9–25.5 μg/mL) (Table 2). Lung doxorubicin concentration reached a plateau at a perfusate concentration of 255.2 ± 12.8 μg/mL of doxorubicin. Extraction ratio, the percent of doxorubicin extracted by the lung from the perfusate, appeared to be related to perfusate concentration, ranging from 38% to 58% (Table 2). The optimal perfusate and other pharmacokinetic factors for ILP using doxorubicin were also investigated in rats (13). The mean lung concentrations of doxorubicin were < 100 and < 300 μg/g, respectively, for perfusate concentrations of 80 μg/mL and 320 μg/mL. Extraction ratios were 5.5 and 4.3, respectively, which were lower than those reported (12). The study also suggested that the dose per kilogram or per square meter of body surface area, the total infused dose of doxorubicin, and the rate of infusion were not important in the final lung concentration of doxorubicin. The results indicated that the

Table 3
Concentration of FUDR, Melphalan, and Paclitaxel in Perfusate and Lung Tissue

Drug	Animals	Route	Dose or initial conc.	Perfusate (μg/mL)	Lung (μg/g)	$AUC_{(0-4.5 h)}$ (μg·h^{-1}·mg^{-1})	Reference
FUDR	Rat	ILP	7 mg/mL		116.3 (21.1)		8
		ILP	14 mg/mL		299.1 (44.8)		
		ILP	21 mg/mL		508.5 (96.4)		
		IV	1 mg/kg/d		7.5 (4.1)		
Melphalan	Rat	ILP	0.5 mg		40.9 (3.8)		15
		ILP	1 mg		50.5 (2.6)		
		IV	0.5 mg		0.8 (0.5)		
		IV	1 mg		1.7 (0.2)		
Paclitaxel	Sheep	ILP	40 mg	11.9[a]	15[b]	26.2	16
		ILP	200 mg	69[a]	59.9[b]	78.9	
		ILP	800 mg	289.8[a]	90.1[b]	183.8	
		IV	200 mg		25.4[b]	73	

Numbered in parentheses are standard deviations. ILP, Isolated lung perfusion; IV, intravenous infusion; FUDR, 2'-deoxy-5-fluorouridine.

[a] Initial concentration.
[b] Peak concentration.

doxorubicin perfusate concentration and the duration of perfusion are the only factors deter-mining the final lung concentration of doxorubicin *(13)*. An equation to predict final lung concentration of doxorubicin in rats was proposed: $\log (FLC) = 1.9 + 0.0071P + 0.186T$, where FLC is final lung concentration, P is measured perfusate doxorubicin concentration, and T is perfusion time in minutes ($r^2 = 0.91$).

Furrer et al. performed a study of ILP with doxorubicin in pigs by two different systems *(14)*. Doxorubicin lung tissue concentrations were 17.5 μg/g to 21.9 μg/g at a dose of 50 mg/m^2 and were approximately six- to sevenfold higher than after intravenous administration at a dose of 10 mg/kg (3 μg/g).

2.4. Melphalan

Hendriks et al. studied ILP with melphalan and tumor necrosis factor for metastatic pulmonary adenocarcinoma in rats *(15)*. Pharmacokinetic results demonstrated that ILP with melphalan was superior to intravenous injection. Lung melphalan levels in ILP groups were 30–50 times higher than in the intravenous groups, for both 0.5 and 1.0 mg of melphalan (Table 3). No significant elevation of melphalan tissue levels could be detected when the dose was doubled from 0.5 mg to 1.0 mg (Table 3). The concentration–time profiles were nearly identical and the decrease in metastatic nodules was similar between the two groups. The results may suggest that lower doses of melphalan may be used.

2.5. Paclitaxel

Pharmacokinetics of paclitaxel administered by ILP was first evaluated by Schrump et al. *(16)*. Nine adult sheep underwent ILP and one sheep received paclitaxel by 1-h intravenous infusion. Paclitaxel concentrations in lung tissues increased nonlinearly with escalating doses ranging from 2 to 800 mg and peaked between 60 and 90 min. Drug tissue levels rapidly declined during washout. In this study, lung tissue samples were collected at different time intervals for pharmacokinetic analysis. Paclitaxel peak concentration (C_{max}) and area under the concentration–time curve (AUC) in lung tissue increased with dose, gradually approaching a plateau (Table 3). The average C_{max} in lung tissues following ILP at 200 mg was approximately twofold higher than that observed after systemic infusion of the same dose of paclitaxel over 1 h. Tissue AUCs under these conditions were relatively comparable. Higher C_{max} and AUC were achieved with increased dose (800 mg), and were higher than those with 1-h intravenous infusion (200 mg) (C_{max}: 90 vs 25.4 µg/g; AUC: 184 vs 73 µg·mg^{-1}·h^{-1}). The continued increase of C_{max} and AUC without reaching a plateau indicates that the transport of paclitaxel into lung tissue was not fully saturated. The results confirm the profound pharmacokinetic advantage for paclitaxel administered by ILP and provide a rationale for considering paclitaxel for ILP administration in clinical trials.

3. CLINICAL PHARMACOKINETIC STUDIES OF ILP WITH ANTITUMOR AGENTS

Pharmacokinetic studies of isolated lung perfusion with different antitumor agents have been evaluated in preclinical animal models. These animal studies have demonstrated that ILP with these drugs are superior pharmacokinetically to systemic administration, providing higher lung tissue (tumor) levels and lower systemic exposure. The results indicate a pharmacologic rationale for ILP in humans. Several clinical studies have been reported or are under evaluation. Some of the reported studies with pharmacokinetic results are discussed here.

3.1. Cisplatin

Johnston et al. reported ILP with cisplatin in patients with metastatic lung sarcoma or diffuse bronchioloalveolar carcinoma (17). Two patients received perfusate with cisplatin at concentrations of 14 and 20 µg/mL. The drug concentrations in the tumor were about twofold higher than those in normal lung tissue (Table 4). The drug was detectable in the mediastinal lymph nodes for one patient.

Ratto et al. reported administering cisplatin by ILP for the treatment of pulmonary metastases from soft tissue sarcoma in six patients (18). Cisplatin at a dose of 200 mg/m^2 was administered. The AUC (0–60 min) values in pulmonary plasma were about 43 times greater than those in systemic plasma (12.8 ± 5.6 vs 0.3 ± 0.2 mg·mL^{-1}·min^{-1}). Cisplatin concentration in mediastinal lymph nodes (the diameter < 1 cm) was 2.57 µg/g, and was similar to those achieved in normal lung tissue. In this study, cisplatin concentration in larger metastases was not investigated as they were removed during the operation.

In a clinical study of hyperthermic (41°C) ILP with cisplatin for the treatment of lung sarcoma metastasis, four patients were treated with high doses of cisplatin (70 mg/m^2) (19). Initial cisplatin concentrations in the perfusate were higher than 100 µg/mL. At the end of the perfusion, a lung tissue sample was found to have a cisplatin concentration of 93.8 µg/g of tissue. This is the highest cisplatin lung concentration reported. However, cisplatin tumor concentrations were not reported in this study.

3.2. Doxorubicin

Minchin et al. first evaluated the pharmacokinetics of doxorubicin in isolated lung samples from humans and dogs (10). Three patients with sarcoma lung metastases were perfused at 25°C with doxorubicin perfusate concentration of 0.56–0.98 µg/mL. Drug concentrations in lung tissue increased steadily with time. Tumor concentrations of doxorubicin were consis-

Table 4
Doxorubicin and Cisplatin Concentrations in Perfusate, Lung, and Tumor Tissue in Patients

Drug	Dose or initial conc.	Perfusate (μg/mL)	N	Lung (μg/g of tissue)	Tumor (μg/g of tissue)	Reference
Doxorubicin	1 μg/mL	0.56[a]	1	0.72	0.64	17
	1 μg/mL	0.56[a]	1	0.79	0.25	17
	1.5 μg/mL	0.98[a]	1	2.58	0.62	17
	3 μg/mL	1.46[a]	1	1.58	2.19	17
	5 μg/mL	2.76[a]	1	2.13	1.56	17
	10 μg/mL	3.08[a]	1	2.81	2.81	17
	40 mg/m²	4.52[b]	1	0.58	NA	20
	40 mg/m²	3.76[b]	1	4.64	5.03	20
	40 mg/m²	8.48[b]	1	10.10	6.62	20
	40 mg/m²	12.9[b]	1	18.60	14.5	20
	80 mg/m²	27.95	1	57.30	33.5	20
Cisplatin	14 μg/mL		1	0.69	1.42	17
	20 μg/mL		1	0.68	1.09	17
	70 mg/m²	>100[a]	4	≤98.30		19
	200 mg/m²		6		2.57	18

[a] Perfusate peak concentration during the perfusion.

[b] Mean perfusate concentration.

tently lower than in the lung tissue in all three patients, possibly owing to poor vascularity of the tumor tissue. Lung tissue doxorubicin concentrations in these patients were considerably lower than those seen in dogs treated with similar drug concentrations (10).

ILP with doxorubicin in patients with metastatic lung sarcoma or diffuse bronchioloalveolar carcinoma was reported by Johnston et al. (17). Escalating doses of doxorubicin ranging from 1 to 10 μg/mL were administered in six patients. Although showing much variability, drug concentrations in tumor and lung tissue immediately after perfusion generally increased with higher doses. Doxorubicin concentration in tumor tissue appeared lower than in lung tissue, although there was no statistical difference (Table 4) (17).

Another Phase I trial of ILP with doxorubicin in patients with metastatic sarcoma was reported by Burt et al. (20). Seven patients were treated with doxorubicin at a dose of 40 mg/m² or less, and one patient received 80 mg/m². The mean perfusate level of doxorubicin was 5.9 μg/mL in the group of patients receiving 40 mg/m² or less. The mean lung tissue level of doxorubicin in this group was 6.5 μg/g. Doxorubicin concentrations in lung and tumor appear to correlate with the amount of doxorubicin in the perfusate. In general, tumors took up less drug than the healthy lung tissues (Table 4). Thirteen percent of the drug (10 mg) was extracted during ILP.

4. DRUG PENETRATION IN TUMOR TISSUE AND ISOLATED LUNG PERFUSION

Many solid tumors are rather resistant to chemotherapy. The mechanisms of genetically determined factors expressed in individual tumor cells includes the existence of drug efflux pumps (such as P-glycoprotein or multidrug resistance-associated proteins), changes in the expression of topoisomerase, alterations of drug metabolism, DNA repair, and apoptosis.

Other areas of potential causes for drug resistance in solid tumors are those related to the solid tumor microenvironment and the problems relating to the drug delivery into the tumor cells *(21)*.

With regional chemotherapy such as ILP, the maximum tolerated dose is given to achieve high concentrations at tumor site and kill all tumor cells. However, for the effective treatment of solid tumors, anticancer drugs must penetrate through the extravascular space to achieve a lethal concentration in all of the target cancer cells. The limited penetration of anticancer drugs through tumor tissue may be a very important cause of clinical resistance of solid tumors to chemotherapy, especially regional chemotherapy such as ILP.

Blood flow in tumors is often irregular. Blood vascular systems may be poorly formed, with variable rates of blood flow, and the intercapillary distance may be relatively large when compared with normal tissue. For drug to be effective, it must penetrate through multiple layers of solid tissue to reach all cells in a tumor. Thus, tissue penetration of anticancer drugs is likely more limited in tumors than in normal tissue. It is more difficult to predict pharmacokinetic behavior of the drugs. Many other factors would also affect drug distribution in tumors, such as drug delivery by the vascular system, the rate of diffusion through tissue, drug metabolism, and binding to tissue components. Tumor cell density, tumor blood supply, and the distance from tumor nodule surface all could have an impact on tumor tissue pharmacokinetic results *(21,22)*. More variability of pharmacokinetic results could be expected with ILP.

The concentration of anticancer drugs in lung tissue and tumors has been compared in many preclinical and clinical ILP studies. Some studies show that high concentrations of anticancer drugs are achieved in normal tissue but not in tumors. Saeki et al. evaluated tumor size and weight with pharmacokinetic characteristics of ILP in tumor tissues *(23)*. They found that the total platinum concentrations in tumor nodules were correlated inversely with the tumor weight (total platinum concentration in tumor = 1.167 × 1/tumor wt; $r^2 = 0.981$; $p < 0.001$). The results suggested that ILP may be more effective against small tumors than large ones. The results showed that large tumor legions may need to be debulked before utilizing ILP in patients with an unresectable lung tumor. To increase intracellular platinum concentration and enhance the antitumor effect of ILP with cisplatin, a combination study with cisplatin and digitonin, a detergent to increase cell permeability, was performed in rat *(24)*. The rats underwent ILP with 100 μg/mL of cisplatin after 20 μmol/L of digitonin was injected. However, pharmacokinetic results showed that cisplatin concentration of tumor nodules in the rats treated with digitonin–cisplatin increased slightly, only 20% higher than in the cisplatin-only rats ($5.48 ± 0.64$ vs $4.5 ± 1.09$ μg/g; $p = 0.067$), although the number of pulmonary nodules decreased significantly by digitonin use ($1.3 ± 1.5$ vs $9.7 ± 2$) *(24)*.

5. SUMMARY

Preclinical and clinical studies indicate that ILP can deliver high concentrations of antitumor drugs to lung tissue with minimal systemic toxicity. High drug concentrations in lung and tumor tissue are achievable. The studies indicate there are pharmacokinetic differences in tumor and lung tissues following ILP with different anticancer agents. Perfusate concentration and perfusion time are important factors influencing drug pharmacokinetics in lung and tumor tissue. Other contributing factors may include tumor size, tumor types, poorly formed blood vascular system in tumor, site of biopsy, animal models, and so forth. Some of studies show that the drug concentrations are generally lower in tumor tissue than in normal lung tissue. The strategies to improve the penetration of anticancer drugs through poorly vascularized tumor tissue have considerable potential to improve the outcome of isolated lung perfusion for solid tumors.

ACKNOWLEDGMENTS

I would like to thank Dr. Michael C. Cox and Dr. Juliana Chan for their editorial assistance.

REFERENCES

1. Weksler B, Burt M. Isolated lung perfusion with antineoplastic agents for pulmonary metastases. Chest Surg Clin N Am 1998; 8:157–182.
2. Hendriks JM, Van Schil PE. Isolated lung perfusion for the treatment of pulmonary metastases. Surg Oncol 1998; 7:59–63.
3. Upton RN, Doolette DJ. Kinetic aspects of drug disposition in the lungs. Clin Exp Pharmacol Physiol 1999; 26:381–391.
4. Pacifici GM, Franchi M, Bencini C, Repetti F, Di Lascio N, Muraro GB. Tissue distribution of drug-metabolizing enzymes in humans. Xenobiotica 1988; 18:849–856.
5. Li TS, Sugi K, Ueda K, Nawata K, Nawata S, Esato K. Isolated lung perfusion with cisplatin in a rat lung solitary tumor nodule model. Anticancer Res 1998; 18:4171–4176.
6. Wang HY, Hochwald S, Ng B, Burt M. Regional chemotherapy via pulmonary artery with blood flow occlusion in a solitary tumor nodule model. Anticancer Res 1996; 16:3749–753.
7. Li TS, Kaneda Y, Saeki K, Ueda K, Zempo N, Esato K. Pharmacokinetic differences between rat tumour and lung tissues following isolated lung perfusion with cisplatin. Eur J Cancer 1999; 35:1846–1850.
8. Port JL, Ng B, Ellis JL, Nawata S, Lenert JT, Burt ME. Isolated lung perfusion with FUDR in the rat: pharmacokinetics and survival. Ann Thorac Surg 1996; 62:848–852.
9. Minchin RF, Boyd MR. Uptake and metabolism of doxorubicin in isolated perfused rat lung. Biochem Pharmacol 1983; 32:2829–2832.
10. Minchin RF, Johnston MR, Aiken MA, Boyd MR. Pharmacokinetics of doxorubicin in isolated lung of dogs and humans perfused in vivo. J Pharmacol Exp Ther 1984; 229:193–198.
11. Baciewicz FA Jr, Arredondo M, Chaudhuri B, et al. Pharmacokinetics and toxicity of isolated perfusion of lung with doxorubicin. J Surg Res 1991; 50:124–128.
12. Weksler B, Ng B, Lenert JT, Burt ME. Isolated single-lung perfusion with doxorubicin is pharmacokinetically superior to intravenous injection. Ann Thorac Surg 1993; 56:209–214.
13. Weksler B, Ng B, Lenert JT, Burt ME. Isolated single-lung perfusion: a study of the optimal perfusate and other pharmacokinetic factors. Ann Thorac Surg 1995; 60:624–629.
14. Furrer M, Lardinois D, Thormann W, et al. Isolated lung perfusion: single-pass system versus recirculating blood perfusion in pigs. Ann Thorac Surg 1998; 65:1420–1425.
15. Hendriks JM, Van Schil PE, De Boeck G, et al. Isolated lung perfusion with melphalan and tumor necrosis factor for metastatic pulmonary adenocarcinoma. Ann Thorac Surg 1998; 66:2164.
16. Schrump DS, Zhai S, Nguyen DM, et al. Pharmacokinetics of paclitaxel administered by hyperthermic retrograde isolated lung perfusion techniques. J Thorac Cardiovasc Surg 2002; 123:686–694.
17. Johnston MR, Minchen RF, Dawson CA. Lung perfusion with chemotherapy in patients with unresectable metastatic sarcoma to the lung or diffuse bronchioloalveolar carcinoma. J Thorac Cardiovasc Surg 1995; 110:368–373.
18. Ratto GB, Toma S, Civalleri D, et al. Isolated lung perfusion with platinum in the treatment of pulmonary metastases from soft tissue sarcomas. J Thorac Cardiovasc Surg 1996; 112:614–622.
19. Schroder C, Fisher S, Pieck AC, et al. Technique and results of hyperthermic (41 degrees C) isolated lung perfusion with high-doses of cisplatin for the treatment of surgically relapsing or unresectable lung sarcoma metastasis. Eur J Cardiothorac Surg 2002; 22:41–46.
20. Burt ME, Liu D, Abolhoda A, et al. Isolated lung perfusion for patients with unresectable metastases from sarcoma: a phase I trial. Ann Thorac Surg 2000; 69:1542–1549.
21. Tannock IF, Lee CM, Tunggal JK, Cowan DS, Egorin MJ. Limited penetration of anticancer drugs through tumor tissue: a potential cause of resistance of solid tumors to chemotherapy. Clin Cancer Res 2002; 8:878–884.
22. Kuh HJ, Jang SH, Wientjes MG, Weaver JR, Au JL. Determinants of paclitaxel penetration and accumulation in human solid tumor. J Pharmacol Exp Ther 1999; 290:871–880.
23. Saeki K, Kaneda Y, Li TS, Ueda K, Esato K. Relationship between the concentration of CDDP in tumor and tumor size after isolated lung perfusion treatment experimental study on a solitary pulmonary sarcoma model in rats. J Surg Oncol 2000; 75:193–196.
24. Tanaka T, Kaneda Y, Li TS, Matsuoka T, Zempo N, Esato K. Digitonin enhances the antitumor effect of cisplatin during isolated lung perfusion. Ann Thorac Surg 2001; 72:1173–1178.

23 Central Nervous System Malignancy and Clinical Pharmacology

Steve Y. Cho, MD and Howard A. Fine, MD

CONTENTS

1. INTRODUCTION

The brain is a frequent site of primary and metastatic tumors. It is estimated that approx 16,800 new cases of primary brain tumors (<1.5% of all malignant diseases) and 170,000 new cases of new brain metastases are diagnosed annually in the United States (1,2). In the pediatric population primary brain tumors are the most common solid tumor, second only to leukemia in overall tumor frequency in this age group (3).

The prognosis of patients with the most common types of malignant brain tumors, anaplastic astrocytoma and glioblastoma multiforme, remains poor despite current treatment strategies. Despite significant advances in neuroimaging, microsurgery, and radiation therapy, the median survival for patients with malignant gliomas is still less than 1 yr. Conventional therapy for the most common form of malignant glioma, glioblastoma multiforme, consists primarily of surgical debulking followed by radiation therapy. Unfortunately, the median survival after surgical intervention alone is 6 mo, with only 7.5% of patients surviving for 2 yr, and fewer than 5% are alive by 3 yr. The addition of systemic chemotherapy may extend survival slightly but is associated with significant toxicity. A meta-analysis concluded that a significant but limited survival benefit exists for adjuvant chemotherapy in glioblastoma multiforme (4). Eighty percent of malignant gliomas are known to recur within 2 cm of the original tumor site and are due to the presence of locally invasive glioma cells, whereas distant metastases are exceedingly rare (5,6). New therapies and novel approaches are clearly needed to treat gliomas.

Handbook of Anticancer Pharmacokinetics and Pharmacodynamics
Edited by: W. D. Figg and H. L. McLeod © Humana Press Inc., Totowa, NJ

The problems in treating brain tumors are inherent in the unique environment of the brain including its distinct anatomical compartment, surrounding cerebrospinal fluid (CSF), the presence of the blood–brain barrier (BBB) and blood–tumor barrier (BTB), and exquisite sensitivity of normal brain tissue to chemical or physical intervention. The delivery of therapeutic agents past the BBB is a major factor limiting progress in translational molecular oncology to the development of clinically effective antibrain tumor agents (7).

2. CELL BIOLOGY/ANATOMY OF THE BBB

The BBB is a physical and metabolic barrier between the central nervous system (CNS) and the systemic circulation, which serves to regulate and protect the microenvironment of the brain. Whereas the BBB protects and regulates the microenvironment of the brain and spinal cord to allow the CNS to function optimally under diverse conditions during health, these very same mechanisms thwart our ability to intervene during disease, encumbering our corrective measures (8).

Cerebral capillaries differ from other capillaries. The endothelial cells lack fenestrations, are not pinocytotic, and consist of cerebrovascular endothelial cells interconnected by continuous belts of tight junctions. Tight junctions are enveloped by astrocytic foot processes that further regulate entry past the BBB. The presence of these tight junctions, which characterize the BBB, results in high transendothelial electrical resistance (1500–2000 ohms/cm^2) and decreased paracellular resistance (9). Astrocytes also confer a protective role on the BBB against hypoxia and hypoglycemia (9,10). Passive transport across the BBB therefore is highly dependent on the physicochemical features of the drug. Excluding some hydrophilic and large molecules, which are actively transported, only lipophilic drugs can enter the brain to varying degrees (10).

The BBB selectively transports nutrients into the brain via a number of surface transporters to maintain brain homeostasis. There are reported to be as much as 20 or more active or facilitated carrier systems expressed in brain capillaries at high levels (11). Alterations in the levels or distribution of transporters can be seen in various disease states. Tight junctions limit *paracellular diffusion* of molecules and the formation of extracellular fluid. Several markers have been used to demonstrate tight junction alterations during disease, including sucrose, and gadolinium diethylenetriamine pentaacetic acid. The BBB blocks paracellular transport of polar, hydrophilic drugs. By contrast, *transcellular diffusion* allows the transport of lipophilic substances and small molecules such as O_2 and CO_2. *Carrier systems* are essential to shuttle nutrients (e.g., glucose, amino acids), vitamins, hormones, monocarboxylic acids, and amines to the brain. The insulin-independent GLUT-1 transporter is responsible for transporting glucose, the main energy source for the brain, and increased expression of GLUT-1 has been observed on the luminal surface during hypoglycemia and hypoxia. *Pinocytotic vesicles*, although reduced in the BBB, are an important mechanism for transporting molecules such as transferrin, insulin and leptin via receptor-mediated endocytosis (9).

There is an eight-log difference in the rate at which an immunoglobulin will cross a liver capillary vs the rate at which one will cross a capillary in the brain (12). The hydraulic conductivity coefficient of brain capillaries is 500 times less than in heart muscle, 1000 times less than in peripheral muscle, and 3000 times less than intestinal capillaries. The oncotic reflection of this coefficient impedes protein delivery (10).

Drugs must utilize transcellular pathways to cross the BBB and enter the brain. Ways in which one can theoretically increase permeability of the BBB to a particular drug include (1) increasing the lipophilicity of the drug thereby allowing greater passive diffusion, (2) increasing carrier-mediated influx via facilitated transport across the cell membrane by increasing the affinity of BBB endogenous transporters, and/or (3) decreasing carrier-mediated efflux of the drug at the BBB through inhibition of the relevant transporter *(7,8)*.

2.1. Characteristics of the Brain–Tumor Barrier

In primary or metastatic brain tumors, a number of alterations in the brain capillary ultrastructure have been described. These vary from subtle alteration in tight junction structure, with enlargement of the perivascular space and slight swelling of the basal lamina, to a very irregular appearance of the endothelium, with many fenestrations and an increase in the number and size of pinocytic vacuoles and a totally irregular basal lamina. Some of these alterations may be explained by the lack of normal astrocytes supporting the cerebral endothelium within the tumor *(10)*.

The vascular permeability within a brain tumor is a function of both the microarchitecture of the tumor-associated vascular endothelial cells and the spatial distribution of the associated capillaries. There are three distinct microvessel populations in brain tumors: (1) continuous, nonfenestrated capillaries (seen in normal brain and low-grade gliomas), (2) continuous, fenestrated capillaries (seen in some brain tumor animal models) with increased permeability to small molecules, and (3) vasculature containing interendothelial gaps that measure as much as 1 μm (also seen in animal models). Although this latter type of vasculature does allow permeability of some larger molecules, the degree of permeability is still 2–3 logs less than in liver or lung *(13,14)*.

The spatial distribution of brain tumor capillaries is also a determinant of the degree of permeability of a given tumor or area within a tumor. The degree of vascular permeability and capillary density varies not only within a given tumor but also by the type of tumor. For example, there is great heterogeneity in intratumor vascular permeability in high-grade gliomas. The central areas of large malignant gliomas tend to have low capillary density (so much so that central areas are often severely hypoxic and necrotic), and thus, although the individual capillaries are highly permeable, the overall permeability within this central area of the tumor is low. Alternately, the outer highly proliferative rim of a malignant tumor contains many angiogenic vessels that are highly permeable, thus resulting in a region of high permeability and extravasation of intravascular content. By contrast, the area of brain surrounding the tumor mass that contains the leading zone of the infiltrative glioma cells has relatively normal vascular permeability and density *(12)*. These variable degrees of permeability within a given high-grade glioma can be differentiated clinically by the contrast-enhancing patterns seen on computed axial tomography (CAT) and magnetic resonance imaging (MRI) scans, as only areas of relatively high perfusion and permeability will allow extravasation of the contrast material (i.e., gadolinium for MRI scans). The low perfusion central areas of these tumors are usually seen as non-contrast-enhancing, necrotic regions, whereas the outer rim of tumor is avidly contrast enhancing. The area of brain surrounding the tumor, although edematous, does not generally contrast enhance *(13)*. Thus, drug delivery can be a difficult problem to the central area of a malignant glioma and to infiltrative glioma cells in the brain around such a tumor.

The situation for low-grade gliomas is quite different than that in higher-grade tumors in that most non-contrast-enhancing low-grade tumors contain a relatively intact BBB, significantly complicating drug delivery. On the other end of the spectrum are brain metastases that have essentially no intact BBB or even a BTB once they reach a certain size. This is the reason that brain metastasis from chemosensitive systemic tumors (i.e., breast carcinoma, small lung cancer) can respond to drugs that do not usually cross the BBB or even the BTB.

The reason most brain metastases do not respond to systemic chemotherapy is less a matter of drug delivery and more a function of the chemotherapy-resistant nature of the systemic cancer to gave rise to the brain metastases.

2.2. Blood–CSF Barrier

Another important feature relative to pharmacokinetic issues within the CNS is the presence of the blood–CSF barrier (BCB). This barrier is formed by the endothelial microarchitecture of the BBB within the arachnoid lining of the brain and spinal cord and the tightly bound choroidal epithelial cells, which are responsible for the production of CSF. The BCB closely regulates the exchange of molecules between the blood and CSF and thus it can control the penetration of molecules within the interstitial fluid of the brain parenchyma. Furthermore, the BCB is fortified by an active organic acid transport system. Thus, it can actively remove a number of agents, such as methotrexate, from the CSF and thereby prevent the diffusion of chemotherapeutic agents directly into the brain parenchyma *(5)*. Because the surface area of the BBB is estimated to be 5000-fold lager than that of the BCB, the BBB is the main route for the uptake of endogenous substances into the brain parenchyma *(11)*.

In essence, the BCB is the product of junctions between the choroidal epithelial cells and the endothelial cells that form the BBB. There is a concentration diffusion gradient favoring passage of substances from the extracellular fluid in the brain parenchyma to the CSF, secondary to the fact that the CSF constantly circulates, thereby carrying substances away. Thus, the CSF may act as a perpetual sink to the brain. Because the CSF is relatively easily accessible for in vivo pharmacokinetic sampling, CSF drug levels are often used as surrogate markers for brain drug levels. Unfortunately, this is an oversimplification and in the best of circumstances the CSF drug levels only partially reflect the intraparenchymal drug levels. In some drugs or disease states (i.e., neoplastic meningitis) CSF drug levels have little correlation to brain parenchymal levels *(13)*.

2.3. Pharmacokinetics of Crossing the BBB

As previously mentioned, the greater the lipid solubility of a drug, the greater its ability to penetrate the BBB through simple diffusion. Nevertheless, the percentage of a drug that enters a tumor, compared to that circulating through the entire body, is miniscule (generally <1%) regardless of the drug's permeability and regardless of changes in capillary permeability. Therefore, any method that is used to increase brain tumor permeability will still have to deal with the reality that most of the administered drug is distributed to the rest of the body, and therefore does not reach the brain tumor. Thus, systemic administration will usually be limited by systemic toxicity, making dose intensification a less viable option than it is for systemic tumors. Alternative methods for increasing the fraction of drug that reaches the brain tumor will need to be devised.

Once a drug gets into the brain it experiences rather complicated pharmacodynamic forces. Steady-state brain distribution in vivo is not only a function of passive diffusion across the BBB, but also depends on the relative affinity of the drug for plasma proteins and brain tissue. Ionization at physiologic pH (pK_a), the affinity and capacity of transport systems, potential BBB/cerebral metabolism, and egress through the CSF route are also important factors. Furthermore, there are a number of active efflux transport mechanisms present in the CNS, located both in the BBB and in the choroid plexus *(15)*.

Understanding the pharmacokinetic properties governing the steady-state drug concentrations within the brain is complicated by the fact that other, as yet ill-defined barrier mechanisms, may be at work in the BBB. The octanol/buffer partition coefficient is a measure of the ability of a compound to partition into an organic solvent relative to a physiologic buffer. It is a well-established method of predicting the probability of passive transport of molecules with a molecular weight < 400–600 kDa across a lipophilic membrane. Recent studies of several lipophilic drugs show lower brain concentrations than expected on the basis of their octanol/buffer coefficient, suggesting that other functional barrier mechanisms (i.e., transmembrane efflux pumps) may be operative in the intra-CNS pharmacology of these agents *(10)*. Nevertheless, the overall hydrophilic/lipophilic balance of a molecule still appears to be a generally useful guide to the penetrability of a given drug through the BBB.

Plasma protein binding is another factor thought to play a role in drug delivery to the brain. The time course and concentration of the free drug within the circulation is an important factor in determining the amount of drug that is available for diffusion or transport into the brain. There are a number of macromolecules within blood that can avidly bind lipophilic drugs including albumin, α_1-acid glycoprotein, lipoproteins, immunoglobulins, and even whole erythrocytes *(11)*.

3. DRUG RESISTANCE

While many primary brain tumors are intrinsically chemoresistant, limited penetration of cytotoxic drugs across the BBB may also contribute to the poor response of brain tumors to chemotherapy secondary to inadequate dose. Furthermore, sublethal concentrations of drug exposure to tumor cells, secondary to the BBB, can lead to the generation of drug-resistant clones despite an initial response to therapy.

Brain metastases often respond poorly to chemotherapy; however, as discussed above, this has less to do with the BBB or BTB then it does for primary brain tumors since the BBB is almost fully disrupted in brain metastases (at least within the center of the tumor). Rather, the chemotherapy resistance seen with brain metastases is more a reflection of the intrinsic chemotherapy resistance of the types of tumors that tend to metastasize to the brain (i.e., non-small-cell lung cancer, melanoma) and/or the advanced nature of the systemic disease by the time the tumor metastasizes to the brain (i.e., breast cancer, gastrointestinal cancers) *(15)*.

3.1. Drug Pumps

Once resistant tumor cells are generated, the resistance phenotype may be restricted to a certain anticancer agent or a class of related drugs rather than individual drug resistance. One specific mechanism of resistance results from overexpression of enzymes involved in a specific cellular drug metabolism or DNA repair. In other cases, however, the pattern of drug resistance is much more general with tumor-cell resistance to a particular cytotoxic agent being associated with the development of cross-resistance to many other drugs that have little or no structural or target similarity *(16)*. This phenomenon is known as multidrug resistance (MDR). The mechanism of MDR is generally one of a transport-mediated efflux of many endogenous substances and xenobiotics by either the tumor cell itself or the endothelium that makes up the BBB, thereby effectively reducing the effective concentration of the drug within the CNS. In this line of research, much attention has been focused on the multidrug transporters P-glycoprotein (Pgp) and the MDR-associated protein (MRP) *(15)*.

3.1.1. P-GLYCOPROTEIN

Pgp is a 170-kDa glycosylated membrane protein encoded by the *MDR1* (multiple drug resistance 1) gene. Pgp functions as an ATP-driven transmembrane bidirectional drug transporter participating in both drug uptake and drug efflux. Specific chemotherapeutic agents are excellent substrates for Pgp-mediated intracellular drug efflux including the vinca alkaloids, epipodophyllotoxins, anthracyclines, and taxanes. Thus, these agents are particularly vulnerable to *MDR1*-mediated drug resistance *(16)*. The most common types of brain tumors express the *MDR1* gene including gliomas, ependymomas, and primitive neuroectodermal tumors (PNETs). Some evidence points to an association between expression and prognosis in glioblastoma and medulloblastoma (a type of PNET).

To date, the site of action of Pgps in brain neoplasms remains uncertain. Pgp is seen as an early marker of the BBB in the microvessels of the developing brain and strongly expressed by endothelial cells at the BBB and BCB sites. Pgps are also thought to be present in the cell membranes of tumor cells or in the luminal membranes of tumor vessels, contributing to the formation of the BTB. Thus there appear to be two levels of Pgp drug resistance operative in mediating brain tumor resistance to chemotherapy *(17–19)*.

3.1.2. MRP

MRP is 180–195-kDa family of membrane proteins with at least seven members, belonging to the ATP-binding-cassette transmembrane transporter C subfamily. By contrast to Pgp, MRP decreases intracellular drug accumulation preferentially by unidirectional, ATP-driven export of the target molecule. Vinca alkaloids, epipodophyllotoxins, platinum DNA compounds, and anthracyclines are all susceptible to this resistance mechanism. There is growing evidence that increased MRP expression may be a factor in intrinsic or acquired drug resistance in a subset of brain tumors, especially gliomas. In addition, a link between MRP and survival of patients has recently been defined for neuroblastoma, with high expression signifying a worse clinical outcome *(16)*.

3.1.3. OTHER TRANSPORTERS

Two newly discovered categories of transporters are the organic anion transporter (OAT) family and the organic cation transporter (*OCT*) family. In both families, three homologs have been identified (OAT1, OAT2, OAT3, OCT1, OCT2, OCT3). OAT1, which appears to exchange organic anions with HCO_3^-, is present on the brush border of the choroid plexus, and OAT3 appears to be present in the BBB based on an in vitro model of the BBB using cultured mouse brain endothelial cells *(10)*. It remains unclear, however, if OATs are involved in the uptake into the brain or efflux of substances from the brain. For example, in rat brains, OAT2 has been demonstrated to transport digoxin against a concentration gradient from blood to brain, resulting in an accumulation of digoxin in the brain.

3.1.4. THERAPEUTIC ROLE OF DRUG PUMPS

Because drug pumps such as Pgp and MRP may play a role in the chemoresistance of some brain tumors, modulation or inhibition of such pumps represents a potentially promising therapeutic strategy for rendering tumors more sensitive to chemotherapeutic agents. Nevertheless, non-tumor-selective modulation of drug transporters would likely lead to increased drug exposure of normal brain issue, as well as tumor tissue, increasing the chance for significant neurotoxicity. This potential for neurotoxicity, the chance for increased systemic toxicity, and the continued uncertainly of the true clinical importance of drug pumps to tumor chemoresistance, have led many drug manufacturers to shy away from the clinical development of pump-inhibiting compounds *(16)*.

3.2. Glutathione and Glutathione-Linked Enzyme System

Glutathione and its related enzyme complex are known to protect tumor cells against chemotherapy-induced damage. This system includes glutathione, glutathione-related enzymes (mainly glutathione *S*-transferase), and transporters that export glutathione–drug complexes. The combination of glutathione with anticancer agents leads to a conjugation reaction that is catalyzed by glutathione *S*-transferase, leading to the formation of less toxic and more water-soluble conjugates. Drug families known to be susceptible to this resistance system include the chloroethylnitrosoureas, platinum compounds, anthracyclines, and phosphamides *(16)*.

The glutathione/glutathione *S*-transferase system has been shown to play a role in drug resistance of gliomas, medulloblastomas, and meningiomas, through a change in glutathione *S*-transferase, altered intracellular glutathione concentrations, or a combination of both. An increasing number of studies have demonstrated that the level of the π isoform of glutathione *S*-transferase is a predictor of survival, suggesting its importance in brain tumor biology and potentially drug resistance. A potential relationship exists between survival and the level of expression and subcellular localization of glutathione *S*-transferase in patients with high-grade gliomas *(20,21)*.

Apart from quantitative changes in the intracellular concentrations of glutathione and glutathione *S*-transferase isoenzymes, genetic polymorphisms of individual glutathione *S*-transferase alleles may significantly impact the rate and efficiency of *de novo* or salvage glutathione synthesis, thereby also impacting on the relative chemosensitivity of individual tumors *(22)*.

Methods to deplete glutathione pharmacologically (i.e., using buthionine sulfoximine) have been explored in the preclinical and clinical setting. Although one such study demonstrated increased chemosensitivity of biopsy-derived human malignant gliomas cells to carmustine and platinum compounds, these findings did not translate to a better clinical outcome *(23)*.

3.3. *O^6-Methylguanine-DNA Methyltransferase (MGMT)*

An important mechanism of individual drug resistance results from changes in MGMT (also O^6-alkylguanine-DNA alkyltransferase) contributing to clinical resistance to alkylating chloronitrosoureas (e.g., BCNU) and temozolomide, the leading chemotherapeutic agents currently used for high-grade gliomas. MGMT acts to remove cytotoxic alkyl adducts from the O^6 position of DNA-guanine and prevents the formation of DNA interstrand crosslinks by accepting the alkyl group at an active cysteine moiety within its own sequence. Resistance to chloronitrosoureas has been linked to MGMT-mediated DNA repair in several different CNS tumor types in adults and children, including high-grade gliomas, primitive neuroectodermal tumors, and ependymomas *(24,25)*. There are preclinical and clinical research efforts directed toward attempting to modulate genetically and pharmacologically MGMT activity in brain neoplasms. O^6-Alkylguanine derivatives, thioguanine, and streptozotocin are well known inhibitors of MGMT and have shown effectiveness in vitro and in brain tumor animal models. A new MGMT inhibitor, O^6-benzylguanine, has demonstrated significant activity in preclinical models and is currently undergoing Phase I and II testing in combination with nitosoureas and temozolomide for patients with primary brain tumors *(16)*.

3.4. *Topoisomerase II*

Topoisomerase II, consisting of α and β isoenzymes, is involved in negative supercoiling of superhelical DNA, allowing for replication, recombination, and transcription of nuclear DNA. Alteration of the topological state of DNA by topoisomerase II also allows accessibility of DNA to drug-mediated platination or alkylation. Topoisomerase IIα causes drug resistance to a number of chemotherapeutic agents including both those directly affecting topoisomerase II (i.e., epipodophyllotoxins) and those that do not (i.e., doxorubicin, mitoxantrone, amsacrine, cisplatin, and BCNU). The mechanisms by which topoisomerase II can affect drug sensitivity include: (1) reduction in topoisomerase II concentration, resulting in decreased access of DNA to the effects of chemotherapy, (2) altered topoisomerase

II subcellular localization, and (3) mutations in the structural topoisomerase II gene leading to drug-resistant variants.

Altered activity of this enzyme seems to be involved in the development of drug resistance in a subset of intracranial tumors, particularly high-grade gliomas and medulloblastomas *(27,28)*. Also, topoisomerase IIα expression has previously been reported to be predictive of both favorable and poor outcome in patients with glioma *(16)*. These contrasting results may stem from the dual role of topoisomerase IIα in tumor-cell proliferation and drug resistance, resulting in more biologically aggressive tumor and chemotherapy sensitivity, respectively. Clearly, further investigation is needed to study the role of this enzyme in drug sensitivity and tumor prognosis.

4. FACTORS TO CONSIDER FOR BRAIN TUMOR DELIVERY

4.1 Factors that Determine Drug Delivery and Time-Dependent Concentration in the Brain

There is a complex interchange of factors that determine the amount of a drug that can be delivered to and maintained within the brain. Discussions of these factors can be found in several authoritative reviews *(8,29,30,31)*. Several of the more important factors include:

1. The time-dependent plasma concentration profile of a drug. This governs the amount of drug available to enter the brain while the drug's plasma concentration depends on its absorption, volume of distribution, metabolism, and elimination.
2. The binding of the drug to plasma and brain constituents, and related binding off-rates. The binding of a drug to plasma proteins can be either restrictive or nonrestrictive to brain uptake, increasing with its lipophilicity. In the restrictive case, only the free fraction of the drug is available to enter the brain, whereas in the nonrestrictive case, drug stripping from the plasma protein occurs during the transit of the agent through the brain circulation *(32)*.
3. Drug permeability at the BBB. The BBB solubility of a drug in the lipid component of the endothelial cell membrane determines its permeability across the cell and therefore its ability to penetrate into the brain. The octanol/water partition coefficient, a physicochemical measure of a compound's "lipophilicity," is one measure of the permeability of a drug at the BBB *(33)*. In general, if a drug's octanol/water partition coefficient is >1 ($\log p > 0$) then its rate of transfer across the BBB is rapid and mainly limited by the availability of the drug, or the blood flow rate. On the other hand, if a drug's octanol/water partition coefficient is <0.1 ($\log p < -1$) its permeability across the BBB is low and is limited from entering the brain. Both permeability and the rate of cerebral blood flow control the rate of transfer of drugs whose octanol/water partition coefficient lie between 1 and 0.1 *(8)*.
4. Facilitated transport systems. The permeability coefficient of drugs that utilize a transport mechanism at the BBB does not correlate proportionally with either the cerebrovascular permeability or the octanol/water partition coefficient. Such systems can either augment drug entry into the brain (e.g., amino acids and d-glucose) or potentially limit brain uptake by expelling drug (e.g., Pgp and MRP substrates) *(8)*.
5. BBB metabolic/degradative enzymes. There are a number of metabolic or degradative enzymes located at the BBB that have the potential to metabolize lipophilic drugs to more hydrophilic compounds, thereby reducing their BBB permeability and entry into the brain. These enzymes are similar to those involved in hepatic phase I and II metabolic processes *(34)*.

6. Cerebral blood flow for lipophilic agents. For lipophilic agents, the cerebral blood flow rather than cerebrovascular permeability is the main factor that can limit brain delivery. In addition, different regions of the brain can vary relative to blood flow rate by as much as twofold and therefore cause a substantial difference in the brain distribution of the drug *(35,36)*.

The physicochemical characteristics of a compound, derived from its chemical structure, will determine its penetrability at the BBB. The effective brain tumor drug will possess a "balance" between lipo/hydrophilicity, providing it with solubility in the hydrophilic phases of the plasma and extracellular fluid, as well as in the lipophilic component of the cell membrane to cross the BBB and diffuse through the extracellular compartment to its target. Although experimental validation of BBB permeability is crucial, there do exist computational programs that may be useful in predicting a drug's delivery. A quantitative prediction of a drug's BBB permeability that encompasses the critical physical chemistry issues is found within the Abraham solvation equations *(37,38)*. Several commercial computer programs are also available to predict log P values from a compound's molecular structure (e.g., Pallas, Compudrug, CA).

4.2. Pharmacological Principles Related to CNS Drug Delivery and Action

Several factors must be considered when attempting to augment drug delivery to the brain. These factors have been discussed by Grieg et al. *(8)* and are summarized below:

1. Is the target on a sufficiently linear part of the dose–response curve to improve drug action by increasing drug concentration? If a maximal pharmacological response has already been achieved, improvements in drug delivery will likely be inconsequential.
2. What factor preferentially limits drug therapeutic action in the disease of interest? Specific pharmacokinetic factors such as subtherapeutic concentration, insufficient time-dependent concentration ($C \times T$, integral), or rather poor pharmacodynamics (e.g., drug insensitivity or poor selectivity to the target) can affect efficacy. In reality, however, some combination of all three of these factors limits the final efficacy of most drugs.
3. Exactly where in the CNS is the target located? Different regions of the brain have different rates of blood flow and different BBB properties (i.e., areas around the choroid plexus and pineal gland tend to have more open barriers) .
4. What is the optimal pharmacokinetic profile for maximal drug action? Understanding the mechanism of action and metabolism of the drug (i.e., active and toxic species) is crucial for understanding how best to optimize its therapeutic effectiveness.
5. What part of the drug is essential for pharmacological activity? Very often a charged moiety on a compound is essential for drug–target binding and biological activity. This knowledge may allow for the production of prodrugs that contain reversible chemical modifications that optimize transport across the BBB prior to converting to the active drug form within the brain.

4.3. Methods of Evaluating Drug Delivery to Brain Tumors and the CNS

The pharmacokinetic and pharmacodynamic properties of any new anticancer agent being developed for brain tumors are an important consideration in the clinical evaluation of the drug. Serum pharmacokinetics alone will give little information regarding what is happening with the drug within the brain and brain tumor. Such assessments require serial measurements of drug levels, directly or indirectly, in the actual region of interest. The principal experimental methods currently available to assess drug delivery to the brain include CSF sampling, brain biopsy, microdialysis, positron emission tomography (PET), and magnetic resonance spectroscopy (MRS) *(6)*.

5. INTRAVASCULAR METHODS FOR INCREASING DRUG DELIVERY ACROSS THE BBB AND BTB

5.1. High-Dose Systemic Chemotherapy

High-dose chemotherapy has been considered as a means to increase the amount of drug that crosses the BBB into the brain. Several studies of high-dose chemotherapy with autologous bone marrow transplantation or peripheral stem cell rescue for treatment of newly diagnosed or recurrent anaplastic glioma have been conducted that used high-dose (HD) BCNU, HD BCNU plus intraarterial cisplatin, or some combination of BCNU, carboplatin, etoposide, and thiotepa. Although a few durable responses have been reported, limited sample size and selection bias make it difficult to compare treatment outcomes for high-dose chemotherapy vs standard dosing regimens. It is also difficult to draw firm conclusions regarding the potential of this technique for malignant gliomas because local tumor concentrations of the drugs were not measured in any of these trials. The potential benefit of high-dose chemotherapy must also be balanced against the 5–20% reported incidences of toxic deaths and potential for delayed neurotoxicity from HD BCNU or thiotepa *(40,41)*. In general, the data over the last decade suggest that the use of high-dose chemotherapy for a tumor type that is generally chemotherapy resistant, such as most gliomas, is unwarranted. The strategy of high-dose chemotherapy followed by stem-cell rescue holds more promise for chemosensitive brain tumors such as anaplastic oligodendrogliomas, embryonal tumors (i.e., medulloblastomas), and primary CNS lymphomas.

5.2. Modification of Existing Drugs

Chemical modification of existing drugs has been a strategy utilized to increase its delivery into the brain. Examples of this approach include modifying the chemical structure of the drug to fit a transport receptor in the BBB (i.e., melphalan), linking the drug to an antibody targeted to a BBB receptor (i.e., growth factor), or making the drug more lipophilic. Synthesis of a prodrug requires that the drug be chemically modified to increase its capillary permeability. Once in the brain, the prodrug undergoes an enzymatic reaction that returns the drug to its active state and with reduced BBB permeability, thereby trapping the active drug within the brain behind the BBB. Increasingly accurate means to predict physicochemical properties of drugs, such as membrane permeability, may mean wider use of this method to develop brain tumor drugs in the future *(12)*.

5.3. Intraarterial Administration

Intraarterial injection allows the tissue (i.e., tumor) perfused by that arterial supply to receive a higher serum concentration during the first passage through the circulation than can be obtained following standard intravenous administration. In a series of studies, Fenstermacher and colleagues have evaluated the efficacy of intraarterial delivery to the brain and brain tumor *(41,42)*. They concluded that there were significant delivery advantages to intraarterial administration in the setting where the rate of tumor blood flow is very low or where the rate of systemic transformation or excretion is very high. Once past the target tissue, the pharmacokinetics of the intraarterially administered agent is the same as it is following systemic administration. The ideal intraarterially delivered drug is one that rapidly crosses the BBB or BTB and is either bound to tissue elements or locally metabolized to its active metabolites. Unfortunately, most drugs used to treat brain tumors do not have these characteristics, possibly accounting for the fact that most clinical trials of intraarterial chemotherapy in brain tumors show no improvement over systemic delivery. Furthermore, as the area supplied by the artery is never restricted solely to the tumor, but rather to normal brain as well, most studies demonstrate minimal to significant neurotoxicity from such treatment (43–45).

5.4. Hyperosmolar BBB Disruption

The BBB can be opened to water-soluble drugs and macromolecules in vivo by infusing a hypertonic solution of arabinose or mannitol into a cerebral artery followed by the intraarterial administration of a drug. The principal feature of this method, originally proposed by Rapoport (46,47), is to take advantage of the first-pass principle of intraarterial infusion with the added theoretical benefit of greater intrabrain drug delivery following transient breakdown of the BBB. Under osmotic stress, tight junctions at the cerebrovascular endothelium can be reversibly opened by osmotic stress, allowing blood-borne drugs, proteins, and other solutes into the brain (48). The parameter determining the opening threshold is the product of infusate osmolality and duration of infusion, which is essentially the quantity of water that must be removed acutely from brain (proportional to time of exposure × osmotic pressure difference across capillary × capillary hydraulic conductivity) (49,50). Acute removal of water causes cerebral vasodilatation with subsequent stretching of the vasculature, producing opening of the tight junctions. Opening of the BBB therefore involves widening of tight junctions between endothelial cells of the BBB mediated by endothelial cell shrinkage and vascular dilation associated with removal of water from the brain. In addition to endothelial cell shrinkage and vasodilatation, tight junctional opening appears to involve calcium-mediated modulation of the endothelial cytoskeleton and junctional proteins (1). Cytoskeletal modulation mediated by calcium may also contribute to BBB opening by hypertension, bradykinin, histamine, serotonin, and other inflammatory response mediators as well as trauma (12,48).

The effect of hypertonic infusion can cause an initial 10-fold increment in the "effective" capillary permeability–surface product (PA^{eff}) of small water-soluble solutes that lasts for approx 10 min following osmotic exposure. Recent evidence indicates that the duration of peak BBB opening can be extended beyond 30 min, without producing brain damage in animal studies, by pretreatment with a Na^+/Ca^{2+} channel blocker (52). The high osmotically induced increment in PA^{eff} arises not only because of increased diffusion of solute across widened interendothelial tight junctions but also because additional solute is carried by fluid (bulk) flow from blood to brain. In rat studies, the pore radius, which normally has a mean radius of 7–8 Å, increases to 200 Å following infusion of hypertonic mannitol. Iron oxide nanoparticles, with a radius of 100 Å can readily enter the brain after osmotic treatment. There have been reports that particles as large as adenoviral viral vectors (radius of 350 Å) as well as herpes simplex vectors (radius 600 Å) may also enter an osmotically disrupted BBB, although passage of such large molecules may actually represent damage or breakdown of the BBB (53).

Individual brain tumors can have significant intratumoral heterogeneity relative to vascular permeability, varying between permeabilities that approximate those found in the systemic circulation (i.e., no BBB) to those that are equal to that found in normal brain. In rat brain tumor models, osmotically induced increases in vascular permeability are greater for tumors with initially low rather than high permeabilities given that the vasculature of the high-permeablitiy tumors is already leaky. PET imaging has been used in patients with malignant astrocytomas to study the time course of BBB permeability following osmotic disruption of the BBB. The data showed that BBB permeability was increased 1000% and 60% in normal brain and in tumor, respectively. The half-time of the osmotic effect was 8.1 min in brain and 4.2 min in tumor (54). Thus, theoretical, preclinical, and clinical data suggest that osmotic-induced increments in BBB permeability are greater in intact brain than in tumor. If osmotic BBB disruption leads to an increase in normal brain tissue drug delivery over that seen in the tumor, one must again be concerned for increased neurotoxicity.

5.5. Biochemical Disruption of the BBB and BTB

Biochemical opening of the BBB is a relatively new method in which agents, mostly derivatives of normal vasoactive compounds, are pharmacologically used to open up the BBB transiently. Such agents include bradykinin, interleukin-2, leukotriene C4, histamine, and others that are administered intraarterially followed by intraarterial dosing of a chemotherapeutic agent. Biochemical-mediated opening of the BBB may have preferential effects on tumor-associated BBB and the BTB compared to normal BBB. The reasons for this are not entirely clear; however, the effect may be related to the ability of an intact BBB to naturally inactivate vasoactive compounds (55).

RMP-7 is a nine-amino-acid peptide bradykinin analogue that is selective for the bradykinin B2 receptor and has a longer plasma half-life than bradykinin itself. Initial proof of principle studies using electron microscopy demonstrated that intravenous RMP-7 increased the permeability of the BBB by disengaging the tight junctions of the endothelium that make up the BBB. Intravenous or intraarterial RMP-7 increases the uptake of many different radiolabeled tracers and chemotherapeutic agents into the tumor in a dose-related fashion (56). The increase in permeability is very rapid but transient, with the BBB being restored 2–5 min following cessation of infusion. Increased chemotherapeutic concentrations remained elevated for at least 90 min in the tumor; however, even with continuous infusion of RMP-7, spontaneous restoration of the BBB occurred in 10–20 min. Nine malignant glioma patients evaluated with clinical PET studies were shown to have increased permeability of malignant gliomas to ^{68}Ga-EDTA after intracarotid infusion of RMP-7. Increased transport into tumor regions was increased an average of 46% whereas permeability in normal tissue regions was not significantly increased (57).

Initial adult Phase I clinical trials evaluating RMP-7 with carboplatin reported only transient side effects including flushing, nausea, headache, and mild increase in heart rate (58). A pediatric Phase I clinical trial of RMP-7 and carboplatin in children also reported only reversible side effects including hypotension, flushing, headache, and gastrointestinal complaints and one episode of seizure during drug infusion at the highest dose level (59). A Phase II study of RMP-7 and carboplatin in the treatment of recurrent high-grade glioma reported a 79% response rate (stable, partial, or complete response) in the chemotherapy-naive group and 24% response for previous chemotherapy treated patients by radiological evaluation. The median duration of response was 30.3 wk in the chemotherapy-naive group and 19.6 wk in the previous chemotherapy treated group (60). Despite these somewhat positive findings, a multiinstitutional, randomized, placebo-controlled Phase II trial of carboplatin with or without RMP-7 for adults with recurrent high-grade gliomas did not reveal a significant difference between treatment arms.

5.6. Receptor-Mediated Transport

The kinetics of receptor-mediated drug transport are significantly different from the kinetics of simple diffusion. This can be characterized by the Michaelis–Menten constants, K_m (the concentration at which the reaction velocity is half-maximal) and V_{max} (the limiting velocity as the concentration approaches infinity). One strategic approach to increase the transport of certain molecules into the brain is to modify drugs such that they can utilize one of these endogenous transport systems localized to the brain capillary endothelial membrane. Most of the available transport receptors are thought to be low-affinity, low-capacity systems, such as those for nucleosides, various peptides, transferring, and insulin *(12)*. Thus, an important factor to consider in this drug delivery strategy is the plasma concentration and binding affinity of the native substrate for the receptor compared to that of the modified drug of interest (i.e., phenylalanine vs melphalan).

There are three major classes of endogenous transport systems within the BBB that potentially could be exploited for drug delivery: (1) carrier-mediated transport systems (e.g., glucose and amino acid carriers), (2) active efflux transporters (e.g., Pgp), and (3) receptor-mediated transcytosis systems. Whereas the carrier-mediated transport and active efflux transporters are portals of entry or egress for small molecules, the receptor-mediated transcytosis system naturally transports larger molecules such as peptides *(61)*. The chimeric peptide strategy couples therapeutic but nontransportable peptides or proteins to a BBB drug transport vector *(62)*. Transport vectors are proteins such as cationized albumin or the OX26 monoclonal antibody to the transferrin receptor that will undergo absorptive-mediated and receptor-mediated transcytosis through the BBB, respectively. In addition to vector construction, the development of mechanisms to couple drugs directly to the vector with high efficiency and with effective cleavable linkers is an important developmental component for this delivery strategy. Although there are a number of recent papers describing the successful use of this strategy in various preclinical models, to date there have been no clinical trials utilizing chimeric peptide to traverse the BBB.

A number of novel methods of intravascular drug delivery are being developed and may ultimately be applied toward brain tumors. Theses methods include biodegradable nanoparticles, liposomes, magnetic microspheres, and monoglyceride-based systems *(12)*.

6. NEWER METHODS FOR BYPASSING THE BBB AND BTB

There is a growing interest in the direct administration of drugs into the brain, thereby bypassing the problem of the BBB. One or more of four forces will affect drug movement within the brain depending on the particular mode of drug administration: (1) bulk flow of CSF, (2) bulk flow of brain interstitial fluid, (3) bulk flow due to the infusion of a solution into the brain or CSF, and (4) diffusion. Drug movement will also be variably affected by the amount of white matter in the target area as it moves from the highly tortuous environment of gray matter structure (isotropic) to the highly oriented fiber pathways of white matter (anisotropic) *(12)*.

The potential benefits of direct drug injection into the CNS include bypassing the BBB, delivery of 100% of the dose to the target site, maintenance of elevated drug concentration into target tissue, and minimized systemic drug exposure and systemic toxicity. There are, however, major limitations to this general method of drug delivery including: invasiveness, unpredictable drug distribution, and neurotoxicity *(13)*.

6.1. Intrathecal and Intraventricular Drug Administration

Intrathecal drug administration refers to injection of the drug into the lumbar subarachnoid space and *intraventricular* administration refers to injection or infusion into the lateral ventricle. In humans, the normal volume of CSF produced is between 400 and 500 mL per day. Since the volume of CSF within CNS is about 150 mL, there is considerable bulk flow within the system and significant variability in the velocity of CSF flow from region to region. As a result of these bulk flow pathways, materials injected into the CSF will attain initial concentrations that are directly proportional to the concentration in the infusate. Historically, all drugs directly injected into the CSF had to be administered through an intrathecal injection. With the advent of the Ommaya reservoir (and now other similar reservoir systems) drugs can be efficiently and safely injected directly into the lateral ven-

tricle through a permanently indwelling intraventricular catheter that connects to a subcutaneous reservoir that can be easily accessed by a small-gauge needle. Studies have shown
that intraventricularly administered drugs result in a more homogeneous concentration and
distribution of the drug than does intrathecal injections where much of the drug often settles
to the lower part of the thecal sac. The intra-CSF route of administration is ideal for situations
in which the target is within the subarachnoid space or close to the CSF–brain interface such
as in the prevention and treatment of leptomeningeal seeding of malignant tumors. However,
the capacity of drugs to enter the brain extracellular space from the CSF is limited. There
have been a number of studies that have shown that entry into the brain is diffusional and that
concentrations decline exponentially from the brain surface, making this route of administration both impractical and inefficient for intraparenchymal targets (i.e., primary brain
tumors) (66,67).

6.2. Intratumoral and Intracavitary Injection

The distribution of drug following intratumoral and intracavitary injection is determined
by the rate and duration of the injection as well as tissue bulk flow pathways and diffusion.
This method has been used clinically for the purpose of delivering both drugs and large
molecules such as viral vectors (68). Unfortunately, distribution of these agents following
direct intratumor injection tends to be quite limited and the direction of distribution is
unpredictable.

6.3. Biodegradable Polymers

The concept of implantable polymers able to release chemotherapeutic agents directly
into the CNS was first described by Langer and Folkman (69). They reported the sustained
and predictable release of macromolecules from a nonbiodegradable ethylene vinyl acetate
(EVAc) copolymer. A drug incorporated into this polymer was released by means of diffusion through the micropores of its matrix. The EVAc polymer has found application in
various clinical settings (e.g., glaucoma, contraceptive devices) as well as application in the
treatment of gliomas (70). This polymer delivery system was limited by its permanence at
the site of implantation in the body, although these polymers have now been replaced with
biodegradable polymer systems.

The polyanhydride poly(bis[p-carboxyphenoxy] propane sebacic acid) (PCPP-SA)
matrix is one such biodegradable polymer that will break down to dicarboxylic acids by
spontaneous reaction with water. The spectrum of drugs that can be released has been
broadened by newer biodegradable polymers such as the fatty acid dimer–sebacic acid
(FAD-SA) copolymer, which allows the incorporation of more hydrophilic agents or
hydrolytically unstable compounds (e.g., methotrexate and carboplatin). Another system
is a poly(lactide-coglycolide) polymer that can be formed into microspheres and stereo-
tactically injected into the brain. When covalently linked to a polyethylene glycol coating,
this polymer matrix has also been shown to reduce opsonization and elimination by the
immune system. Others systems include polyethylene-coated liposomes that encapsulate
anthracyclines, and gelatin-chondroitin sulfate-coated microspheres, which have been
used to release cytokines in vivo (71–73).

The main strategy behind polymer-mediated drug delivery is that multiple drug-impreg-
nated polymers can be implanted into the brain, allowing for local distribution of the drug
at high concentration by diffusion, with variable contribution from the inherent bulk flow
pathways of the brain. One of the principal advantages of polymer-mediated drug delivery
is the minimization of systemic drug exposure. The advantage of biodegradable polymers
vs nonbiodegradable polymers are that the biodegradable polymer can be made to release

drug at a nearly constant rate and the breakdown rate can be altered by changing the ratio of the polymer components (from 3 wk to 3 yr for complete degradation in the PCPP-SA matrix) *(5)*.

The main limiting feature of this method of drug delivery is that drug distribution occurs mainly by diffusion, whereby drug concentrations fall away exponentially from the point of administration. For most drugs, experimental evidence has demonstrated that this diffusion results in a distribution of drug limited to a few millimeters of tissue. Most patients with gliomas have infiltrating tumors cells at a distant of many centimeters away from the primary tumor site, making the ultimate utility of a diffusion-based delivery system suspect. Wang et al. used a surgical model to predict that implantation of BCNU-impregnated polymers after resection of 80% of the tumor would be more effective than direct wafer implantation without surgical resection *(74,75)*. In vivo primate studies showed that BCNU-impregnated polymers were able to release clinically significant levels of BCNU (0.1–7.5 μM) 1–2 cm from the polymer implant up to 30 d after polymer implantation, although other studies in rodent demonstrated a much smaller area of distribution *(74)*.

Phase I and II clinical trials were conducted to evaluate different variations of BCNU loaded in PCPP-SA polymers in 21 patients with recurrent malignant gliomas. Previously surgically resected patients were implanted with eight BCNU-loaded polymers into the tumor cavity. The treatment was well tolerated and no patient experienced any local or systemic toxicity. The 3.85% BCNU-loaded polymers were chosen for further clinical study *(76)*. A Phase III prospective, randomized, double-blind, placebo-controlled clinical trial of PCPP-SA polymer with 3.8% BCNU was conducted with 222 patients with recurrent malignant glioma who have failed standard therapy and needed reoperation at 27 medical centers in the United States and Canada *(77)*. Whereas the BCNU polymer-treated group had a median survival of 31 wk, the median survival of the control group was 23 wk, which was statistically significant ($p = 0.005$). In the glioblastoma multiforme group, patients treated with the BCNU polymers had a 50% greater survival at 6 mo compared to patients treated with placebo alone ($p = 0.02$). In 1996, the US Food and Drug Administration approved BCNU biodegradable polymers (Gliadel, Aventis Pharmaceutical) as safe and effective in the treatment of recurrent gliomas, the first FDA-approved new treatment against malignant brain tumors in 23 yr *(5)*. Nevertheless, the fact that they can be used only in patients capable of undergoing an extensive surgical debulking, the marginal benefit for those treated, and the significant expense of the Gliadel Wafers have limited their use.

A variety of other drugs have been incorporated into the polymer matrix such as taxol (a microtubule binding agent) and camptothecin (an inhibitor of DNA-replicating enzyme topoisomerase I), and clinical trials involving brain tumors are planned. Other chemotherapeutic agents, including carboplatin, 4-HC, methotrexate, 5-fluorouracil (5-FU), and adriamycin, have demonstrated potent local activity against intracranial tumors *(78–81)*.

6.4. Convection-Enhanced Delivery (CED)

Under normal physiologic conditions, brain interstitial fluid moves by both convection and diffusion. Unlike diffusion, convection is affected by a pressure gradient that produces a fluid bulk flow and is independent of the molecular weight of the infusate. The distribution of the infused drug is highly dependent on whether the drug is infused into a homogeneous gray matter structure or a structure containing fiber pathways. In a homogeneous brain tissue, the infusion will produce a spherical volume in which the concentration of the drug is directly proportional to that of the infusate. The infusion reaches equilibrium when the amount of drug leaving across brain capillaries is equal to the amount being infused.

At this point the drug begins to diffuse away from the edge of the sphere at concentrations that decline exponentially by diffusion. If the infusion encounters an organized white matter pathway, the rate of movement is either increased or decreased depending on the direction of the inherent bulk flow within the pathway (12). Thus, CED allows for the homogeneous targeted delivery of high concentrations of macromolecules with a volume of distribution that is linearly proportional to the volume of infusion. CED is best suited for delivery of large compounds with low efflux rates. In contrast to intravascularly administered drugs, in which increased capillary permeability results in increased tissue concentrations, increased efflux across permeable tumor capillaries will reduce both the extracellular drug concentration and volume of distribution following CED (74).

An important feature of CED is that distribution of the drug is determined by the infusion parameters (i.e., rate, volume) and the physical/chemical properties of the drug being infused, whereas the concentration of drug in the infusate has no effect on distribution. Although one of the primary advantages of CED is that the concentration of the infused molecule is generally homogeneous within the central volume of infusion, there will be variability at the edge of the convection boundary where diffusion is occurring. Concentrations of the infused molecules are 50–100 times lower in the diffusional boundary than in the central infused volume (12). Oldfield and co-workers have studied the factors that influence the optimization of CED in various preclinical models. They evaluated the effect of infusion rate, cannula size, concentration of the infusion, and preinfusion sealing time on convection delivery by using quantitative autoradiography of ^{14}C-labeled albumin. They found that the rate of infusion and cannula size significantly affected the convection distribution of the molecules. The infusion rate determined the volume of the infusate, and larger cannulae sizes were associated with back flow of the infusate along the catheter track at higher infusion rates, as increases in diameter facilitate the formation of a low-resistance pathway along the surface of the catheter (82).

For convection-enhanced delivery to be effective in the clinical treatment of brain tumors, a high drug concentration must be maintained in the brain or brain tumor tissue for extended periods of time. Groothius compared the delivery of $[^{14}C]$sucrose to rat brain by bolus intravenous, chronic intraventricular, and chronic convection-enhanced cerebral infusion (from 1 h to 7 d) using quantitative autoradiography. Intraventricular administration produced sucrose concentrations that decreased exponentially with distance away from the ventricular wall. Chronic convection-enhanced delivery resulted in focal concentrations of sucrose up to 10,000 times higher than those concentrations in the intravenous group (83). By using convection to supplement simple diffusion, enhanced distribution of large and small molecules can be obtained in the brain while achieving drug concentrations orders of magnitude greater than systemic levels.

Convection-enhanced delivery has been used to ablate the globus pallidus internus selectively by administration of an excitotoxin, quinolinic acid, in a primate model of Parkinson's disease. Safe lesioning of neuronal subpopulations by this methodology resulted in dramatic improvement in Parkinsonian symptoms in nonhuman primates (84). Oldfield et al. recently reported the use of convection to deliver an immunotoxin in patients with recurrent high-grade gliomas. The convection infusions were generally well tolerated and a number of radiographic responses were documented, suggesting that the immunotoxin was successfully convected at a distance away from the site of infusion (85). Thus, CED represents a very promising strategy for delivering both small and large therapeutic agents, particularly those that are normally impermeable across the BBB. Nevertheless, much work remains to be done to determine the specific CED parameters that are necessary for optimizing the delivery of agents into the white and gray mater of brains with infiltrating tumor.

7. CNS TUMOR CHEMOTHERAPY AND DRUG INTERACTIONS

7.1. Anticonvulsants

Anticonvulsants drugs are commonly prescribed for brain tumor patients and can often have significant pharmacokinetic interactions with other concurrently administered agents such as chemotherapeutic drugs. Although it has been know for many years that anticonvulsants agents such as phenytoin, phenobarbital, and carbamazepine induce hepatic cytochrome P450 (P450 or CYP) isoenzymes, it was not until a lower than expected frequency of toxicity was seen in brain tumor patients who were being treated on a Phase I/II study of paclitaxel that investigators began to appreciate the importance of these drug interactions. It has subsequently been demonstrated that enzyme-inducing antiepileptic drugs (EIAED) alter the P450-mediated metabolism of paclitaxel resulting in significantly (2–3 times) lower plasma steady-state concentrations of the drug compared to patients not on EIAEDs *(86)*. Other studies have demonstrated lower than expected plasma concentrations of additional anticancer agents, including 9-aminocampothecin, vincristine, teniposide, and irinotecan in association with EIAEDs *(87–90)*. Recognition of these interactions have resulted in the adoption of brain tumor-specific Phase I pharmacokinetic trials of new chemotherapeutic agents that involve independent dose-escalation arms for patients who are, and those who are not, undergoing chronic treatment with EIAEDs *(6)*.

Practice parameters, based on a meta-analysis of 12 studies, for the use of anticonvulsant prophylaxis in patients with newly diagnosed brain tumors were recently published. The authors found that anticonvulsant medications were not effective at preventing first seizures in patients with newly diagnosed brain tumors and recommend that prophylactic anticonvulsants should not be used routinely in this patient population. They also recommend tapering and discontinuing anticonvulsants after the first postoperative week in brain tumor patients who have not had seizures *(91)*.

7.2. Glucocorticoids

Glucocorticoids are commonly used to treat cerebral edema and the symptoms associated with increased intracranial pressure associated with brain tumors. Some investigators have suggested that because glucocorticoids may play a role in restoration of the normal physiological properties of the BBB, concurrent administration of chemotherapy with glucocorticoids may decrease the amount of drug that passes through the BBB into the brain tumor. Animal experiments have shown that pretreatment with dexamethasone decreases cisplatin concentration in normal tissue adjacent to the tumor. Dexamethasone, however, does not decrease the concentration of topotecan or cisplatin in brain tumor or normal brain tissue *(92,93)*. It is known that glucocorticoids can induce components of the cytochrome P450 enzyme system as well. Preclinical studies have shown that the metabolism of paclitaxel, cyclophosphamide, and ifosfamide is increased by dexamethasone pretreatment in rodents *(6)*. The clinical implications of these interactions are uncertain at this point but further studies are proposed given the highly prevalent use of glucocorticoids in patients with brain tumors.

8. CONCLUSIONS

The treatment of tumors of the CNS with drugs is complicated not only by the usual issues related to the systemic pharmacology, but also by the very specific pharmacological/pharmacokinetic issues related to the CNS. As a separate body compartment, encased by a physiological barrier that is relatively impermeable to most intravascular agents, and surrounded by a constantly replenishing fluid stream, the CNS has a very complex and dynamic pharmacodynamic profile of its own. Currently the relative ineffectiveness of most chemo-therapeutic agents against primary brain tumors is more a function of both intrinsic and acquired drug resistance. Nevertheless, as new targeted and rational therapeutic agents are developed over the next decade, impaired and inefficient drug delivery to intracerebral neoplasms may become the limiting factor to effective treatment. If we do not begin to understand better the pharmacodynamic principles that govern drug entry and distribution within the CNS, and devise better ways to deliver these agents to the CNS, most patient with primary brain tumors will still die of their tumors. Furthermore, as these new therapeutic agents are utilized to treat systemic tumors we will see a significant increase in the number of patients who ultimately succumb to metastatic disease within the CNS unless but we can devise improved strategies to delivery these new agents to the CNS where micrometastatic disease often exists.

REFERENCES

1. Madajewicz S, Chowhan N, Tfayli A, et al. Therapy for patients with high grade astrocytoma using intraarterial chemotherapy and radiation therapy. Cancer 2000; 88:2350–2356.
2. Olivi A, DiMeco F, Bohan E, Brem H. Developing new methods for the treatment of malignant brain tumours: local delivery of anti-neoplastic agents using biodegradable polymers. Trends Exp Clin Med 2000; 10:152–163.
3. Davis FG, McCarthy BJ. Epidemiology of brain tumors. Curr Opin Neurol 2000; 13:635–640.
4. Fine HA, Dear KBG, Loeffler JS, Black P, Canellos GP. Meta-analysis of radiation therapy with and without adjuvant chemotherapy for malignant gliomas in adults. Cancer 1993; 71:2585–2597.
5. Lesniak MS, Langer R, Brem H. Drug delivery to tumors of the central nervous system. Curr Neurol Neurosci Rep 2001; 1:210–216.
6. Ciordia R, Supko J, Gatineau M, Batchelor T. Cytotoxic chemotherapy: advances in delivery, pharma-cology, and testing. Curr Oncol Rep 2000; 2:445–453.
7. Terasaki T, Pardridge WM. Preface: Targeted drug delivery to the brain. J Drug Target 2000; 8:353–355.
8. Greig NH, Yu QS, Utsuki T, et al. Optimizing drugs for brain action. In: Kobiler D, Lustig DS, Shapira S (eds). Blood–Brain Barrier. New York, NY: Kluwer Academic/Plenum, 2001.
9. Huber JD, Egleton RD, Davis TP. Molecular physiology and pathophysiology of tight junctions in the blood–brain barrier. Trends Neurosci 2001; 24719–725.
10. Bart J, Groen HJM, Hendrikse NH, van der Graaf WTA, Vaalburg W, de Vries EGE. The blood–brain barrier and oncology: new insights into function and modulation. Cancer Treat Rev 2000; 26:449–462.
11. Smith QR, Fisher C, Allen DD. The role of plasma protein binding in drug delivery to brain. In: Kobiler D, Lustig DS, Shapira S (eds). Blood–Brain Barrier. New York, NY: Kluwer Academic/Plenum, 2001.
12. Groothuis DR. The blood–brain and blood–tumor barriers: a review of strategies for increasing drug delivery. J Neurooncol 2000; 2:45–59.
13. Siegal T. Strategies for increasing drug delivery to the brain. In: Kobiler D, Lustig DS, Shapira S (eds). Blood–Brain Barrier. New York: Kluwer Academic/Plenum, 2001.
14. Schlageter KE, Molnar P, Lapin GD, Groothius DR. Microvessel organization and structure in experi-mental brain tumors: microvessel populations with distinctive structural and functional properties. Microvasc Res 1999; 58:312–328.
15. Regina A, Demeule M, Laplante A, et al. Multidrug resistance in brain tumors: roles of the blood–brain barrier. Cancer Metastasis Rev 2001; 20:13–25.
16. Bredel M, Zentner J. Brain–tumor drug resistance: the bare essentials. Lancet Oncology 2002; 3:397–406.
17. Henson JW, Cordon-Cardo C, Posner JB. P-Glycoprotein expression in brain tumors. J Neurooncol 1992; 14:37–43.
18. Korshunov A, Golanov A, Sycheva R. Prognostic value of the immunoexpression of chemoresistance-related proteins in cerebral glioblastomas: an analysis of 168 cases. Neuropathology 1999; 19:143–149.
19. Toth K, Vaughn MM, Peress NS. MDR1 P-glycoprotein is expressed by endothelial cells of the neovasculature in central nervous system tumors. Brain Tumor Pathol 1999;16:23–27.
20. Friedman HS, Colvin OM, Kaufmann SH. Cyclophosphamide resistance in medulloblastoma. Cancer Res 1992; 52:5373–5378.

21. Kudo H, Mio T, Kokunoai T. Quantitative analysis of glutathione in human brain tumors. J Neurosurg 1990; 72:610–615.
22. Lo HW, Ali-Osman F. Genomic cloning of hGSTP1*C, an allelic Pi class glutathione S-transferase gene variant and functional characterization of its retinoic acid response elements. J Biol Chem 1997; 272:32,743–32,749.
23. Lida M, Asamoto S, Sugiyama H. Effects of glutathione-modulating compounds on platinum compounds-induced cytotoxicity in human glioma cells. Anticancer Res 1999; 19:5383–5384.
24. Hongeng S, Brent TP, Sanford PA. O^6-Methylguanine-DNA methyltransferase protein levels in pediatric brain tumors. Clin Cancer Res 1997; 3:2459–2463.
25. Silber JR, Bobola MS, Ghatan S. O^6-Methylguanine-DNA methyltransferase activity in adult gliomas: relation to patient and tumor characteristics. Cancer Res 1998; 58:1068–1073.
26. Tomlinson FH, Lihou MG, Smith PJ. Comparison of in vitro activity of epipodophyllotoxins with other chemotherapeutic agents in human medulloblastomas. Br J Cancer 1991; 64:1051–1059.
27. Bredel M, Slavc I, Birner P. Topoisomerase IIα expression in optic pathway gliomas of childhood. Eur J Cancer 2002; 38:393–400.
28. Bredel M, Gatterbauer B, Birner P, et al. Expression of DNA topoisomerase IIα in oligodendroglioma. Anticancer Res 2002; 22:1301–1304.
29. Greig NH. Drug entry into the brain and its pharmacologic manipulation. In: Bradbury MWB (ed). Physiology and Pharmacology of the Blood–Brain Barrier, Handbook of Experimental Pharmacology, Vol. 103. Berlin, Germany: Springer-Verlag, 1992, pp. 489–523.
30. Pardridge WM. Blood–brain barrier biology and methodology. J Neurovirol 1999; 5:556–569.
31. Habgood MD, Begley DJ, Abbott NJ. Determinants of passive drug entry into the central nervous system. Cell Mol Neurobiol 2000; 20:231–253.
32. Greig NH. Drug delivery to the brain by blood–brain barrier and its modification. In: Neuwelt EA (ed). Implications of the Blood–Brain Barrier and Its Modification, Vol. 1. New York, NY: Plenum Press, 1989, pp. 311–367.
33. Levin VA. Relation of octanol/water partition and molecular weight to rat brain capillary permeability. J Med Chem 1980; 23:682–684.
34. Hardebo JE, Owman C. Enzymatic barrier mechanisms for neurotransmitter monoamines and their precursors at the blood–brain barrier. In: Johansson BB, Owman C, Widner H (eds). Pathophysiology of the Blood–Brain Barrier. Amsterdam, The Netherlands: Elsevier, 1991, pp. 71–82.
35. Fenstermacher JD, Gross P, Sposito N, Acuff V, Petersen S, Gruber K. Structural and functional variations in capillary systems within the brain. Ann NY Acad Sci 1988; 529:21–30.
36. Fenstermacher JD. The blood–brain barrier is not a barrier for many drugs. NIDA Res Monogr 1992; 120:108–120.
37. Abraham MH. Scales of solute hydrogen bonding: their construction and application to physicochemical and biochemical processes. Chem Soc Rev 1993; 22:73–83.
38. Abraham MH, Chadha HS. Applications of solvation equations to drug transport properties. In: Pliska V, Testa B, Van de Waterbeem E (eds). Lipophilicity in Drug Action and Toxicity. Weinheim, Germany: VCH, 1996, pp. 311–337.
39. Dropcho EJ. Novel chemotherapeutic approaches to brain tumors. Hematol/Oncol Clin North Am 2001; 15:1027–1052.
40. Fine HA, Antman KH. High-dose chemotherapy with autologous bone marrow transplantation in the treatment of high grade astrocytomas in adults: therapeutic rationale and clinical experience. Bone Marrow Transplant 1992; 10:315–321.
41. Fenstermacher J, Gazendam J. Intra-arterial infusions of drugs and hyperosmotic solutions as ways of enhancing CNS chemotherapy. Cancer Treat Rep 1981; 65(Suppl 2):27–37.
42. Fenstermacher JD, Cowles AL. Theoretic limitations of intracarotid infusions in brain tumor chemotherapy. Cancer Treat Rep 1977; 61:519–526.
43. Arafat T, Hentschel P, Madajewicz S, et al. Toxicities related to intraarterial infusion of cisplatin and etoposide in patients with brain tumors. J Neurooncol 1999; 42:73–77.
44. Dropcho EJ, Rosenfeld SS, Vitek J, Guthrie BL, Morawetz RB. Phase II study of intracarotid or selective intracerebral infusion of cisplatin for treatment of recurrent anaplastic gliomas. J Neurooncol 1998; 36:191–198.
45. Hirano Y, Mineura K, Mizoi K, Tomura N. Therapeutic results of intraarterial chemotherapy in patients with malignant glioma. Int J Oncol 1998; 13:537–542.
46. Rapoport SJ, Thompson HK. Osmotic opening of the blood–brain barrier in the monkey without associated neurological deficits. Science 1973; 180:971.

47. Kroll RA, Neuwelt EA. Outwitting the blood–brain barrier for therapeutic purposes: Osmotic opening and other means. Neurosurgery 1998; 42:1083–1100.
48. Doolittle ND, Miner ME, Hall WA, et al. Safety and efficacy of a multicenter study using intraarterial chemotherapy in conjunction with osmotic opening of the blood-brain barrier for the treatment of patients with malignant brain tumors. Cancer 2000; 88:637–647.
49. Rapoport SI. Mathematical model for brain edema. J Theoret Biol 1978; 74:439–467.
50. Rapoport SI. A model for brain edema. In: Inaba Y, Klatzo I, Spatz M (eds). Brain Edema: Proceedings of the Sixth International Symposium. Berlin, Germany: Springer-Verlag, 1985, pp. 59–71.
51. Rapoport SI. Osmotic opening of the blood–brain barrier: principles, mechanism and therapeutic applications. Cell Mol Neurobiol 2000; 20:217–230.
52. Bhattacharjee AK, Nagashima T, Kondoh T, Tamaki N. The effects of the Na^+/Ca^{++} exchange blocker on osmotic blood–brain barrier disruption. Brain Res 2001; 900:157–162.
53. Muldoon LL, Nilaver G, Kroll RA. Comparison of intracerebral inoculation and osmotic blood–brain barrier disruption for delivery of adenovirus, herpes virus, and iron oxide particles to normal rat brain. Am J Pathol 1995; 147:1840–1851.
54. Zunkeler B, Carson RE, Olson J, et al. Quantification and pharmacokinetics of blood–brain barrier disruption in humans. J Neurosurg 1996; 85:1056–1065.
55. Cloughesy TF, Black KL. Pharmacological blood–brain barrier modification for selective drug delivery. J Neurooncol 1995; 26:125–32.
56. Emerich DF, Dean RL, Osborn C, Bartus RT. The development of the bradykinin agonist labradimil as a means to increase the permeability of the blood–brain barrier: from concept to clinical evaluation. Clin Pharmacokinet 2001; 40:105–123.
57. Black KL, Cloughesy T, Huang SC, et al. Intracarotid infusion of RMP-7, a bradykinin analog, and transport of gallium-68 ethylenediamine tetraacetic acid into human gliomas. J Neurosurg 1997; 86: 603–609.
58. Ford J, Osborn C, Barton J, Bleenhen NM. A Phase I study of intravenous RMP-7 with carboplatin in patients with progression of malignant glioma. Eur J Cancer 1998; 34:1807–1811.
59. Warren KE, Patel MC, Aikin AA, et al. Phase I trial of lobradimil (RMP-7) and carboplatin in children with brain tumors. Cancer Chemother Pharmacol 2001; 48:275–282.
60. Gergor A, Lind M, Newman H, et al. Phase II studies of RMP-7 and carboplatin in the treatment of recurrent high grade glioma. RMP-7 European Study Group. J Neurooncol 1999; 44:137–145.
61. Pardridge WM. Targeting neurotherapeutic agents through the blood-brain barrier. Arch Neurol 2002; 59:35–40.
62. Pardridge WM. Brain Drug Targeting: The Future of Brain Drug Development. Cambridge, UK: Cambridge University Press, 2001, pp. 1–353.
63. Li JY, Sugimura K, Boado RJ. Genetically engineered brain drug delivery vectors: cloning, expression, and in vivo application of an anti-transferrin receptor single chain antibody–streptavidin fusion gene and protein. Protein Engin 1999; 12:787–796.
64. Penichet ML, Kang Y-S, Pardridge WM, Morrison SL, Shin S-U. An anti-transferrin receptor antibody–avidin fusion protein serves as a delivery vehicle for effective brain targeting in an animal model: initial applications in antisense drug delivery to the brain. J Immunol 1999; 163:4421–4426.
65. Lee HJ, Engelhardt B, Lesley L, Bickel U, Pardridge WM. Targeting rat anti-mouse transferring receptor monoclonal antibodies through the blood-brain barrier in the mouse. J Pharmacol Exper Ther 2000; 292:1048–1052.
66. Blasberg RG. Methotrexate, cytosine arabinoside, and BCNU concentration in brain after ventriculocisternal perfusion. Cancer Treat Rep 1977; 61:625–631.
67. Groothuis DR, Levy RM. The entry of antiviral and antiretroviral drugs into the central nervous system. J Neurovirol 1997; 3:387–400.
68. Tomita T. Interstitial chemotherapy for brain tumors: review. J Neurooncol 1991; 10:57–74.
69. Langer R, Folkman J. Polymers for the sustained release of proteins and other macromolecules. Nature 1976; 263:797–800.
70. Tamargo RJ, Myseros JS, Epstein JI. Interstitial chemotherapy of the 9L gliosarcoma: controlled release polymers for drug delivery in the brain. Cancer Res 1993; 53:329–333.
71. Leong KW, Brott BC, Langer R. Bioerodible polyanhydrides as drug-carrier matrices. I. Characterization, degradation, and release characteristics. J Biomed Mater Res 1985; 19:941–955.
72. Chasin M. Polyanhydrides as drug delivery systems. In: Chasin M, Langer R (eds). Biodegradable Polymers as Drug Delivery Systems. New York, NY: Marcel Dekker, 1990, pp. 43–70.

73. Leong KW, D'Amore PD, Marletta M, Langer R. Bioerodible polyanhydrides as drug-carrier matrices. II. Biocompatibility and chemical reactivity. J Biomed Mater Res 1986; 20:51–64.
74. Haroun RI, Brem H. Local drug delivery. Curr Opin Oncol 2000; 12:187–193.
75. Wang C, Li J, Teo CS, Lee T. The delivery of BCNU to brain tumors. J Control Rel 1999; 61:21–41.
76. Brem H, Mahaley MS Jr, Vick NA, et al. Interstitial chemotherapy with drug polymer implants for the treatment of recurrent gliomas. J Neurosurg 1991; 74:441–446.
77. Brem H, Piantadosi S, Burger PC, et al. Placebo-controlled trial of safety and efficacy of intraoperative controlled delivery of biodegradable polymers of chemotherapy for recurrent gliomas. Lancet 1995; 345:1008–1012.
78. Dang W, Colvin OM, Brem H, Saltzman WM. Covalent coupling of methotrexate to dextran enhances the penetrations of cytotoxicity into tissue-like matrix. Cancer Res 1994; 54:1729–1735.
79. Judy K, Olivi A, Buahin KG, et al. Effectiveness of controlled release of a cyclophosphamide derivative with polymers against rat glioma. J Neurosurg 1995; 82:481–486.
80. Menei P, Boisdron-Celle M, Croue A, et al. Effect of stereotactic implantation of biodegradable 5-fluorouracil-loaded microspheres into healthy and C6 glioma-bearing rats. Neurosurgery 1996; 39:117–124.
81. Olivi A, Gilbert M, Duncan KL, et al. Direct delivery of platinum-based antineoplastics to the central nervous system: a toxicity and ultrastructural study. Cancer Chemother Pharmacol 1993; 31:449–454.
82. Chen MY, Lonser RR, Morrison PF, Governale LS, Oldfield EH. Variables affecting convection-enhanced delivery to the striatum: a systemic examination of rate of infusion, cannula size, infusate concentration, and tissue-cannula sealing time. J Neurosurg 1999; 90:315–320.
83. Bobo RH, Laske DW, Akbasak A, Morrison PF, Dedrick RL, Oldfield EH. Convection-enhanced delivery of macromolecules in the brain. Proc Natl Acad Sci USA 1994; 91:2076–2080.
84. Lonser RR, Corthesy ME, Morrison PF, Gogate N, Oldfield EH. Convection-enhanced selective excitotoxic ablation of the neurons of the globus pallidus internus for treatment of parkinsonism in nonhuman primates. J Neurosurg 1999; 91:294–302.
85. Pace JR, Lonser RR, Kirby RD, Jeffries N, Rogawski MA, Oldfield EH. Epileptiform activity extinguished by amygdala infusion of the neurotoxin ibotenate in a rat model of temporal lobe epilepsy. J Neurosurg 2002; 97:450–454.
86. Fetell MR, Grossman SA, Fisher JD, et al. Preirradiation paclitaxel in glioblastoma multiforme: efficacy, pharmacology, and drug interactions. New Approaches to Brain Tumor Therapy Central Nervous System Consortium. J Clin Oncol 1997; 15:3121–3128.
87. Grossman SA, Hochberg F, Fisher J, et al. Increased 9-aminocamptothecin dose requirements in patients on anticonvulsants. Cancer Chemother Pharmacol 1998; 42:118–126.
88. Villikka K, Kivisto KT, Maenpaa H, et al. Cytochrome P450-inducing antiepileptics increase the clearance of vincristine in patients with brain tumors. Clin Pharmacol Ther 1999; 66:589–593.
89. Baker DK, Relling MV, Pui CH, et al. Increased teniposide clearance with concomitant anticonvulsant therapy. J Clin Oncol 1992; 10:311–315.
90. Friedman HS, Petros WP, Friedman AH, et al. Irinotecan therapy in adults with recurrent or progressive malignant glioma. J Clin Oncol 1999; 17:1516–1525.
91. Glantz MJ, Cole BF, Forsyth PA, et al. Practice parameter: anticonvulsant prophylaxis in patients with newly diagnosed brain tumors. Neurology 2000; 54:1886–1893.
92. Straathof CSM, van den Bent MJ, Ma J, et al. The effect of dexamethasone on the uptake of cisplatin in 9L glioma and the area of brain around tumor. J Neurooncol 1998; 37:1–8.
93. Straathof CSM, van den Bent, Loos WJ, et al. The accumulation of topotecan in 9L glioma and in the brain parenchyma with and without dexamethasone administration. J Neurooncol 1999; 42:117–122.

24 Pharmacokinetics of Anticancer Drugs in Children

Lisa C. Iacono, Pharm D, P. Kellie Turner, Pharm D, and Clinton F. Stewart, Pharm D,

Contents

1. INTRODUCTION

Several comprehensive reviews of the disposition of anticancer drugs in children with cancer have been published *(1–7)*. However, recent advances in cellular and molecular biology techniques have led to the design and analysis of clinical pharmacology studies, which have increased our understanding of the age-related changes that govern drug disposition: absorption, distribution, metabolism, and elimination. Moreover, recent studies have characterized the disposition of new anticancer drugs in children, as well as contributed new insights into the use of currently available anticancer drugs. Thus, an update on pediatric pharmacokinetics of anticancer drugs in children is warranted.

In the past the US Food and Drug Administration (FDA) used data from adult clinical trials when making decisions about approval of a drug for pediatric use. However, in April 1999, the FDA instituted a rule mandating the conduct of clinical trials of new drugs or biologics intended for use in children *(8)*. The rule also mandates studies of drugs or biologics already approved by the FDA and used in a substantial number of pediatric patients for which insufficient labeling could pose significant risks. In addition, the rule mandates studies in children if an approved drug would provide meaningful therapeutic benefit over existing treatments for children, and the absence of adequate labeling could pose significant risks to children. Before 1999, the FDA required studies of drugs in children only if information about pediatric use was included in the product labeling. However, clinical pharmacology studies are now performed in children on a more routine basis, and those data are used in the

Handbook of Anticancer Pharmacokinetics and Pharmacodynamics
Edited by: W. D. Figg and H. L. McLeod © Humana Press Inc., Totowa, NJ

review and approval process. This change has occurred only after significant work by many individuals to clarify that it is critical to understand the relationship between drug disposition and drug effect in children. Furthermore, the relation between pharmacokinetics and pharmacodynamics of anticancer drugs in children cannot be extrapolated from what is known about the adult population for many reasons, including the different spectra of malignancies acquired by children and adults. Moreover, many age-related changes in drug disposition occur in children, which are the subject of this chapter.

In addition to age-related changes in physiology that contribute to the differences in pharmacokinetics between children and adults, wide interindividual variability has been well documented in the pharmacokinetics of many drugs in children. This interindividual variability that characterizes the pharmacokinetic parameters of many anticancer drugs in the pediatric population has significant clinical implications. For example, when standardized dosages are administered to children, some with relatively low levels of clearance will have increased systemic exposure, which can lead to toxicity. Conversely, those children with more rapid clearance may not have toxicity, but they may have unacceptable antitumor activity *(1)*.

Differences in drug disposition among children can be attributed not only to developmental changes in physiology but also to variation in genetic composition of individuals. The genotype of drug metabolizing enzymes or drug transport proteins can often be correlated with a pharmacokinetic phenotype, further explaining a source of the variability in pharmacokinetics observed among individuals. Interindividual variation in disposition of anticancer drugs often results in interindividual variation in drug systemic exposure (i.e., uniform dosages can yield different systemic exposures in different children). Evaluation of the relationship between systemic exposure and drug effect (e.g., toxicity and efficacy) has become an important aspect of new drug development in children, as many clinical pharmacology studies have reported a relationship between systemic exposure and response *(3,5,9–13)*. Understanding the pharmacokinetics of anticancer drugs in children is essential to develop new drugs and new combination regimens and to define rational dosing schedules for these drugs. The first section of this chapter reviews the basic principles of drug absorption, distribution, metabolism, and elimination in children and adolescents. Subsequent sections address the appropriate method to select drug dosages in children, practical issues associated with clinical pharmacokinetic studies in children with cancer, and the pharmacokinetics of specific anticancer drugs in children.

2. EFFECT OF MATURATION ON DETERMINANTS OF DRUG DISPOSITION

2.1. Influence of Age on Drug Absorption

Although many anticancer drugs are administered parenterally, several of the currently available drugs are administered orally, such as methotrexate, 6-mercaptopurine, etoposide, and temozolomide. Also, many agents that are administered intravenously are now being evaluated as the intravenous solution given orally. Knowledge of the age-related changes in factors associated with drug absorption will enhance the ability of the clinician to use oral anticancer drugs appropriately in children. Moreover, because many young children are unable to swallow whole tablets or capsules, a clinician must consider that crushing or dissolving tablets may alter oral absorption. Whether absorption will be increased or decreased depends on the physicochemical properties of the drug, and the clinician is advised to consult appropriate references prior to altering commercially manufactured dosage formulations.

Oral drug absorption is dependent on both physicochemical and physiological factors. Physicochemical factors, which can vary among individual agents and formulations, consist of molecular weight, size and shape, degree of ionization under physiologic conditions, and solubility at the site of absorption. Because these characteristics are drug specific they are not subject to maturational changes; however, they are relevant when one considers the practical implications of crushing or dissolving tablets for extemporaneous administration to children. Physiological factors can vary among individuals as well as with maturation. These factors include gastric emptying time, gastric pH, bile salt production, bacterial colonization of the gastrointestinal tract, gastrointestinal transit time, and pancreatic function.

Gastric emptying time is prolonged in children relative to adults (14), and this can reduce or delay the peak concentration of drugs administered orally. Moreover, the rate of gastric emptying is directly related to gestational and postnatal age and the type of feeding (15-17). Furthermore, meals with high caloric density can increase gastric emptying time further in premature infants (18). Gastric emptying time approaches values comparable to adults within the first 6–8 mo of life.

Gastrointestinal transit time, which can also affect the absorption of orally administered drugs, has been less extensively studied in children than gastric emptying time. Intestinal transit times of 3–13.1 h have been reported for full-term neonates aged 3–5 days (19,20). After 45 d, breast-fed infants had a longer transit time (>10 h) than infants who were fed formula (<10 h) (21). In comparison to adults, who usually have an intestinal transit time of about 24 h, it is possible that infants could have reduced absorption of some agents. The frequency of defecation decreases with age, so that 85% of children 1–4 yr of age defecate once or twice daily. A proportionate decrease of high-amplitude propagating contractions occurs in toddlers compared to adults (22).

Gastric acid secretion and pH strongly influence gastrointestinal absorption. At birth gastric pH is neutral because of the presence of amniotic fluid in the stomach. However, within hours pH rapidly falls to 1.5–3.0. Acid secretion peaks during the first 10 d of life and decreases from 10 to 30 d after birth (23). Gastric pH usually reaches adult values by 2 yr of age. The volume of gastric acid secretions approaches adult values by 3 mo of age. The lack of acidity in the gut could decrease the absorption (and hence bioavailability) of anticancer drugs that are weak acids and increase the absorption of weak bases. For example, methotrexate absorption is reduced by coadministration with milk, which effectively reduces the acidity of the gut (24).

Both the rate of bile acid synthesis and the bile acid pool size are decreased in neonates compared to adults (25,26). These changes may alter the disposition of drugs that undergo enterohepatic recirculation, such as irinotecan. Also, the absorption of lipid soluble drugs may be decreased in neonates. However, within the first year of life bile acid synthesis and pool size increase to adult values.

Pancreatic enzyme activity is low at birth and is even lower in premature infants (26). Lipase activity is low in the neonate, and in combination with low bile acid production could reduce the gastrointestinal absorption of lipid soluble drugs. However, even with low pancreatic lipase, the neonate is able to absorb 90–95% of dietary fat through gastric and intestinal lipases (27). Lipase activity increases 20-fold during the first 9 mo of life to reach adult values (15,28,29). The secretion of both amylase and trypsin remains low for the first year of life (16,30,31).

Colonization of the gastrointestinal tract by bacterial flora varies with respect to age, type of delivery, and type of feeding. Before birth, the gut lacks bacterial flora; thereafter, the gut acquires bacteria from the environment. For example, a vaginal birth would lead to colonization of the gut by the mother's vaginal and large intestinal flora (32). Owing to the presence of certain antibodies in the breast milk, an infant who is fed breast milk will acquire different types of bacteria compared to an infant who is fed formula *(32)*. These age-related changes in bacterial colonization of the gastrointestinal tract have theoretical implications for drug absorption and metabolism, as discussed later in the section on irinotecan.

2.2. Influence of Age on Drug Distribution

The volume of distribution (V_d) is a pharmacokinetic parameter that relates the drug dosage to the plasma concentration. Although V_d is a pharmacokinetic parameter and a theoretical term, for many drugs the value is similar to physiological volumes. As such, clinicians often attach physiological relevance to this term, and similar to gastrointestinal absorption, drug distribution in children is dependent on physicochemical and physiological factors. As with physiochemical factors associated with gastrointestinal absorption of drugs, those associated with the volume of distribution remain relatively constant from patient to patient. However, the physiological factors that can change with age include body composition, extent of protein binding, tissue binding characteristics, and vascular perfusion.

Body composition, which can be expressed as the relative proportion of total body water, total extracellular water, and total body fat, varies widely from neonates to teenagers *(33,34)*. Total body water (as a percentage of total body weight) falls from 85% and 77% in the premature and full-term neonate, respectively, to 73% at 3 mo, 59% at 1 yr, and to 55% by 12 yr of age *(35)*. The clinical relevance of this observation is that relatively water-soluble drugs (e.g., topotecan) will have a larger volume of the central compartment in infants compared with adults, whereas lipid-soluble drugs (e.g., etoposide or SN-38, the active metabolite of irinotecan) will have a smaller volume of the central compartment. Similarly, extracellular water falls from 45% of total body weight in the full-term neonate to 33% at 3 mo, 28% at 1 yr, and 20% in the adult *(35)*. Also, total body fat increases from infancy to about 10 yr of age. In boys during puberty, the percentage of total body weight that is fat begins to decrease at about age 17 to a mean of 12%. Conversely, in girls, the percentage of body weight that is fat rapidly increases during puberty to as much as 25% *(36)*. These changes suggest that during adolescence, sex-related differences in volume of distribution play a more important role than they do in younger children or adults.

Drug distribution in children may also be affected by age-related changes in plasma proteins. Extent of protein binding depends on a variety of factors such as amount of plasma proteins and the presence of endogenous substances that may compete for binding (e.g., bilirubin). Protein binding is reduced in infants owing to the presence of fetal albumin and decreased albumin, γ-globulin, and α_1-acid glycoprotein. The concentrations of these proteins do not approach adult values until about 1 yr of life *(34)*; thus, an infant given highly protein-bound drugs (e.g., etoposide or SN-38) will likely have decreased protein binding and an increased fraction unbound. This could lead to an increase in the systemic exposure to the unbound and putatively active drug. For anticancer drugs that have a very narrow therapeutic range, this could potentially be associated with toxicity. Theoretically, increases in the unbound fraction of a drug could also potentiate antitumor activity; therefore, the predicted changes in toxicity and efficacy resulting from changes in the unbound-drug fraction should be balanced when selecting appropriate dosages of highly protein-bound drugs in children. Even though protein concentrations are relatively stable from 2 yr to adulthood, other factors such as disease or malnutrition can decrease plasma protein concentrations and create similar circumstances potentiating both toxicity and efficacy of protein-bound drugs.

Tissue binding also affects drug distribution and changes with maturation. The absolute mass of tissue available for binding in each organ will increase with age. Therefore, younger children who have smaller organs have less tissue available for drugs to bind. This could lead to a greater amount of free drug in the plasma and a greater exposure to the drug. Each tissue has a different affinity for drug binding based on the physicochemical properties of the drug, and the maturational changes in the amount and composition of such tissues may significantly alter drug distribution.

To develop physiologically based pharmacokinetic (PB-PK) models that are age-specific, Haddad and colleagues performed a literature search to obtain previously published data on age-related changes in body weight and tissue weight *(37)*. The authors were not comprehensive in their literature search and instead relied on two previously published databases to cover age groups between birth and 18 yr. Empirical relationships were then developed based on the body and tissue weight data found in these references, sometimes using one reference to develop equations for multiple organs and other times combining data from different sources to develop an equation for one organ/tissue. The authors suggest that the relationships/equations developed in this study can ultimately be used to estimate organ size in children when generating PB-PK models. Although the authors suggest that the equations may provide reasonable initial estimates for PB-PK models, one must be aware of the numerous limitations to this quasi-population analysis. For example, the demographics of the study population are not defined, the statistical analysis lacks sophistication, and the method for determination of body weight (i.e., lean body mass vs ideal body weight) was not specified. In the absence of these details the use of these equations cannot be recommended.

2.3. Influence of Age on Drug Metabolism

The cytochrome P450 enzyme system is a crucial pathway in the metabolism of xenobiotics, including many anticancer drugs. Furthermore, numerous medications used in the supportive care of the children with cancer are substrates, inducers, or inhibitors of CYP450 enzymes, which alter the metabolism, efficacy, and toxicity of anticancer agents that are metabolized via this pathway. Children exhibit higher clearance than adults for many drugs metabolized by the liver (e.g., busulfan *[38,39]* and cyclophosphamide *[40]*). This phenomenon has been ascribed, possibly falsely, to greater activity of the CYP450 enzyme system in children than adults; however, current data do not support this observation.

The literature regarding age-related changes in drug metabolism is rife with inconsistencies between activity of CYP450 enzymes, the level of expression of CYP450 protein or mRNA, and the clearance of CYP450 substrates. Consequently, it has not been possible to establish a link between the age-related changes in the CYP450 enzyme system and the age-related changes in drug metabolism. It has been demonstrated that antipyrine, which is a substrate of CYP450 3A4, 1A2, and 2C9, exhibits higher clearance in children than adults when normalized to body weight. However, no difference was observed in antipyrine clearance between children and adults on normalization to body surface area *(41)*. Blanco and colleagues subsequently showed that in a panel of 52 normal human livers from individuals ranging in age from 0.5 to 93 yr, catalytic activity of CYP 1A2, 3A4/5, 2E1, 2C8, and 2C9 was not affected by age *(42)*. Likewise, a panel of human livers from donors ranging in age from 9 to 89 yr demonstrated weak and insignificant correlation between age and total CYP450 content or activity of microsomes *(43)*. Although a relationship has not been defined between CYP450 catalytic activity or content and the differences in clearance observed in children and adults, perhaps variation in oxygen tension or other currently unknown factors determine the maturational changes in drug metabolism responsible for the maturational changes in drug clearance.

de Wildt and colleagues reviewed the literature on the CYP3A family, which is the most abundant CYP450 subfamily in the liver. They noted the absence of a correlation between liver size and hepatic microsomal enzyme activity and hepatic CYP activity and microsomal protein amount. Therefore, plasma drug clearance may not be informative in determining the relationship between maturation and CYP3A activity. Furthermore, they cautioned against the use of corrections for body weight or body surface area to obtain a relationship between CYP3A substrate pharmacokinetics and age-related changes in metabolism of CYP3A substrates *(44)*. Because a definitive relationship between development of drug-metabolizing enzymes and anticancer drug metabolism has not been established, the clinician who treats children with anticancer drugs must rely on the reports of metabolism of individual anticancer drugs in children of all ages rather than a paradigm of developmental physiology to predict the metabolism of an anticancer drug in a child of any given age.

Despite the controversy about the determination of age-related changes in CYP450 expression or catalytic activity, the use of isoform specific probes has allowed for the characterization of the ontogeny of CYP3A4 and 3A7. In the developing child, the catalytic activity of CYP3A7 reaches peak levels in the first week of life when CYP3A4 catalytic activity is very low. As CYP3A7 catalytic activity declines from 3 mo to 1 yr, there is a corresponding increase in that of CYP3A4. At approx 1 yr, CYP3A7 catalytic activity is negligible, and CYP3A4 has reached peak levels of catalytic activity *(44)*.

In addition to the phase I oxidative metabolism reactions that are important in the disposition of drugs, phase II conjugation reactions are also important in the disposition of some drugs used in children with cancer. For example, the anticancer drug irinotecan, the opioid analgesic morphine, and the antipyretic/analgesic acetaminophen are all glucuronidated by uridine 5'-diphosphase glucuronosyltransferase (UGT). However, at least 10 different isoforms of UGT have been identified. Moreover, some UGT isoforms are polymorphic, which may affect the interindividual variability in the disposition of UGT substrates. Irinotecan *(45–47)* and acetaminophen are metabolized by isoforms in the UGT1A family, which is subject to genetic polymorphism and undergoes maturational changes. UGT1A1 is virtually undetectable in the fetus, its activity increases immediately after birth, and adult levels are attained by 3–6 mo of life. The activity of UGT1A3 is approx 30% of adult levels in neonates. UGT1A6 (for which acetaminophen is a substrate) activity slowly increases after birth to 50% of adult levels at 6 mo and does not reach adult levels prior to 10 yr of age. The implications of these developmental changes in the expression and activity of the UGT1A for the metabolism of irinotecan in children are discussed later in this chapter.

UGT2B7, which catalyzes the metabolism of morphine to morphine-6-glucuronide (100 time more potent analgesic than morphine), has approx 10–20% of adult activity by 15–27 wk of fetal life. Adult levels of UGT2B7 activity are reached by 2–30 mo of life *(48)*. However, the complete ontogeny of all of the UGT isoforms has not yet been determined, so the full impact of the development of UGT on drug metabolism, especially anticancer drugs, is unknown.

2.4. Influence of Age on Renal Excretion

In the treatment of children with cancer many of the anticancer drugs and their metabolites are excreted renally; thus, it is important to understand the effect of maturation on renal function. As with adults, anticancer drugs and supportive therapy (e.g., cisplatin, radiocontrast dye, aminoglycosides, or amphotericin B) can alter renal function. Also, the presence of disease (e.g., from high burden of leukemic blasts, renal obstruction) can impair renal function. Thus, the clinician must accurately measure renal function in the pediatric patient; however, accurate measurement of renal function in this population presents challenges.

Table 1
Methods to Evaluate Renal Function in Children with Cancer

Method	Advantages	Disadvantages
Nomogram (e.g., Schwartz: plasma creatinine) *(51,169)*	1. Avoids urine collection 2. Rapid 3. Robust for children of normal body habitus *(170)* 4. Relatively inexpensive	1. Maternal creatinine present in neonates 2. Reflects GFR only under steady-state conditions 3. Clinician must recall many proportionality constants for specific demographics 4. Invasive sampling required
24-H urine collection for creatinine clearance	1. Accurate if entire urine volume in a 24-h sample can be collected and quantified 2. Noninvasive 3. Relatively inexpensive	1. Difficult to collect and quantify 2. Impractical to measure urine volume accurately for young child (e.g., diapers) 3. Time delay (at least a 24-h turnaround time from initiation of test)
Radionuclide clearance (^{99m}Tc-DTPA or ^{51}Cr-EDTA)	1. Sensitive marker of GFR even in the presence of impaired renal function *(57)* 2. Rapid 3. Avoids urine collection	1. Expensive 2. Requires administration of radiopharmaceutical 3. Invasive sampling required

At birth, the glomerular filtration rate (GFR) in full-term infants is 40 mL/min/1.73 m^2 *(49,50)*, and it reaches adult values (90–140 mL/min/1.73 m^2) by 3 yr of age *(51)*. Miall and colleagues have demonstrated that plasma creatinine rises in preterm infants during the first 48 h after birth, and the greatest absolute increase and the longest time to the mean peak in plasma creatinine occurred in infants 23–26 wk compared to ≥27 wk gestational age *(52)*. The elevated plasma creatinine observed in the preterm infant population for approx 2 d after birth could be attributed to reabsorption of creatinine by the renal tubule *(53)* or a delay in the establishment of a normal GFR. In the preterm infant population studied, all of the patients had respiratory distress syndrome, which could have contributed to a decreased GFR. Furthermore, preterm infants are predisposed to a delay in the development of a normal GFR secondary to incomplete nephrogenesis, which reaches completion at approx 34 wk postconception *(54,55)*. Although such young infants are rarely treated for cancer, the clinician must consider not only postnatal age but also postconceptional age to determine appropriate dosages of renally excreted anticancer drugs in light of the development of GFR.

Schwartz and colleagues *(51)* have demonstrated that the mean GFR for neonates 5–7 d of age is 50.6 mL/min/1.73 m^2. During the first year of life, GFR increases exponentially *(56)* to a mean of 87 mL/min/1.73 m^2 *(51)*. Because the growth of lean body mass increases more rapidly than GFR after 1 yr of life, serum creatinine gradually increases during childhood to reach the normal adult values of 1.0–1.5 mg/dL during adolescence *(55)*.

Although a detailed discussion of all of the available methods for evaluation of renal function in children is beyond the scope of this chapter, the major advantages and disadvantages of some of the most commonly used methods are outlined in Table 1. Despite its limitations (e.g., cost and radioactivity), ^{99m}Tc-DTPA clearance is the best method for assessing GFR in children with cancer *(57)*. In an uncomplicated pediatric patient the clinician might depend on a paradigm of renal developmental physiology to predict the capacity to eliminate a renally excreted drug. However, in a child with altered renal function due to multiple factors (e.g., maturational changes, malignancy, anticancer drugs, supportive care drugs, sepsis), the clinician cannot rely solely on this paradigm and must measure renal function. Although it is recommended that ^{99m}Tc-DTPA clearance be determined, in those institutions not able to perform these studies the clinician must utilize the best available method to assess renal function when dosing renally excreted drugs in children with altered renal function.

3. SELECTING THE APPROPRIATE METHOD TO DOSE ANTICANCER DRUGS IN CHILDREN

Several reviews have recently addressed the question of the selection of the appropriate method to dose anticancer drugs *(58–60)*. Although many of the issues regarding dosing anticancer drugs in adults that were addressed in these reviews may be relevant in children, many of the issues are different. A potential source of variability in calculation of drug doses in children arises from the different methods used to calculate body surface area (BSA). Although the initial approaches to measuring BSA utilized direct measurement techniques, current practices rely instead on nomograms developed from early studies. In 1916, the DuBois formula for calculation of BSA was developed by measuring the BSA of nine subjects (one child) and conducting regression analysis of the known height and weight of subjects to yield $BSA = W^{0.425} \times H^{0.725} \times 71.84$. Height (or supine length) in centimeters and weight in kilograms are the major components of the most frequently used formulas for calculating BSA. Therefore, one of the primary determinants of accurate assessment of BSA is accurate measurement of height and weight, which can be difficult to obtain in children. Calculation of BSA from regression is limited further by the potential for either over- or underestimation of true BSA in a proportion of the population.

It is common practice to normalize drug doses to a measure of body size (e.g., total body weight, BSA) with the intention of reducing interindividual variability in drug systemic exposure and thus response (i.e., efficacy and toxicity). In 287 adults, Grochow and colleagues *(61)* examined the correlation between the pharmacokinetic parameters of nine anticancer drugs and weight, BSA, or height. The clearance of only one drug, paclitaxel, was highly correlated with one measure of body size, height. Thus, normalizing doses of the studied drugs did not reduce interindividual variability in drug exposure, leading the authors to recommend the use of fixed doses. Since the letter by Grochow and colleagues, numerous drugs have been examined in adults for a correlation between dosage normalization and variability in pharmacokinetic parameters. Gurney and colleagues summarized these reports and found that only 4 drugs out of 20 had a possible correlation of BSA and a pharmacokinetic parameter *(58)*. Sawyer and Ratain recently reviewed the question of whether BSA or body weight is more appropriate to determine the dose of anticancer drugs in adults *(59)*. The use of BSA was originally introduced into clinical medicine to translate data from preclinical animal studies to starting dosages for first-time human clinical trials. As these authors correctly note, many discrepancies have been suggested among the formulas used to calculate BSA in adults. Also the authors noted that BSA was selected for its perceived correlation with organ function associated with drug elimination, which is not supported by the analysis of Grochow et al. *(61)* or Gurney *(58)*. Although liver volume measured by magnetic resonance imaging (MRI) in children with cancer correlated with BSA, owing to the inconsistencies in the results of studies of liver volume, body weight, BSA, and clearance of hepatically eliminated drugs, hepatic oxidative metabolism is unlikely to correlate with BSA *(59,62)*. Moreover, creatinine clearance has not been shown to correlate with BSA. Lean body weight correlates more strongly than BSA with physiologic volumes. No correlation of BSA with the pharmacokinetics of epirubicin, carboplatin, and etoposide has been found. Sawyer and Ratain suggest that the use of BSA in the dosing of anticancer agents has not been sufficiently validated, and they recommend that BSA be evaluated prospectively along with age, renal and hepatic function, albumin, and other covariates in future pharmacokinetic studies of anticancer drugs to determine which covariate(s) most appropriately reduce the interpatient variability in response (e.g., efficacy, toxicity, systemic exposure). Although several experts in the pharmacokinetics of anticancer drugs in adults have recommended that the convention of calculating doses solely based on BSA be abandoned, the evidence to support completely abandoning this convention for children is still lacking. However, for selected drugs in some pediatric populations, dosing anticancer drugs based on body weight is more appropriate than dosing based on BSA.

Infants have proportionately higher BSA to weight than older children, so drug dosages based on BSA rather than weight may be too large for infants. Evans and colleagues have demonstrated a statistically significant difference in doxorubicin clearance when normalized to BSA between children < 2 yr old and children > 2 yr old; however, between these two groups a statistically significant difference was not observed in doxorubicin clearance normalized to weight *(2)*. To minimize anthracycline-induced cardiotoxicity, it has been suggested to use either lower milligram per meter squared doses of doxorubicin in young children or to dose doxorubicin in young children in terms of milligram per kilogram, but no further studies have been published to validate this recommendation. Conversely, when comparing children < 1 yr ($n = 2$) and > 1 yr ($n = 23$), the same investigators *(2)* demonstrated a statistically significant difference in etoposide systemic clearance between the age groups when normalized to body weight but not when normalized to BSA. Although this study contained a small number of subjects, a relationship between total body weight and clearance was defined. However, further studies have presented conflicting data and are reviewed below in the section on etoposide. In addition, specific dosing recommendations based on body size are discussed for individual drugs later in this chapter.

4. PRACTICAL ISSUES INVOLVED WITH CLINICAL PHARMACOKINETIC STUDIES IN CHILDREN WITH CANCER

In addition to the effect of maturation leading to differences between children and adults in drug disposition, the clinician must also consider the practical aspects of pharmacokinetic studies conducted in children. Often children will have indwelling venous access for administration of anticancer drugs; however, this site is not practical for obtaining pharmacokinetic samples because of the need for repeated use of the line and infection concerns, excessive blood loss due to flushing of the line, and potential for drug adsorption, which might lead to falsely high plasma concentrations. Therefore, children enrolled in pharmacokinetic studies often need two separate lines, a central line from which blood is drawn and a peripheral line where the anticancer agent is administered. Another potential option for the patient with a double-lumen Hickman or Broviac central line is to use the same line for drug administration and sample acquisition; however, this must be done with appropriate attention to catheter care (e.g,. proper flushing and nursing care) and careful attention to the results of the pharmacokinetic study to determine if adsorption has occurred.

As noted previously, children have a smaller intravascular volume than adults, which places a practical limit on the volume of blood that can be safely collected from each subject for pharmacokinetic studies. Currently, no formal recommendation is available for the amount of blood that can be obtained from children for pharmacokinetic studies. However, the FDA has published guidelines for industry that state that the volume of blood withdrawn should be "minimized" in pediatric studies and institutional review boards/independent ethics committees should review and may define the maximum amount of blood (usually on a milliliters per kilogram or percentage of total blood volume basis) that may be used for pharmacokinetic studies. Some institutions use 5–7% of total blood volume in 24 h or 3–5 mL blood/kg over 8 wk as a guideline for the maximum amount of blood that can be withdrawn from a child for pharmacokinetic studies. Selection of the most informative sample times for pharmacokinetic studies in children is critical. However, even with appropriate selection of plasma sample times for pharmacokinetic studies the clinician should consider that for the individual child blood will be collected not only for pharmacokinetic studies but also for routine laboratory tests including serum chemistries, complete blood counts, bacterial cultures, and blood gases. In neonates and infants, even the discard volume from routine blood draws may be significant. Therefore, the clinician must coordinate pharmacokinetic studies with the clinical pharmacologist.

Population pharmacokinetic modeling and limited sampling models can help maximize the information obtained from pharmacokinetic studies in children with cancer. For example, for a given drug, data sets from a large population of patients can be analyzed to determine if any patient specific factors, such as age, weight, or renal function, correlate with the pharmacokinetic parameters (e.g., systemic clearance). These correlations between patient specific parameters and pharmacokinetic parameters can be useful to refine dosage selection as exemplified by carboplatin dosing based on a patient's renal function and desired carboplatin systemic exposure. Similarly, with analysis of concentration–time profiles collected from serial plasma samples, a limited sampling model can be derived that will minimize the number of plasma samples necessary for a pharmacokinetic study, yet maximize the information yielded from those samples. Thus, with the application of these techniques the clinician can derive much information from a child with cancer regarding the clinical pharmacology of a drug, while remaining attentive to the volume of blood taken from the patient.

5. PHARMACOKINETICS OF SPECIFIC ANTICANCER DRUGS IN CHILDREN

5.1. Methotrexate

Methotrexate is a folate acid antagonist used as an antileukemic agent since the 1940s. Methotrexate competitively inhibits dihydrofolate reductase (DHFR), the enzyme responsible for converting folic acid to reduced folate cofactors, and interferes with several critical biosynthetic pathways including DNA and RNA synthesis. Methotrexate is FDA approved for use in the treatment of acute lymphocytic leukemia (ALL) and osteosarcoma in adults and children. Furthermore, methotrexate is used extensively in both adults and children for nonmalignant diseases such as rheumatoid arthritis. New regimens containing methotrexate are currently being evaluated in pediatric clinical trials for the treatment of ALL and osteosarcoma. Pharmacokinetic monitoring of patients receiving methotrexate has been shown to reduce morbidity and mortality associated with this drug (63,64).

The oral bioavailability of methotrexate is highly variable in adults and children, with reports ranging from 36–83% (65) to 25–95% (66–68). Because some children who have received larger doses of oral methotrexate absorbed a smaller fraction of the dose, it is possible that the mechanism of methotrexate absorption may be saturable *(66)*. Certainly, this trend can be seen when comparing studies with a range of dosages *(6)*. Balis and colleagues observed a 30% higher methotrexate area under the concentration–time curve (AUC) in girls than boys after oral dosing and suggested that gender-related absorption mechanisms might be related *(68)*. Also, it has been shown that when methotrexate is administered with milk a delay occurs in the time to peak methotrexate concentration as well as a decrease in the AUC *(24)*. In addition, more recently Dupuis and colleagues *(69)* have shown that time to peak methotrexate concentration was increased and bioavailability was decreased when it was administered orally after a meal.

The volume of distribution of methotrexate is approx 0.18 L/kg *(70)*; however, its steady-state volume of distribution has been studied more recently and ranges from 0.4 to 0.8 L/kg *(71–75)*. Methotrexate is approx 50% bound to albumin in plasma *(76)*. Organs with the greatest distribution of methotrexate are kidney, gall bladder, bone marrow, small intestine, and liver *(77–79)*. Methotrexate also distributes into pleural fluid and ascites, Even though concentrations in these "third spaces" reach only about 10% maximum serum concentrations *(80)*, the movement of methotrexate from third spaces into the central compartment is slow, leading to a prolonged systemic clearance. Thus, the presence of ascites or pleural effusions should be documented so that a sufficient duration of leucovorin rescue can be provided.

Methotrexate cerebrospinal fluid (CSF) concentrations range about 1.5–2.5% of serum concentrations after a 24-h infusion *(81–83)*. However, if higher dosages are used (≥ 5 g/m^2 over 24 h), it is possible to achieve cytotoxic concentrations (≥ 0.01 μmol/L) despite poor distribution into CSF *(81–83)*. To attain putatively cytotoxic CSF concentrations methotrexate has been administered via the intrathecal route. Intrathecal dosage regimens based on body surface area underdose children < 8 yr old because they have larger CSF volumes relative to their body surface area *(84)*. Because of these age-related changes in CSF volume, it has been suggested that intrathecal methotrexate dose should be based on age *(85)*. However, Strother and colleagues did not find age to be significantly correlated with methotrexate dose in a group of patients treated with intra-Ommaya methotrexate *(86)*.

The metabolism of methotrexate in children is primarily catalyzed by hepatic aldehyde oxidase, which yields the less active metabolite, 7-hydroxymethotrexate, which has been found in low concentrations (0.1–0.3 μM) *(66)*. However, the ontogeny of hepatic aldehyde oxidase has not been well characterized. Even though 7-hydroxymethotrexate is 40–200 times less active then methotrexate against DHFR it could still have clinical consequences. Because this metabolite is less soluble than methotrexate at physiologic pH, it may contribute to renal toxicity through precipitation in renal tubules *(87)*. Bacteria in the gastrointestinal tract also metabolize both oral and enterohepatically recycled methotrexate to 4-amino-4-deoxy-N^{10}-methylpteroic acid (DAMPA). This metabolite is rarely detectable in patients and is 200 times less active than methotrexate. Also in both adults and children, folyl polyglutamate synthetase metabolizes intracellular methotrexate to methotrexate-polyglutamates *(88)*, which are more toxic to cells than methotrexate, because the polyglutamates are retained by cells for longer periods of time than methotrexate *(89)*. Methotrexate-polyglutamates are at least as active as methotrexate, and therefore have a major role in the cytotoxicity of methotrexate.

Renal excretion of methotrexate is a primary route of methotrexate elimination, with approx 80% excreted unchanged in the urine in 24 h through renal tubular secretion and glomerular filtration *(66)*. Less than 10% of a dose is excreted as the 7-hydroxymethotrexate metabolite in the urine *(90,91)*; however, this has been shown to increase when methotrexate is administered as a prolonged infusion *(71)*. Furthermore, methotrexate systemic clearance, which includes renal and nonrenal pathways, is higher in children than in adults (92) and decreases with age (93,94). However, this can be due to a variety of factors that can alter the disposition of methotrexate such as renal function, pleural effusion, and gastrointestinal obstruction.

Hydration and urinary alkalinization can increase the renal clearance of methotrexate as shown in the study by Sand and Jacobsen (95). It is therefore recommended that patients are well hydrated with intravenous fluids and treated with sodium bicarbonate to alkalinize the urine prior to high dose methotrexate therapy (i.e., intravenous fluid [with 40 mEq $NaHCO_3/L$] administered at the rate of 200 mL/m^2/h for at least 2 h before the start of high-dose methotrexate). Urinary pH should also be monitored during infusion and additional sodium bicarbonate therapy be administered if the pH is ≤ 6.0. Acetazolamide may be used if systemic alkalosis limits the administration of bicarbonate for urinary alkalinization.

Murry and colleagues evaluated the effects of the variability in GFR on the pharmacokinetic variability of methotrexate clearance in children receiving remission-induction therapy for ALL (96). Because GFR accounted for only 37% of the variability in methotrexate clearance, the investigators concluded that tubular secretion and reabsorption, hydration, volume status, urinary alkalinization, and nonrenal clearance might also contribute significantly to methotrexate pharmacokinetic variability. In addition, they demonstrated that remission-induction therapy that included methotrexate, leucovorin rescue, prednisone, vincristine, daunorubicin, asparaginase, etoposide, and cytarabine was not associated with a significant reduction in GFR when compared to pretreatment values.

Methotrexate is also excreted into the bile, however, to a much smaller extent (approx 10%) than other routes of elimination. Although biliary excretion is not a major route of elimination, methotrexate can be reabsorbed from the gastrointestinal tract, which can prolong its terminal half-life (97).

5.2. Cyclophosphamide and Ifosfamide

The oxazophosphorine alkylating agents cyclophosphamide and ifosfamide are prodrugs that are activated by 4-hydroxylation via the CYP450 system to 4-hydroxycyclophosphamide and 4-hydroxyifosfamide, respectively. Cyclophosphamide is approved for acute nonlymphocytic leukemia (ANLL), ALL, neuroblastoma, retinoblastoma, and Wilms' tumor. However, cyclophosphamide is also used in bone marrow transplantation, childhood germ cell tumors, Ewing's sarcoma, osteosarcoma, and rhabdomyosarcoma. Ifosfamide is used in Hodgkin's lymphoma, non-Hodgkin's lymphoma, Ewing's sarcoma, osteosarcoma, rhabdomyosarcoma, and Wilms' tumor.

Metabolic deactivation of ifosfamide to 2- and 3-dechloroethylifosfamide by CYP3A4 and 2B6 also yields an equimolar amount of chloroacetaldehyde, which has been implicated in the neurotoxicity associated with ifosfamide (98,99). Kerbusch and colleagues have demonstrated that coadministration of ketoconazole with ifosfamide can reduce the formation of the active metabolite 4-hydroxyifosfamide, which may lead to reduced antitumor efficacy. They also showed that coadministration of rifampin with ifosfamide increases the metabolism of ifosfamide to both the active metabolite and the two inactive metabolites 2- and 3-dechloroethylifosfamide, as well as the neurotoxic byproduct chloracetaldehyde. Thus, they concluded that administration of either the CYP inhibitor ketoconazole or the CYP inducer rifampin can reduce the therapeutic benefit of ifosfamide (98).

Yule and colleagues have evaluated the pharmacokinetics of cyclophosphamide in pediatric patients and reported a wide interpatient variability in drug disposition (100). The cyclophosphamide clearance varied from 1.2 to 10.6 L/h/m^2. The half-life varied from 1.1 to 16.8 h, and was significantly prolonged at high dosage levels. In a more recent study, Yule and colleagues have demonstrated that fluconazole inhibits the first step in the activation of cyclophosphamide in vitro *(101)*. Moreover, in a group of 22 children ranging in age from 2 mo to 18 yr, they have demonstrated a statistically significant reduction in clearance and increase in half-life of cyclophosphamide when fluconazole is coadministered.

Because pharmacologically induced changes in the expression and/or activity of the cytochrome P450 system resulted in changes in the metabolism and clearance of cyclophosphamide and ifosfamide, similar variations could be observed in children of different ages treated with cyclophosphamide or ifosfamide owing to the maturational changes in the CYP450 system. Therefore, not only should the clinician be aware of specific CYP450 drug interactions (actual or potential) with cyclophosphamide and ifosfamide, but also the clinician should anticipate different patterns of metabolism of these drugs in children of various ages.

5.3. Vincristine

Vincristine is a naturally occurring alkaloid, which exerts its cytotoxic effects by binding to tubulin, thus stopping mitosis and leading to apoptosis. Vincristine has been approved by the FDA as part of a combination regimen to treat a variety of adult and pediatric malignancies, including, ALL, Hodgkin's disease, and Wilms' tumor. Because it lacks myelosuppression as a dose-limiting toxicity, vincristine is an attractive anticancer agent for use in combination with other myelosuppressive agents. In general, vincristine pharmacokinetics are associated with high intra- and interindividual variability in children; however, intraindividual variability is usually smaller than interindividual variability *(102,103)*.

Vincristine is administered as an intravenous infusion or bolus dose due to poor oral absorption. Gidding and colleagues demonstrated that the vincristine volume of distribution at steady state is variable in children with acute lymphoblastic leukemia, non-Hodgkin's lymphoma, or Wilms' tumor (range: 56–1165 L/m^2) *(103)*. Within 15–30 min after intravenous administration vincristine is rapidly distributed, and > 90% distributes from the blood to the tissue where it is tightly (but not irreversibly) bound *(104)*. Although CSF penetration of vincristine is poor *(105)*, intrathecal administration is strictly contraindicated because of associated lethality.

Vincristine is metabolized by the CYP3A family into a variety of poorly characterized metabolites that are considered devoid of antitumor activity *(106,107)*. Because coexpression of CYP3A4 and NADPH-P450 (hOR) in a Chinese hamster ovary (CHO) cell line decreased the cytotoxicity of vincristine compared to the parental CHO line, Yao and colleagues conclude that vincristine metabolism by the P450 system leads to inactivation *(108)*. Furthermore, vincristine systemic clearance was significantly increased with a consequent significant decrease in the AUC in patients with brain tumors who were receiving the CYP3A4-inducing antiepileptic drugs carbamazepine or phenytoin compared to control patients who did not receive any CYP3A4 inducing agents *(109)*. While it is unknown whether the induction of the clearance of the vinca alkaloids has a clinically significant consequence (i.e., reduction in efficacy or toxicity), inhibition of vincristine clearance has been shown to augment toxicity *(110)*. Furthermore, age-related changes in the CYP3A system could contribute to the high interindividual variability in vincristine pharmacokinetics among children.

Conflicting reports about the similarities or differences in the pharmacokinetics of vincristine between pediatric and adult populations may reflect increased sophistication of assay methods with time. An early report of vincristine pharmacokinetics in children showed similar disposition in adults and children *(111)*; however, this study was conducted in only four children using a radioimmunoassay rather than the more specific high-performance liquid chromatography (HPLC) method. Woods and colleagues *(112)* demonstrated that a high incidence of neurotoxity in infants smaller than 0.5 m² and recommended that children with a BSA of < 1 m² receive dosages based on body weight. Delayed hepatic conjugation and clearance of vincristine and the large ratio of BSA to weight in infants could cause the observed increase in toxicity. A more recent study *(113)* used a specific HPLC assay for vincristine and showed that the vincristine clearance in children with acute lymphoblastic leukemia was higher than in adults with lung cancer (431 vs 189 mL/min/m2). This study, however, did not account for concomitant medications, such as steroids and antibiotics, which may have accounted for the increased vincristine clearance. Crom and colleagues *(104)* used this same HPLC method, and in 54 children aged 2–18 yr reported a vincristine clearance similar to that reported by de Graaf (482 mL/min/m²); however, in the Crom study only two patients received CYP450 inducers, so it is likely that children do have a higher vincristine clearance than adults.

Two recent reports *(102,103)* discuss aspects of interindividual variability in vincristine pharmacokinetics in children. Gidding and colleagues showed that age had a weak positive correlation with vincristine clearance when normalized to body surface area, but a weak negative correlation when normalized to body weight. Their findings are consistent with the reports of Woods et al. *(112)*and Crom et al. *(104)*, which also describe a significant relationship between weight and vincristine clearance. Drug–drug interactions also contribute to the interindividual variability seen with vincristine pharmacokinetics, as observed by Gidding and colleagues when they showed that children who received steroids, which induce CYP3A isoenzymes, had a significantly higher vincristine clearance ($p = 0.0092$) *(103)*. Groninger and colleagues administered vincristine as a single agent to children ages 1–16 yr and reported a clearance of 228 mL/min/m² *(102)*. This value, which is lower than that reported by other investigators, could be due to exclusion of very young children and the absence of enzyme-inducing drugs. However, they did find that $t_{1/2}\beta$ was significantly smaller and clearance was significantly higher in children who received cephalosporins, but did not offer any further pharmacological explanation (including details of cephalosporin therapy). The relationship between vincristine disposition and measures of biliary function have been investigated, as vincristine is eliminated mainly in the bile. Two authors *(102,114)* found vincristine clearance to be inversely related to alkaline phosphatase and gamma-glutamyltransferase; however, these enzymes are not specific to biliary function. Other investigators have seen no correlation between vincristine clearance and total bilirubin, alkaline phosphatase, or albumin level *(103)*.

5.4. Etoposide

Etoposide, a topoisomerase II inhibitor that can be administered orally or intravenously, is used in the treatment of children with ALL, AML, ANLL, Ewing's sarcoma, non-Hodgkin's lymphoma, neuroblastoma, retinoblastoma, rhabdomyosarcoma, and Wilms' tumor. High-dose etoposide is also used in conditioning regimens for bone marrow transplantation.

Chen and colleagues determined that the mean (range) bioavailability of etoposide in 12 children with relapsed ALL is 60.6% (17.6–91.2%) *(115)*. By evaluating the disposition of oral etoposide in 16 patients ranging in age from 3 to 73 yr in comparison to intravenous etoposide in 18 different children ranging in age from 0.8 to 17 yr, Wurthwein and colleagues determined a similar mean apparent bioavailability of 59% *(116)*.

In children with ALL, Relling and colleagues have studied the penetration of intravenous and oral etoposide into the CSF *(117)*. Although only approx 0.3% of the concentrations of etoposide that are attained in plasma are reached in the CSF, it is thought that even these low levels of etoposide can be cytotoxic to leukemic blasts, depending on the inherent sensitivity of each individual child's disease to etoposide. The ratio of etoposide CSF and plasma concentrations in children with ALL are comparable to those observed in adults with brain tumors without tumor invasion of the ventricles or subarachnoid space (0.7%) *(118)*. Therefore, it is unlikely that age-related changes exist in the penetration of etoposide into the CSF; changes in CSF penetration are more likely due to the effects of specific disease (e.g., disruption of the blood–brain barrier).

Etoposide is extensively plasma protein bound (90–94%) *(119)*. In eight children ranging in age from 4.2 to 22 yr with refractory solid tumors, 45% of the parent drug was excreted unchanged in the urine. In children with refractory solid tumors investigators reported an inverse relationship between albumin concentration and etoposide renal clearance, which suggests that a changes in albumin concentration might influence the amount of free drug available for renal clearance *(120)*.

In vitro, CYP3A4 catalyzes 3'-demethylation of etoposide, and CYP1A2 and 2E1 also have minor catalytic activity in this metabolic pathway. Ketoconazole, troleandomycin, verapamil, cyclosporin, vincristine, and prednisolone inhibited etoposide 3'-demethylation in human liver microsomes *(121)*. CYP3A4 also catalyzes the *O*-demethylation of etoposide in vitro in human hepatic microsomes and heterologous expression systems, which can be inhibited by erythromycin, cyclosporin, dexamethasone, prednisone, midazolam, nifedipine, and troleandomycin *(122,123)*. Furthermore, a high degree of variability was observed in the maximal microsomal activity among individual livers, which may account for some of the interindividual variation in the disposition of etoposide *(122)*.

Wurthwein and colleagues have reported a population pharmacokinetic model of the disposition of high-dose etoposide in children ranging in age from 9.6 mo to 23.7 yr *(124)*. The concentration–time data were best fit by a three-compartment model with a volume of distribution, clearance, AUC, and terminal half-life of 0.067 L/kg, 15.5 mL/min/m^2, 1175 mg/L·h, and 44.2 h, respectively. These values are similar to those reported by Evans and colleagues *(120,125)*. High inter- and intraindividual variability in protein binding was observed in this study *(124)*. Furthermore, they demonstrated a negative correlation between age and etoposide clearance normalized to body weight; however, they found no correlation between age and clearance normalized to BSA. However, Boos and colleagues demonstrated that etoposide clearance adjusted neither for weight or BSA was correlated with age *(126)*. Thus, no relationship has been reported between etoposide clearance (normalized to weight) and age.

5.5. Topotecan

Topotecan, a water-soluble camptothecin analog, is a topoisomerase I inhibitor. Topotecan undergoes a reversible, pH-dependent conversion from the lactone form to carboxylate form at physiologic pH *(127–129)*. Topotecan has been approved by the FDA as second-line treatment of small-cell lung cancer and ovarian cancer in adults; however, it has been shown to be effective in a variety of pediatric solid tumors and leukemias. Topotecan is currently being evaluated as a single agent or in combination in clinical trials in children to treat neuroblastoma, medulloblastoma, glioblastoma, ALL, and other childhood cancers *(130–132)*.

The oral bioavailability of the intravenous solution of topotecan in children is approx 30% *(133)*, which is similar to that reported in adults *(134)*. After oral administration topotecan peak lactone plasma concentrations occurred from 0.75 to 2 h. The absorption half-life of topotecan lactone was 0.78 ± 0.54 h. Large interpatient variability was noted in oral topotecan pharmacokinetics, whereas intrapatient variability was relatively small.

The topotecan volume of distribution (V_{dss}) has shown high interindividual variability. In adults it is as large as 160 L; however, in children it has been reported to be 73 ± 27 L/m^2

(135) and 13–458 L/m^2 *(130)*. A study in adults showed that topotecan also distributes into third spaces and pleural effusions without sequestration *(136)*. Furthermore, these authors demonstrated that distribution into third spaces had no effect on topotecan disposition, but inadequate data were presented to evaluate fully the conclusion of the authors. Plasma protein binding of topotecan is 7–35% in adults and children *(137)*, which is reasonably low. Alterations in plasma proteins in children, whether age-related or disease-related, will likely not alter topotecan disposition or pharmacologic effect.

Topotecan is metabolized by the CYP450 enzyme system to an active metabolite, *N*-desmethyl topotecan, and has also been found to exist as an *O*-glucuronide *(138–140)*. However, topotecan primarily undergoes renal elimination, with 49–70% of a dose recovered in the urine as unchanged drug *(141)*.

The renal excretion of topotecan includes both glomerular filtration and tubular secretion *(142)*. A study of adults receiving topotecan demonstrated that patients with impaired glomerular filtration, as measured by creatinine clearance, had decreased topotecan renal clearance. Thus it is recommended that adult patients with creatinine clearance <39 mL/min receive topotecan at reduced dosages. However, renal dysfunction in children receiving topotecan did not alter topotecan renal or systemic clearance *(143)*. In a study of six children with unilateral nephrectomies due to Wilms' tumor, a topotecan clearance of 25.7 L/h/m^2 was reported *(144)*. When compared with an age-, SrCR-, and BSA-matched cohort of patients the topotecan clearance was not statistically different ($p = 0.08$) although the Wilms' tumor patients had significantly reduced GFR ($p = 0.03$), as measured by ^{99m}Tc-DTPA clearance. It is likely that other mechanisms (i.e., increase in drug transporters, other unspecified metabolic pathways) may have compensated for the anticipated decrease in topotecan renal clearance. Based on these data, it is therefore not recommended that topotecan dosage be altered in children with decreased renal function as measured by ^{99m}Tc-DTPA clearance.

The disposition of topotecan in infants <2 yr has been evaluated and results have shown that clearance correlated with weight better than BSA. This finding supports the practice of dosing infants (<2 yr of age) by weight instead of BSA *(145)*. Multiple studies of pharmacokinetically guided dosing to attain discrete target AUC have also been conducted. Thus far, we have been successful in adjusting individual patients' topotecan systemic exposure to reduce interindividual variability in drug exposure *(146)*.

5.6. Irinotecan

Irinotecan also inhibits topoisomerase I and is a prodrug that must be activated by carboxylesterase to form SN-38, the active moiety of irinotecan. Similar to topotecan, irinotecan undergoes reversible pH-dependent hydrolysis from lactone to carboxylate at physiologic pH. The FDA has approved irinotecan for use in adults with colorectal cancer. Although irinotecan has not yet been approved for pediatric use, preclinical studies have shown that neuroblastoma is sensitive to both oral and intravenous irinotecan *(147,148)*. Furthermore, in Phase I trials in children, irinotecan is active in a variety of solid tumors including neuroblastoma, hepatocellular carcinoma, pineoblastoma, glioblastoma, brainstem glioma, osteosarcoma, hepatoblastoma, rhabdomyosarcoma, and squamous cell carcinoma of the larynx *(149,150)*.

Although irinotecan is only 8% bioavailable, in children (2–19 yr) with solid tumors, the relative extent of conversion of irinotecan to SN-38 is greater for oral administration (0.38 ± 0.31) than for intravenous administration (0.11 ± 0.06), suggesting that SN-38 is formed presystemically after oral irinotecan *(151)*. Thus oral administration is a reasonable alternative to intravenous, and Phase I studies of oral irinotecan are ongoing.

The age-related changes in bacterial colonization of the gastrointestinal tract have theoretical implications for drug absorption and metabolism as exemplified by irinotecan. Irinotecan-associated diarrhea can be ameliorated in a rat model by administration of penicillin and streptomycin. These antibiotics can in effect inhibit the cleavage of SN-38 glucuronide to SN-38 in the gut by elimination of the β-glucuronidase-producing bacteria *(152)*. In a follow-up study, the same group demonstrated that inhibition of β-glucuronidase increased the exposure of the large intestinal luminal tissue to SN-38 glucuronide and decreased the exposure of this tissue to SN-38 *(153)*. Furthermore, inhibition of β-glucuronidase did not alter the systemic pharmacokinetics or small intestinal luminal exposure of irinotecan, SN-38 glucuronide, or SN-38. These results have important implications for irinotecan-associated diarrhea. Because bacterial flora change with age, one should be aware of developmental stage when administering anticancer drugs for which the parent drug or the metabolite is a substrate of β-glucuronidase. In theory, very young children in whom gastrointestinal flora are not fully established would be less susceptible than adults or older children to irinotecan-induced diarrhea owing to a relative lack of β-glucuronidase, which increases the local exposure of the large intestine to the putative toxic moiety, SN-38.

SN-38 is highly protein bound. Children with serum albumin within normal limits (3.0–4.4 g/dL) exhibited approx 3.4% unbound SN-38 (range 0.7–6.5%) *(150,154)*. Thus, the clinician must be aware of possible interactions between irinotecan and other highly protein-bound drugs and pathophysiological changes that can alter a child's serum albumin. The clearance of irinotecan lactone in children is approx 55.5 L/h/m^2 *(154,155)*, which is similar to that observed in adults *(156,157)*.

Irinotecan is extensively metabolized in the liver by carboxylesterase to form the active metabolite SN-38, which is subsequently metabolized by hepatic UDP-glucuronyltransferase (UGT) *(158)* and CYP450 *(159,160)*. SN-38 is glucuronidated by the UGT1 family. Ciotti and colleagues *(45)* have demonstrated that COS-1 cells transfected with UGT1A7 were 12- to 40-fold more active at pH 7.6 in the conjugation of SN-38 to glucuronide than nine other isoforms of the UGT1A family, including UGT1A1, which had been previously demonstrated to be the predominant isoform responsible for this reaction *(46)*. In addition, Hanioka and colleagues have demonstrated that recombinant human UGT1A3, UGT1A6, and UGT1A9 expressed in microsomes of insect cells catalyze the glucuronidation of SN-38 *(47)*. Because the expression of the UGT1A family increases as a child matures and because this family of enzymes detoxifies SN-38, children may be subject to an increased risk of SN-38 toxicity compared to adults until the expression of UGT1A isoforms reaches adult levels. SN-38 is also metabolized by CYP3A to NPC *(160)* and APC *(159)*. NPC can be metabolized by carboxylesterase to SN-38; whereas APC is not converted to SN-38 in the presence of carboxylesterase *(161)*. Although NPC appeared to induce topoisomerase I-mediated DNA cleavage, it is thought that this pharmacologic property is due to contamination with SN-38 rather than activity of NPC itself. Even though NPC is likely an inactive metabolite, it can be converted to the active SN-38; therefore, alterations in CYP3A metabolism through pharmacologic induction or inhibition, developmental stage, or genetic polymorphism could impact the pharmacokinetics of irinotecan and its metabolites and thus the clinical response to this anticancer drug.

Enzyme-inducing anticonvulsants (EIAs) have been shown to alter pharmacokinetics of irinotecan in children (age range 3–21 yr) with high grade glioma *(155)*. Patients who received EIAs exhibited greater clearance of irinotecan lactone and lower SN-38 lactone AUCs than those who did not receive EIAs. Because those who received EIAs did not have a significantly greater median AUC of APC than those who did not receive EIAs, induction of CYP3A4 may not explain the alteration in the pharmacokinetics of irinotecan in the presence of EIAs. The mechanism for the increase in the systemic clearance of irinotecan without a consequent increase in the AUC of its metabolites has yet to be elucidated, but it is thought that EIAs may increase the biliary excretion of irinotecan through induction of MRP2 (ABCC2) and Pgp (ABCB1). When possible, EIAs should be avoided in children receiving irinotecan; if anticonvulsants are required, the newer non-enzyme-inducing anticonvulsants should be considered *(155)*.

5.7. Temozolomide

Temozolomide is a methylating agent that is approved for treatment of refractory anaplastic astrocytoma in adults *(162,163)* and is undergoing evaluation for use in pediatrics to treat high-grade gliomas and sarcomas. This highly bioavailable compound undergoes spontaneous base-catalyzed hydrolysis to form the methyl triazene, MTIC, which is the final active methylating species. MTIC is believed to exert its toxic effects through acid catalysis, forming the methyldiazonium ion, which ultimately leads to O^6-methylguanine formation in DNA plus the inactive metabolite, AIC *(164–166)*.

Only one pediatric pharmacokinetic study has been published that evaluated temozolomide disposition *(167)*. After oral administration temozolomide was rapidly absorbed, with maximal concentrations observed within 60 min. Based on the assumption of 0.98 oral bioavailability, the total body clearance of temozolomide was $100 \, mL/min/m^2$ and the plasma elimination half-life was approx 100 min. The AUC seen with the $200 \, mg/m^2/dose$ was the same for a single dose or after repeated doses (d 1 vs d 5). Plasma elimination half-life and apparent total body clearance values were constant over the dose range of $100–260 \, mg/m^2$.

Beale and colleagues showed that, although a theoretical possibility, increasing gastric pH by administration of an H_2-receptor antagonist did not alter the bioavailability of temozolomide *(168)*. In the case of children who are unable or are too young to swallow temozolomide capsules, temozolomide capsules can be opened carefully and reconstituted in applesauce, apple juice, or orange juice. No clinically relevant difference has been observed in temozolomide pharmacokinetic parameters using this method of administration.

6. SUMMARY AND CONCLUSIONS

Recent advances in cellular and molecular biology techniques have led to an increased understanding of pediatric clinical pharmacology, and in many instances a more rational approach to dosing drugs in children. As described in this chapter, a stronger scientific basis for dosing drugs in children will be derived from an increased understanding of the effects of maturation on the physiological processes affecting drug disposition, concomitant drug therapy, and disease states. Moreover, a further evaluation of the most appropriate dosing approach (e.g., dose per weight, height, BSA, age) in the pediatric population is warranted. Because the importance of pharmacokinetic and pharmacodynamic studies in this age group has been highlighted, an improved understanding of the clinical pharmacology of many anticancer drugs in children has been gained. In addition, computer hardware and software has become readily available to enhance the conduct of pharmacokinetic studies. This improvement in technology has encouraged investigators to pursue additional aspects of clinical pharmacokinetic studies, including pharmacokinetically guided dosing, on a more routine basis in this age group. This approach is viewed as one method to reduce the wide interindividual variability that so often characterizes pediatric pharmacokinetic parameters. Finally, pharmacogenomic analysis in children with cancer will further explain the observed interindividual variability in pharmacokinetics, toxicity, and efficacy. Establishing phenotype–genotype correlations will improve the care of children with cancer.

REFERENCES

1. Knoester PD, Underberg WJ, Beijnen JH. Clinical pharmacokinetics and pharmacodynamics of anticancer agents in pediatric patients (review). Anticancer Res 1993; 13:1795–1808.
2. McLeod HL, Relling MV, Crom WR, et al. Disposition of antineoplastic agents in the very young child. Br J Cancer 1992; 66:S23–S29.
3. Petros WP, Evans WE. Pharmacokinetics and pharmacodynamics of anticancer agents: contributions to the therapy of childhood cancer. Pharmacotherapy 1990; 10:313–325.
4. Evans WE, Petros WP, Relling MV, et al. Clinical pharmacology of cancer chemotherapy in children. Pediatr Clin North Am 1989; 36:1199–1230.
5. Evans WE, Relling MV. Clinical pharmacokinetics–pharmacodynamics of anticancer drugs. Clin Pharmacokinet 1989; 16:327–336.
6. Crom WR, Glynn-Barnhart AM, Rodman JH, et al. Pharmacokinetics of anticancer drugs in children. Clin Pharmacokinet 1987; 12:168–213.
7. Evans WE, Crom WR, Sinkule JA, Yee GC, Stewart CF, Hutson PR. Pharmacokinetics of anticancer drugs in children. Drug Metab Rev 1983; 14:847–886.
8. FDA HHS. Regulations requiring manufacturers to assess the safety and effectiveness of new drugs and biological products in pediatric patients. Fed Regist 1998; 63:66,632–66,672.
9. Relling MV, McLeod HL, Bowman LC, Santana VM. Etoposide pharmacokinetics and pharmacodynamics after acute and chronic exposure to cisplatin. Clin Pharmacol Ther 1994; 56:503–511.
10. Rodman JH, Relling MV, Stewart CF, et al. Clinical pharmacokinetics and pharmacodynamics of anticancer drugs in children. Semin Oncol 1993; 20:18–29.
11. Rodman JH, Abromowitch M, Sinkule JA, Hayes FA, Rivera GK, Evans WE. Clinical pharmacodynamics of continuous infusion teniposide: systematic exposure as a determinant of response in a phase I trial. J Clin Oncol 1987; 5:1007–1014.
12. Sonnichsen DS, Ribeiro RC, Luo X, Mathew P, Relling MV. Pharmacokinetics and pharmacodynamics of 21-day continuous oral etoposide in pediatric patients with solid tumors. Clin Pharmacol Ther 1995; 58:99–107.
13. Stewart CF, Baker SD, Heideman RL, Jones D, Crom WR, Pratt CB. Clinical pharmacodynamics of continuous infusion topotecan in children: systemic exposure predicts hematologic toxicity. J Clin Oncol 1994; 12:1946–1954.
14. Kearns GL, Reed MD. Clinical pharmacokinetics in infants and children—a reappraisal. Clin Pharmacokinet 1989; 17:29–67.
15. Cavell B. Gastric emptying in preterm infants. Acta Paediatr Scand 1979; 68:725–730.
16. Grand RJ, Watkins JB, Torti FM. Development of the human gastrointestinal tract. A review. Gastroenterology 1976; 70(5 Pt.1):790–810.
17. Gupta M, Brans YW. Gastric retention in neonates. Pediatrics 1978; 62:26–29.
18. Siegel M, Lebenthal E, Krantz B. Effect of caloric density on gastric emptying in premature infants. J Pediatr 1984; 104:118–122.
19. Rubaltelli FF, Largajolli G. Effect of light exposure on gut transit time in jaundiced newborns. Acta Paediatr Scand 1973; 62:146–148.
20. Fomon SJ. Nutritional requirements in relation to growth. Monatsschr Kinderheilkd 1974; 122 (5 Suppl):236–239.
21. Lebenthal E, Lee PC, Heitlinger LA. Impact of development of the gastrointestinal tract on infant feeding. J Pediatr 1983; 102:1–9.
22. Di Lorenzo C, Flores AF, Hyman PE. Age-related changes in colon motility. J Pediatr 1995; 127:593–596.
23. Ulshen M. Stomach and intestines: Normal development, structure, and function. In: Nelson WE, Behrman RE, Kliegman RM, Jenson HB (eds). Nelson Textbook of Pediatrics. Philadelphia, PA: WB Saunders, 2000, pp. 1128–1129.
24. Pinkerton CR, Welshman SG, Glasgow JF, Bridges JM. Can food influence the absorption of methotrexate in children with acute lymphoblastic leukaemia? Lancet 1980; 2:944–946.
25. Heubi JE, Balistreri WF, Suchy FJ. Bile salt metabolism in the first year of life. J Lab Clin Med 1982; 100:127–136.
26 Watkins JB. Mechanisms of fat absorption and the development of gastrointestinal function. Pediatr Clin North Am 1975; 22:721–730.
27. Hamosh M. Lipid metabolism in premature infants. Biol Neonate 1987; 52(Suppl 1):50–64.

28. Besunder JB, Reed MD, Blumer JL. Principles of drug biodisposition in the neonate. A critical evaluation of the pharmacokinetic-pharmacodynamic interface (Part II). Clin Pharmacokinet 1988; 14:261–286.
29. Besunder JB, Reed MD, Blumer JL. Principles of drug biodisposition in the neonate. A critical evaluation of the pharmacokinetic–pharmacodynamic interface (Part I). Clin Pharmacokinet 1988; 14:189–216.
30 Hadorn B, Zoppi G, Shmerling DH, Prader A, McIntyre I, Anderson CM. Quantitative assessment of exocrine pancreatic function in infants and children. J Pediatr 1968; 73:39–50.
31. Zoppi G, Andreotti G, Pajno-Ferrara F, Njai DM, Gaburro D. Exocrine pancreas function in premature and full term neonates. Pediatr Res 1972; 6:880–886.
32. Harmsen HJ, Wildeboer-Veloo AC, Raangs GC, et al. Analysis of intestinal flora development in breast-fed and formula-fed infants by using molecular identification and detection methods. J Pediatr Gastroenterol Nutr 2000; 30(1):61–67.
33. Crom WR. Pharmacokinetics in the child. Environ Health Perspect 1994;102:111–118.
34. Milsap RL, Jusko WJ. Pharmacokinetics in the infant. Environ Health Perspect 1994; 102(Suppl 11): 107–110.
35. Friis-Hansen B. Body composition during growth. In vivo measurements and biochemical data correlated to differential anatomical growth. Pediatrics 1971; 47(Suppl):264.
36. Finkelstein JW. The effect of developmental changes in adolescence on drug disposition. J Adolesc Health 1994; 15:612–618.
37. Haddad S, Restieri C, Krishnan K. Characterization of age-related changes in body weight and organ weights from birth to adolescence in humans. J Toxicol Environ Health A 2001; 64:453–464.
38. Grochow LB, Krivit W, Whitley CB, Blazar B. Busulfan disposition in children. Blood 1990; 75:1723–1727.
39. Hassan M, Oberg G, Bekassy AN, et al. Pharmacokinetics of high-dose busulphan in relation to age and chronopharmacology. Cancer Chemother Pharmacol 1991; 28:130–134.
40. Tasso MJ, Boddy AV, Price L, Wyllie RA, Pearson AD, Idle JR. Pharmacokinetics and metabolism of cyclophosphamide in paediatric patients. Cancer Chemother Pharmacol 1992; 30:207–211.
41. Crom WR, Relling MV, Christensen ML, Rivera GK, Evans WE. Age-related differences in hepatic drug clearance in children: studies with lorazepam and antipyrine. Clin Pharmacol Ther 1991; 50: 132–140.
42. Blanco JG, Harrison PL, Evans WE, Relling MV. Human cytochrome P450 maximal activities in pediatric versus adult liver. Drug Metab Dispos 2000; 28:379–382.
43. Schmucker DL, Woodhouse KW, Wang RK, et al. Effects of age and gender on in vitro properties of human liver microsomal monooxygenases. Clin Pharmacol Ther 1990; 48:365–374.
44. de Wildt SN, Kearns GL, Leeder JS, van den Anker JN. Cytochrome P450 3A: ontogeny and drug disposition. Clin Pharmacokinet 1999; 37:485–505.
45. Ciotti M, Basu N, Brangi M, Owens IS. Glucuronidation of 7-ethyl-10-hydroxycamptothecin (SN-38) by the human UDP-glucuronosyltransferases encoded at the UGT1 locus. Biochem Biophys Res Commun 1999; 260:199–202.
46. Iyer L, King CD, Whitington PF, Green MD, Roy SK, Tephly TR et al. Genetic predisposition to the metabolism of irinotecan (CPT-11). Role of uridine diphosphate glucuronosyltransferase isoform 1A1 in the glucuronidation of its active metabolite (SN-38) in human liver microsomes. J Clin Invest 1998; 101:847–854.
47. Hanioka N, Ozawa S, Jinno H, Ando M, Saito Y, Sawada J. Human liver UDP-glucuronosyltransferase isoforms involved in the glucuronidation of 7-ethyl-10-hydroxycamptothecin. Xenobiotica 2001; 31: 687–699.
48. de Wildt SN, Kearns GL, Leeder JS, van den Anker JN. Glucuronidation in humans. Pharmacogenetic and developmental aspects. Clin Pharmacokinet 1999; 36:439–452.
49. Grochow LB, Baker SD. The Relationship of Age to the Disposition and Effects of Anticancer Drugs. In: Grochow LB, Ames MM (eds). A Clinician's Guide to Chemotherapy Pharmacokinetics and Pharmacokinetics. Baltimore, MD: Williams & Wilkins, 1998, pp. 35–53.
50. Milsap RL, Hill MR, Szefler SJ. Special Pharmacokinetic considerations in children. In: Evans WE, Schentag JJ, Jusko WJ, (eds.) Applied Pharmacokinetics: Principles of Therapeutic Drug Monitoring. Vancouver, WA: Applied Therapeutics, 1992, pp. 10-1–10-32.
51. Schwartz GJ, Feld LG, Langford DJ. A simple estimate of glomerular filtration rate in full-term infants during the first year of life. J Pediatr 1984; 104:849–854.
52. Miall LS, Henderson MJ, Turner AJ, et al. Plasma creatinine rises dramatically in the first 48 hours of life in preterm infants. Pediatrics 1999; 104:e76.

53. Guignard JP, Drukker A. Why do newborn infants have a high plasma creatinine? Pediatrics 1999; 103:e49.

54. Wilkins BH. Renal function in sick very low birthweight infants: 1. Glomerular filtration rate. Arch Dis Child 1992; 67(Spec Issue [10]):1140–1145.

55. Arant BS, Jr. Postnatal development of renal function during the first year of life. Pediatr Nephrol 1987; 1:308–313.

56. Aperia A, Broberger O, Thodenius K, Zetterstrom R. Development of renal control of salt and fluid homeostasis during the first year of life. Acta Paediatr Scand 1975; 64:393–398.

57. Rodman JH, Maneval DC, Magill HL, Sunderland M. Measurement of Tc-99m DTPA serum clearance for estimating glomerular filtration rate in children with cancer. Pharmacotherapy 1993; 13:10–16.

58. Gurney H. Dose calculation of anticancer drugs: a review of the current practice and introduction of an alternative. J Clin Oncol 1996; 14:2590–2611.

59. Sawyer M, Ratain MJ. Body surface area as a determinant of pharmacokinetics and drug dosing. Invest New Drugs 2001; 19:171–177.

60. Gurney H. How to calculate the dose of chemotherapy. Br J Cancer 2002; 86:1297–1302.

61. Grochow LB, Baraldi C, Noe D. Is dose normalization to weight or body surface area useful in adults? J Natl Cancer Inst 1990; 82:323–325.

62. Murry DJ, Crom WR, Reddick WE, Bhargava R, Evans WE. Liver volume as a determinant of drug clearance in children and adolescents. Drug Metab Dispos 1995; 23:1110–1116.

63. Evans WE, Pratt CB, Taylor RH, Barker LF, Crom WR. Pharmacokinetic monitoring of high-dose methotrexate. Early recognition of high-risk patients. Cancer Chemother Pharmacol 1979; 3:161–166.

64. Galpin AJ, Evans WE. Therapeutic drug monitoring in cancer management. Clin Chem 1993; 39: 2419–2430.

65. Schornagel JH, Van Engelen ME, De Vos D. Bioavailability of methotrexate tablets. Pharm Weekbl Sci 1982; 4:89–90.

66. Balis FM, Savitch JL, Bleyer WA. Pharmacokinetics of oral methotrexate in children. Cancer Res 1983; 43:2342–2345.

67. Ravelli A, Di Fuccia G, Molinaro M, et al. Plasma levels after oral methotrexate in children with juvenile rheumatoid arthritis. J Rheumatol 1993; 20:1573–1577.

68. Balis FM, Holcenberg JS, Poplack DG, et al. Pharmacokinetics and pharmacodynamics of oral methotrexate and mercaptopurine in children with lower risk acute lymphoblastic leukemia: a joint children's cancer group and pediatric oncology branch study. Blood 1998; 92:3569–3577.

69. Dupuis LL, Koren G, Silverman ED, Laxer RM. Influence of food on the bioavailability of oral methotrexate in children. J Rheumatol 1995; 22:1570–1573.

70. Leme PR, Creaven PJ, Allen LM, Berman M. Kinetic model for the disposition and metabolism of moderate and high-dose methotrexate (NSC-740) in man. Cancer Chemother Rep 1975; 59: 811–817.

71. Evans WE, Stewart CF, Hutson PR, Cairnes DA, Bowman WP, Yee GC et al. Disposition of intermediate-dose methotrexate in children with acute lymphocytic leukemia. Drug Intell Clin Pharm 1982; 16:839–842.

72. Henderson ES, Adamson RH, Oliverio VT. The metabolic fate of tritiated methotrexate. II. Absorption and excretion in man. Cancer Res 1965; 25:1018–1024.

73. Huffman DH, Wan SH, Azarnoff DL, Hogstraten B. Pharmacokinetics of methotrexate. Clin Pharmacol Ther 1973; 14:572–579.

74. Raude E, Oellerich M, Weinel P, et al. High-dose methotrexate: pharmacokinetics in children and young adults. Int J Clin Pharmacol Ther Toxicol 1988; 26:364–370.

75. Pratt CB, Howarth C, Ransom JL, Bowles D, Green AA, Kumar AP et al. High-dose methotrexate used alone and in combination for measurable primary or metastatic osteosarcoma. Cancer Treat Rep 1980; 64:11–20.

76. Taylor JR, Halprin KM. Effect of sodium salicylate and indomethacin on methotrexate-serum albumin binding. Arch Dermatol 1977; 113:588–591.

77. Iqbal MP. Accumulation of methotrexate in human tissues following high-dose methotrexate therapy. J Pak Med Assoc 1998; 48:341–343.

78. Bischoff KB, Dedrick RL, Zaharko DS, Longstreth JA. Methotrexate pharmacokinetics. J Pharm Sci 1971; 60:1128–1133.

79. Zaharko DS, Dedrick RL, Bischoff KB, Longstreth JA, Oliverio VT. Methotrexate tissue distribution: prediction by a mathematical model. J Natl Cancer Inst 1971; 46:775–784.

80. Evans WE, Pratt CB. Effect of pleural effusion on high-dose methotrexate kinetics. Clin Pharmacol Ther 1978; 23:68–72.

81. Evans WE, Hutson PR, Stewart CF, Cairnes DA, Bowman WP, Rivera G et al. Methotrexate cerebrospinal fluid and serum concentrations after intermediate-dose methotrexate infusion. Clin Pharmacol Ther 1983; 33:301–307.

82. Millot F, Rubie H, Mazingue F, Mechinaud F, Thyss A. Cerebrospinal fluid drug levels of leukemic children receiving intravenous 5 g/m^2 methotrexate. Leuk Lymphoma 1994; 14:141–144.

83. Seidel H, Andersen A, Kvaloy JT, et al. Variability in methotrexate serum and cerebrospinal fluid pharmacokinetics in children with acute lymphocytic leukemia: relation to assay methodology and physiological variables. Leuk Res 2000; 24:193–199.

84. Bleyer AW. Clinical pharmacology of intrathecal methotrexate. II. An improved dosage regimen derived from age-related pharmacokinetics. Cancer Treat Rep 1977; 61:1419–1425.

85. Ruggiero A, Conter V, Milani M, et al. Intrathecal chemotherapy with antineoplastic agents in children. Paediatr Drugs 2001; 3:237–246.

86. Strother DR, Glynn-Barnhart A, Kovnar E, Gregory RE, Murphy SB. Variability in the disposition of intraventricular methotrexate: a proposal for rational dosing. J Clin Oncol 1989; 7:1741–1747.

87. Bertino JR. Clinical use of methotrexate—with emphasis on use of high doses. Cancer Treat Rep 1981; 65(Suppl 1):131–135.

88. McGuire JJ, Bertino JR. Enzymatic synthesis and function of folylpolyglutamates. Mol Cell Biochem 1981; 38(Spec Issue [Pt 1]:19–48.

89. Galivan J. Evidence for the cytotoxic activity of polyglutamate derivatives of methotrexate. Mol Pharmacol 1980; 17:105–110.

90. Breithaupt H, Kuenzlen E. Pharmacokinetics of methotrexate and 7-hydroxymethotrexate following infusions of high-dose methotrexate. Cancer Treat Rep 1982; 66:1733–1741.

91. Shen DD, Azarnoff DL. Clinical pharmacokinetics of methotrexate. Clin Pharmacokinet 1978; 3:1–13.

92. Wang YM, Sutow WW, Romsdahl MM, Perez C. Age-related pharmacokinetics of high-dose methotrexate in patients with osteosarcoma. Cancer Treat Rep 1979; 63:405–410.

93. Kerr IG, Jolivet J, Collins JM, Drake JC, Chabner BA. Test dose for predicting high-dose methotrexate infusions. Clin Pharmacol Ther 1983; 33:44–51.

94. Bressolle F, Bologna C, Kinowski JM, Arcos B, Sany J, Combe B. Total and free methotrexate pharmacokinetics in elderly patients with rheumatoid arthritis. A comparison with young patients. J Rheumatol 1997; 24:1903–1909.

95. Sand TE, Jacobsen S. Effect of urine pH and flow on renal clearance of methotrexate. Eur J Clin Pharmacol 1981; 19:453–456.

96. Murry DJ, Synold TW, Pui CH, Rodman JH. Renal function and methotrexate clearance in children with newly diagnosed leukemia. Pharmacotherapy 1995; 15:144–149.

97. Evans WE, Tsiatis A, Crom WR, Brodeur GM, Coburn TC, Pratt CB. Pharmacokinetics of sustained serum methotrexate concentrations secondary to gastrointestinal obstruction. J Pharm Sci 1981; 70:1194–1198.

98. Kerbusch T, Jansen RL, Mathot RA, et al. Modulation of the cytochrome P450-mediated metabolism of ifosfamide by ketoconazole and rifampin. Clin Pharmacol Ther 2001; 70:132–141.

99. Cerny T, Kupfer A. The enigma of ifosfamide encephalopathy. Ann Oncol 1992; 3:679–681.

100. Yule SM, Boddy AV, Cole M, et al. Cyclophosphamide pharmacokinetics in children. Br J Clin Pharmacol 1996; 41:13–19.

101. Yule SM, Walker D, Cole M, et al. The effect of fluconazole on cyclophosphamide metabolism in children. Drug Metab Dispos 1999; 27:417–421.

102. Groninger E, Meeuwsen-De Boar T, Koopmans P, Uges D, Sluiter W, Veerman A et al. Pharmacokinetics of vincristine monotherapy in childhood acute lymphoblastic leukemia. Pediatr Res 2002; 52:113–118.

103. Gidding CE, Meeuwsen-de Boer GJ, Koopmans P, Uges DR, Kamps WA, de Graaf SS. Vincristine pharmacokinetics after repetitive dosing in children. Cancer Chemother Pharmacol 1999; 44:203–209.

104. Crom WR, de Graaf SSN, Synold T, et al. Pharmacokinetics of vincristine in children and adolescents with acute lymphocytic leukemia. J Pediatr 1994; 125:642–649.

105. Jackson DV Jr, Sethi VS, Spurr CL, McWhorter JM. Pharmacokinetics of vincristine in the cerebrospinal fluid of humans. Cancer Res 1981; 41:1466–1468.

106. Zhou-Pan XR, Seree E, Zhou XJ, et al. Involvement of human liver cytochrome P450 3A in vinblastine metabolism: drug interactions. Cancer Res 1993; 53:5121–5126.

107. Zhou XJ, Zhou-Pan XR, Gauthier T, Placidi M, Maurel P, Rahmani R. Human liver microsomal cytochrome P450 3A isozymes mediated vindesine biotransformation. Metabolic drug interactions. Biochem Pharmacol 1993; 45:853–861.

108. Yao D, Ding S, Burchell B, Wolf CR, Friedberg T. Detoxication of vinca alkaloids by human P450 CYP3A4-mediated metabolism: implications for the development of drug resistance. J Pharmacol Exp Ther 2000; 294:387–395.

109. Villikka K, Kivisto KT, Maenpaa H, Joensuu H, Neuvonen PJ. Cytochrome P450-inducing antiepileptics increase the clearance of vincristine in patients with brain tumors. Clin Pharmacol Ther 1999; 66:589–593.

110. Chan JD. Pharmacokinetic drug interactions of vinca alkaloids: summary of case reports. Pharmacotherapy 1998; 18:1304–1307.

111. Sethi VS, Kimball JC. Pharmacokinetics of vincristine sulfate in children. Cancer Chemother Pharmacol 1981; 6:111–115.

112. Woods WG, O'Leary M, Nesbit ME. Life-threatening neuropathy and hepatotoxicity in infants during induction therapy for acute lymphoblastic leukemia. J Pediatr 1981; 98:642–645.

113. de Graaf SSN, Bloemhof H, Vendrig DEMM, Uges DRA. Vincristine disposition in children with acute lymphoblastic leukemia. Med Ped Oncol 1995; 24:235–240.

114. van den Berg HW, Desai ZR, Wilson R, Kennedy G, Bridges JM, Shanks RG. The pharmacokinetics of vincristine in man: reduced drug clearance associated with raised serum alkaline phosphatase and dose-limited elimination. Cancer Chemother Pharmacol 1982; 8:215–219.

115. Chen CL, Rawwas J, Sorrell A, Eddy L, Uckun FM. Bioavailability and pharmacokinetic features of etoposide in childhood acute lymphoblastic leukemia patients. Leuk Lymphoma 2001; 42:317–327.

116. Wurthwein G, Krumpelmann S, Tillmann B, et al. Population pharmacokinetic approach to compare oral and i.v. administration of etoposide. Anticancer Drugs 1999; 10:807–814.

117. Relling MV, Mahmoud H, Pui C-H, et al. Etoposide achieves potentially cytotoxic concentrations in cerebrospinal fluid of children with acute lymphoblastic leukemia. J Clin Oncol 1996; 14:399–404.

118. Kiya K, Uozumi T, Ogasawara H, et al. Penetration of etoposide into human malignant brain tumors after intravenous and oral administration. Cancer Chemother Pharmacol 1992; 29:339–342.

119. Allen LM, Creaven PJ. Comparison of the human pharmacokinetics of VM-26 and VP-16, two antineoplastic epipodophyllotoxin glucopyranoside derivatives. Eur J Cancer 1975; 11:697–707.

120. Sinkule JA, Hutson P, Hayes FA, Etcubanas E, Evans WE. Pharmacokinetics of etoposide (VP-16) in children and adolescents with refractory solid tumors. Cancer Res 1984; 44:3109–3113.

121. Kawashiro T, Yamashita K, Zhao XJ, et al. A study on the metabolism of etoposide and possible interactions with antitumor or supporting agents by human liver microsomes. J Pharmacol Exp Ther 1998; 286:1294–1300.

122. Relling MV, Evans R, Dass C, Desiderio DM, Nemec J. Human cytochrome P450 metabolism of teniposide and etoposide. J Pharmacol Exp Ther 1992; 261:491–496.

123. Relling MV, Nemec J, Schuetz EG, Schuetz JD, Gonzalez FJ, Korzekwa KR. O-Demethylation of epipodophyllotoxins is catalyzed by human cytochrome P450 3A4. Mol Pharmacol 1994; 45:352–358.

124. Wurthwein G, Klingebiel T, Krumpelmann S, Metz M, Schwenker K, Kranz K et al. Population pharmacokinetics of high-dose etoposide in children receiving different conditioning regimens. Anticancer Drugs 2002; 13:101–110.

125. Evans WE, Sinkule JA, Crom WR, Dow L, Look AT, Rivera G. Pharmacokinetics of teniposide (VM-26) and etoposide (VP16-213) in children with cancer. Cancer Chemother Pharmacol 1982; 7:147–150.

126. Boos J, Krumpelmann S, Schulze-Westhoff P, Euting T, Berthold F, Jurgens H. Steady-state levels and bone marrow toxicity of etoposide in children and infants: does etoposide require age-dependent dose calculation? J Clin Oncol 1995; 13:2954–2960.

127. Pommier Y, Leteurtre F, Fesen MR, et al. Cellular determinants of sensitivity and resistance to DNA topoisomerase inhibitors. Cancer Investig 1994; 12:530–542.

128. Tanizawa A, Fujimori A, Fujimori Y, Pommier Y. Comparison of topoisomerase I inhibition, DNA damage, and cytotoxicity of camptothecin derivatives presently in clinical trials. J Natl Cancer Inst 1994; 86:836–842.

129. Hertzberg RP, Caranfa MJ, Holdern KG, Jakas DR, Gallagher G, Mattern MG. Modification of the hydroxy lactone ring of camptothecin: inhibition of mammalian topoisomerase I and biological activity. J Med Chem 1989; 32:715–720.

130. Athale UH, Stewart C, Kuttesch JF, et al. Phase I study of combination topotecan and carboplatin in pediatric solid tumors. J Clin Oncol 2002; 20:88–95.

131. Saylors RL III, Stine KC, Sullivan J, Kepner JL, Wall DA, Bernstein ML et al. Cyclophosphamide plus topotecan in children with recurrent or refractory solid tumors: a Pediatric Oncology Group phase II study. J Clin Oncol 2001; 19:3463–3469.

132. Park JR, Slattery J, Gooley T, et al. Phase I topotecan preparative regimen for high-risk neuroblastoma, high-grade glioma, and refractory/recurrent pediatric solid tumors. Med Pediatr Oncol 2000; 35:719–723.

133. Zamboni WC, Bowman LC, Tan M, Santana VM, Houghton PJ, Meyer WH et al. Interpatient variability in bioavailability of the intravenous formulation of topotecan given orally to children with recurrent solid tumors. Cancer Chemother Pharmacol 1999; 43:454–460.

134. Schellens JHM, Creemers GJ, Beijnen JH, et al. Bioavailibility and pharmacokinetics of oral topotecan: a new topoisomerase I inhibitor. Br J Cancer 1996; 73:1268–1271.

135. Verweij J, Lund B, Beijnen J, P et al. Phase I and pharmacokinetics study of topotecan, a new topoisomerase I inhibitor. Ann Oncol 1993;4:673–678.

136. Gelderblom H, Loos WJ, Verweij J, de Jonge MJ, Sparreboom A. Topotecan lacks third space sequestration. Clin Cancer Res 2000; 6:1288–1292.

137. Dennis MJ, Beijnen JH, Grochow LB, van Warmerdam LJ. An overview of the clinical pharmacology of topotecan. Semin Oncol 1997; 24(1 Suppl 5):S5.

138. Rosing H, Herben VMM, van Gortel-van Zomeren DM, et al. Isolation and structural confirmation of N-desmethyl topotecan, a metabolite of topotecan. Cancer Chemother Pharmacol 1997; 39: 498–504.

139. Rosing H, van Zomeren DM, Doyle E, Bult A, Beijnen JH. O-Glucuronidation, a newly identified metabolic pathway for topotecan and N-desmethyl topotecan. Anticancer Drugs 1998; 9:587–592.

140. Rosing H, van Zomeren DM, Doyle E, et al. Quantification of topotecan and its metabolite N-desmethyltopotecan in human plasma, urine and faeces by high-performance liquid chromatographic methods. J Chromatogr B Biomed Sci Appl 1999; 727:191–203.

141. Herben VMM, Schoemaker NE, Rosing H, et al. Urinary and fecal excretion of topotecan in patients with malignant solid tumors. Cancer Chemother Pharmacol 2002; 50:59–64.

142. Zamboni WC, Houghton PJ, Johnson RK, et al. Probenecid alters topotecan systemic and renal disposition by inhibiting tubular secretion. J Pharmacol Exp Ther 1998; 284:89–94.

143. Zamboni WC, Heideman RL, Meyer WH, Gajjar AJ, Crom WR, Stewart CF. Pharmacokinetics (PK) of topotecan in pediatric patients with normal and altered renal function. Proc Am Soc Clin Oncol 1996; 15:371.

144. Iacono LC, Dome JS, Panetta CP, Stewart CF. Topotecan pharmacokinetics in children with Wilm Tumor and unilateral nephrectomy. American College of Clinical Pharmacy Spring Practice and Research Forum. Palm Springs, CA. April 2003. Pharmacotherapy; 23(3), 410:127.

145. Kirstein MN, Santana VM, Furman WL, Gajjar A, Liu T, Tan M, Bai F, Iacono LC, Stewart CF. Disposition of topotecan in the very young child. Also Abstact 494, 2002.

146. Santana VM, Zamboni WC, Kirstein MN, et al. A pilot study of protracted topotecan dosing using a pharmacokinetically guided dosing approach in children with solid tumors. Clin Cancer Res 2003; 9:633–640.

147. Thompson J, Zamboni WC, Cheshire PJ, et al. Efficacy of oral administration of irinotecan against neuroblastoma xenografts. Anticancer Drugs 1997; 8:313–322.

148. Thompson J, Zamboni WC, Cheshire PJ, et al. Efficacy of systemic administration of irinotecan against neuroblastoma xenografts. Clin Cancer Res 1997; 3:423–431.

149. Blaney S, Berg SL, Pratt C, et al. A Phase I study of irinotecan in pediatric patients: a pediatric oncology group study. Clin Cancer Res 2001; 7:32–37.

150. Furman WL, Stewart CF, Poquette CA, et al. Direct translation of a protracted irinotecan schedule from a xenograft model to a phase I trial in children. J Clin Oncol 1999; 17:1815–1824.

151. Radomski KM, Stewart CF, Panetta JC, Houghton PJ, Furman WL. Phase I and pharmacokinetic study of oral irinotecan in pediatric patients with solid tumors. Proc Annu Meet Am Soc Clin Oncol 2000; 19:593a.

152. Takasuna K, Hagiwara T, Hirohashi M, et al. Involvement of beta-glucuronidase in intestinal microflora in the intestinal toxicity of the antitumor camptothecin derivative irinotecan hydrochloride (CPT-11) in rats. Cancer Res 1996; 56:3752–3757.

153. Takasuna K, Hagiwara T, Hirohashi M, et al. Inhibition of intestinal microflora beta-glucuronidase modifies the distribution of the active metabolite of the antitumor agent, irinotecan hydrochloride (CPT-11) in rats. Cancer Chemother Pharmacol 1998; 42:280–286.

154. Ma MK, Zamboni WC, Radomski KM, et al. Pharmacokinetics of irinotecan and its metabolites SN-38 and APC in children with recurrent solid tumors after protracted low-dose irinotecan. Clin Cancer Res 2000; 6:813–819.

155. Crews K, Stewart CF, Jones-Wallace D, Thompson SJ, Houghton PJ, Heideman RL et al. Altered irinotecan pharmacokinetics in pediatric high-grade glioma patients receiving enzyme-inducing anti-convulsant therapy. Clin Cancer Res 2002; 8:2202–2209.

156. Rowinsky EK, Grochow LB, Ettinger DS, Sartorius SE, Lubejko BG, Chen T. Phase I and pharmacological study of the novel topoisomerase I inhibitor 7-ethyl-10-[4-1-(1-piperidino)-1-piperdino]carbonyloxycamptothecin (CPT-11) administered as a ninety-minute infusion every 3 weeks. Cancer Res 1994; 54:427–436.

157. Xie R, Mathijssen RHJ, Sparreboom A, Verweij J, Karlsson MO. Clinical pharmacokinetics of irinotecan and its metabolites: a population analysis. J Clin Oncol 2002; 20:3293–3301.

158. Haaz MC, Rivory L, Jantet S, Ratanasavanh D, Robert J. Glucuronidation of SN-38, the active metabolite of irinotecan, by human hepatic microsomes. Pharmacol Toxicol 1997; 80:91–96.

159. Haaz MC, Rivory LP, Riche C, Vernillet L, Robert J. Metabolism of irinotecan (CPT-11) by human hepatic microsomes: participation of cytochrome P-450 3A and drug interactions. Cancer Res 1998; 58:468–472.

160. Haaz MC, Riche C, Rivory LP, Robert J. Biosynthesis of an aminopiperidino metabolite of irinotecan [7-ethyl-10-[4-(1-piperidino)-1-piperidino] carbonyloxycamptothecine] by human hepatic microsomes. Drug Metab Dispos 1998; 26:769–774.

161. Dodds HM, Haaz MC, Riou JF, Robert J, Rivory LP. Identification of a new metabolite of CPT-11 (irinotecan): pharmacological properties and activation to SN-38. J Pharmacol Exp Ther 1998; 286: 578–583.

162. Brandes AA, Pasetto LM, Monfardini S. New drugs in recurrent high grade gliomas. Anticancer Res 2000; 20:1913–1920.

163. Prados MD. Future directions in the treatment of malignant gliomas with temozolomide. Semin Oncol 2000; 27(3 Suppl 6):41–46.

164. Baker SD, Wirth M, Statkevich P, et al. Absorption, metabolism, and excretion of ^{14}C-temozolomide following oral administration to patients with advanced cancer. Clin Cancer Res 1999; 5:309–317.

165. Newlands ES, Blackledge GRP, Slack JA, et al. Phase I trial of temozolomide (CCRG 81045: M&B 39831: NSC 362856). Br J Cancer 1992; 65:287–291.

166. Reid JM, Stevens DC, Rubin J, Ames MM. Pharmacokinetics of 3-methyl-(triazen-1-yl)imidazole-4-carboximide following the administration of temozolomide to patients with advanced cancer. Clin Cancer Res 1997; 3:2393–2398.

167. Estlin EJ, Lashford L, Ablett S, et al. Phase I study of temozolomide in paediatric patients with advanced cancer. United Kingdom Children's Cancer Study Group. Br J Cancer 1998; 78:652–661.

168. Beale P, Judson I, Moore S, et al. Effect of gastric pH on the relative oral bioavailability and pharmacokinetics of temozolomide. Cancer Chemother Pharmacol 1999; 44:389–394.

169. Schwartz GJ, Haycock GB, Edelmann CM Jr, Spitzer A. A simple estimate of glomerular filtration rate in children derived from body length and plasma creatinine. Pediatrics 1976; 58:259–263.

170. Schwartz GJ, Brion LP, Spitzer A. The use of plasma creatinine concentration for estimating glomerular filtration rate in infants, children, and adolescents. Pediatr Clin North Am 1987; 34:571–590.

25 Clinical Pharmacokinetics in the Elderly

Patricia W. Slattum, Pharm D, PhD
and Jürgen Venitz, MD, PhD

Contents

INTRODUCTION
GENERAL PHARMACOKINETIC CHANGES ASSOCIATED WITH AGING
EFFECTS OF AGE ON THE PHARMACOKINETICS
  OF CHEMOTHERAPEUTIC AGENTS

1. INTRODUCTION

Clinical response to medication in an individual patient is the net result of the interaction of a number of complex processes. These processes can be categorized into two broad areas: those affecting pharmacokinetics or the relationship between the administered dose and the concentrations of the drug in the systemic circulation, and those affecting pharmacodynamics or the relationship between concentrations of the drug in the systemic circulation and the observed pharmacologic response. Absorption, distribution, metabolism, and excretion of a drug determine its pharmacokinetics. Drug–receptor interactions, concentrations of the drug at the receptor, and homeostatic compensatory mechanisms determine a drug's pharmacodynamics. Pharmacokinetics and pharmacodynamics are affected by a number of patient-specific factors including age, sex, ethnicity, genetics, disease processes, and prior and present drug exposure. This chapter focuses on the effects of advanced age on pharmacokinetics.

In clinical decision-making for the elderly patient it is important to recognize that the elderly may also experience an unexpected clinical response to a medication owing to the impact of factors other than their age, such as concurrent diseases and coadministered medications. Despite the fact that much less is known about pharmacodynamic changes in the elderly than changes in pharmacokinetics, the potential for altered pharmacodynamics must also be considered.

1.1. Definition of "Elderly"

"Elderly" has generally been defined as age 65 yr or older, although many other chronological definitions have been applied. Some researchers have enrolled patients as young as 50 yr old as "elderly" whereas others have studied only those patients in their 80s or older as "elderly." Although a chronological age is most often used to define elderly, it is important to recognize that the elderly are a heterogeneous group, with individuals aging

Handbook of Anticancer Pharmacokinetics and Pharmacodynamics
Edited by: W. D. Figg and H. L. McLeod © Humana Press Inc., Totowa, NJ

421

at varying rates. Interindividual variation is much larger in the elderly than in the young *(1)*. The aging process has been described as a condition of "incipient disease" with a variety of deteriorative changes taking place *(2)*. When decline occurs more obviously in one organ system than another, a disease is diagnosed. It is therefore difficult to distinguish between normal age-related changes and pathological states. Biological or physiological definitions of elderly have proved difficult to formulate, so chronological definitions of elderly remain the standard. The Food and Drug Administration's "Guideline for Industry Studies in Support of Special Populations: Geriatrics" arbitrarily defines the geriatric population as comprising patients aged 65 yr or older, although the inclusion of older patients is encouraged to the extent possible *(3)*.

1.2. The Elderly Patient

Although many older adults age successfully and lead healthy, productive lives well into their later years, the elderly as a group are more likely to suffer from chronic diseases and take more medications than their younger counterparts. The aging process itself is associated with changes in physiology that may alter drug pharmacokinetics and pharmacodynamics. When applying general knowledge of pharmacokinetic alterations in the elderly to the care of an individual patient in the clinical setting, it is necessary to consider the patient's overall condition, "physiologic age," disease states, and concurrent medications.

The elderly are especially vulnerable to adverse reactions to medications. The incidence of adverse drug reactions is two to three times that found in younger adults but may be underestimated because of lack of detection and underreporting *(4)*. Many adverse reactions are preventable. Examples of preventable adverse effects include consequences of known drug–drug interactions or prescribing an inappropriate dosage for the elderly. The increased incidence of adverse reactions in the elderly results from altered pharmacokinetics, altered pharmacodynamics, increased opportunity for drug interactions, and inappropriate prescribing. While the changes in pharmacokinetics and pharmacodynamics are well recognized, age-related differences in dosing often are not noted in compendia such as the *Physician's Desk Reference* (*PDR*) that are used by prescribers. One recent study *(5)* found many examples of evidence-based recommendations for dose alterations in the elderly that were reported in the literature but were not noted in the product labeling included in the *PDR*. This could explain, in part, the significant increase in adverse events in the elderly. Knowledge of basic pharmacokinetic differences in the elderly associated with age-related changes in physiology can be used to choose appropriate dosing regimens for the elderly and avoid preventable adverse drug reactions.

1.3. Pharmacokinetic Studies in the Elderly

Almost all of the information known about age-related changes in humans, including pharmacokinetics, has been obtained from cross-sectional studies. In these studies, the variable under investigation is measured in groups of subjects of different ages at a single point in time. Age differences are then inferred from a comparison of the mean values for each group or from a regression of the variable on age. The cross-sectional approach assumes that average differences between age groups reflect the change that occurs in an individual with the passage of time, which may or may not be valid.

When studying chronological changes in a particular variable, there are three primary time-related factors that must be considered: the effects of age, the effects of an environmental change or historical event at a specified period in time (period effects), and the effects of being part of the group or cohort of individuals born at a particular time (birth cohort). Cross-sectional studies often confound age effects with birth cohort effects. Findings in a group of individuals aged 65 today may differ from those in a group of 65-yr-olds studied 25 yr from now. These groups would be the same age but from different birth cohorts with different group experiences. Cross-sectional studies can also suffer from selective mortality effects, because the oldest study cohorts include only those individuals who survived to reach old age, and these individuals may be unique regarding the variable of interest.

Another approach to studying age-related changes is longitudinal studies. In these studies repeated measurements of a variable are made on the same individual at various points in time. This approach measures individual rates of aging for the specified variable, rather than differences between age groups as in cross-sectional studies. Although the results of longitudinal studies may be a more reliable approach to studying age-related changes, longitudinal studies tend to confound age effects with the effects of an environmental change or historical event at a specified period in time (period effects). These studies are also very difficult to conduct, taking many years to complete. For this reason, pharmacokinetic studies are virtually always cross-sectional in design *(6)*.

Two general cross-sectional approaches are used to study pharmacokinetics in the elderly. The first is a formal pharmacokinetic study conducted either in healthy geriatric subjects or in elderly patient volunteers with the disease the drug is intended to treat. A relatively small group of subjects is studied using intensive blood sampling in each individual. In this approach, very healthy elderly people are selected for participation in an attempt to ensure that advanced age, and not disease, is the primary factor under investigation. Often these studies include only relatively young geriatric subjects that can meet the stringent inclusion criteria, limiting the generalizability of the results to the very old or frail patient. Results of these studies must be considered along with pharmacokinetic studies in other populations, such as patients with renal impairment, when making therapy decisions for individual patients.

The second cross-sectional approach is the pharmacokinetic screening or population pharmacokinetic study. These studies are typically conducted in conjunction with the main Phase III (or Phase II) clinical trials program. Under steady-state conditions, a small number of samples for drug level determinations are collected and analyzed. When appropriately designed, the influence of demographic and disease factors on pharmacokinetics can be examined in this type of study. Although the data analysis is more difficult, the advantage to this approach is that age and other factors, as well as their interactions, can be evaluated.

2. GENERAL PHARMACOKINETIC CHANGES ASSOCIATED WITH AGING

Normal aging is associated with changes in human physiology, and many of these changes contribute to altered pharmacokinetics in the elderly. These changes are even more evident in frail or very old patients. Drug absorption and bioavailability, distribution, metabolism, and renal excretion may be altered in geriatric patients. If these changes are not considered when dosing elderly patients, preventable medication-related problems may result.

2.1. Absorption and Bioavailability

The bioavailability of a drug is defined as the fraction of drug reaching the systemic circulation after drug administration. Age-related changes in bioavailability depend on the route of drug administration, age-associated changes in the gastrointestinal tract and other organs of drug absorption, and age-associated changes in metabolism during the first pass through the liver or intestine. Despite changes in physiology with age, oral absorption and bioavailability of most drugs appear to remain unchanged in the elderly owing in part to the large functional reserve capacity of the gastrointestinal tract.

Gastric pH, gastrointestinal blood flow, active transport processes, and gastrointestinal motility have been reported to be altered in the elderly to a variable extent *(7)*. Atrophic changes in the gastric mucosa may result in decreased acid secretion. The resulting increase in gastric pH could affect the ionization and solubility of some drugs *(8)*. Decreased perfusion of the gastrointestinal tract and diminished active membrane transport processes could result in decreased rate or extent of drug absorption. These effects may be offset, however, by longer gastrointestinal transit times, with decreased gastrointestinal motility resulting in increased contact time for drug absorption *(7)*. Most drug absorption in the gastrointestinal tract occurs by passive diffusion, and the majority of studies indicate that there are no clinically significant changes in the rate or extent of drug absorption from the gastrointestinal tract.

Intragastric metabolism and hepatic first-pass metabolism may be reduced in the elderly, resulting in increased drug bioavailability. Studies with levodopa, for example, have shown that the elderly experience a threefold increase in availability of levodopa related to a reduction in gastric wall content of dopa decarboxylase *(9)*. Intestinal metabolism of verapamil, however, was well preserved in the elderly *(10)*. Drugs that undergo a high rate of first-pass metabolism, such as propranolol, demonstrate increased bioavailability owing to decreased first-pass extraction *(11)*.

Absorption and bioavailability for nonoral routes of administration (intramuscular, rectal, buccal, transdermal) and sustained release dosage forms have not been as well studied in the elderly. The rate of intramuscular absorption of antibiotics may be reduced in the elderly, but there are insufficient data to draw conclusions regarding the potential for age-related changes in drug absorption and bioavailability by these routes *(7)*.

2.2. Distribution

Age-related changes in body composition and plasma protein binding may affect drug distribution in the elderly. The elderly tend to have decreased lean body mass, increased body fat, and decreased total body water *(8)*. Interestingly, elderly individuals with high levels of physical activity are not different from those with low activity levels with respect to fat-free mass and fat mass *(12)*. Lipid-soluble drugs may show an increased volume of distribution and water-soluble drugs may show a decreased volume of distribution in elderly patients related to these changes in body composition. For example, the elderly have an approx 20% lower volume of distribution for ethanol, which distributes in body water, than young individuals *(13,14)*. Changes in body composition resulting in changes in volume of distribution may necessitate changes in loading doses of some drugs for the elderly.

Age-related changes in protein binding do not generally result in clinically significant changes in drug therapy for elderly patients. Generally, plasma protein binding of drugs remains unchanged or is decreased in the elderly. Serum albumin concentrations may be decreased in the elderly by 15–20%, but this is often related to renal dysfunction, hepatic disease, or frailty *(15)*.

2.3. Hepatic Metabolism

Hepatic metabolism is one of the major routes of drug clearance in humans. The rate and extent of hepatic drug biotransformation depend on hepatic blood flow and hepatic enzyme content, affinity, and activity rate. Hepatic inactivation of drugs and environmental toxins occurs through phase I oxidative pathways (oxidation, deamination, or hydroxylation) or phase II conjugative pathways (acetylation, glucuronidation, or sulfation). Not all pathways of hepatic drug metabolism are equally efficient. Hepatic biotransformation results in a metabolite, which may be pharmacologically active or inactive, and may be eliminated from the body or further metabolized before elimination.

Interest in potential age-associated changes in drug metabolism is significant because of the need to reduce the risk of adverse drug reactions and drug interactions in the elderly. A number of age-related changes in physiology that may impact hepatic drug metabolism in elderly patients have been reported, but the effect of age on hepatic metabolism remains controversial. Much of the literature in this area has been conflicting. Early studies attributed observed changes in drug clearance in the elderly to changes in hepatic enzyme activity, and more recently to decreased liver size and hepatic blood flow. In vitro tests of enzyme have been inconsistent with results of in vivo studies. Despite these controversies, several generally accepted principles of the affect of aging on hepatic drug metabolism have emerged.

Hepatic blood flow has been shown to decline by approx 40% with age, in parallel with a decline in cardiac output *(16,17)*. For drugs with a high hepatic extraction ratio, where clearance depends primarily on the rate of drug presentation to the liver through hepatic blood flow, aging is associated with decreased drug clearance *(16)*. Phase I oxidative metabolism of some drugs appears to decline with aging *(7,18)*, despite the fact that in vitro hepatic enzyme activity does not appear to be altered by age. Reduction in hepatic oxygen diffusion resulting from age-related changes in hepatocyte volume and surface membrane permeability and conformation is one proposed explanation for reduced oxidative drug metabolism observed with aging *(16)*. Hepatic enzymes can be inhibited and induced by drugs and other compounds. Changes in hepatic enzyme induction with aging remain controversial. Phase II conjugative metabolic pathways appear to be unchanged with aging.

When prescribing for the elderly patient, age-related changes in drug metabolism should be considered. From a pharmacokinetic point of view, drugs that are metabolized exclusively by phase II conjugative mechanisms are preferred in the elderly. For oxidatively metabolized drugs with a high extraction ratio (high clearance drugs), dosages should generally be reduced owing to decreased hepatic blood flow *(16)*. Dosages for drugs with a low extraction ratio (low clearance drugs) should be reduced as well *(16)*. After initial dosing, doses can be adjusted based on patient response and tolerability. The potential for significant drug interactions, particularly resulting from hepatic enzyme inhibition in elderly patients on multiple medications, must be carefully considered.

2.4. Renal Excretion

Altered renal elimination of drugs is the most clinically important pharmacokinetic difference between elderly and young patients. Renal clearance depends, in part, on renal blood flow, which delivers drugs and metabolites to the kidneys for elimination. Elimination from the kidneys then occurs through glomerular filtration, tubular secretion, and tubular reabsorption. With aging, renal blood flow declines as cardiac output declines, resulting in decreased glomerular filtration rate as measured by creatinine clearance in the elderly. Although there is considerable interindividual variability, declining creatinine clearance with age (about 10% per decade after age 20) is consistently reported in the literature *(7,19)*. Changes in the kidneys that occur with aging include a decrease in kidney weight, a thickening of the intrarenal vascular intima, sclerogenous changes of the glomeruli, and fibrosis and infiltration of chronic inflammatory cells in the stroma *(19)*. Altered tubular function may also be present in advanced age.

The most important aspect of renal function to monitor clinically is the glomerular filtration rate (GFR). Most decisions about drug dosing for renally excreted drugs can be made based on the estimated GFR. Clinically, creatinine clearance is used to estimate GFR.

Serum creatinine alone is not a good indicator of renal function in the elderly population because muscle mass, and therefore creatinine production, declines with age. A normal serum creatinine can result when both creatinine formation and elimination are reduced. Several algorithms have been proposed to estimate creatinine clearance. One frequently used method was developed by Cockcroft and Gault *(20)*, where creatinine clearance (CL_{cr}) is calculated based on the patient's age, weight, and serum creatinine concentration:

$$CL_{cr} = \frac{(140 - \text{age in yr}) \times \text{weight (kg)}}{72 \times \text{serum creatine (mg/100 mL)}} \tag{1}$$

For women, the result is multiplied by 0.85. This formula is less accurate for estimates in the very high or low range and when renal function is changing rapidly. For frail elderly patients with chronic muscle atrophy, an alternative formula has been proposed *(21)* that takes into account serum albumin levels as well.

For men:

$$CL_{cr} = \frac{\left\{ \left[19 \times \text{serum albumin (g/dL)} \right] + 32 \right\} \times \text{body weight (kg)}}{100 \times \text{serum creatine (mg/dL)}} \tag{2}$$

For women:

$$CL_{cr} = \frac{\left\{ \left[13 \times \text{serum albumin (g/dL)} \right] + 29 \right\} \times \text{body weight (kg)}}{100 \times \text{serum creatine (mg/dL)}} \tag{3}$$

This approach provides more accurate and less biased estimates of CL_{cr} than the Cockcroft and Gault *(20)* method in elderly patients with renal insufficiency or serum albumin levels < 2.8 g/dL.

3. EFFECTS OF AGE ON THE PHARMACOKINETICS OF CHEMOTHERAPEUTIC AGENTS

3.1. Introduction

Old age is playing an increasing role in the treatment of cancer, as the prevalence of cancer in elderly patients is high and increasing *(22)*: 60% of all cancers occur in patients aged 65 yr and above, and the elderly constitute a growing portion of the overall population, with 20% of the population expected to be > 65 yr by the year 2030.

This will lead to an increased use of anticancer agents by elderly patients. In addition to the physiological effects that aging may have on the pharmacokinetic characteristics of these agents, it has to be noted that the likelihood of polypharmacy due to noncancer, age-related chronic illnesses may lead to an increased incidence of drug–drug interactions *(23)*. Quite a few of these interactions are pharmacokinetically based, for example, inhibition of hepatic metabolism (cytochrome P450-dependent, CYP) by concurrent medications.

3.2. Examples

Previous articles *(22–28)* have reviewed the primary literature describing the effects of aging on the pharmacokinetic properties of chemotherapeutic agents. Most of these clinical studies were small, cross-sectional trials and assess plasma concentrations of the drug of interest, and in some cases, their active metabolites. A large portion of these studies reports

Table 1
General Properties of Anticancer Drugs

Drug class	Route of elimination	Dose-limiting toxicity
Antimetabolites	Renal excretion	Myelosuppression and mucositis
Alkylating agents	Hepatic metabolism and renal excretion of metabolites	Myelosuppression, cardiac, renal, CNS
Platinum analogues	Renal excretion	Renal, neurotoxicity, myelosuppression
Anthracyclines	Hepatic metabolism and biliary excretion	Cardiac
Vinca alkaloids	Hepatic metabolism and biliary excretion	Peripheral neurotoxicity
Taxanes	Hepatic metabolism and biliary excretion	Neutropenia and neurotoxicity
Camptothecins	Chemical conversion and renal or biliary excretion	Diarrhea

Adapted from ref. *26*.

changes in systemic exposure (e.g., peak plasma concentration, area under the curve, and terminal half-life) rather than more meaningful pharmacokinetic parameters such as volume of distribution, specific organ clearances, and oral bioavailability, if appropriate. Therefore, as pointed out earlier, it is sometimes difficult to assess whether physiological aging, concurrent medications or other confounding covariates are responsible for the observed age differences in systemic exposure. In addition, it is sometimes very difficult to interpret the results mechanistically, that is, what pharmacokinetic process is affected by age-related changes.

Table 1 lists the major routes of elimination and dose-limiting toxicities for commonly used classes of anticancer drugs.

Based on these general properties, Table 2 lists individual drugs whose pharmacokinetics are known to be affected by age, the likely mechanism of that age effect, and the need for dose modification in the elderly *(24–30)*. Note that f_e indicates the fraction of the total dose renally eliminated unchanged (see Subheading 2.4.).

As can be seen from Table 2, the major reason for dose modification in the elderly is the age-related impairment in renal excretory function. Therefore, Table 3 illustrates the dose modifications based on renal function for selected anticancer agents (see Subheading 2.3.).

Overall, it is apparent that age-related renal impairment is the major cause of dose modifications in the elderly, and the (estimated) creatinine clearance serves as a good predictor for a patient-individualized dosing regimen. Apparent age-related effects on hepatic metabolism/biliary excretion have been observed, but usually do not lead to dose adjustments. Age-related effects on absorption are rare since most agents are given intravenously, while age effects on drug distribution are difficult to observe and are unlikely to result in dose modifications.

This overall conclusion may change in the future when cancer treatment will involve chemoprevention and disease modification, with the agents given orally and less likely to be

Table 2
Age Effects on the Pharmacokinetics of Specific Anticancer Drugs

Drug	Mechanism of age effect	Dose modification
Antimetabolites		
Methotrexate	Renal elimination (f_e: 44–100%)	Yes
5-FU in the presence of a DPD inhibitor only	Renal elimination (f_e: 77%)	Yes
Fludarabine	Renal elimination (f_e: 60%)	Yes
Gemcitabine	Hepatic metabolism	No
Alkylating agents		
Ifosfamide	Distribution into body fat reduced	No
Melphalan	Renal elimination	Yes
Platinum compounds		
Cisplatin	Renal elimination (f_e: 90%)	Yes
Carboplatin	Renal elimination (f_e: 100%)	Yes
Oxaliplatin	Renal elimination	No, severe renal failure only
Anthracyclines		
Idarubicine	Accumulation of renally eliminated metabolites	Yes (ref. 29)
Mitoxantrone	Hepatic metabolism (f_e: 10%)	No, hepatic failure only
Vinca alkaloids		
Vinblastine	Hepatic metabolism	Yes (ref. 28)
Vinorelbine	Biliary excretion	No, severe hepatic failure only
Taxanes		
Paclitaxel	Hepatic metabolism	No, but potential for drug inter-
Docetaxel	(CYP3A4)	actions; severe hepatic failure
Topoisomerase inhibitors		
Topotecan	Renal elimination (f_e: 30%)	No, moderate/severe renal failure only
Irinotecan	Metabolism/biliary excretion of active metabolite (SN38)	No
Etoposide	Renal elimination	Yes

Table 3
Dose Modification Algorithms for Selected Drugs Based on Renal Function

	Renal function (creatinine clearance)		
Drug	<60 mL/min	<45 mL/min	<30 mL/min
Bleomycin	0.70	0.60	Unknown
Carboplatin	Use Calvert formula based on glomerular filtration rate.		
Carmustin	0.80	0.75	Unknown
Cisplatin	0.75	0.50	Unknown
Cytarabine	0.80	0.50	Unknown
Dacarbazine	0.80	0.75	0.65
Fludarabine	0.80	0.75	0.65
Ifosfamide	0.80	0.75	0.70
Melphalan	0.65	0.50	Unknown
Methotrexate	0.85	0.75	0.70

Adapted from ref. 25.
The values listed indicate the dose-multiple relative to a standard dose for a patient with normal renal function, for example, 0.75 means 75% of the standard dose.

renally eliminated. Furthermore, owing to polypharmacy the likelihood of clinically significant drug–drug interactions at the level of drug absorption, first-pass, and systemic metabolism will increase.

REFERENCES

1. Kinirons MT, Crome P. Clinical pharmacokinetic considerations in the elderly: an update. Clin Pharmacokinet 1997; 33:302–312.
2. Holliday, R. Understanding Ageing. Cambridge, UK: Cambridge University Press, 1995.
3. Federal Register. Tuesday, August 2, 1994; 59(102):39398–39400.
4. Hanlon JT, Schmader KE, Ruby CM, Weinberger M. Suboptimal prescribing in older inpatients and outpatients. J Am Geriatr Soc 2001; 49:200–209.
5. Cohen JS. Dose discrepancies between the Physicians' Desk Reference and the medical literature and their possible role in the high incidence of dose-related adverse drug events. Arch Intern Med 2001; 161:957–964.
6. Abernethy DR, Azarnoff DL. Pharmacokinetic investigations in elderly patients: clinical and ethical considerations. Clin Pharmacokinet 1990; 19:88–93.
7. Schwartz JB: Clinical pharmacology. In: Hazzard WR, Blass JP, Ettinger WH, Halter JB, Ouslander JG (eds). Principles of Geriatric Medicine and Gerontology, 4th Edit. New York, NY: McGraw-Hill, 1999.
8. Hämmerlein A, Derendorf H, Lowenthal DT. Pharmacokinetic and pharmacodynamic changes in the elderly: clinical implications. Clin Pharmacokinet 1998; 35:49–64.
9. Evans M, Triggs E, Broe G, et al. Systemic availability of orally administered L-dopa in the elderly parkinsonian patient. Eur J Clin Pharmacol 1980; 17:215–221.
10. Klotz U. Effect of age on pharmacokinetics and pharmacodynamics in man. Int J Clin Pharmacol Ther 1998; 36:581–585.
11. Casteldon C, George C. The effect of aging on the hepatic clearance of propranolol. Br J Clin Pharmacol 1979; 7:49–54.
12. Westerterp KR, Meijer EP. Physical activity and parameters of aging: a physiological perspective. J Gerontol 2001; 56A (Special Issue [Pt II]):7–12.
13. Vestal RE, McGuire EA, Tobin JD, et al. Aging and ethanol metabolism. Clin Pharmacol Ther 1976; 21:343–354.
14. Pozzato G, Moretti M, Franzin F, et al. Ethanol metabolism and aging: the role of "first pass metabolism" and gastric alcohol dehydrogenase activity. J Gerontol 1995; 50A:B135–B141.
15. Grandison MK, Boudinot FD. Age-related changes in protein binding of drugs: implications for therapy. Clin Pharmacokinet 2000; 38:271–290.
16. Le Couteur DG, McLean AJ. The aging liver: drug clearance and an oxygen diffusion barrier hypothesis. Clin Pharmacokinet 1998; 34:359–373.
17. Durnas C, Loi CM, Cusack BJ. Hepatic drug metabolism and aging. Clin Pharmacokinet 1990; 19:359–389.
18. Sotaniemi EA, Arranto AJ, Pelkonen O, Pasanen M. Age and cytochrome P450-linked drug metabolism in humans: an analysis of 226 subjects with equal histopathologic conditions. Clin Pharmacol Ther 1997; 61:331–339.
19. Mühlberg W, Platt D. Age-dependent changes of the kidneys: pharmacological implications. Gerontology 1999; 45:243–253.
20. Cockcroft DW, Gault MH. Prediction of creatinine clearance from serum creatinine. Nephron 1976; 16:31–41.
21. Sanaka M, Kikuo T, Shimakura K, Koike Y, Mineshita S. Serum albumin for estimating creatinine clearance in the elderly with muscle atrophy. Nephron 1996; 73:137–144.
22. Balducci L, Extermann M. A practical approach to the older patient with cancer. Curr Prob Cancer 2001;25(1):6–76.
23. Vestal RE. Aging and pharmacology. Cancer 1997; 80:1302–1310.
24. Lichtman SM, Villani G. Chemotherapy in the elderly: pharmacologic considerations. Cancer Cont 2000; 7:548–556.
25. Lichtman SM, Skirvin JA. Pharmacology of antineoplastic agents in older cancer patients. Oncology 2000; 14:1743–1752.
26. Baker SD, Grochow LB. Pharmacology of cancer chemotherapy in the older person. Clin Geriatr Med 1997; 13:169–183.

27. Sekine I, Fukuda H, Kunitoh H, Saijo N. Cancer chemotherapy in the elderly. Jpn J Clin Onc 1995; 28:463–473.

28. Balducci L, Corcoran MB. Antineoplastic chemotherapy of the older cancer patient. Hematol Oncol Clin North Am 2000; 14:193–212.

29. Leoni F, Ciolli S, Giulianin G, et al. Attenuated-dose idarubicin in acute myeloid leukaemia of the elderly: pharmacokinetic study and clinical results. Br J Haematol 1995; 90:169–174.

30. Bonetti A, Franceschi T, Apostoli P, et al. Cisplatin pharmacokinetics in elderly patients. Ther Drug Monit 1994; 16:477–482.

26   The Combination of Angiogenesis Inhibitors and Radiotherapy for the Treatment of Primary Tumors

Kevin Camphausen, MD *and Cynthia Ménard,* MD

CONTENTS

1. INTRODUCTION

There were about 1.2 million nonskin cancers diagnosed in North America in 2002. Conventional cancer therapeutic regimens include surgery, chemotherapy, and radiotherapy. Modern oncology has brought immunotherapy, hyperthermia, cryotherapy, radiofrequency ablation, and molecularly targeted drug therapy to the investigational front. Historically, these therapies have been focused on tumor cell kill. More recently, however, cancer research has begun to examine the permissive environment in which the cancer cell survives. This has led to extensive research in the fields of invasion and metastases, extracellular matrix biology, and angiogenesis. Some of the most powerful antitumor agents include molecules in that inhibit angiogenesis. It is the objective of this chapter to review the evidence and rationale for treating primary tumors with a combined regimen of angiogenesis inhibitors and radiotherapy *(1)*.

2. THE TWO-CELL COMPARTMENT MODEL OF TUMORS

Angiogenesis is the growth of blood vessels that are necessary for the progression and survival of tumors *(2)*. Most solid tumors begin as an avascular nodule, and remain < 1–2 mm

Handbook of Anticancer Pharmacokinetics and Pharmacodynamics
Edited by: W. D. Figg and H. L. McLeod © Humana Press Inc., Totowa, NJ

in diameter. Nutrients are supplied and wastes are removed by passive diffusion. A permissive environment allows an angiogenic "switch," whereby a previously dormant tumor becomes vascularized by undergoing this process termed angiogenesis (3). The newly vascularized tumor can be conceptualized as a two-compartment model (4). The tumor cells receive nutrients and survival factors from the vasculature, and the endothelium receives stimulus from the tumor, for example, vascular endothelial growth factor (VEGF), for endothelial proliferation and migration. To achieve tumor "cure" one of two things must happen: either the tumor cells or the supporting stromal cells must be targeted. Endothelial cell kill can lead to tumor cell death through starvation. Combination therapy directed against either compartment theoretically should lead to more successful cure rates.

This two-compartment model, in which the endothelial cell supports the tumor cell, led to the discovery of a class of compounds called angiogenesis inhibitors. There are multiple subclasses of antiangiogenic agents including growth factor inhibitors such as VEGF blockers, small molecules including thalidomide and TNP-470, and natural protein fragments such as angiostatin. Many naturally produced angiogenesis inhibitors are fragments of larger proteins that are normally intimately involved with the vasculature. For example, angiostatin is a fragment of plasminogen, endostatin is a fragment of collagen XVIII, and antiangiogenic antithrombin III is a fragment of antithrombin III (5–7). These drugs are highly potent, work against a variety of tumor types, and are minimally toxic in preclinical animal trials.

3. CHANGING VIEWS OF THE RADIOTHERAPY TARGET

Radiation therapy has been used for more than 100 yr in the treatment of cancer. The "radiation effect" against tumor cells is conventionally thought to occur through DNA damage caused by ionizing radiation, resulting in reproductive cell death. With fractionated regimens, tumor cells are more sensitive to radiation than normal tissues (8). Radiation-induced side effects and complications are thought to result from unrepaired DNA damage within normal cells. For example, acute radiation damage to the small intestine is thought to result from DNA damage in epithelial stem cells located in the intestinal crypts of Lieberkühn.

A recent article by Paris et al. challenges this hypothesis. By using supratherapeutic doses of radiotherapy, they demonstrated that endothelial apoptosis leads to secondary gut stem cell apoptosis (9). Therefore, the target for radiation-induced small bowel toxicity was the gut endothelium and not the gut epithelial stem cell. This effect could be abrogated by the administration of basic fibroblast growth factor, acting as an endothelial survival factor, which prevented endothelial cell apoptosis. The authors also demonstrated that in a transgenic knockout mouse model of acid sphingomyelinase, in which the endothelium is resistant to radiation-induced apoptosis, the gut epithelial stem cells survived a larger dose of radiation before undergoing apoptosis. In this transgenic mouse model, in which the normal signaling pathways in endothelial cells were altered, the gut endothelium and not the intestinal epithelial stem cell pool was the primary target for acute radiation-induced gastrointestinal syndrome.

Targeting of the endothelium with radiotherapy is not a new idea. In 1982 Denekamp described the differential proliferation rates between the endothelial cells found in tumors and those found in normal tissues (10). The tumor endothelium had a proliferation rate 20 times greater than the proliferation rate of the normal vasculature. The proliferating endothelium seemed to be a perfect target for an emerging technology at the time, radiolabeled monoclonal antibodies (MAbs). MAbs against antigens found on proliferating endothelial cells would allow a very high dose of radiation to be selectively targeted to the tumor endothelium. As yet, MAbs have had limited success in the clinic in part due to their large size and heterogeneous distribution. Modern techniques utilizing phage display technology are now being used to the discover receptors or antigens that might be differentially expressed between tumor endothelium and normal endothelium (11). The identification of such a differential expression could lead to novel molecular therapeutic strategies specifically targeted to tumor endothelial cells.

4. THE ENDOTHELIUM AS A TARGET FOR ANGIOGENESIS INHIBITORS

As early as 1971, publications by Folkman emphasized that tumors need a constant blood supply to survive. Early work was successful at finding a stimulator of angiogenesis, termed tumor angiogenesis factor (TAF) (12), but much effort was spent on isolating and characterizing a tumor-derived inhibitor of angiogenesis. The key to finding this inhibitor was the observation of a unique clinical pattern of metastases in 10–15% of all surgical patients (13). A patient with this pattern of metastases would have a primary tumor without evidence of metastases but following surgery would demonstrate an immediate and rapid growth of previously undetectable metastases. If the primary tumor was producing an inhibitor of angiogenesis, and the removal of the primary tumor resulted in the growth of metastases, then the inhibitor should be detectable in either urine or blood.

It was this model that O'Reilly and colleagues studied with the Lewis lung carcinoma cell line. By selecting a tumor cell line variant that suppressed growth of its own metastases, they had selected a tumor cell line that was producing an inhibitor of angiogenesis. After many years of work and laboratory analysis from hundreds of liters of mouse urine, a protein was purified that could inhibit endothelial cell proliferation in vitro and prevent the growth of the metastases in vivo when given exogenously. This protein was called angiostatin, a fragment of the larger molecule plasminogen (5). The unique and significant feature of this molecule was its ability to inhibit endothelial cell proliferation (in three different endothelial cell lines) without inhibiting the proliferation of nonendothelial cells (nine different cell lines tested).

Finding an inhibitor of angiogenesis that was a fragment of a larger molecule already found within the vasculature gave credence to the hypothesis that angiogenesis, even in tumors, is a highly regulated process. This process is also quite complex, as demonstrated in attempts to elucidate the mechanism of angiostatin production from plasminogen. Other molecules, which were thought to be strictly involved in cellular invasion and metastases, such as metalloelastase and matrix metalloproteinase-2, have now been implicated in the production of angiostatin (14,15).

It is with a similar experimental method, in this case using a hemangioendothelioma cell line that suppressed the growth of its own metastases, that O'Reilly was able to purify another inhibitor of angiogenesis, endostatin (6). Endostatin, a fragment of collagen XVIII, is a specific inhibitor of endothelial cell proliferation and has little effect on the proliferation of six other nonendothelial cell lines. The production of endostatin from its precursor molecule can be regulated by either elastase or cathepsin-L (16,17). A wide range of other molecules have now been identified as having antiangiogenic properties. To be classified in this category, a molecule must inhibit endothelial proliferation in more than one of the standard assays: endothelial cell proliferation, chick chorioallantoic membrane assay, matrigel migration assay, or corneal micropocket assay, while not inhibiting the proliferation of other nonendothelial cell lines.

5. COMBINATION OF RADIATION AND ANTIANGIOGENIC THERAPY: IMPACT ON LOCAL CONTROL OF PRIMARY TUMORS

The oxygen effect on the radioresistance of hypoxic tumor cells has been well demonstrated (8). It may be counterintuitive to some that the use of antiangiogenic therapy may augment local control with radiotherapy. Classic dogma teaches that if the tumor bed is rendered more hypoxic with antiangiogenic therapy, then the tumor cells must be less radiosensitive. Generating hypoxia with antiangiogenic therapies may select cancer cells that have acquired hypoxia resistance and have a higher metastatic and invasive potential. Paradoxically, three preclinical studies have shown that the treatment of tumors with antiangiogenic drugs actually increases the tumor partial pressure of oxygen (pO_2) (18–20).

In 1992, Teicher published the seminal paper describing a combination of antiangiogenic therapy and radiotherapy against a primary tumor (18,21). She demonstrated, in a tumor growth delay study, that the combination of minocycline (a weak metalloproteinase inhibitor), TNP-470, and radiotherapy was superadditive against Lewis lung carcinoma cells in mice. The growth delay observed with radiotherapy alone was 4.4 d while the delay with combination therapy was 12.6 d ($p < 0.0001$). These results triggered a paradigm shift in the rationale for combining antiangiogenic therapy with radiotherapy.

Why do we see this greater than additive effect? Radiotherapy can reduce the number of 5–15 µm diameter vessels in a dose-dependent fashion with no change in the tumor volume (22). Yet, the numbers of 20–50 µm diameter vessels are unchanged. This has led to speculation that although the quantity of the vessels has decreased, the quality, as measured by oxygen carrying capacity, has actually increased (20). Anti-VEGF therapy has also been shown to decrease microvessel density and tumor interstitial fluid pressure, yet increase the measured pO_2 (20). Therefore, the combination of radiotherapy and antiangiogenic therapy may result in more oxygenated and radiosensitive tumors.

6. ANGIOSTATIN OR ENDOSTATIN AND RADIOTHERAPY

The surprising results presented by Teicher, combined with the high potency and low toxicity of naturally occurring antiangiogenic protein fragments, led to the experimental combination of radiotherapy and angiostatin by Weichselbaum's group at the University of Chicago (23). They treated four different tumor cell lines, one mouse and three human, with a dose of angiostatin that reduced the tumor volume by 38%. When they combined angiostatin with radiotherapy, they observed an additive effect. Tumor volume reduction was greater than with either angiostatin or radiotherapy alone. When the tumors were examined histologically, microvessel density was lower in tumors treated with combination therapy, compared to either angiostatin or radiation treatments alone. They concluded that radiotherapy and angiostatin both targeted the tumor endothelium in an additive fashion.

The same group followed up on this early work by looking at the timing of angiostatin administration when used in combination with radiotherapy (24). In this case, they gave angiostatin in three different combination schedules with radiotherapy. Radiotherapy was given on d 0 and 1 and angiostatin was given on d 0 and 1, d 0–13, or d 2–13. They were able to demonstrate that concurrent schedules resulted in a greater effect than sequential administrations. It was also interesting to note that in the two groups that received concurrent angiostatin administrations, similar tumor growth inhibition was observed. Adjuvant administration of angiostatin alone had no effect, consistent with a radiosensitizing mechanism of action.

Later experiments with recombinant endostatin confirmed a significant benefit to combination therapy compared to either modality alone. It was also demonstrated, similar to their results with angiostatin, that the microvessel density in endostatin-treated mice was 40 vessels/area vs 14 vessels/area in endostatin plus radiotherapy treated mice.

7. VEGF INHIBITION AND RADIOTHERAPY

VEGF, or vascular permeability factor, is a heparin binding angiogenic growth factor that was first discovered by Dvorak in 1983 *(25)*. VEGF can stimulate endothelial cells to proliferate or migrate through its interaction with VEFGR-1 (flt-1) or VEGFR-2 (KDR/flk-1) and is up-regulated by hypoxia *(26)*. This VEGF up-regulation by hypoxia is mediated through an up-regulation of hypoxia-inducible factor 1 (HIF-1), which binds upstream of the VEGF promoter *(18)*.

The first study using an anti-VEGF drug in combination with radiotherapy was published in 1999, in this case with a soluble antibody against VEGF-165 *(27)*. VEGF levels in irradiated tumors were three- to fourfold higher than in nonirradiated controls as measured by enzyme-linked immunosorbent assay (ELISA) and Northern blotting. In four separate tumor model experiments, the investigators were able to demonstrate a more significant tumor growth delay with combined therapy compared to either anti-VEGF therapy or radiotherapy alone. This group concluded that radiation up-regulates endothelial cell production of VEGF which in turn acts as a survival factor, and that VEGF inhibition counters this survival effect.

Another group of investigators were able to demonstrate a similar effect in 2000 *(20)*. Using a MAb against human VEGF, they measured several interesting tumor parameters including microvessel density (MVD), pO_2, and interstitial fluid pressure (IFP). They hypothesized that anti-VEGF therapy should decrease IFP resulting in radiosensitization. Results indeed showed a significant reduction in MVD (36–60%) and IFP (approx 75%), and an increase in pO_2 with anti-VEGF therapy compared to controls. The increase in pO_2 may have been due to an improvement in the quality of oxygen delivery, partly owing to a decreased IFP.

Their subsequent work investigated the effects of a VEGF-receptor blocking peptide, DC101, on tumor control probability in combination with radiotherapy *(28)*. For each cell line tested, they observed an additive effect. Surprisingly, tumor oxygen levels measured with an Eppendorf polarographic probe did not reveal a change in pO_2. One should note that although both studies were performed by the same group of investigators, different experimental techniques were employed, which could account for the difference seen in pO_2 measurements. It is interesting to speculate that inhibition of VEGF receptor binding with a peptide and antibody binding of the VEGF-R may result in different physiological effects.

A second and possibly more appealing method of inhibiting VEGF-R is to block the tyrosine kinase (TK) portion of the receptor with a small molecule such as SU-5416, SU-6668, or PTK787/ZK222548 *(29)*. These small molecules have been shown in mouse tumor models to have significant antitumor effect *(30,31)*. They have also been found to act synergistically with radiotherapy *(32)*. The first paper addressing this question tested SU5416, a TK inhibitor specific for flk-1 (K_i of 0.16 μM) in combination with radiotherapy. Several parameters were measured, including vascular ultrasound (US) measurements, tumor window measurements, and tumor growth delay. They found that combined therapy with SU5416 decreased the number and length of vessels measured in the dorsal chamber window, which correlated with the drop in US flow measurements. They also found a greater than additive effect in tumor growth delay with combined therapy compared to either SU5416 or radiotherapy alone.

These results were confirmed by two additional groups, using both SU5416 and SU6668, a broader TK antagonist of VEGF, fibroblast growth factor (FGF), and platelet-derived growth factor (PDGF) *(19,33)*. Both groups found a greater than additive effect on tumor growth delay with combined therapy using SU6668, and one group confirmed an increase in pO_2 after treatment with SU6668. Furthermore, SU6668 was found to have a greater therapeutic effect than SU5416 by almost doubling the tumor growth delay from 6.5 d to 11.9 d. The authors speculated that this more pronounced effect might be due to the inhibition of multiple growth factor receptors with SU6668 compared to the more specific inhibition of VEGF-R with SU5416.

By examining the entire anti-VEGF strategy, several general conclusions can be drawn. The first is that combination therapy with VEGF inhibitors is more effective than radio-therapy alone. The second is that the effect appears to be at least partly due to an elevation in pO_2, which may be mediated through a change in MVD and/or IFP. As VEGF is a growth factor that is up-regulated by radiotherapy and acting as a survival factor for endothelial cells, it is plausible that VEGF-R inhibition results in blockade of this survival signal, leading to a greater radiation effect.

8. COMBINATION THERAPY TO ADDRESS MICROMETASTATIC DISEASE OUTSIDE THE RADIATION FIELD

Angiostatin and endostatin cure tumors in mice, and early Phase I clinical trials demonstrate little toxicity; however, they also demonstrate little efficacy. It is currently felt by the oncology community that antiangiogenic agents, as a class, are cytostatic and not cytotoxic. This accounts for the very low toxicity observed thus far. Therefore, to reap the most benefit from a cytostatic agent, one needs to combine these compounds with cytotoxic agents such as radiotherapy.

An alternate explanation for the lack of efficacy in the early trials is that cytostatic agents are not effective in a widely metastatic setting, which is the cohort of patients so far recruited to Phase I trials. Another patient cohort theoretically worthy of investigation would be locally controlled patients who have a high risk of distant failure. For example, a patient with limited stage small-cell lung cancer has a 30% risk of brain metastasis after complete regression of his or her thoracic disease. In such a patient, antiangiogenic agents could be administered following successful primary therapy and followed for a change in the incidence of growth of already metastatic microscopic disease.

9. IMAGING ANGIOGENESIS

The rapidly proliferating endothelium is an appealing target for antiangiogenic therapy and for molecular imaging techniques *(34,35)*. As the number of compounds targeting the endothelium continues to increase, the need for noninvasively monitoring tumor microvasculature is becoming more critical. Multiple modalities including US, computed tomography (CT), magnetic resonance imaging (MRI), and radionuclide imaging such as positron emission tomography (PET) are currently being investigated to image the tumor microvasculature and the endothelium. US, CT, and MRI make use of the differences in vascular flow and permeability between normal and tumor tissues utilizing Doppler color images and/or contrast materials *(36,37)*. MRI and PET scanning can potentially image very specific molecules engineered to bind to endothelial cells *(38)*. Clinical trials that investigate antiangiogenic treatments should consider incorporating a detailed imaging protocol as part of the evaluation process, especially in the context of radiation therapy which is always designed and delivered with image reference.

10. CONCLUSION

Classic tumor biology has focused on a method of damaging malignant cells to eradicate tumors. As the fields of angiogenesis and vascular biology mature, new drugs with new targets can be investigated in combination with classical therapies. Antiangiogenic strategies focus on inhibiting the proliferation of endothelial cells, while antivascular strategies target more mature vascular structures. Each field perceives the support structure of a tumor as a potential site of intervention. It should be remembered that antiangiogenic and antivascular treatments are not mutually exclusive and will likely be used in combination in the future.

A thorough review of the literature has shown that many antiangiogenic agents administered concurrently with radiotherapy result in synergistic cell killing. Early warnings of a theoretical disadvantage to this combined approach due to hypoxia have been disproved. However, much still needs to be learned in both preclinical and clinical trials. For example, timing of drug administration, duration of drug exposure, and combination antiangiogenic drug therapies must be investigated. Of concern is that there are no data concerning the late effects in normal tissues of antiangiogenic agents alone or in combination with radiotherapy. Future clinical studies should address this important issue and closely monitor untoward normal tissue late effects.

REFERENCES

1. Camphausen K, Menard C. Angiogenesis inhibitors and radiotherapy of primary tumors. Expert Opin Biol Ther 2002; 2:477–481.
2. Folkman J. Tumor angiogenesis: therapeutic implications. N Engl J Med 1971; 285:1182–1186.
3. Fang J, Shing Y, Wiederschain D, et al. Matrix metalloproteinase-2 is required for the switch to the angiogenic phenotype in a tumor model. Proc Natl Acad Sci 2000; 97:3884–3889.
4. Folkman J. Tumor angiogenesis. In: Holland JF, Frei E, Bast R, et al. (eds). Cancer Medicine. Baltimore, MD: Williams & Wilkins, 1996, pp. 181–204.
5. O'Reilly MS, Holmgren L, Shing Y, et al. Angiostatin: a novel angiogenisis inhibitor that mediates the suppression of metastases by Lewis lung carcinoma. Cell 1994; 79:315–328.
6. O'Reilly MS, Boehm T, Shing Y, et al. Endostatin: an endogenous inhibitor of angiogenesis and tumor growth. Cell 1997; 88:277–285.
7. O'Reilly M, et al. Antiangiogenic activity of the cleaved conformation of the serpin antithrombin. Science 1999; 285:1926–1928.
8. Hall E. Radiobiology for the Radiologist, 5th Edit. Philadelphia, PA: Lippincott, Williams & Wilkins, 2000, p. 588.
9. Paris F, Fuks Z, Kang A, et al. Endothelial apoptosis as the primary lesion initiating intestinal radiation damage in mice. Science 2001; 293:293–297.
10. Denekamp J. Endothelial cell proliferation as a novel approach to targeting tumour therapy. Br J Cancer 1982; 45:136–141.
11. Arap W. Targeting the prostate for destruction through a vascular address. Proc Natl Acad Sci USA 2002; 99:1527–1531.
12. Folkman J. Tumor angiogenesis factor. Cancer Res 1974; 34:2109–2113.
13. Folkman J. Angiogenesis in cancer, vascular, rheumatoid and other disease. Nat Med 1995; 1:27–31.
14. Dong Z, Kumar R, Yang X, Fidler IJ. Macrophage-derived metalloelastase is responsible for the generation of angiostatin in Lewis lung carcinoma. Cell 1997; 88:801–810.
15. O'Reilly MS, Wiederschain D, Stetler-Stevenson WG, Folkman J, Moses MA. Regulation of angiostatin production by matrix metalloproteinase-2 in a model of concomitant resistance. J Biol Chem 1999; 274:29,568–29,571.
16. Wen W, Moses MA, Wiederschain D, Arbiser JL, Folkman J. The generation of endostatin is mediated by elastase. Cancer Res 1999; 59:6052–6056.
17. Felbor U, Dreier L, Bryant RA, Ploegh HL, Olsen BR, Mothes W. Secreted cathepsin L generates endostatin from collagen XVIII. Eur Mol Biol Org J 2000; 19:1187–1194.

18. Teicher B, et al. Antiangiogenic agents can increase tumor oxygenation and response to radiation therapy. Radiat Oncol Invest 1995; 2:269–276.
19. Griffin RJ, Williams BW, Wild R, Cherrington JM, Park H, Song CW. Simultaneous inhibition of the receptor kinase activity of vascular endothelial, fibroblast, and platelet-derived growth factors suppresses tumor growth and enhances tumor radiation responses. Cancer Res 2002; 62:1702–1706.
20. Lee CG, Heijn M, di Tomaso E, et al. Anti-vascular endothelial growth factor treatment augments tumor radiation response under normoxic or hypoxic conditions. Cancer Res 2000; 60:5565–5570.
21. Teicher BA, Holden SA, Ara G, et al. Potentiation of cytotoxic cancer therapies by TNP-470 alone and with other anti-angiogenic agents. Int J Cancer 1994; 57:920–925.
22. Solesvik O, Rofstad E, Brustad T. Vascular changes in a human malignant melanoma xenograft following single-dose irradiation. Radiat Res 1984; 98:115–128.
23. Mauceri HJ, Hanna NN, Beckett MA, et al. Combined effects of angiostatin and ionizing radiation in antitumor therapy. Nature 1998; 394:287–291.
24. Gorski DH, Mauceri HJ, Salloum RM, et al. Potentiation of the antitumor effect of ionizing radiation by brief concomitant exposures to angiostatin. Cancer Res 1998; 58:5686–5689.
25. Senger DR, Galli SJ, Dvorak AM, Perruzzi CA, Harvey VS, Dvorak HF. Tumor cells secrete a vascular permeability factor that promotes accumulation of ascites fluid. Science 1983; 219:1296–1299.
26. Neufeld G, Cohen T, Gengrinovitch S, Poltorak Z. Vascular endothelial growth factor (VEGF) and its receptors. FASEB J 1999; 13:9–22.
27. Gorski DH, Beckett MA, Jaskowiak NT, et al. Blockade of the vascular endothelial growth factor stress response increases the antitumor effects of ionizing radiation. Cancer Res 1999; 59:3374–3378.
28. Kozin SV, Boucher Y, Hicklin DJ, Bohlen P, Jain RK, Suit HD. Vascular endothelial growth factor receptor-2-blocking antibody potentiates radiation-induced long-term control of human tumor xenografts. Cancer Res 2001; 61:39–44.
29. Hennequin LF, Thomas AP, Johnstone C, et al. Design and structure–activity relationship of a new class of potent VEGF receptor tyrosine inhibitors. J Med Chem 1999; 42:5369–5389.
30. Shaheen RM, Davis DW, Liu W, et al. Antiangiogenic therapy targeting the tyrosine kinase receptor for vascular endothelial growth factor receptor inhibits the growth of colon cancer liver metastasis and induces tumor and endothelial cell apoptosis. Cancer Res 1999; 59:5412–5416.
31. Shaheen RM, Tseng WW, Davis DW, et al. Tyrosine kinase inhibition of multiple angiogenic growth factor receptors improves survival in mice bearing colon cancer liver metastases by inhibition of endothelial cell survival mechanisms. Cancer Res 2001; 61:1464–1468.
32. Geng L, Donnelly E, McMahon G, et al. Inhibition of vascular endothelial growth factor receptor signaling leads to reversal of tumor resistance to radiotherapy. Cancer Res 2001; 61:2413–2419.
33. Ning S, Laird D, Cherrington JM, Knox SJ. The antiangiogenic agents SU5416 and SU6668 increase the antitumor effects of fractionated irradiation. Radiat Res 2002; 157:45–51.
34. Denekamp J. Vascular attack as a therapeutic strategy for cancer. Cancer Metastasis Reviews 1990; 9: 267–282.
35. Tatum J, Hoffman J. Role of imaging in clinical trials of antiangiogenesis therapy in oncology. Acad Radiol 2000; 7:798–799.
36. Cheng WF, Lee CN, Chu JS, et al. Vascularity index as a novel parameter for the in vivo assessment of angiogenesis in patients with cervical carcinoma. Cancer 1999; 85:651–657.
37. Miles K. Tumor angiogenesis and its relation to contrast enhancement on computed tomography: a review. Eur J Radiol 1999; 30:198–205.
38. Sipkins DA, Cheresh DA, Kazemi MR, Nevin LM, Bednarski MD, Li KC. Detection of tumor angiogenesis in vivo by alphaV-beta3 targeted magnetic resonance imaging. Nat Med 1998; 4:623–626.

27 Gene Therapy for the Treatment of Cancer

H. Trent Spencer, PhD and Jacques Galipeau, MD

CONTENTS

1. INTRODUCTION

Since the initial confirmation that genetic alterations cause disease, the pervasive outlook has been that the future for gene therapy is very promising, but curing diseases by the transfer of specific nucleic acid sequences has been problematic. It should be recognized, however, that the hurdles facing investigators in the field of gene therapy can be defined and are likely not insurmountable. The major limitations facing gene therapy investigators are the inability to genetically modify sufficient numbers of target cells and the inability to express the transferred gene(s) over prolonged periods *(1,2)*. With respect to the application of gene therapy for the treatment of cancer, in many aspects the fundamental cause of these hurdles is not different than those faced by pioneers of other treatments, for example, in the development of chemotherapy agents, which is mainly a lack of understanding of the biological systems being manipulated. Even so, great strides and accomplishments have been achieved during the last decade, not only with respect to the physical transfer of genes into target cells but also in the clinical practice of gene therapy *(3)*. The purpose of this chapter is to provide a general background on how genes are transferred as well as a specific example focusing on the translation of a gene therapy study from inception through a completed Phase III clinical trial.

Although it was initially envisioned that gene therapy would be used to cure monogenetic inherited disorders, numerous ingenious applications have been developed to treat a wide variety of diseases. As of September 2001, there are more than 600 gene therapy clinical trials registered worldwide (www.wiley.co.uk/genetherapy/clinical). Of these more than 60% are focused on cancer as the target illness and have enrolled more than 2300 patients (Fig. 1). Classic gene therapy strategies seeking to reprogram tumor cells in vivo by direct

Handbook of Anticancer Pharmacokinetics and Pharmacodynamics
Edited by: W. D. Figg and H. L. McLeod © Humana Press Inc., Totowa, NJ

transgene delivery are now being complemented by a growing array of studies exploring the use of engineered autologous immunocompetent cells, engineered oncolytic viruses, cancer vaccines, and others, as biopharmaceuticals. When compared with mature fields of cancer clinical research, gene therapy is rich in potential but weak in accomplishments. This is reflected by the very high proportion of Phase I and Phase II studies (>550) underway worldwide, with fewer than 2% of all trials being Phase III. Interestingly, the first human gene therapy trial, performed in May of 1989, involved the treatment of melanoma *(4)*; a year later a second trial was initiated that was designed to treat the genetic defect of adenosine deaminase deficiency.

2. GENE TRANSFER TECHNIQUES

A hope for gene therapy is to be able to supply a physician with a vial containing material that can easily be administered and that efficiently alters cellular functions by incorporating new genetic sequences. Although this scenario is far from reality, the transfer of genetic material is currently accomplished using a variety of techniques, with the majority of transfer techniques being classified as either viral or nonviral delivery systems, both of which are being developed for the treatment of cancer. There are also many strategies that are under development to target specific cells for genetic modification, which can be classified as (1) systemic in vivo administration of the genetic delivery system; (2) *in situ* delivery, in which the material is delivered only to a local area, such as a tumor; and (3) ex vivo delivery, in which target cells are removed from the affected patient or from a suitable donor and genetically modified before reinfusion into the patient. The number of ideas conceived to treat cancer using gene transfer techniques is astounding. The majority of these investigations can be grouped into one of the following categories:

1. Transfer of genes into target cells that affect drug sensitivity:

    a. Confer protection to chemotherapy-sensitive noncancerous tissues by transferring genes that encode drug-resistance proteins. The encoded proteins serve to protect the sensitive tissues and thereby allow for altered dosing, and possibly more aggressive treatment, of chemotherapy agents.
    b. Transfer of genes into cancerous tissues that confer drug sensitivity to the modified cells. The encoded proteins serve to sensitize cancer cells to specific drugs that increase the selectivity of chemotherapy.

2. Transfer of genes into cancer cells that inhibit or alter specific cellular functions:

    a. Transfer of genes that encode complementary nucleic acid sequences that can hybridize to specific RNA sequences and block the expression of cancer-promoting gene products.
    b. Transfer of genes that encode antibodies that specifically recognize proteins critical to tumor cell proliferation.
    c. Transfer of genes that encode proteins that replace or augment missing gene products of tumor suppressor genes.

3. Transfer of genes that affect the immune response against cancer cells:

    a. Transfer of genes that encode missing or down-regulated costimulatory molecules into cancer cells for the purpose of increasing the immune recognition of cancer cells.
    b. Transfer of genes that encode proteins uniquely expressed or overexpressed in cancer cells into antigen-presenting cells to activate cytotoxic T cells against the cancer.
    c. Transfer of genes that encode specific cytokines that stimulate an immune response against cancerous cells.

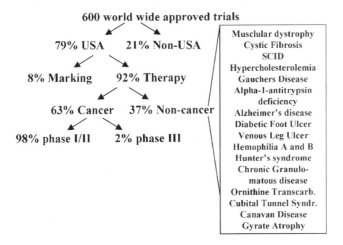

Fig. 1. Summary of gene therapy clinical trials.

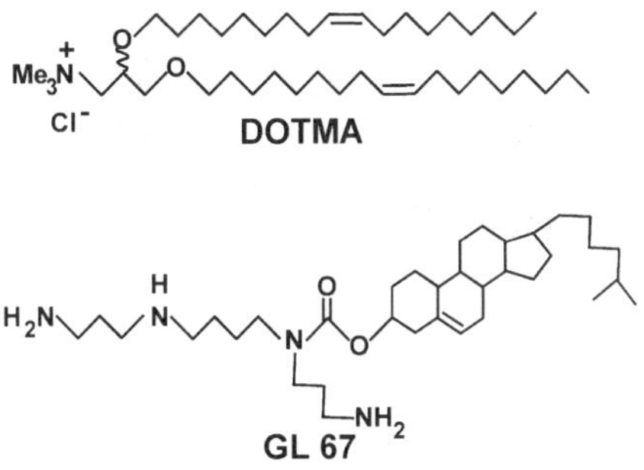

Fig. 2. Structures of two cationic liposomes used in nonviral gene transfer.

2.1. Nonviral Gene Transfer

Depending on the specific requirements of the gene transfer vehicle, the physical transfer of nucleic acid sequences can be achieved by several methods. The use of nonviral gene transfer is very attractive because the components of the delivery system can be chemically synthesized and can be very well regulated. A well-regulated system is certainly more appealing for FDA approval compared to the use of viral transfer systems that, as discussed below, require a number of components that are more difficult to standardize. But compared to viral gene transfer, the use of nonviral gene transfer reagents is very inefficient. It is anticipated, however, that studies aimed at understanding the mechanisms involved in the entry of nucleic acids into cells will result in the generation of improved compounds. Indeed, the use of cationic liposomes has shown some promise and has been used clinically (5). In general, the formation of a liposome/DNA delivery vehicle requires a synthetic cationic amphiphile such as DOTMA or GL67, the structures of which are shown in Fig. 2, and a neutral lipid, such as dioleoyl L-α-phosphatidylethanolamine (DOPE). The key to efficient gene transfer is to determine the exact molar ratio of each component that will allow the greatest amount of DNA to be transfected into the target cells. In addition to liposome/DNA delivery systems, cationic polymers such as poly-L-lysine and various peptide complexes have been used to deliver plasmid DNA (6,7).

The gene being transferred is typically contained in a plasmid, and its expression can be driven by a variety of promoters. Because large quantities of highly purified plasmid DNA can be obtained by growing relatively small bacterial cultures, the isolation of the genetic material to be transferred is relatively straightforward. The success of many of these new agents is encouraging in the fact that several have mediated high-level gene transfer in vitro, but the lack of in vivo success has been discouraging.

2.2. Viral Gene Transfer

Although it is hoped that the efficiency of gene transfer using synthetically derived compounds can be sufficiently increased for general use, if high transduction efficiencies are needed recombinant viruses are typically used. Because of the early success and high transduction levels achieved with viral transfer systems, vast amounts of resources have been expended to develop novel viral delivery systems as well as to understand better the basic biology of viral gene transfer. In general, a basic concept for creating recombinant viruses is the use of a viral-packaging cell line. Recombinant retroviral packaging cell lines are derived by specifically controlling the expression of wild-type viral sequences. For example, Fig. 3A shows a schematic of the genome of a wild-type murine leukemia retrovirus. The virus contains two long-terminal-repeat (LTR) regions, the 5' and 3'-LTRs. The 5'-LTR contains an enhancer region and a promoter that drives the expression of the viral RNA transcript. From the processed RNA transcript the proteins necessary for the assembly of an infectious viral particle are translated from the *gag*, *pol*, and *env* sequences. The *gag* gene translates a single polyprotein that is subsequently cleaved into three proteins—the matrix, capsid, and nucleic acid-binding protein. The *pol* gene encodes both the reverse transcriptase and integrase proteins. Importantly, the Ψ region of the preprocessed RNA transcript is recognized by and incorporated into the viral particle. So the genome of the viral particle contains the full-length RNA transcript. The viral particle is then released by budding from the cell membrane. The envelope proteins are encoded by *env* and recognize specific cell surface proteins on target cells, which dictate viral tropism. On recognizing specific cellular receptors, the viral particles bind to the target cells and the RNA transcript is deposited into the cell. The RNA is reverse transcribed into DNA and then incorporated into the genome of the target cell. Once the viral sequence becomes part of the genome of the target cell (or proviral sequence), more infectious virus can be generated. Because the viral sequence integrates into the genome of the target cell, as the host cell divides the viral sequence is also replicated and the genome of both resulting cells contains the viral sequence.

To produce recombinant viruses that can be used in gene therapy applications, the generation of packaging cells was paramount *(8–10)*. Packaging cells are generated from cell lines that are easily grown in the laboratory, such as NIH 3T3 or 293T cells *(11)*. As shown in Fig. 3B, to generate a packing cell that produces replication incompetent virus, that is, viruses that can infect target cells but do not contain the necessary elements to make more virus, specific sequences of a wild-type virus were cloned into expression cassettes and transferred into tissue culture cell lines. Safe packaging cells have been generated by expressing the *gag* and *pol* sequences from one promoter and *env* by a separate promoter on a second expression cassette. Expression of these sequences is sufficient to generate a viral particle. However, because the Ψ region is eliminated from these expression constructs there is no viral RNA transcript packaged into the viral particle. The packaging cell line is, therefore, capable of producing viral particles but the particles being produced are void of RNA. The RNA to be packaged is supplied by retroviral vectors. Retroviral vectors contain 5'- and 3'-LTRs, the Ψ region, and the cDNA sequence necessary to encode a therapeutic protein (Fig. 3B). By transfecting the retroviral vector into a packaging cell

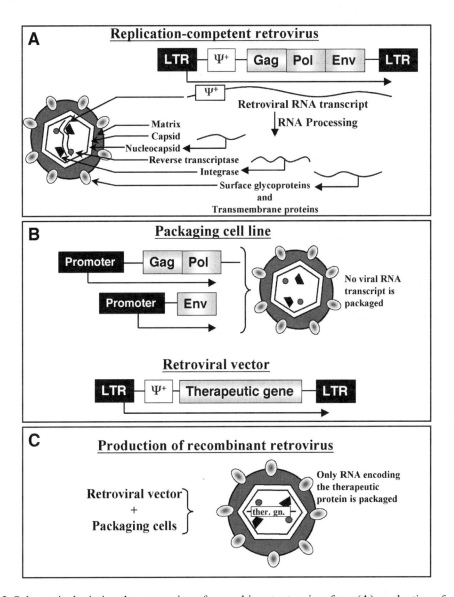

Fig. 3. Schematic depicting the generation of recombinant retrovirus from (**A**) production of wild-type virus to (**B**) generation of packaging cell lines to (**C**) transfection of recombinant retroviral vectors into packaging cells to generate recombinant retroviruses.

line, the 5'-LTR drives the production of the retroviral vector RNA. Because the retroviral vector RNA contains the Ψ region, the RNA sequence will be recognized by the viral particle and packaged, generating a recombinant virus (Fig. 3C). The recombinant virus is composed of all the protein components of the wild-type virus but the packaged RNA sequence is supplied by the retroviral vector. The recombinant virus can be collected from the supernatant of the packaging cells and used to infect target cells. Using the cellular entry mechanisms of a wild-type virus, the RNA sequence is introduced into the target cell, is reverse-transcribed into DNA, and integrates into the genome of the infected cell. The only nucleic acid sequence transferred is the sequence that encodes the therapeutic protein. Because the viral genome is not transferred, the targeted cells do not produce infectious virus. Noncompetent recombinant retroviruses can therefore be used to introduce specific gene sequences safely into target cells.

A useful feature of the murine leukemia virus transfer system is the ability to switch easily the *env* sequences to produce pseudotyped virus *(9,10,12)*. Pseudotyped viruses have altered receptor usage owing to the expression of the different envelope proteins. For example, if the gene encoding the gp70 envelope is used, ecotropic virus is produced that will infect only mouse and rat cells because this envelope recognizes the mCAT1 receptor specific for mice and rats. But if the A2070A envelope is expressed, amphotropic virus is produced that can infect many mammalian cell types because this envelope recognizes the PIT-2 receptor that is present on many types of cells. Recent studies have shown that the degree of PIT-2 expression on target cells determines the efficiency of viral transduction. Cells that have low-level amphotropic receptor RNA expression, such as human hematopoietic stem and progenitor cells, are inefficiently transduced with amphotropic pseudotyped virus, whereas subpopulations of cells with high amphotropic receptor RNA expression are more efficiently transduced *(13)*. The G-protein from the vesicular stomatitis virus (VSV-G) is also used for viral pseudotyping because this envelope protein mediates viral entry through association with anionic phospholipids *(12)*. VSV-G pseudotyped viral particles have the added advantage of being more physically stable, which allows the virus to be concentrated by centrifugation. More recently, the envelope of the RD114/type D retrovirus, which recognizes a neutral amino acid transporter, has been used for gene transfer into human and nonhuman primates with relatively high efficiency *(10,12,14)*.

In addition, retroviruses other than the murine leukemia virus (MLV) have also been develolped. Although much more complicated in molecular structure, lentiviruses such as the human immunodeficiency virus have been genetically altered to create safe gene packaging vehicles *(8,15)*. A major limitation to the use of MLVs is the requirement that the target cell must proceed through at least one round of replication. Many cell types that are possible targets for gene therapy are quiescent and therefore resistant to MLV transduction. Lentiviruses can infect mitotically inactive cells, and recombinant viruses generated from the HIV genome also appear to infect nondividing cells. Pseudotyping recombinant lentivirus with VSV-G expands the viral host range and allows for targeting of a broad range of cell types *(12)*. Because lentiviruses are extremely efficient gene transfer vehicles, tremendous effort has been directed at making safe transfer systems using the lentiviral genome. In addition to lentiviruses, ecombinant retroviruses derived from foamy viruses have also shown potential as vehicles for gene transfer *(16)*. The genome of foamy viruses is similar to that of the MLV, that is, *gag, pol,* and *env* genes, but several accessory proteins are also encoded that are referred to as *bel* genes. Although the exact function of each *bel* gene product is unknown, packaging cells have been generated that encode the necessary proteins required for viral particle formation. Advantages of using recombinant foamy viruses are their broad host range and their ability to package large retroviral vectors.

The ability to transfer specific nucleic acid sequences reproducibly made recombinant retroviruses the choice for many investigators. However, the limelight is now being shared by viral transfer systems that are more complex and for many applications superior to retroviral transfer. DNA virus vectors such as adenovirus, adeno-associated virus, and herpes simplex virus are finding their own niches in the field of gene therapy. Adeno-associated virus type 2 (AAV) is a human parvovirus having several features that make it a very attractive vehicle for gene transfer *(17,18)*. Although 80% of adults are seropositive for AAV-2, the wild-type virus is not associated with any disease, and unlike retroviruses that integrate randomly into the genome, recombinant adeno-associated virus can be engineered to integrate into the long arm of human chromosome 19. However, a major limitation to the development of recombinant AAV gene therapy products is the difficulty in producing highly purified virus. One reason for this is because AAV-2 is in the genus *Dependovirus*, meaning it requires a helper virus for replication. Wild-type adenovirus is its helper virus and is a major contaminant of recombinant AAV-2.

Wild-type AAV-2 is a nonenveloped virus with an icosahedral capsid composed of three proteins—VP-1, VP-2, and VP-3—in a 1:1:10 ratio. Two rep proteins, Rep 78 and Rep 68, have DNA helicase and DNA nicking activities and are required for site-specific integration of the AAV-2 genome. The wild-type genome of AAV-2 is a 4681 single DNA strand that has a 145 nucleotide inverted terminal repeat (ITR) at each end, which are required for DNA encapsulation. Between the two ITRs are the genes that encode the rep and VP proteins. Similar to the production of recombinant retroviruses, a vector plasmid was developed by removing the rep and VP sequences and replacing them with a therapeutic gene. The rep and VP sequences are expressed from a separate plasmid that does not contain the ITR packaging signal, similar to the controlled expression described above for *gag/pol* and *env* for recombinant retroviral production. To generate recombinant AAV-2 the two plasmids, that is, vector plasmid and rep-cap expressing plasmid, are cotransfected into a suitable cell line. Unlike the production of recombinant retrovirus, transfection of the AAV genome into tissue culture cells does not produce recombinant virus. Transfectants must then be infected with adenovirus to help stimulate AAV-2 expression *(17,18)*. Recombinant AAV-2 is produced and a single strand of DNA sequence encoded by the vector plasmid is packaged. In addition, wild-type adenovirus is also produced. The wild-type virus can be heat inactivated and removed by cesium chloride density gradient centrifugation. Alternatively, affinity chromatography methods have been developed to increase the speed and purity of recombinant AAV-2 isolation. The ability to isolate purified AAV-2 has increased the feasibility of using AAV-derived vectors in gene therapy applications.

Recombinant adenovirus has also been used extensively in preclinical and clinical cancer gene therapy applications *(19,20)*. Adenovirus virions are composed of a protein-only capsid consisting of three main proteins: the hexon, penton, and fiber. The hexon proteins compose the structural framework of the virion and the penton and fiber proteins compose the infectious machinery. The fiber proteins mediate the initial association with the membrane of the target cell, and the penton proteins mediate viral internalization by secondary interactions with specific membrane proteins such as integrins. The genome of the adenovirus is a single double-stranded DNA molecule of approx 36,000 basepairs. Once the adenovirus genome enters the nucleus of an infected cell, the viral DNA does not integrate into the cell's genome but replicates in an extrachromosomal state. A serious of "timed" transcription events occur that initiate formation of new virions. Several genes are initially transcribed, termed early genes, one of which is *E1A*. Because the function of *E1A* is to initiate transcription of other early genes, nonreplication competent recombinant adenoviruses were first generated by deleting *E1A* from the viral genome. The technology for generating recombinant adenoviruses has now advanced to the point at which most of the adenovirus genome is deleted and the genes necessary to encode a functionally infectious virion are supplied by a helper genome *(21–23)*. By gutting the wild-type genome of all but regions necessary for replication and packaging, adenoviral vectors can accommodate extremely large nucleic acid sequences. For efficient packaging the adenoviral vector must be between 27,000 and 38,000 basepairs, which is sufficiently large for most gene transfer purposes *(24)*.

However, as described more fully below, the limiting aspect for using adenoviruses is the pronounced immunogenicity of the capsid proteins and the transient expression of the transferred gene. Initial administration of recombinant adenovirus generates immune responses that limit the effectiveness of subsequent virus administrations *(25,26)*. Although not typically observed with the use of adenoviruses for the treatment of cancers, immune responses can be so significant as to result in severe complications.

As shown in the previous subheadings, there are a number of methods available to transfer therapeutic nucleic acid sequences into target cells. With respect to the clinical practice of gene therapy, although almost 20% of patients are treated using nonviral gene transfer methods, approx 35% of gene therapy protocols use recombinant retroviruses, and about 50% of patients in gene therapy trials are treated using recombinant retroviruses (www.wiley.co.uk/genetherapy/clinical). Protocols using adenovirus constitute an additional 27% of gene therapy protocols, and 18% of patients in gene therapy trials receive recombinant adenovirus. Therefore, the majority of gene therapy is being conducted using recombinant viral gene transfer. Because a comprehensive review of all strategies would be encyclopedic, and because excellent reviews are available *(27–30)*, in the next sections a model study is described by considering preclinical investigations that generated enthusiasm for a clinical trial that culminated in a phase III study.

3. PHASE III STUDIES IN CANCER GENE THERAPY

There were seven cancer gene therapy phase III studies posted worldwide as of September 2001 (www.wiley.co.uk/genetherapy/clinical). They can be segregated into two broad categories: (1) use of p53-expressing adenoviral vectors *(31)* in combination with chemotherapy for treatment of ovarian, non-small-cell lung cancer (NSCLC) and squamous cell carcinoma of the head and neck (SCCHN) and (2) use of retroviral vectors encoding *HSVtk* for treatment of glioma. The latter strategy is the first cancer gene therapy biopharmaceutical that has completed scientific analysis and Phase III clinical trial scrutiny and will serve as a paradigm for discussion. The common denominator of all these approaches is the use of replication-defective viral vectors for tumor-targeted tumoricidal transgene delivery and sponsorship by large pharmaceutical interests.

3.1. HSVtk *and Cancer Gene Therapy/*HSVtk *as a Tumoricidal Transgene*

The "suicide" gene approach was originally developed to act as a fail-safe mechanism for replacement gene therapy *(32)*. It was later reasoned that the same "suicide" gene, inserted into malignant cells, should also induce cell death when activated. The concept of suicide gene therapy is thus based on the paradigm that gene transfer can confer new properties to tumor cells, enabling them to activate a given prodrug *(33,34)*. The best characterized and most widely used suicide gene is by far the *HSVtk* gene. It encodes a viral enzyme that converts the nontoxic guanosine analog ganciclovir (GCV) into a monophosphorylated metabolite, which is subsequently converted by cellular granylate kinases to a toxic triphosphorylated form *(35,36)*. Because GCV is a relatively poor substrate for mammalian thymidine kinase, plasma concentrations can be achieved in vivo that are lethal to cells expressing the *HSVtk* gene but nontoxic to normal mammalian cells. Triphosphorylated GCV acts as a DNA polymerase inhibitor and a chain terminator, eventually leading to cell death *(37,38)*. In vitro and in vivo treatment of *HSVtk*-positive tumor cells with GCV has also been shown to induce apoptosis *(39,40)* and/or necrosis *(41,42)*. Craperi et al. *(43)* examined the molecular process leading to the in vitro cell death of C6 rat glioma expressing *HSVtk* following exposure to GCV. They demonstrated that GCV triggered cell cycle arrest in the

S phase, which was followed by apoptosis. They found that this cytotoxic effect was independent of p53 and Bcl-xL expression, but associated with Bax induction. They showed that GCV treatment up-regulates the level of Bax protein. Given that Bax can antagonize the antiapoptotic protein Bcl-xL *(44)*, it is conceivable that the balance between Bax and Bcl-xL may be a critical determinant. This is consistent with earlier observations that cell death could be inhibited by Bcl-2 expression *(45)*.

3.2. The "Bystander Effect"

Moolten and Wells *(46)* demonstrated that tumor cells expressing the *HSVtk* gene could be killed in vitro and in vivo after administration of GCV. Freeman et al. *(39)* further demonstrated that the toxic effect of GCV is not limited only to *HSVtk* gene modified tumor cells, but also affected adjacent nontransduced tumor cells. When a mixed population of tumor cells containing only 10% *HSVtk*-positive cells was exposed to GCV, the entire population was eradicated. This phenomenon, in which a minority of *HSVtk* expressing cells leads to the death and elimination of adjacent tumor cells not expressing *HSVtk* is known as the "bystander effect" *(47–49)*.

Understanding the mechanism of this bystander effect is crucial because it would be almost impossible to gene modify all the cells of a tumor in vivo using available gene transfer techniques. When *HSVtk*-positive and -negative murine sarcoma cells were cultured in Transwell plates separated by a filter membrane, the bystander effect was abolished, suggesting that this phenomenon was dependent, in part, on cell–cell contact *(39)*. In their autoradiography studies using [³H]GCV, Bi et al. *(50)* further showed in vitro the apparent cell to cell transfer of radioactivity that correlated with the observed bystander effect. Ishii-Morita et al. *(51)* later demonstrated unequivocally the presence of the three phosphorylated metabolites of GCV in *HSVtk*-negative cells. Because different studies showed that phosphorylated GCV cannot pass through the cell membrane *(50)*, this suggests that the bystander effect is dependent in part on intercellular communications through gap junctions *(52)*. This is in accordance with other observations in different cell types that nonimmune bystander killing requires cell-to-cell contact through gap junctions *(53–55)*.

Clearly, gap junctions play a crucial role in the bystander effect. However, it is obvious that other mechanisms are also involved in distinct cell types *(56)*. There is evidence that the uptake of apoptotic vesicles by adjacent *HSVtk*-negative cells can lead to cell death *(39)*. In another study, Princen et al. *(57)* demonstrated that the transfer of filtered supernatant from *HSVtk*-positive DHD/K12 GCV-treated cells to *HSVtk*-negative cells killed these cells in a concentration-dependent manner, clearly evoking a gap junction independent bystander effect.

3.2.1. IMMUNE BYSTANDER EFFECT

If in vitro exposure of *HSVtk*-positive cells to GCV can induce apoptosis, several independent studies demonstrated, on the other hand, that different animal tumors expressing the *HSVtk* gene predominantly die by necrosis when GCV is administered in vivo. Vile et al. *(42)* showed that in vivo GCV ablation of *HSVtk*-positive B16 murine melanoma cells converted the tumor in an immunostimulatory environment characterized by the induction of the cytokines interleukin-2 (IL-2), IL-12, interferon-γ (INF-γ), tumor necrosis factor-α (TNF-α), and GM-CSF accompanied by a pronounced tumor infiltrate consisting of macrophages as well as CD4+ and CD8+ T cells. Several other in vivo experiments with different cancer cell lines have also shown that the host immune system was implicated in the observed bystander effect *(58–60)*. The current model is that rapid necrotic cell death of *HSVtk* cells after GCV administration can provide an initial stimulus for the recruitment of immune cells to the tumor site, leading to effective presentation of tumor antigens to immune cells infiltrating the tumor in response to the cytokines released. This immune bystander effect is not specific to *HSVtk* because it has also been described for another suicide gene, encoding for the *E. coli* cytosine deaminase, which activates 5-fluorocytosine (5-FC) *(61)*. These observations suggest that "suicide" activity leads to release of tumor antigens previously unrecognizable by immune cells and that these antigens are distinct from *HSVtk (62,63)*.

In sum, the "bystander" effect is dependent, in part, on: cell–cell contact *(39,51)*; phagocytosis of gancyclovir phosphate laden cell debris *(39)*; an antiangiogenic effect *(64)*; cytokine-mediated hemorrhagic necrosis in local, but noncontiguous, tumor deposits *(65)*; and immune recognition and rejection of tumor *(66,67)*. CD4$^+$ lymphocytes, CD8$^+$ lymphocytes, natural killer (NK) cells, and antigen presenting cells *(67,68)* take part in a tumor-specific immune response which is an important component of the local *(62,63,68,70)* as well as the distant antitumor immune bystander effect *(59,71)*.

4. PROS AND CONS OF REPLICATION-DEFECTIVE VIRAL VECTORS FOR TUMOR-TARGETED SUICIDE GENE DELIVERY

As described earlier, viral vectors, such as adenoviral vectors and retroviral vectors, remain the most efficient and most studied means to introduce genetic material in tumor cells in vivo. This is usually achieved by direct intratumoral injection of viral particle suspension *(62,72)*. Clinical trials examining the safety and utility of tumor-targeted gene delivery have been hampered by diametrically opposite problems depending on the gene vehicle used. First, as previously discussed, nonviral vectors are inefficient as tumor-targeted gene delivery vehicles in animals *(73)*. Conversely, viral vectors, such as adenoviral vectors, are very potent for gene delivery. However, adenoviral vectors will efficiently modify cancer and normal tissue. This is of significant concern if toxic genes are delivered. Also, murine recombinant retroviruses modify only actively dividing cells, a characteristic of cancer cells, but their efficiency in doing so is very low. In sum, current technology for tumor-targeted gene delivery is plagued by nonspecific or inefficient gene delivery. Both scenarios may lead to either intolerable toxicity or ineffectiveness.

4.1. HSVtk *Adenoviral Vectors: Trials and Tribulations*

Replication-defective adenoviral vectors (AVs) are nonintegrating vectors that can infect both dividing and nondividing cells *(74)* that express the coxsackie-adenoviral receptor (CAR) *(75)*. Among viral vector delivery platforms, adenoviruses are among the most studied because they can be concentrated to high titers (>10^{10} pfu/mL), which facilitate pharmacological delivery of a large viral dose at tumor sites. AVs are very efficient at transducing normal tissue that express CAR and this can create problems when AVs encode for a toxic, "cancer-killing" transgene. Furthermore, first-generation AVs can evoke an early and late cellular and humoral reaction by the host that eventually leads to the elimination of all transduced cells—malignant and normal—by cytotoxic T lymphocytes and macrophages *(76)*. This poses a formidable, even lethal, dose-limiting obstacle when AVs are given systemically for nonmalignant illnesses *(77–79)*. The same problem may also arise in cancer therapy applications.

In brain cancer models, AVs can, however, disseminate and genetically modify contiguous normal brain cells *(80,81)*. For instance, Dewey et al. have demonstrated that an adenovector coding for herpes simplex virus thymidine kinase (HSVtk) injected intratumorally in rodents with brain cancer led to regression of tumor following gancyclovir treatment

(82). However, the "cancer cured" animals developed demyelinating encephalitis as a consequence of an immune reaction to AV-driven expression of HSVtk in normal neurons. Thus, the use of AVs may theoretically lead to toxicity in patients, limiting their application.

Phase I clinical trials using recombinant adenovirus to deliver the *HSVtk* gene were conducted in patients with advanced non-central nervous system (CNS) cancers revealed some systemic toxicities. Delivery of the *HSVtk* gene by means of AVs was performed in 21 patients with malignant mesothelioma *(83)*. The treatment consisted of a single intrapleural injection of AVs ranging from 1×10^9 to 1×10^{12} pfu followed by intravenous GCV twice daily for 14 d. Eleven patients out of 20 analyzed had evidence of *HSVtk* gene transfer in a dose-related fashion. Side effects reported included fever, anemia, transient liver enzyme elevations, and skin eruptions. A transient systemic inflammatory response was seen in all patients receiving the highest dosages. Three of the treated patients remained clinically stable for at least 26 mo after the trial. In a prostate cancer Phase I trial, 18 patients with local recurrence were intratumorally injected with *HSVtk* AVs ranging from 1×10^8 to 1×10^{11} pfu *(84)*. Three patients were reported to have achieved an objective response (one for each of the highest dose levels). However, one patient developed reversible grade 4 thrombocytopenia and grade 3 hepatotoxicity at the highest dose level. Alvarez et al. *(85)* reported the absence of dose-limiting toxicity when adenovectors encoding *HSVtk* (up to 10^{12} pfu) were injected intraperitoneally in women with recurrent ovarian cancer. It is conceivable that the peritoneal cavity is more tolerant of viral vectors compared to other closed compartments *(86)*. In contrast to the above studies, Trask et al. *(87)* treated 13 glioblastoma patients with a single intracranial injection of replication-defective adenoviral vectors (up to 10^{12} pfu) followed by intravenous injection of GCV. They observed a stabilization of the disease in one patient for at least 29 mo, while 11 patients died from tumor progression. Of note is that the highest dose treatment induced CNS toxicity with confusion and seizures in all patients. In sum, the use of adenovectors for in vivo gene delivery targeting normal or malignant tissue may be associated with significant side effects that can limit their clinical utility and the impetus to initiate Phase III studies.

4.2. HSVtk Retroviral Producer Cells as a Biopharmaceutical for Therapy of Gliomas

Recombinant retroviral vectors are well characterized as vehicles for tumor-targeted gene delivery *(72)*. Moloney-based retroviruses can integrate only in cells undergoing mitosis *(88)*. Because uncontrolled mitotic activity defines the basic nature of cancer, Moloney-based retrovectors are expected to restrict gene transfer to proliferating malignant cells when injected directly into a tumor mass. In contradistinction to adenovectors, quiescent cells—such as normal tissue adjacent to a targeted tumor deposit—will be refractory to retroviral gene transfer and spared from subsequent toxicity *(47,89)*. The concept has been robustly validated, repeatedly, in animal models of cancer, including brain cancer. Further, experimental brain tumor implants consisting of a mixture of unmodified tumor cells with *HSVtk*-expressing cells will also regress following gancyclovir treatment without harm to adjacent normal tissue *(47)*. Retroviral vectors have been extensively used in human clinical trials studying suicide gene delivery to malignant brain tumors, as discussed below. Limitations to the use of retroviruses are their inability to infect cells that do not express the retroviral receptor *(69)* and the low particle concentration($<10^6$ cfu/mL) in clinical grade viral preparations. The logistical impediment to low titer retroparticle delivery to tumor was addressed experimentally in clinical trials by injecting retroviral vector producing cells directly into glioma. The idea was that constant production of viral particles could transduce cancer cells more efficiently than low-titer, cell-free retrovector injections.

With this purpose at hand, Genetic Therapy Inc. (Gaithesberg, MD, subsequently acquired by Novartis) developed a novel cancer gene therapy biopharmaceutical. The platform is based upon the PA317 retroviral packaging cell line originally designed by Miller et al. *(90)*. This cell line is derived from murine NIH3T3 cells transfected to express continuously the Moloney oncoretroviral gag-pol polyprotein as well as the MLV amphotropic envelope protein. These cells were subsequently transfected with a plasmid retroviral vector construct encoding for *HSVtk* within a replication-defective retroviral genome construct. A resulting retroviral producer clonal cell line (PA317/G1TkSvNa.53) was characterized and validated as a biopharmaceutical for clinical trials. This clonal vector producing cell (VPC) line was shown to generate a titer of 10^4–10^5 cfu/mL *(91)*, which roughly translates to a few infectious retroviral particles generated per producer cell per day.

In 1997, Ram et al. published the results of a Phase I–II study in which 15 patients suffering from primary or metastatic brain cancer received up to 10^9 PA317/G1TkSvNa.53 VPCs intratumorally by computed tomography (CT)-guided stereotactic injections *(91)*. All patients were given high-dose dexamethasone and GCV intravenously (5 mg/kg) for 2 wk following VPC injection. Four patients with radiological evidence of regression received a second treatment. Four patients had a PR that lasted from 4 to 11 wk, including one patient with apparent absence of any tumor growth for more than 2 yr after treatment. Two patients had elective resection of their VPC-injected glioma prior to GCV treatment. *In situ* hybridization for *HSVtk* mRNA on histological specimens revealed low-level gene transfer to tumor along needle tracks, especially in regions of angiogenesis where transduction of endothelial cells occurred, a phenomena also observed by others *(92)*. Further, in some patients in whom a PR was noted in the injected lesion, other contemporaneous brain lesions continued to progress, suggesting that a distant bystander effect was absent. Interestingly, 10 of 15 patients developed humoral immunity to the VPCs. It was concluded that no safety hazards attributable to the use of xenogenic VPCs in brain tumor were identified.

An international Phase II study of VPCs for glioma was performed by the GLI328 European–Canadian Study Group and their results published in 1999 *(93)*. This group utilized an improved biopharmaceutical generated by Genetic Therapy Inc. The PA317/ G1TkSvNa.7 clonal producer (GLI-328) had a 100-fold higher titer than the VPCs used in the trial by Ram et al. An important clinical trial design distinction was the use of GLI328 immediately following surgical debulking of recurrent glioblastoma, as opposed to direct injection into unresected primary cancer. Following surgical removal of the tumor, 10^9 VPCs where injected in the resection cavity in as many as 60 distinct injection sites to ensure wide distribution of VPCs. GCV was given intravenously for 2 wk without systemic steroids. One patient remained disease-free 31 mo post-therapy; however 46 of 48 patients died of progressive disease or complications related to glioma. Interestingly, 17 patients tested polymerase chain reaction (PCR)-positive for vector sequences in peripheral blood leukocyte DNA, and all except one became negative at 12 mo post-therapy. As observed in the previous study, five patients developed an antiretrovector humoral response. The results were corroborated by the Study Group on Gene Therapy for Glioblastoma *(94)* that explored the use of the conceptually related biopharmaceutical M11 HSVTK retroviral vector-producing cell line (Génopoiétic, Paris, France). In sum, 12 patients were enrolled in a Phase II study with a design similar to that of the GLI328 Study Group, and comparable conclusions of tolerability and a perception of improved survival was noted.

A Phase III randomized controlled trial of GLI-328 VPCs gene therapy was therefore initatied by the GLI328 International Study Group *(95)* on 248 patients with previously untreated glioblastoma multiform and the results published in November 2000 *(96)*. Treatments consisted either of standard therapy alone—gross resection of tumor with radiation therapy—or standard therapy plus intratumoral implantation of *HSVtk* encoding VPCs followed by GCV administration. There was no severe neurological side effects during treatment, comparable to the previous Phase I–II studies. After more than 2 yr of follow-up, this extensive trial failed to show that the addition of VPC gene therapy provided any advantage in regard to tumor progression or overall survival. The median survival was 365 vs 354 d in the gene therapy and control groups, respectively. The main cause of failure of this therapeutic strategy is presumably low tumor gene transfer efficiency. A follow-up study performed on autopsy material collected from 32 patients determined that retroviral DNA was detected in 55% of brain tumor samples, albeit at a very low <0.03% transduction efficiency *(97)*. As observed in the Phase II studies, vector DNA sequences were transiently detected in peripheral blood of nine patients, possibly from transduced lymphocytes at the time of implantation.

Thus, the greatest impediment to retrovector VPCs suicide gene therapy seems to be the very low efficiency of in vivo gene transfer to cancer cells, possibly compounded by a specific immune response against VPCs *(91)*. Although "suicide" retrovectors are "safe," implantation of VPCs as a means to deliver *HSVtk* to glioma is of limited efficacy *(94)*. It remains to be seen whether the *HSVtk* gene—if it were delivered in a sufficiently high tumor fraction—will lead to a therapeutic effect following GCV administration in humans.

5. FAILURE ANALYSIS

In a strictly formal sense, it is still unknown whether *HSVtk* gene expression in human cancer is of use or not. Until gene transfer efficiencies exceeding 10% are achieved in a tumor-restricted manner, this question will remain unanswered. Possible remedies likely lie in refinement of gene delivery platforms. Possible candidate remedies could include helper-dependent (gutless) adenoviral vectors *(98)* or adeno-associated vectors *(99)* that incorporate robust tumor-specific promoters *(100)*; oncolytic viruses *(101)* engineered to express an exogenous suicide gene *(102)*, or even concentrated pseudotyped suicide retrovectors *(103)*. Furthermore, the use of more potent suicide genes *(104)* and clinically tolerable variants of GCV could be of use. In a sense, the issue of safe, high-efficiency and durable tumor-specific gene transfer is one that plagues the field of cancer gene therapy as a whole and is not solely an idiosyncratic problem of "suicide" gene therapy.

6. OF MICE AND MEN

Gene therapy readily and easily cures "artificial" cancers in inbred rodents. Unfortunately, the biology of spontaneous cancer in outbred mammals is very distinct, much to the regret of cancer gene therapists. The ability to deliver, the gene and the biology of the gene, once delivered, can be quite difficult to ascertain in clinical trials. Ethical considerations, such as repeated invasive biopsies and the like, markedly reduce our ability to perform failure analysis in humans suffering of cancer. Indeed, it has not always been clear which (or both) of the two has failed: inappropriate gene transfer or unsatisfactory anticancer transgene biology. Creative use of small mammals, such as cats and dogs, suffering from spontaneous malignancies may be a complementary and informative way of testing complex biopharmaceuticals such as gene therapy stratagems *(105,106)*. Roland Scollay, chief scientific officer of a california gene therapy company, shared his view that "...therapies going to the clinic are not always the very best available; rather, they are those for which licenses are held, another factor contributing to the high failure rate of gene therapy trials to date" *(107)*.

Indeed, pressure to develop gene therapy for large-market indications (i.e., profitable), unrealistic appraisal of sometimes unproven intellectual property value, and the perverse effect of "royalty stacking" all conspire to a competitive rather than a cooperative spirit. This may, in part, explain the multiplicity of similar, ineffective and iterative early phase studies in cancer gene therapy. The societal aim of science—improvement of man's condition through reason—can be directly translated in the applied science that is gene therapy. Effective and safe cancer gene therapy biopharmaceuticals can be creatively developed only if there is ongoing cooperative arrangements between diverse interests: academic, medical, and commercial.

REFERENCES

1. Culver KW, Blease RM. Gene therapy and cancer. Trends Genet 1994; 10:174–178.
2. Hanazono Y, Terao K, Ozawa K. Gene transfer into nonhuman primate hematopoietic stem cells: implications for gene therapy. Stem Cells 2001; 19:12–23.
3. Valere T. Gene therapy in the clinic: human trials of gene therapy. In: Lemoine NR (ed). Understanding Gene Therapy. New York, NY: Springer-Verlag, 1999, pp. 141–154.
4. Rosenberg SA, Aebergold P, Cornetta K, et al. Gene transfer into humans—immunotherapy of patients with advanced melanoma, using tumor-infiltrating lymphocytes modified by retroviral gene transduction. N Engl J Med 1990; 323:570–578.
5. Alton EWFW, Stern M, Farley R, et al. Cationic lipid-mediated CFTR gene transfer to the lungs and nose of patients with cystic fibrosis: a double-blind placebo-controlled trial. Lancet 1999; 353:947–954.
6. Miller AD. Cationic liposomes systems in gene therapy. Curr Res Mol Ther 1998; 1:494–503.
7. Felgner PL, Barenholz Y, Behr J-P, et al. Nomenclature for synthetic gene delivery systems. Hum Gene Ther 1997; 8:511–512.
8. Chang LJ, He J. Retroviral vectors for gene therapy of AIDS and cancer. Curr Opin Mol Ther 2001; 3:468–475.
9. Ory D, Neugeboren BA, Mulligan CR. A stable human-derived packaging cell line for production of high titer retrovirus/vesicular stomatitis virus G pseudotypes. Proc Natl Acad Sci USA 1996; 93: 11,400–11,406.
10. Rasko J, Battini JL, Gottschalk RJ, Mazo I, Miller DA. The RD114/simian type D retrovirus receptor is a neutral amino acid transporter. Proc Natl Acad Sci USA 1999; 96:2129–2134.
11. Miller AD. Retrovirus packaging cells. Hum Gene Ther 1990; 1:5–14.
12. Hanawa H, Kelly PF, Nathwani AC, et al. Comparison of various envelope proteins for their ability to pseudotype lentiviral vectors and transduce primitive hematopoietic cells from human blood. Mol Ther 2002; 5:242–251.
13. Orlic D, Girard LJ, Anderson SM, et al. Transduction efficiency of cell lines and hematopoietic stem cells correlates with retrovirus receptor mRNA levels. Stem Cells 1997; 15(Suppl 1):23–28.
14. Cosset FL, Takeuchi Y, Battini JL, Weiss RA, Collins, MK. High-titer packaging cells producing recombinant retroviruses resistant to human serum. J Virol 1995; 69:7430–7436.
15. Buchschacher GL, Wong-Staal F. Development of lentiviral vectors for gene therapy for human disease. Blood 2000; 95:2499–2504.
16. Hill CL, Mcclure MO. Foamy viruses: molecular features and therapeutic potential. In: Cid-Arregui A, Garcia-Carranca A (eds). Viral Vectors: Basic Science and Gene Therapy. Natick, MA: MA Eaton Publishing/BioTechniques Books, 2000, pp. 503–514.
17. Paonnazhagan S, Curiel DT, Shaw DR, Alvarez RD, Siegal GP. Adeno-associated virus for cancer gene therapy. Cancer Res 2001; 61:6313–6321.
18. Srivastava A. Gene transfer with adeno-associated vectors. In: Cid-Arregui A, Garcia-Carranca A (eds). Viral Vectors: Basic Science and Gene Therapy, MA: Eaton Publishing/BioTechniques Books, 2000, pp. 11–26.
19. Zhang WW. Review: adenovirus vectors: development and application. Exp Opin Invest Drugs 1997; 6:1419–1457.
20. Garble M, Hearing P. Cis and trans requirements for the selective packaging of adenovirus type-5 DNA. J Virol 1992; 66:723–731.
21. Parks RJ, Graham FL. A helper-dependent system for adenovirus vector production helps define a lower limit for efficient DNA packaging. J Virol 1997; 71:3293–3298.

22. Haecker SE, Stedman H, Balice-Gordan RJ, et al. In vivo expression of full-length dystrophin from adenoviral vectors deleted of all viral genes. Hum Gene Ther 1996; 7:1907–1914.
23. Parks RJ, Chen L, Anton M, Sankar U, Rudnicki A, Graham FL. A helper-dependent adenovirus vector system: removal of helper virus by Cre-mediated excision of the viral packaging signal. Proc Natl Acad Sci USA 1996; 93:13,565–13,570.
24. Bett AJ, Prevec L, Graham FL. Packaging capacity and stability of human adenovirus type 5 vectors. J Virol 1993; 67:5911–5921.
25. Yang Y, Jooss KU, Su Q, Ertl HCJ, Wilson JM. Immune response to viral antigens versus transgene product in the elimination of recombinant adenovirus-infected hepatocytes in vivo. Gene Ther 1996; 3:137–144.
26. Dai Y, Schwarz E, Gu D, Zhang W, Sarvetnick N, Verma I. Cellular and immune responses to adenoviral vectors containing factor IX gene: tolerization of factor IX and vector antigens allows for long-term expression. Proc Natl Acad Sci USA 1995; 92:1401–1405.
27. Buchsbaum DJ, Curiel DT. Gene therapy for the treatment of cancer. Cancer Biother Radiopharmaceut 2001; 16:275–288.
28. Galanis E, Russell S. Cancer gene therapy clinical trials: lessons for the future. Br J Cancer 2001; 85:1432–1436.
29. Beltinger C, Uckert W, Debatin KM. Suicide gene therapy for pediatric tumors. J Mol Med 2001; 78:598–612.
30. Kouraklis G. Progress in cancer gene therapy. Acta Oncol 1999; 38:675–683.
31. Merritt JA, Roth JA, Logothetis CJ. Clinical evaluation of adenoviral-mediated p53 gene transfer: review of INGN 201 studies. Semin Oncol 2001; 28:105–114.
32. Anderson WF. Prospects for human gene therapy. Science 1984; 226:401–409.
33. Moolten FL. Drug sensitivity ("suicide") genes for selective cancer chemotherapy. Cancer Gene Ther 1994; 1:279–287.
34. Freeman SM. Suicide gene therapy. (Review). Adv Exp Med Biol 2000; 465:411–422.
35. Smith KO, Galloway KS, Kennell WL, Ogilvie KK, Radatus, BK. A new nucleoside analog, 9-[[2-hydroxy-1-(hydroxymethyl)ethoxyl]methyl]guanine, highly active in vitro against herpes simplex virus types 1 and 2. Antimicrob Agents Chemother 1982; 22:55–61.
36. Smee DF, Martin JC, Verheyden JP, Matthews TR. Anti-herpesvirus activity of the acyclic nucleoside 9-(1,3-dihydroxy-2-propoxymethyl)guanine. Antimicrob Agents Chemother 1983; 23:676–682.
37. Moolten FL. Tumor chemosensitivity conferred by inserted herpes thymidine kinase genes: paradigm for a prospective cancer control strategy. Cancer Res 1986; 46:5276–5281.
38. Fyfe JA, Keller PM, Furman PA, Miller RL, Elion GB. Thymidine kinase from herpes simplex virus phosphorylates the new antiviral compound, 9-(2-hydroxyethoxymethyl)guanine. J Biol Chem 1978; 253:8721–8727.
39. Freeman SM, Abboud CN, Whartenby KA, et al. The "bystander effect": tumor regression when a fraction of the tumor mass is genetically modified. Cancer Res 1993; 53:5274–5283.
40. Colombo BM, Benedetti S, Ottolenghi S, et al. The "bystander effect": association of U-87 cell death with ganciclovir-mediated apoptosis of nearby cells and lack of effect in athymic mice. Hum Gene Ther 1995; 6:763–772.
41. Kaneko Y, Tsukamoto A. Gene therapy of hepatoma: bystander effects and nonapoptotic cell death induced by thymidine kinase and ganciclovir. Cancer Lett 1995; 96:105–110.
42. Vile RG, Castleden S, Marshall J, Camplejohn R, Upton C, Chong H. Generation of an anti-tumour immune response in a non-immunogenic tumour: HSVtk killing in vivo stimulates a mononuclear cell infiltrate and a Th1-like profile of intratumoural cytokine expression. Int J Cancer 1997; 71:267–274.
43. Craperi D, Vicat JM, Nissou MF, et al. Increased bax expression is associated with cell death induced by ganciclovir in a herpes thymidine kinase gene-expressing glioma cell line. Hum Gene Ther 1999; 10:679–688.
44. Simonian PL, Grillot DM, Merino R, Nunez G. Bax can antagonize Bcl-XL during etoposide and cisplatin-induced cell death independently of its heterodimerization with Bcl-XL. J Biol Chem 1996; 271:22,764–.
45. Hamel W, Magnelli L, Chiarugi VP, Israel MA. Herpes simplex virus thymidine kinase/ganciclovir-mediated apoptotic death of bystander cells. Cancer Res 1996; 56:2697–2702.
46. Moolten FL, Wells JM. Curability of tumors bearing herpes thymidine kinase genes transferred by retroviral vectors. J Natl Cancer Inst 1990; 82:297–300.

47. Culver KW, Ram Z, Wallbridge S, Ishii H, Oldfield EH, Blaese RM. In vivo gene transfer with retroviral vector-producer cells for treatment of experimental brain tumors (see comments). Science 1992; 256:1550–1552.

48. Caruso M, Panis Y, Gagandeep S, Houssin D, Salzmann JL, Klatzmann D. Regression of established macroscopic liver metastases after in situ transduction of a suicide gene. Proc Natl Acad Sci USA 1993; 90:7024–7028.

49. Barba D, Hardin J, Ray J, Gage FH. Thymidine kinase-mediated killing of rat brain tumors. J Neurosurg 1993; 79:729–735.

50. Bi WL, Parysek LM, Warnick R, Stambrook PJ. In vitro evidence that metabolic cooperation is responsible for the bystander effect observed with HSV tk retroviral gene therapy. Hum Gene Ther 1993; 4:725–731.

51. Ishii-Morita H, Agbaria R, Mullen CA, et al. Mechanism of 'bystander effect' killing in the herpes simplex thymidine kinase gene therapy model of cancer treatment. Gene Ther 1997; 4:244–251.

52. Fick J, Barker FG, Dazin P, Westphale EM, Beyer EC, Israel MA. The extent of heterocellular communication mediated by gap junctions is predictive of bystander tumor cytotoxicity in vitro. Proc Natl Acad Sci USA 1995; 92:11,071.

53. Mesnil M, Piccoli C, Tiraby G, Willecke K, Yamasaki H. Bystander killing of cancer cells by herpes simplex virus thymidine kinase gene is mediated by connexins. Proc Natl Acad Sci USA 1996; 93:1831–1835.

54. Vrionis FD, Wu JK, Qi P, Waltzman M, Cherington V, Spray DC. The bystander effect exerted by tumor cells expressing the herpes simplex virus thymidine kinase (HSVtk) gene is dependent on connexin expression and cell communication via gap junctions. Gene Ther 1997; 4:577–585.

55. Touraine RL, Ishii-Morita H, Ramsey WJ, Blaese RM. The bystander effect in the HSVtk/ganciclovir system and its relationship to gap junctional communication. Gene Ther 1998; 5:1705–1711.

56. Imaizumi K, Hasegawa Y, Kawabe T, et al. Bystander tumoricidal effect and gap junctional communication in lung cancer cell lines. Am J Respir Cell Mol Biol 1998; 18:205–212.

57. Princen F, Robe P, Lechanteur C, et al. A cell type-specific and gap junction-independent mechanism for the herpes simplex virus-1 thymidine kinase gene/ganciclovir-mediated bystander effect. Clin Cancer Res 1999; 5:3639–3644.

58. Barba D, Hardin J, Sadelain M, Gage FH. Development of anti-tumor immunity following thymidine kinase-mediated killing of experimental brain tumors. Proc Natl Acad Sci USA 1994; 91:4348–4352.

59. Wei MX, Bougnoux P, Sacre-Salem B, et al. Suicide gene therapy of chemically induced mammary tumor in rat: efficacy and distant bystander effect. Cancer Res 1998; 58:3529–3532-.

60. Kuriyama S, Kikukawa M, Masui K, et al. Cancer gene therapy with HSV-tk/GCV system depends on T-cell-mediated immune responses and causes apoptotic death of tumor cells in vivo. Int J Cancer 1999; 83:374–380.

61. Consalvo M, Mullen CA, Modesti A, et al. 5-Fluorocytosine-induced eradication of murine adenocarcinomas engineered to express the cytosine deaminase suicide gene requires host immune competence and leaves an efficient memory. J Immunol 1995; 154:5302–5312.

62. Vile RG, Nelson JA, Castleden S, Chong H, Hart IR. Systemic gene therapy of murine melanoma using tissue specific expression of the *HSVtk* gene involves an immune component. Cancer Res 1994; 54:6228–6234.

63. Ramesh R, Marrogi AJ, Munshi A, Abboud CN, Freeman SM: In vivo analysis of the 'bystander effect': a cytokine cascade. Exp Hematol 1996; 24:829–838.

64. Ram Z, Culver KW, Walbridge S, Blaese RM, Oldfield EH. In situ retroviral-mediated gene transfer for the treatment of brain tumors in rats (see comments). Cancer Res 1993; 53:83–88.

65. Ram Z, Walbridge S, Shawker T, Culver KW, Blaese RM, Oldfield EH. The effect of thymidine kinase transduction and ganciclovir therapy on tumor vasculature and growth of 9L gliomas in rats. J Neurosurg 1994; 81:256–260.

66. Melcher A, Todryk S, Hardwick N, Ford M, Jacobson M, Vile RG. Tumor immunogenicity is determined by the mechanism of cell death via induction of heat shock protein expression. Nat Med 1998; 4:581–587.

67. Mullen CA, Anderson L, Woods K, Nishino M, Petropoulos D. Ganciclovir chemoablation of herpes thymidine kinase suicide gene-modified tumors produces tumor necrosis and induces systemic immune responses. Hum Gene Ther 1998; 9:2019–2030.

68. Chen SH, Kosai K, Xu B, et al. Combination suicide and cytokine gene therapy for hepatic metastases of colon carcinoma: sustained antitumor immunity prolongs animal survival. Cancer Res 1996; 56:3758–3762.

69. Freeman SM, Ramesh R, Marrogi AJ. Immune system in suicide-gene therapy. Lancet 1997; 349:2–3.
70. Gagandeep S, Brew R, Green B, et al. Prodrug-activated gene therapy: involvement of an immunological component in the "bystander effect." Cancer Gene Ther 1996; 3:83.
71. Kianmanesh AR, Perrin H, Panis Y, et al. A "distant" bystander effect of suicide gene therapy: regression of nontransduced tumors together with a distant transduced tumor. Hum Gene Ther 1997; 8:1807.
72. Hurford RKJ, Dranoff G, Mulligan RC, Tepper RI. Gene therapy of metastatic cancer by in vivo retroviral gene targeting. Nat Genet 1995; 10:430.
73. Roth JA, Cristiano RJ. Gene therapy for cancer: what have we done and where are we going? J Natl Cancer Inst 1997; 89:21.
74. Yoshii Y, Maki Y, Tsuboi K, Tomono Y, Nakagawa K, Hoshino T. Estimation of growth fraction with bromodeoxyuridine in human central nervous system tumors. J Neurosurg 1986; 65:659.
75. Karpati G, Lochmuller H, Nalbantoglu J, Durham H. The principles of gene therapy for the nervous system. Trends Neurosci 1996; 19:49.
76. Lochmuller H, Petrof BJ, Allen C, Prescott S, Massie B, Karpati G. Immunosuppression by FK506 markedly prolongs expression of adenovirus-delivered transgene in skeletal muscles of adult dystrophic (mdx) mice. Biochem Biophys Res Commun 1995; 213:569.
77. Miller HI. Gene therapy on trial. Science 2000; 287:591.
78. Wadman M. NIH under fire over gene-therapy trials. Nature 2000; 403:237.
79. Jenks S. Gene therapy death—"Everyone has to share in the guilt." J Natl Cancer Inst 2000; 92:98.
80. Maron A, Gustin T, Le RA, et al. Gene therapy of rat C6 glioma using adenovirus-mediated transfer of the herpes simplex virus thymidine kinase gene: long-term follow-up by magnetic resonance imaging. Gene Ther 1996; 3:315.
81. Parr MJ, Manome Y, Tanaka T, et al. Tumor-selective transgene expression in vivo mediated by an E2F-responsive adenoviral vector. Nat Med 1997; 3:1145.
82. Dewey RA, Morrissey G, Cowsill CM, et al. Chronic brain inflammation and persistent herpes simplex virus 1 thymidine kinase expression in survivors of syngeneic glioma treated by adenovirus-mediated gene therapy: implications for clinical trials. Nat Med 1999; 5:1256.
83. Sterman DH, Treat J, Litzky LA, et al. Adenovirus-mediated herpes simplex virus thymidine kinase/ganciclovir gene therapy in patients with localized malignancy: results of a phase I clinical trial in malignant mesothelioma. Hum Gene Ther 1998; 9:1083.
84. Herman JR, Adler HL, Aguilar-Cordova E, et al. In situ gene therapy for adenocarcinoma of the prostate: a phase I clinical trial. Human Gene Ther 1999; 10:1239.
85. Alvarez RD, Gomez-Navarro J, Wang M, et al. Adenoviral-mediated suicide gene therapy for ovarian cancer. Mol Ther J Am Soc Gene Ther 2000; 2:524.
86. Alvarez RD, Barnes MN, Gomez-Navarro J, et al. A cancer gene therapy approach utilizing an anti-erbB-2 single-chain antibody-encoding adenovirus (AD21): a phase I trial. Clin Cancer Res 2000; 6:3081.
87. Trask TW, Trask RP, Aguilar-Cordova E, et al. Phase I study of adenoviral delivery of the HSV-tk gene and ganciclovir administration in patients with current malignant brain tumors. Mol Ther J Am Soc Gene Ther 2000; 1:195.
88. Miller DG, Adam MA, Miller AD: Gene transfer by retrovirus vectors occurs only in cells that are actively replicating at the time of the infection (published erratum appears in Mol Cell Biol 1992; 12:433). Mol Cell Biol 1990; 10:4239.
89. Kavanaugh MP, Miller DG, Zhang W, et al. Cell-surface receptors for gibbon ape leukemia virus and amphotropic murine retrovirus are inducible sodium-dependent phosphate symporters. Proc Natl Acad Sci USA 1994; 91:7071.
90. Miller AD, Buttimore C. Redesign of retrovirus packaging cell lines to avoid recombination leading to helper virus production. Mol Cell Biol 1986; 6:2895.
91. Ram Z, Culver KW, Oshiro EM, et al. Therapy of malignant brain tumors by intratumoral implantation of retroviral vector-producing cells (see comments). Nat Med 1997; 3:1354.
92. Floeth FW, Shand N, Bojar H, et al. Local inflammation and devascularization—in vivo mechanisms of the "bystander effect" in VPC-mediated HSV-Tk/GCV gene therapy for human malignant glioma. Cancer Gene Ther 2001; 8:843.
93. Shand N, Weber F, Mariani L, et al. A phase 1–2 clinical trial of gene therapy for recurrent glioblastoma multiforme by tumor transduction with the herpes simplex thymidine kinase gene followed by ganciclovir. GLI328 European–Canadian Study Group. Hum Gene Ther 1999; 10:2325.

94. Klatzmann D, Valery CA, Bensimon G, et al. A phase I/II study of herpes simplex virus type 1 thymidine kinase "suicide" gene therapy for recurrent glioblastoma. Study Group on Gene Therapy for Glioblastoma. Hum Gene Ther 1998; 9:2595–2604.

95. Stockhammer G, Brotchi J, Leblanc R, et al. Gene therapy for glioblastoma (correction of gliobestome) multiform: in vivo tumor transduction with the herpes simplex thymidine kinase gene followed by ganciclovir. J Mol Med 1997; 75:300–304.

96. Rainov NG. A phase III clinical evaluation of herpes simplex virus type 1 thymidine kinase and ganciclovir gene therapy as an adjuvant to surgical resection and radiation in adults with previously untreated glioblastoma multiforme. Hum Gene Ther 2000; 11:2389.

97. Long Z, Lu P, Grooms T, et al. Molecular evaluation of biopsy and autopsy specimens from patients receiving in vivo retroviral gene therapy. Hum Gene Ther 1999; 10:733–740.

98. Morsy MA, Caskey CT. Expanded-capacity adenoviral vectors—the helper-dependent vectors. Mol Med Today 1999; 5:18–24.

99. Dumon KR, Ishii H, Fong LY, et al. FHIT gene therapy prevents tumor development in Fhit-deficient mice. Proc Natl Acad Sci USA 2001; 98:3346–3351.

100. Akporiaye ET, Hersh E. Clinical aspects of intratumoral gene therapy. Curr Opin Mol Ther 1999; 1:443–453.

101. Gomez-Navarro J, Curiel DT. Conditionally replicative adenoviral vectors for cancer gene therapy. Lancet Oncol 2000; 1:148–158.

102. Zwiebel JA. Cancer gene and oncolytic virus therapy. (Review). Semin Oncol 2001; 28:336.

103. Galipeau J, Li H, Paquin A, Sicilia F, Karpati G, Nalbantoglu J. Vesicular stomatitis virus G pseudotyped retrovector mediates effective in vivo suicide gene delivery in experimental brain cancer. Cancer Res 1999; 59:2384–2394.

104. Spencer DM. Developments in suicide genes for preclinical and clinical applications. Curr Opin Mol Ther 2000; 2:433.

105. Ciftci K, Trovitch P. Applications of genetic engineering in veterinary medicine. Adv Drug Del Rev 2000; 43:57–64.

106. Argyle DJ. Gene therapy in veterinary medicine. Vet Rec 1999; 144:369.

107. Scollay R. Gene therapy: a brief overview of the past, present, and future. Ann NY Acad Sci 2001; 953:26.

28 Vaccines for the Treatment of Cancer

Philip M. Arlen, MD, James Gulley, MD, PhD,
Lauretta Odogwu, MD, and John L. Marshall, MD

CONTENTS

CANCER VACCINE STRATEGIES
PHARMACODYNAMICS: IMMUNOLOGICAL ENDPOINTS
DRUG DEVELOPMENT ISSUES ASSOCIATED WITH VACCINES
CONCLUSION

1. CANCER VACCINE STRATEGIES

The primary goal of cancer vaccines is to activate the immune system to eliminate tumor cells without affecting normal tissues. There are two major approaches to cancer immunotherapy: active immunotherapy and passive immunotherapy (Fig. 1). Active immunotherapy involves the delivery of a substance designed to elicit an immune reaction. The host's immune system must first recognize and then respond to the target. Passive immunotherapy involves the delivery of a substance with intrinsic immunological activity such as an antibody or activated lymphocytes. This chapter focuses on the former approach.

General strategies for vaccine development use either whole cell approaches or vaccines that are based on a specific tumor-associated antigen (TAA).

1.1. Whole Tumor Vaccines

Whole tumor cells (either autologous or allogeneic) rendered safe by radiation and often mixed with an immunological adjuvant were one of the earliest forms of active immunotherapy. Throughout the last five or more decades whole tumor cells have been used in clinical trials for a number of cancers particularly melanoma and renal and colorectal cancers *(1)*.

In early studies whole tumor vaccines were often admixed with nonspecific adjuvants (e.g., bacillus Calmette-Guérin [BCG]) as initial attempts to immunize with irradiated autologous tumor cells were met with little success *(2)*. Following these initial disappointments, new developments with cancer vaccines have led to a resurgence of interest. New technologies now allow for improved immunogenicity of vaccines genetically modified tumor cells to produce cytokines (interleukin [IL]-2 *[52,56]*, IL-4 *[57]*, tumor necrosis factor-α TNF-α *[58]*), growth factors such as granulocyte colony-stimulating factor (G-CSF), *(59,61)*, T-cell costimulatory factors such as CD 80 and CD 86, or a combination thereof. This approach is known as ex vivo gene therapy.

Clinical trials of either autologous tumor cell preparations (from the patients own tumor cells) (Table 1) or allogeneic tumor cell preparations (human tumor cells from another individual or from cell lines) (Table 2) have been reported and results remain inconclusive.

Handbook of Anticancer Pharmacokinetics and Pharmacodynamics
Edited by: W. D. Figg and H. L. McLeod © Humana Press Inc., Totowa, NJ

Table 1
Phase III Clinical Trials with Autologous Tumor Cell Vaccines

Authors	Treatment	Phase	No. of patients	Results
Hoover et al. 1993 Colorectal (62)	ASI with autologous tumor + BCG vs resection alone	III	80	No significance in OS of DFS at 93 mo F/U
Vermoken et al. 1999 Colorectal (63)	ASI with autologous tumor + BCG vs resection alone	III	254	Stage II: 61% of reduced risk of recurrence Stages II and III: 41% reduced risk of recurrence
Harris et al. 2000 Colorectal (64)	ASI with autologous tumor + BCG vs resection alone	III	412	Stages II and III: no significant OS. DTH correlated with improved prognosis

ASI, Active immunotherapy; BCG, bacillus Calmette-Guérin; DFS, disease-free survival; DTH, delayed-type cutaneous hypersensitivity; F/U, follow-up; OS, overall survival.

Table 2
Clinical Trials with Allogeneic Tumor Cell Vaccines in Melanoma

Authors	Treatment	Phase	No. of patients	Results
Morton and Barth 1996 (65)	Polyvalent whole cell vaccine (Cancervax)	II	283	All stage III: DFS >90 mo compared to other adjuvant therapies
Mitchell et al. 1997 (66)	Melacine vs combination chemotherapy	III	106	All stage IV: no difference in OS; tolerability and QOL better with vaccine
Wallack et al. 1998 (67)	Vaccinia virus oncolysate vs virus alone	III	217	All stage III: no difference in OS or DFS; men with 1–5 LN+ and aged 44–57 yr had survival advantage with vaccine
Bystryn et al. 1998 (68)	Polyvalent melanoma shed antigens vs placebo	III	38	All stage III: vaccine vs placebo—RFS 18 mo vs 7.1 mo; 2-yr survival 76% vs 60%; no toxicity

DFS, Disease-free survival; QOL, quality of life; F/U, follow-up; OS, overall survival; RFS, median relapse-free survival.

Active Immunotherapy:
Vaccination Strategies

Whole cells	Tumor antigens
Autologous tumor cells	Proteins
Allogeneic tumor cells	Peptides
Pulsed dendritic cells	Carbohydrates
Dendritic/tumor fusions	DNA
	Viral
	Mimics (anti-id, heat-shock protein)

+/- Genetic modification

Passive Immunotherapy Approaches

Monoclonal antibodies: toxins, radiolabels
Cytokines
Adoptive cellular therapy
Gene therapy

Fig. 1. Cancer immunotherapy approaches.

With the scarcity of fresh autologous tumor material, a number of investigators began using allogeneic cell lines with more frequency. Despite attempts to match allogeneic cell lines in order to have the same HLA class I as autologous tumors, some studies revealed that allogeneic cell lines can confer and enhance antitumor activity compared with autologous cells *(3)*. It was thought that perhaps the allogeneic cells may be inducing some form of graft vs tumor activity. A full understanding of inducing cross-reactive cytotoxic T-lymphocyte (CTL) response may lead to development of more effective allogeneic based vaccines strategy *(4)*.

One major advantage to the whole tumor cell vaccine approach is that the preparations contain multiple undefined antigens and avoid the need for tumor antigen preselection. This approach increases the probability that the vaccine contains unidentified immunogenic antigens that are essential for vaccine activity. However, a major limitation to this approach is that there is a limited supply of vaccine product, limiting repeated treatments. The other disadvantage is that standardizing and characterizing the vaccine product may be problematic, expense is increased, and measuring vaccine-specific immune responses are difficult, if not impossible.

Despite these issues, there remain interesting positive clinical data and continued interest in the whole vaccine approach.

1.1.1. Hybrid Cell Fusion

Hybrid cell vaccination "hybridoma" is a novel approach aimed at recruiting T-cell help for the induction of tumor-specific cytolytic immunity. The patient's tumor cells are fused with allogeneic major histocompatibility class (MHC) II bearing cells *(5,6)*. The theory is that the hybrid cells generated will display the full antigenicity of tumor cell and be highly immunogenic by the effect of those of the allogeneic MHC II and costimulatory contributed by the fusion partner cell. This concept has been tested in animal models for thymoma, hepatocellular carcinoma, and adenocarcinoma of various origins *(7)*. Two small studies with metastatic melanoma and renal cell cancer patients *(8)* demonstrated preliminary evidence of survival benefits with minimal toxic effects *(9)*.

1.1.2. DENDRITIC CELL VACCINES

Antigen presentation is a crucial step in the initiation of an effective immune response, which requires antigens to be presented in order to sensitize naive T cells and to restimulate primed T cells. The most efficient antigen presenting cell (APC) is the dendritic cell (DC). DCs are found in most tissues where they exist in an immature state, unable to stimulate T cells but possessing an exceptional ability to capture and process antigens. These captured antigens can be presented efficiently by both class I and class II MHC molecules. Antigen capture acts as a signal for the DC to mature and mobilize to regional lymph nodes. These cells undergo extensive transformation and antigen capturing decrease while T-cell stimulatory functions increase. The unique capacity of these "mature" DC cells to activate T cells is probably related to the presence of an exceptionally high number of MHC, costimulatory, and adhesion molecules.

Sufficient DCs can now be generated ex vivo using DC growth factors such as GM-CSF and flt-3 ligand. The concept of hybridomas has been applied to DC therapy whereby tumor cells have been infused with DCs to create an APC full of tumor antigens.

Adoptive transfer of autologous or allogeneic DCs pulsed or loaded with tumor antigens prior to reinfusion are now entering clinical trials. In one study *(10)* that was recently updated *(11)*, patients with B-cell lymphoma were vaccinated with idiotype-pulsed DCs cellular and immune responses were noted.

The optimal method to load DC with antigens such as tumor-specific peptides, protein, mRNA, or apoptotic or necrotic cells is currently an area of intensive investigation. DCs can be genetically modified with genes encoding tumor antigens (and/or cytokines). Tumor antigen expression within the DCs should provide the cells with a renewable source of antigen for presentation, and, consequently, more sustained antigen presentation. Recombinant viruses, including adenoviruses and retroviruses, can be used to transduce DCs. Although transduction through this method is highly effective, the expression of viral genes may occur *(12)*. These viral genes may prime antiviral immunity including cytotoxic T-cell lysis, which in turn may rapidly destroy the DCs in subsequent rounds of immunization. Several murine models have shown that preexisting immunity does not prevent successful immunization with adenoviral infected DCs *(13)*. However, there are new vectors ("gutless adenovirus") that don't express viral gene products. In pilot clinical studies in patients with non-Hodgkin's lymphoma, myeloma, and melanoma, vaccination with DC vaccination induced both antitumor immune responses and tumor regression (Table 3).

1.2. Tumor-Associated Antigen (TAA)

Potential advantages of vaccines that are directed against a specific TAA include immune responses that can be reliably measured, standardization in vaccine production, and minimized nonspecific immune activation. The development of TAA-directed vaccine involves identification of a target antigen and selection of a platform (e.g., proteins, peptides, carbohydrates, and DNA-or virus-based vectors) for presentation to the immune system. Potential target candidates are antigens that are expressed only on tumor cells or only those that are relatively overexpressed on tumor cells compared to normal cells. Very few antigens are truly tumor specific to a particular patient's tumor. Some may be limited in expression to a particular tumor type while others have a wide expression on a variety of different tumor types. Molecular techniques such as SERAX analysis, microarrays, serial analysis of gene expression (SAGE), and differential displays have been used recently to identify new antigen targets for vaccine targeting.

1.2.1. VECTOR-DRIVEN TAAS

TAAs are by definition either weakly immunogenic or functionally nonimmunogenic. Vaccine strategies must be developed in which the presentation of these TAAs to the immune system results in far greater activation of T cells than is being achieved naturally in the host. One way to increase the immunogenicity of a TAA is to use a viral vector to deliver the appropriate genetic material. The advantages of using a viral vector include (1) the incorporation of the entire tumor antigen gene, parts of that gene, or multiple genes (including genes for costimulatory molecules and cytokines); (2) the ability of selected vectors to infect APCs allowing them to process the antigens; and (3) the relative cost of viral vector vaccines is low compared with preparation and purification of proteins. Overcoming tolerance to carcinoembryonic antigen (CEA) in CEA transgenic mice was not accomplished with a peptide-based vaccine but was relatively easily accomplished with a vaccinia CEA construct (14).

1.2.2. TYPES OF VECTORS

Viral vectors can be divided into those that are capable of replicating in mammalian species and those that can infect mammalian cells but cannot complete the replication process. There are advantages and disadvantages to each. Some of the viruses that can are replication competent have been extensively studied and have well-defined safety profile. These vectors can continue to infect additional cells, producing more TAA until eradicated by the immune system. Often vaccines associated with these cells are more immunogenic than those using replication-defective vectors. The replication-defective vectors, however, are in theory safer as they can infect mammalian cells only once and therefore cannot cause the rare but in immunocompromised individuals, the potentially life-threatening conditions associated with replication-defective vectors such as vaccinia. One group of vectors extensively studied in tumor vaccines are the pox viruses. These viruses have several advantages including the ability to make stable recombinant vectors with accurate replication and efficient posttranslational processing of the transgene. In addition, as many as seven transgenes have been expressed in a single vaccinia vector (15), making these potentially powerful tools for vaccine gene delivery.

1.2.3. REPLICATION COMPETENT VECTORS

One of the most studied pox viral vectors is vaccinia. This virus has been used since 1796 to vaccinate against smallpox, with more than a billion doses given worldwide. The success of this vaccine in eradiating this disease has led to the discontinuation of the vaccination to the general population. Early of recombinant vaccinia viruses containing human immunodeficiency virus (HIV) transgenes revealed that vaccinia naïve patients had higher antigen specific T-cell responses and antibody responses to a vaccinia vaccine than patients previously vaccinated with vaccinia (16). Subsequent studies have demonstrated that significantly higher doses (e.g., 10^8 plaque-forming units [PFU]) of vaccinia vector given to patients could induce a vigorous response to the transgene. A trial with 26 patients who had advanced colon carcinoma demonstrated a recombinant vaccinia CEA (rV-CEA) vaccine given monthly for 3 mo was well tolerated by patients (17). While there were no clinical responses observed, this was the first demonstrate generation of a human cytolytic T-cell response to specific epitopes of CEA. Other trials with rV-CEA also showed lack of toxicity16, antibody responses (17), and apparent equivalence of subcutaneous and intradermal injections (18).

Table 3
Clinical Trials with Dendritic Cell-Based Vaccines

Authors	Treatment	Phase	No. of patients	Disease and results
Hsu et al. 1996 (69)	Idiotype protein-pulsed DCs	Pilot	4	NHL: RR 75%; cellular antitumor response in all patients, no toxicity
Lim and Bailey-Wood 1999 (70)	Idiotype protein-pulsed DCs	Pilot	6	Myeloma: proliferative response in 5/6 patients
Morse et al. 1999 (71)	CEA peptide-pulsed DCs	I	—	Various: MR, 1; SD, 1; no toxicity
Murphy et al. 1999 (72)	PSM-P1/PSM-P2-pulsed DCs	II	11	Prostate: CR 2, PR 7
Kugler et al. 2000 (73)	Tumor–allogeneic DC heteroconjugate	Pilot	17	Renal: CR 2; PR 2; SD 2

CEA, Carcinoembryonic antigen; CR, complete response; DC, dendritic cell; MR, Minor response; PR, partial response; PSM, prostate-specific membrane antigen; RR, response rate; SD, stable disease.

Table 4
Selected Clinical Trials

Vaccine	No. of patients	Phase	Immune response	Clinical response	Reference
rV-CEA	26	I	Y	N	Tsang 1995 (15)
rV-PSA	33	I	Y	N	Eder et al. 2000 (22)
rV-MCU-1/IL-2					Scholl 2000 (81)
rV-CEA → avi-CEA	18	I	Y	Y	Marshall et al. 2000/Slack et al. 2001 (20,21)
Avi-CEA/B7.1	60	I	Y	N	Von Mehren et al. 2001 (23)
rV-PSA + rV-B7.1 → rF-PSA	27	II	Y	Y[a]	Arlen et al. 2002 (74)
rV-CEA(6D)/TRICOM → avi-CEA(6D)/TRICOM	32	I	Y	Y	Marshall et al. 2002 (25)
Adeno-MART-1 or -gp100	58	I	Y	Y[b]	Rosenberg 1998 (44)

[a]One patient with a sustained PSA decrease from 8.7 ng/dL to 0.2 ng/dL with vaccine alone.
[b]One patient (of 16) 1/16 patient treated with MART-1 without IL-2.

These trials and pre-clinical models demonstrated that further increases in antigen specific immune responses were limited after the second and third vaccination, presumably due to the vigorous immune response to the vaccinia proteins. Avipox vectors, which do not express the late viral antigens in mammalian cells, and thus are replication defective in humans, do not have a significant immune response generated to them. Thus trials using heterologous prime and boost strategies were developed with recombinant vaccinia vectors and recombinant avipox vectors.

1.2.4. REPLICATION-DEFECTIVE VECTOR

Avipox vectors, which do not express the late viral antigens in mammalian cells and thus are replication defective in humans, do not have a significant immune response generated against them. Thus trials using heterologous prime and boost strategies were developed with recombinant vaccinia vectors and recombinant avipox vectors.

Avipox vectors are capable of infecting human cells and expressing their transgene for up to 3 wk before cell death ensues. Avipox vectors include fowlpox and canarypox (ALVAC). Clinical trials with these vectors have shown that these can be given numerous times with a resulting increase in CEA-specific T-cell responses *(19)*. To take advantage of the potency of vaccinia-based vaccines and the lack of immunogenicity of the avipox-based vaccines, prime and boost strategies were developed. In an effort to determine which heterologous prime and boost regimen to use, a small randomized trial was conducted looking at either giving the rV-CEA as the initial priming vaccination followed by boosting with avipox-CEA (VAAA), or giving the three vaccinations with avipox-CEA first followed by rV-CEA (AAAV) *(20)*. This study showed that the immune responses seen in the VAAA arm were much better than in the AAAV arm. Furthermore, continued follow-up of these patients revealed that although there were only nine patients in each arm, at the time of a recent presentation five or nine patients were alive on the VAAA arm (2-yr survival estimate $67 \pm 19\%$) whereas in the AAAV arm zero of nine patients were alive (2-yr survival estimate $0 \pm 0\%$) *(21)*. An ongoing randomized Phase II clinical trial has demonstrated that rV-prostate-specific antigen (rV-PSA) admixed with rV-B7.1 followed by monthly rF-PSA can generate PSA-specific T-cell responses and, in one patient, a sustained PSA decrease from 8.7 ng/dL at the start of the study to 0.19 ng/dL. This vaccine is given with GM-CSF at the vaccine site and low dose IL-2 subcutaneously 1-wk later at a distant site *(74)*. Selected clinical trials are tabulated in Table 4.

2. PHARMACODYNAMICS: IMMUNOLOGICAL ENDPOINTS

A number of different vaccine strategies that activate T-cell responses are now being investigated in clinical trials to evaluate the role of immunotherapy as a modality of anti-tumor therapy. Examples of these approaches include the use of TAAs such as CEA, PSA, and MUC-1, either as full proteins delivered in viral vectors or as peptide pulsed dendritic cells *(22–25)*. Other well known characterized antigens used in cancer vaccine clinical trials include MART-1, gp100, MAGE-1, tyrosinase, and HER2/neu *(26–29)*. It is crucial to evaluate the relative effects of these vaccines on the immune system, in order to develop more potent vaccines that may be used in patients with earlier stages of disease and to combine with other traditional therapeutic modalities such as chemotherapy and/or radiation therapy.

Immune activity can be evaluated by specific responses involving both cell-mediated and humoral immunity. Cell-mediated immunity in general refers to the production of CTL responses against the tumor that the vaccine specifically targets. This involves CD8$^+$ T cells along with mature CD4$^+$ T-helper cells, type 1 (Th1) cells. On the other hand, assays measuring humoral immunity involve antibody production from mature B cells along with B cells that are in part induced by mature CD4$^+$ T-helper cells, type 2 (Th2) cells.

The optimal vaccination strategy in humans using specific TAAs against tumors expressing the antigen won't be determined until large multiarm clinical trials correlating survival, disease-free interval, or tumor regression are completed. In the absence of such data, immunoassays (both T-cell-mediated immunity and antibody-based) may be useful to help define: (1) if a given vaccine can elicit any immune response and (2) the relative potency of such a response.

2.1. Delayed-Type Hypersensitivity Testing (DTH)

DTH is performed by injecting a soluble protein antigen of interest subcutaneously and measuring the area of induration 48–72 h after the antigen has been administered. It is a technically simple test that reflects the development of systemic antigen-specific immunity. Although it has been used commonly to study infectious disease models, such as tetanus toxoid, the significance of this assay is still debatable as a tool for measuring tumor-specific immune responses. It has been shown that selected cancer patients who are anergic to common immunogens by DTH can mount immunologic responses to TAAs. However, recent studies seem to suggest that the DTH response is an accurate indicator of a patient's T-cell response, at least in some populations. Disis et al. looked for the development of tumor antigen-specific DTH responses, using HER-2/neu peptides as the model antigen in patients with advanced stage cancer to test if they would correlate to in vitro measurements of systemic antigen-specific T-cell responses as measured by lymphocytic proliferation. The authors demonstrated that tumor antigen-specific DTH responses ≥ 10 mm^2 correlate significantly to a measurable antigen-specific peripheral blood T-cell response *(28)*.

2.2. Limiting Dilution Assay

Early immunologic monitoring methods to determine precursor frequency analysis of CTL to a particular immunogen were labor intensive and required numerous in vitro stimulations (IVS) of the cell lines *(50)*. The limiting dilution assay (LDA) was used most frequently *(42,51)*. In a recent CEA vaccine clinical trial described by Marshall et al. *(35)*, LDAs were used to determine the CTL precursor frequency to CEA peptide-1 (CEA amino acid position 571–579; YLSGANLNL [CAP-1]) in the prevaccination and postvaccination peripheral blood mononuclear cells (PBMCs) from HLA-A2-positive patients. However, this assay is extremely time consuming and labor intensive. Various numbers of PBMCs were seeded into 96-well flat-bottom plates, with autologous irradiated PBMCs and incubated with . At least 48 cultures were used in this study for each dilution of PBMCs. The 5 d of incubation with peptide plus the 11 d with IL-2 constituted one in vitro stimulation cycle. After two in vitro stimulation cycles, the CTL activity was tested for each well against C1R-A2 target cells with and without incubation with CAP-1, using the procedure described earlier, with unlabeled K562 cells added to each assay at a ratio of 10 unlabeled K562 cells to one target cell, to eliminate the natural killer cell activity. Precursor frequencies were calculated by χ^2 minimization, as described by Taswell et al. *(43)*. Individual counts obtained from each experimental well were compared with the mean counts from the controls on the same plate. LDAs of PBMCs were conducted to quantitate CEA-specific CTL precursors before and after each vaccination per patient. CTL activity that was greater than the mean plus three SDs of the control wells was considered significant.

2.3. Enzyme-Linked Immunosorbent Assay (ELISA)

Other methods such as cytokine production assays by ELISA measure cytokine production of mixed-cell populations. Cytokine production by T cells undergoing in vitro stimulation is considered a well accepted measure of T-cell activation. Various cytokines such as interferon-γ (IFN-γ), IL-2, and TNF-α have been used to monitor numerous tumor immunotherapy studies. Increase levels of IFN-γ and IL-2 would suggest an increase in CTL activity. However, the standard ELISA assay measures overall cytokine levels, which may vary considerably. This assay does not provide a quantitative measurement of TAA-specific T-cells *(29–35)*.

2.4. Tetramers

Newer techniques for analysis of specific T-cell responses to vaccines include tetramers and the Fast Immune assay. Tetramers allow for the identification of a specific T-cell type. Tetramers have been widely used to quantify the number of viruses and bacteria-specific T cells in animal models *(36,37)*. However, this technique can be cumbersome, requiring the preparation and purification of a tetramer for each peptide evaluated. Although tetramers have been developed to several epitopes of human TAAs to phenotype T-cell populations pre- and postvaccination, their sensitivity has not yet been established as an assay to evaluate cancer vaccines.

2.5. Fast Immune

The intracellular cytokine Fast Immune assay can be used to phenotype T-cell responses from vaccinated patients *(38,39)*. This technique incorporates the use of cell flow cytometry to detect intracellular or cell-associated cytokines and allows the examination of multiple cytokines within individual cells. Careful comparison of this assay with the enzyme-linked immunospot (ELISPOT) assay has determined that the sensitivity of this assay is similar to that of the ELISPOT. However, the cost of second antibody reagents and extended fluorescence-activated cell sorter (FACS) scanning time make this assay more expensive and time consuming as compared to the ELISPOT assay.

2.6. ELISPOT Assay

The ELISPOT assay is relatively sensitive and quantitative. By measuring cytokine release on a single-cell basis, the assay can detect a peptide-specific T-cell response against specific HLA class I binding peptides *(40)* (Fig. 2A, B). The level of cytotoxicity determined by the standard chromium release assay after in vitro expansion of specific T cells has been shown to correlate with the number of IFN-γ releasing cells measured by the ELISPOT assay in a study of both healthy donors and melanoma patients *(29)*.

The ELISPOT assay without IVS has been used to monitor two different types of CEA-based cancer-vaccine trials *(24)*. These trials showed that the ELISPOT assay can be performed with previously frozen PBMCs from HLA-A2–positive patients as a source of T cells. C1RA2 cells were used as APCs and were pulsed with Flu matrix peptide (amino acid position 58–66) and a CEA 9-mer peptide.

However, most studies to date have required in vitro stimulations of PBMCs with peptide and IL-2 to monitor immune responses to TAAs *(29,31,43–47)*. A number of variables may alter the results of the ELISPOT assay. The APCs used to conduct the assay may vary. An HLA-A2–positive, Tap-defective T2 cell line has been used by others as the APC. One of the problems reported with T2 cells is the potential for high backgrounds, possibly due to alloreactivity of residual MHC I expression *(48)*. Other studies have used autologous PBMCs

ELISPOT Assay

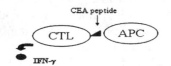

A

T-cells that are specific for CEA will produce IFN-g when activated by CEA (*in vitro*)

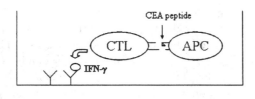

B

**IFN-g secreted by activated T-cells (*in vitro*) is captured
on an anti- IFN-g coated 96-well plate**

Fig. 2. ELISPOT assay.

for peptide presentation. However, autologous PBMCs may not be the ideal APC with which to perform the ELISPOT assay in cancer patients, owing to shifts from the Th1 to Th2 subset *(49)*. In our previous study we used the C1RA2 cell line to circumvent the use of possible defective APCs in cancer patients. Other issues such as the weak signal 1 of the TAAs and the limited number of PBMCs also can contribute to the lack of detection of potential immune responses.

3. DRUG DEVELOPMENT ISSUES ASSOCIATED WITH VACCINES

3.1. Schedule of Administration

Although there has been an explosion of new cancer vaccines being tested in clinical trials, there has been little focus in these trials on the schedule of administration. Because the primary goal of noncancer vaccines is prevention of disease, there is little pressure to create a rapid, powerful immune response. Instead, there is time for priming and boosting over months to years. In contrast, most of the vaccines being tested today for cancer treatment are used in patients with advanced cancer who frequently have rapidly growing, refractory disease. In this patient population, time is of the essence as these patients will have demonstrated progression of their tumors in a very short time (6–12 wk) if effective therapy is not given. By convention, if patients do progress in this time frame, they are removed from the study as treatment failures.

Conventional chemotherapy is given in "cycles," which are typically 3–4 wk long. In the case of cytotoxic agents, the treatment is given and then time away from treatment is built in to allow for recovery from the toxic effects of the treatment. The effects of the chemotherapy are seen acutely, with the antitumor responses observed during the first few treatments. If responses are not seen in the first two or three cycles, then the treatment is unlikely to be of benefit and treatments are stopped and/or changed. However, none of this applies to vaccines. First, we have a very poor understanding of the timing of an optimum immune response. There are no objective data that guide us in deciding when we have achieved an "effective" level of activity, which of course is complicated further by the various ways of measuring an immune response, different types of vaccines, and different vaccination schedules employed. What is an effective/adequate level of T cells, antibodies, and so forth when seeking an anticancer response? How does the time course of an immune response vary when using a viral vector based vaccine compared to a DC approach, and how do cytokines influence this? Should we be giving these vaccines weekly, monthly, or every 3 mo? The truth is that we have very limited insights into the answers to these quite fundamental questions.

Arguably, we do not have the answers to these questions when initially testing novel chemotherapy, but these agents commonly result in toxicity and clinical responses that guide us in designing optimum administration schedules. In the case of cancer vaccines, the absence of toxicity, objective clinical responses, and validated intermediate immune endpoints makes this very difficult. Furthermore our ignorance increases the risk of rejecting a vaccinen not because it does not have potential clinical utility, but because we do not know how to evaluate it's effects properly.

The majority of trials have used an every 2- to 4-wk vaccine administration schedule, often with vaccines given close together at first and then spreading out the subsequent boosting treatments. Some trials have given only a fixed number of vaccines and then stopped, regardless of treatment outcomes. Virtually all of these schedules were designed with regard to convenience, convention, and "best guess" and not based on a firm understanding of the immune response. Of course none of this would matter if frequent anticancer responses were observed in these trials, but unfortunately responses have not been routinely observed. Many vaccines have already been abandoned from further development owing to lack of clinical activity but without a clear understanding concerning the level at which they failed (immune response, administration schedule, dose).

Future vaccine trials must begin to address the issue of administration schedule. To do this, incorporate the best immune monitoring available, optimize the patient selection, and we must test various schedules early in the agent's development. The topic of immune monitoring is covered elsewhere in this chapter, but its importance cannot be overstated. Without the ability to measure a biologic response (specific or nonspecific), we will continue to "fly blind" in our trial designs and conclusions. Optimizing patient selection is critical. The current standard to test vaccines in patients with refractory, advanced cancer adds to our problems. These are not the best patients on whom to test immune-based therapies. These patients have frequently received multiple chemotherapy treatments that might interfere with the immune response, they have larger tumor burdens against which the immune response must fight, and the shortened life expectancy these patients experience limits our ability to understand the long-term effects of these therapies. While it remains extremely important to continue to test novel vaccine approaches in patients with metastatic disease in the hopes of uncovering significant anticancer activity in this patient population, it is also important to recognize that the ultimate target population for these types of therapies is likely to be a much earlier stage patient. Performing early phase clinical trials in patients such as this, however, is more expensive and in some ways riskier. Examples of patients currently being accrued to these types of trials are colon cancer patients following resection of metastases (CALGB 89903), patients with high-risk prostate cancer (Prosvac), and high-risk breast cancer patients (Her-2 based vaccines). Although the results of these studies take longer to mature they are extremely important and worth the wait.

3.2. Combination Therapies Utilizing Vaccines

There is a great deal of excitement about cancer vaccines in clinical trials today, we must recognize that there have only been limited positive objective clinical responses in these studies. At the same time there have been anecdotal reports of clinical activity and frequent reporting of positive immune responses. Based on this it is logical to consider combining vaccine-based approaches with other anticancer treatments in the hopes of capitalizing on the advantages of each approach. The most commonly utilized and most successful form of cancer therapy is cytotoxic chemotherapy. The rationale for combining cytotoxic chemotherapy with immune-based approaches includes evidence supporting a lessening of immune suppression with the potential for enhancing the overall immune response, and the potential that chemotherapy will add to the overall clinical response and allow for adequate disease control to enable the immune system to mount an effective response *(75)*. However, this approach has been tempered by the unknown impact of chemotherapy on the ability to mount an immune response in general.

Preclinical and clinical studies experiments have demonstrated that chemotherapy can modulate the immune response to include enhancement of T-cell activity, tumor vaccines, and macrophages. Machiels et al. demonstrated a positive impact of "immune modulating doses" of cyclophosphamide, doxorubicin, and paclitaxel on the immune response (as measured by ELISPOT and tumor rejection) independent of the cytotoxic anticancer activity of the chemotherapeutic agents alone *(76)*. In another preclinical trial combining an peptide-based vaccine and 5-fluorouracil (5-FU)/leucovorin chemotherapy, Watson et al. demonstrated that the chemotherapy had no effect on the generation of vaccine-specific antibodies and the combination actually had an increased therapeutic effect on tumors in the mouse xenograft model *(77)*.

A series of small clinical trials testing nonspecific immune enhancers (IFN-α, BCG, etc.) in combination with chemotherapy demonstrated no detectable inhibition of the immune responses or clinical outcomes *(78,79)*. Several larger clinical trials have been performed combining immune-based approaches with chemotherapy. The largest of these utilized a monoclonal antibody combined with 5-FU-based chemotherapy in the adjuvant setting *(80)*. This trial was negative and it is unclear whether these results are reflective of an agent that is inactive or a trial design that failed to recognize the potential negative interaction between chemotherapy and immune-based therapies. Recently a Phase II randomized trial was performed in metastatic pancreas cancer utilizing a vaccine alone compared to patients being treated with the combination of gemcitabine and vaccine *(82)*. In this study the chemotherapy did not have a negative influence on the immune response as measured by the detection of target-specific antibodies. Other trials are underway combining vaccines with chemotherapy, many of which with little data to support a positive interaction between the two classes of compounds. When designing trials such as this, the importance of solid preclinical data supporting the combination cannot be underestimated. Future studies should emphasize chemotherapy doses and schedules to optimize the direct anticancer effects and immune modulatory effects of the chemotherapy–vaccine combinations.

3.3. Regulatory Issues for Vaccine-Based Clinical Trials

The last decade of clinical research has been marked by a dramatic increase in regulatory requirements for all trials involving investigational agents, and this increase may have been most dramatic for the so-called "biologic therapies." These agents include viruses, gene therapies, protein therapies, and other "natural" products and, of course, virtually all immune-based therapies fall into one of these categories. The process of protocol review and approval for these agents frequently involves several additional steps not required for more traditional agents.

3.3.1. INSTITUTIONAL REVIEW BOARD REVIEW

Typically, there are no unusual requirements in obtaining IRB approval for these classes of compounds. However, with a heightened awareness of and concern about these agents following a few highly publicized problems with trials using biologic therapies, IRB reviews have become more critical, requiring more safety data and tighter controls on all aspects of the trials. These issues should be accounted for in the writing and design of all trials but are particularly important for biologic agents. In specific, great attention should be focused on the consent form, eligibility criteria, drug storage and handling, and clear reviews of all the known preliminary data that exist supporting the trial and its design.

3.3.2. INSTITUTIONAL BIOSAFETY REVIEWS

The first additional step in the review process for virus- and gene-based therapies is a review by an institution's biosafety committee. The primary purpose of this review is to focus on the proper handling of potentially hazardous biologic products, ensuring that patients and staff are adequately protected from exposure, and that proper documentation is on file detailing the agents in question. This is a frequently overlooked step by investigators and protocol administrators. Often, information requested is not found in investigators' brochures (such as vector maps) but must be obtained and provided. Obviously, different institutions require different information as they interpret the regulations provided by government agencies, so as with all regulatory steps, it is best and most efficient to discuss this early in the process.

3.3.3. FEDERAL REVIEW

Protocols that include gene therapy all must be reviewed at the federal level by two institutions. As with any investigational agent, the US Food and Drug Administration (FDA) must be involved through either the filing of an Investigational New Drug Application (IND) or the cross-filing to an existing IND. More details found on the Web at www.fda.gov. In addition, the protocol must be reviewed by the Recombinant DNA Advisory Committee (RAC), a review group that is responsible for tracking all gene-based therapies in the United States. The RAC was established in 1974 and its major role is to review trials that involve the transfer of recombinant DNA to humans. Currently, the RAC reviews only those trials in which NIH funding is involved. Compliance at the institutional level is the responsibility of the Institutional Biosafety Committees. More details on the RAC can be found at http://www4.od.nih.gov/oba/rac/aboutrdagt.htm.

4. CONCLUSION

In summary, vaccines for the treatment of cancer are an attractive therapeutic adjunct to standard chemotherapy because it represents non-cross-resistant therapy that adds minimal additional toxicities. Currently there are a number of clinical trials using novel vaccine designs and administration that hold promise for the future. However, a considerable amount of work is still required to optimize vaccination regimens, combine vaccines with other cancer treatment modalities, vaccinate populations with early stage disease, and define the most intermediate endpoint assays. The FDA and the public may need to judge whether prolonged time to relapse in the absence of survival difference will justify the approval of vaccines for routine care.

REFERENCES

1. Morton DL, Foshang LJ, Hoon DS, et al. Prolongation of survival in metastatic melanoma after active specific immunotherapy with a new polyvalent melanoma vaccine. Ann Surg 1992; 16:463–482.
2. Browning M, Dagleish AG. Introduction and historical perspective. In: Clinical Science in Practice: Tumor Immunology—Immunotherapy and Cancer Vaccines Cancer. London, UK, and New York, NY: Cambridge University Press, 1996.
3. Knight BC, Souberbielle BE, Rizzardi GP, Ball SE, Dagleish AG. Allogeneic murine melanoma cell vaccine—a model for the development of human allogeneic cancer vaccine. Melan Res 1996; 6:299–306.
4. Kayaga J, Souberbielle BE, Shieke N, et al. Anti-tumor activity against B16-F10 melanoma with a GM-CSF secreting allogeneic tumor cell vaccine. Gene Ther 1996 6:1475–1481.
5. Chen L, Ashe S, Brady WA, et al. Costimulation of antitumor immunity by the B7 counterreceptor for the T-lymphocyte molecules CD28 and CTLA-4. Cell 1992; 71:1093–1102.
6. Guo Y, Wu M, Chen H, et al. Effective tumor vaccine generated by fusion hepatoma cells with activated B cells. Science 1994; 263:518–520.
7. Gong J, Chen D, Kashiwaba M, Kufe D. Induction of antitumor activity by immunization with fusion of dendritic and carcinoma cells. Nat Med 1997; 3:558–561.
8. Hugler A, Stuhler G, Walden P, et al. Regression of human metastatic renal cell carcinoma after vaccination with tumor cell-dendritic cell hybrids. Nat Med 2000; 6:332–336.
9. Renner C, Kubuschok B, Trumper L, Pfreundschuh M. Clinical approaches to vaccination in Oncology. Hematology 2001; 80:255–266.
10. Hsu FJ, Benike C, Fagnoni F, et al. Vaccination of patients with B-cell lymphoma using autologous antigen-pulsed dendritic cells. Nat Med 1996;2:52–58.
11. Timmerman JM, Davis TA, Hsu FJ, et al. Idiotype-pulsed dendritic cell vaccination for B-cell lymphoma: clinical and immunological responses in 26 patients. Blood 1999; 94(Suppl):385a.
12. De Veerman M, Heirman C, Van Meirvenne S, et al. Retrovirally transduced bone marrow-derived dendritic cells require CD4+ T cell help to elicit protective and therapeutic antitumor immunity. J Immunol 1999; 162:144–151.
13. Timmerman JM, Caspar CB, Lambert SL, Syrenglas AD, Levy R. Idio-type encoding recombinant adenovirus provide protective immunity against murine B-cell lymphomas. Blood 2001; 97:1370–1307.
14. Cooney EL, Collier AC, Greenberg PD, et al. Safety of and immunological response to a recombinant vaccinia virus vaccine expressing HIV envelope glycoprotein. Lancet 1991; 337:567–572.
15. Tsang KY, Zaremba S, Nieroda CA, Zhu MZ, Hamilton JM, Schlom J. Generation of human cytotoxic T cells specific for human carcinoembryonic antigen epitopes from patients immunized with recombinant vaccinia-CEA vaccine. J Natl Cancer Inst 1995; 87:982–990.
16. McAneny D, Ryan CA, Beazley RM, Kaufman HL. Results of a Phase I trial of a recombinant vaccinia virus that expresses carcinoembryonic antigen in patients with advanced colorectal cancer. Ann Surg Oncol 1996; 3:495–500.
17. Conry RM, Allen KO, Lee S, Moore SE, Shaw DR, LoBuglio AF. Human autoantibodies to carcinoembryonic antigen (CEA) induced by a vaccinia-CEA vaccine. Clin Cancer Res 2000; 6: 34–41.
18. Conry RM, Khazaeli MB, Saleh MN, et al. Phase I trial of a recombinant vaccinia virus encoding carcinoembryonic antigen in metastatic adenocarcinoma: comparison of intradermal versus subcutaneous administration. Clin Cancer Res 1999; 5:2330–2337.
19. Marshall JL, Hawkins MJ, Tsang KY, et al. Phase I study in cancer patients of a replication-defective avipox recombinant vaccine that expresses human carcinoembryonic antigen. J Clin Oncol 1999; 17:332–337.
20. Marshall JL, Hoyer RJ, Toomey MA, et al. Phase I study in advanced cancer patients of a diversified prime-and-boost vaccination protocol using recombinant vaccinia virus and recombinant non-replicating avipox virus to elicit anti-carcinoembryonic antigen immune responses. J Clin Oncol 2000; 18:3964–3973.
21. Slack R, Ley L, Chang P, et al. Association between CEA-specific T cell responses (TCR) following treatment with vaccinia-CEA (V) and alvac-CEA (A) and survival in patients (Pts) with CEA-bearing cancers. American Society of Clinical Oncology 37th Annual Meeting, San Francisco, CA, 2001: abstract 1086.
22. Eder JP, Kantoff PW, Roper K, et al. A Phase I trial of a recombinant vaccinia virus expressing prostate specific antigen in advanced prostate cancer. Clin Cancer Res 2000; 6:1632–1638.

23. von Mehren M, Arlen P, Rogatko A, et al. Pilot study of a dual gene vector vaccine, ALVAC-CEA B7.1, in patients with recurrent CEA expressing adenocarcinomas. Clin Cancer Res 2000; 6:2219–2228.

24. Arlen P, Tsang KY, Marshall JL, et al. The use of a rapid ELISPOT assay to analyze peptide-specific immune responses in carcinoma patients to peptide vs. recombinant poxvirus vaccines. Cancer Immunol Immunother 2000; 49:517–529.

25. Marshall J, Odogwu L, Hwang J, et al. A phase I study of sequential vaccinations with fowlpox-CEA (6D)-TRICOM (B7.1/CAM-1/:LFA-3) alone, and sequentially with vaccinia-CEA (6D)-TRICOM and GM-CSF in patients with CEA-expressing carcinomas. Program/Proceedings, Am Soc Clin Oncol 2003; 22:662a.

26. Rosenberg SA. A new era for cancer immunotherapy based on the genes that encode cancer antigens. Immunity 1999; 10:281–287.

27. Minev BR, Chavez FL, Mitchell FS. Cancer vaccines: novel approaches and new promise. Pharmacol Ther 1999; 81:121–139.

28. Disis ML, Schiffman K, Gooley TA, McNeel DG, Rinn K, Knutson KL. Delayed-type hypersensitivity response is a predictor of peripheral blood T-cell immunity after HER-2/neu peptide immunization. Clin Cancer Res 2000; 6:1347–1350.

29. Pass HA, Schwarz SL, Wunderlich JR, Rosenberg SA. Immunization of patients with melanoma peptide vaccines: immunologic assessment using the ELISPOT assay. Cancer J Sci Am 1998; 4:316.

30. Merimsky O, Baharav E, Schoenfeld Y, et al. Anti-tyrosinase antibodies in malignant melanoma. Cancer Immunol Immunother 1996; 42:297.

31. Karanikas V, Hwang LA, Pearson J, et al. Antibody and T cell responses of patients with adenocarcinoma immunized with mannan-MUC1 fusion protein. J Clin Invest 1997; 100:2783.

32. Nakao M, Yamana H, Imai Y, Toh Y, Toh U, Kimura A, Yanoma S, Kakegawa T, Itoh K: HLA-A2601-restricted CTLs recognize a peptide antigen expressed on squamous cell carcinoma. Cancer Res 1995; 55:4248.

33. Ressing ME, van Driel WJ, Celis E, et al. Occasional memory cytotoxic T-cell responses of patients with human papillomavirus type 16-positive cervical lesions against a human leukocyte antigen-A*0201-restricted E7-encoded epitope. Cancer Res 1996; 56:582.

34. Bednarek MA, Sauma SY, et al. The minimum peptide epitope from the influenza virus matrix protein. Extra and intracellular loading of HLA-A2. J Immunol 1991; 147:4047–4053.

35. Marshall JL, Hawkins MJ, Tsang KY, et al. Phase I study in cancer patients of a replication-defective avipox recombinant vaccine that expresses human carcinoembryonic antigen. J Clin Oncol 1999; 17:332–337.

36. Bush DH, Pilip IM, Vijh S, Pamer EG. Coordinate regulation of complex T-cell populations responding to bacterial infection. Immunity 1998; 8:353–362.

37. Callan MF, Tan L, Annels N, et al. Direct visualization of antigen-specific CD8+ T cells during the primary immune response to Epstein–Barr virus In vivo. J Exp Med. 1998; 4; 187:1395–1402.

38. Andersson U, Hallden Gk Persson U, Hed J, Moller G, DeLey M. Enumeration of IFN-gamma-producing cells by flow cytometry. Comparison with fluorescence microscopy. J Immunol Methods 1988; 112:139–142.

39. Hallden G, Andersson U, Hed J, Johansson SG. A new membrane permeabilization method for the detection of intracellular antigens by flow cytometry. J Immunol Methods 1989; 124:103–109.

40. Alters SE, Gadea JR, Sorich M, O'Donoghue G, Talib S, Philip R. Dendritic cells pulsed with CEA peptide induce CEA-specific CTL with restricted TCR repertoire. J Immunother 1998; 21:17.

41. Zaremba S, Barzaga E, Zhu MZ, Soares N, Tsang KY, Schlom J: Identification of an enhancer agonist CTL peptide from human carcinoembryonic antigen. Cancer Res 1997; 57:4570.

42. Salazar E, Zaremba S, Tsang KY, Arlen P, Schlom J. Agonist peptide from a cytotoxic T lymphocyte epitope of human carcinoembryonic antigen stimulates production of Tc1-type cytokines and increases tyrosine phosphorylation more efficiently than cognate antigen. Int J Cancer 2000; 86:829.

43. Taswell C. Limiting dilution assays for the determination of immunocompetent cell frequencies. I. Data analysis. J Immunol 1981; 126:1614.

44. Rosenberg, SA, Yang JC, Schwartzentruber DJ, et al. Immunologic and Therapeutic Evaluation of a Synthetic Peptide Vaccine for the Treatment of Patients with Metastatic Melanoma. Nat. Med. 1998; 4:321–327.

45. Tado A, Storkus WJ, Whiteside TL. Evaluation of the modified ELISPOT assay for gamma interferon production in cancer patients receiving antitumor vaccines. Clin Diagn Lab Immunol 2000; 7:145–154.

46. Meidenbauer N, Harris DT, Spitler LE, Whiteside TL. Generation of PSA-reactive effector cells after vaccination with a psa-based vaccine in patients with prostate cancer. Prostate 2000; 43:88–100.

47. Apostolopoulos V, Pietersz GA, McKenzie IF. Cell-mediated immune responses to MUC-1 fusion protein coupled to mannan. Vaccine 1996; 14:930.

48. Scheibenbogen C, Lee KH, Mayer S, et al. A sensitive ELISPOT assay for detection of CD8+ T lymphocytes specific for HLA class I-binding peptide epitopes derived from influenza proteins in the blood of healthy donors and melanoma patients. Clin Cancer Res 1997; 3:221.

49. Pellegrini P, Berghella AM, Del Beato T, Cicia S, Adorno D, Casciani CU. Disregulation of TH1 and TH2 subsets of CD4+ T cells in peripheral blood of colorectal cancer patients and involvement in cancer establishment and progression. Cancer Immunol Immunother 1996; 42:1.

50. Tsang KY, Zaremba S, Nieroda CA, Zhu MZ, Hamilton JM, Schlom J. Generation of human cytotoxic T cells specific for human carcinoembryonic antigen epitopes from patients immunized with recombinant vaccinia-CEA vaccine. J Natl Cancer Inst 1995; 87:982.

51. Coulie PG, Somville M, Lehmann F, et al. Precursor frequency analysis of human cytolytic T lymphocytes directed against autologous melanoma cells. Int J Cancer 1992; 50:289.

52. Arienti F, Sule-Soso J, Belli F, et al. Limited antitumor T cell response in melanoma patients vaccinated with interleukin-2 gene-transduced allogeneic melanoma cells. Hum Gene Ther 1996; 7:1955–1963.

53. Veelken H, Mackensen A, Lahn M, et al. A Phase-I clinical study of autologous tumor cells plus interleukin-2-gene-transfected allogeneic fibroblasts as a vaccine in patients with cancer. Int J Cancer 1997; 70:269–277.

54. Bowman LC, Grossman M, Rill D, et al. Interleukin-2-gene-modified allogeneic tumor cells for the treatment of relapsed neuroblastoma. Hum Gene Ther 1998; 9:1303–1311.

55. Schreiber S, Kampgen E, Wagner E, et al. Immunotherapy of metastatic malignant melanoma by a vaccine consisting of autologous interleukin 2-transfected cancer cells: outcome of a phase I study. Hum Gene Ther 1999; 10:983–993.

56. Sobol RE, Shawler DL, Carson C, et al. Interleukin 2 gene therapy of colorectal carcinoma with autologous irradiated tumor cells and genetically engineered fibroblasts:a phase I study. Clin Cancer Res 1999; 5:2359–2365.

57. Arienti F, Belli F, Napolitano F, et al. Vaccination of melanoma patients with interleukin 4 gene-transduced allogeneic melanoma cells . Hum Gene Ther 1999; 10:2907–2916.

58. Skillings J, Wierzbicki R, Eisenhauer E, et al. A Phase II study or recombinant tumor necrosis factor in renal cell carcinoma: a study of the National Cancer Institute of Canada clinical trials group. J Immunother 1992; 11:67–70.

59. Soiffer R, Lynch T, Mihm M, et al. Vaccination with irradiated autologous melanoma cells engineered to secrete human granulocyte colony stimulating factor generates potent antitumor immunity in patients with metastatic melanoma. Proc Natl Acad Sci USA 1998; 95:13,141–13,146.

60. Simons JW, Mikhak B, Chang JF, et al. Induction of immunity to prostate cancer antigens: results of a clinical trial of vaccination with irradiated prostate tumor cells engineered to secrete granulocyte-macrophage colony-stimulating factor using ex-vivo gene transfer. Cancer Res 1999; 59:5160–5168.

61. Jaffe EM, Hruban Rh, Biedrzycki B, et al. Novel allogeneic granulocyte-colony-stimulating factor-secreting tumor vaccine for pancreatic cancer: a phase I trial of safety and immune activation. J Clin Oncol 2001; 19:145–156.

62. Hoover HC, Jr, Brandhorst JS, Peters LC, et al. Adjuvant active specific immunotherapy for human colorectal cancer: 6.5-year median follow-up of a phase III prospectively randomized trial. J Clin Oncol 1993; 11:390–399.

63. Vermoken JB, Claessen AM, van Tinteren H, et al. Active specific immunotherapy for stage II and stage III human colon: a randomized trial. Lancet 1999; 353:345–350.

64. Harris JE, Ryan L, Hoover HC Jr, et al. Adjuvant active specific immunotherapy for stage II and III colon cancer with an autologous tumor cell vaccine: Eastern Cooperative Oncology Group Study E5283. J Clin Oncol 2000; 18:148–167.

65. Morton DL, Barth A. Vaccine therapy for malignant melanoma. CA Cancer J Clin 1996; 46:225–244.

66. Mitchell MS, Von Eschen KB. Phase III trial of melacine melanoma theracine versus combination chemotherapy in the treatment of stage IV melanoma. Proc Am Soc Clin Oncol 1997; 16:494a: abstract 1778.

67. Wallack MK, Sivanandham M, Balch CM, et al. Surgical adjuvant specific immunotherapy for patients with stage III melanoma: the final analysis of data from a Phase III, randomized, double-blind multicenter vaccinia melanoma oncolysate trial. J Am Coll Surg 1998; 187:69–77.

68. Bystryn J-C, Oratz R, Shapiro RL, et al. Phase 3, double-blind trial of a shed polyvalent, melanoma vaccine in stage III melanoma. Proc Am Soc Clin Oncol 1998; 17:434a: abstract 1673.

69. Hsu FJ, Benike C, Fagoni F, et al. Vaccination of patients with B cell lymphoma using autologous antigen-pulsed dendritic cells. Nat Med 1998; 4:328–332.

70. Lim SH, Bailey-Wood R. Idiotypic protein-pulsed dendritic cell vaccination in multiple myeloma. Int J Cancer 1999; 83:215–222.

71. Morse MA, Deng Y, Coleman D, et al. A Phase I study of active immunotherapy with carcinoembryonic antigen peptide (CAP-1)-pulsed, autologous human cultured dendritic cells in patients with metastatic malignancies expressing carcinoembryonic antigen. Clin Cancer Res 1995; 5:1331–1338.

72. Murphy GP, Tjoa BA, Simmons SJ, et al. Infusion of dendritic cells pulsed with HLA-A2-specific prostate-specific membrane antigen peptides: a Phase II prostate cancer vaccine trial involving patients with hormone-refractory metastatic disease. Prostate 1999; 38:73–78.

73. Kugler A, Stuhler G, Walden P, et al. Regression of human metastatic renal cell carcinoma after vaccination with tumor cell-dendritic cell hybrids. Nat Med 2000; 6:332–337.

74. Arlen PM, Gulley J, Novik L, et al. A randomized phase II trial of either vaccine therapy (recombinant pox viruses expressing PSA and the B7.1 costimulatory molecule) versus hormone therapy (nilutamide) in patients with hormone refractory prostate cancer and no radiographic evidence of disease. Proc Am Soc Clin Oncol 2002; A728.

75. Ben-Efraim S. Cancer immunotherapy: hopes and pitfalls: a review. Anticancer Res 1996; 16:3235–3240.

76. Machiels JP, Reilly RT, Emens LA, et al. Cyclophosphamide, doxorubicin, and paclitaxel enhance the antitumor immune response of granulocyte/macrophage-colony stimulating factor-secreting whole-cell vaccines in HER-2/neu tolerized mice. Cancer Res 2001; 61:3689–3697.

77. Watson SA, Michael D, Justin TA, et al. Pre-clinical evaluation of the Gastrimmune immunogen alone and in combination with 5-fluorouracil/leucovorin in a rat colorectal cancer model. Int J Cancer 1998; 75:873–877.

78. Kaasinen E, Rintala E, Pere AK, et al. Weekly mitomycin C followed by monthly bacillus Calmette-Guerin or alternating monthly interferon-alpha2B and bacillus Calmette-Guerin for prophylaxis of recurrent papillary superficial bladder carcinoma. J Urol 2000; 164:47–52.

79. O'Brien ME, Saini A, Smith IE, et al. A randomized Phase II study of SRL172 (*Mycobacterium vaccae*) combined with chemotherapy in patients with advanced inoperable non-small-cell lung cancer and mesothelioma. Br J Cancer 2000; 83:853–857.

80. Schwartzberg LS. Clinical experience with edrecolomab: a monoclonal antibody therapy for colorectal carcinoma. Crit Rev Oncol Hematol 2001; 40:17–24.

81. Scholl SM, Balloul JM, Le Goc G, et al. Recombinant vaccinia virus endoding human MUC1 and IL2 as immunotheraphy in patients with breast cancer. J Immunother 2000 Sep–Oct; 23:570–580.

82. Iversen P, Marshall J, Blanke C, Yoshihara P, Moulton H, Koren M. Active specific immunotherapy with a B-hCG peptide vaccine in patients with pancreatic cancer. Program/Proceeding, Am Soc Clin Onocol 2001; 20:1083a.

29 Pharmacokinetics of Antibodies and Immunotoxins in Mice and Humans

Victor Ghetie, PhD, E. Sally Ward, PhD, and Ellen S. Vitetta, PhD

CONTENTS

1. THERAPY WITH ANTIBODIES AND IMMUNOTOXINS

Monoclonal antibodies (MAbs) are presently being used to treat malignant and nonmalignant diseases *(1)*. MAb therapy began several years after the development of hybridoma technology in 1975 *(2)*. Early clinical trials using murine MAbs showed that they were immunogenic and, with a few exceptions, had little benefit. Furthermore, they had a short half-life ($t_{1/2}$) in the circulation and poor Fc-mediated effector functions *(3)*. The generation of human anti-murine IgG antibody (HAMA) usually precluded repeated administration because of rapid immune elimination and toxic side effects resulting from the formation of immune complexes. The therapeutic effect of murine MAbs was impaired not only by HAMA but also by their short $t_{1/2}$ before HAMA was elicited. As shown in Fig. 1A, the half-life of murine IgG in humans is 1 d, which is 20-fold shorter than that of human IgG. Conversely, in mice, both human and mouse IgG have $t_{1/2}$s of 5 d (Fig. 1B). The molecular basis of this behavior has recently been elucidated by analyzing the binding of IgG to mouse and human neonatal Fc receptor (FcRn) *(4)* (discussed further below). Data obtained using mice as a model for pharmacokinetics (PK) may therefore not always be relevant to humans.

Handbook of Anticancer Pharmacokinetics and Pharmacodynamics
Edited by: W. D. Figg and H. L. McLeod © Humana Press Inc., Totowa, NJ

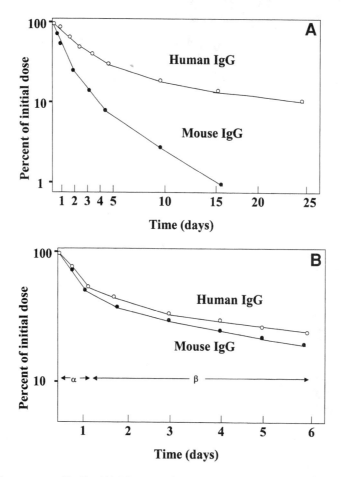

Fig. 1. Elimination curves of IgGs. **(A)** Mouse and human IgGs in humans. **(B)** Mouse and human IgGs in mouse.

To improve the efficacy of murine MAbs, several chemical and genetic approaches have been used to "arm" MAbs with toxic moieties (immunotoxins) (ITs) *(5)*. ITs consist of MAbs linked to toxin or toxin subunits from plants, bacteria, or fungi. ITs are more cytotoxic to targeted cells than "naked" MAbs *(5)*. In this case, the short persistence of the ITs in the circulation is not a drawback but an advantage because the body can rapidly eliminate the unbound cytotoxic IT. For the same reason, ITs constructed with fragments of murine IgG with short half-lives have been successfully used in some clinical trials *(6,7)*. Murine MAbs radiolabeled with ^{131}I or ^{90}Y have been highly successful in the treatment of relapsed lymphoma despite their short half-lives and immunogenicity *(5)*.

The development of chimerized (ch) and humanized (hu) MAbs *(3)* has corrected two of the weaknesses owtmurine MAbs, that is, short $t_{1/2}$ and poor effector functions. The ch and hu MAbs have the same $t_{1/2}$ in the circulation as human IgG (20 d). The longer persistence of ch and hu MAbs results in increased penetration of tumors and better therapeutic activity. Their effector functions (recruiting FcR-bearing effector cells and complement components) are also excellent. The immunogenicity of ch and hu MAbs is considerably diminished, and they have few adverse effects.

Clearly, the structure and PK of the MAbs and ITs have a major impact in their effectiveness in vivo. Therefore, understanding mechanisms that control their persistence in the circulation is of crucial importance.

2. THE MECHANISMS UNDERLYING THE PERSISTENCE OF IGG IN THE CIRCULATION

Following infusion of an IgG antibody, its disappearance from the circulation can be divided into a short period of intravascular distribution, a longer phase of equilibration between intra- and extravascular compartments, and slow removal from the circulation by catabolism. IgG elimination curves can be divided into two phases from which the corresponding PK parameters can be calculated (Fig. 1B). The first is the fast equilibration α-phase and the second is the slow catabolic β-phase. However, some catabolism may also occur during the α-phase. The most documented parameter is the β-phase which is also called the biological $t_{1/2}$. The $t_{1/2}$ of IgG correlates directly with its persistence in the circulation and inversely with its catabolic rate ($= \ln 2/t_{1/2}$). Studies on the PK of IgG in humans have shown that catabolism is accelerated in myeloma patients who have increased levels of serum IgG (short half-life and high catabolic rate) and decreased in hypogammaglobulinemic patients who have low serum concentrations of IgG (long half-life and low catabolic rate) [8]. This catabolism–concentration effect of human IgG has also been reported for mice and other species [9].

To explain the relationship between the catabolic rate of IgG and its serum concentration in mice, Brambell et al. [10] hypothesized that IgG is internalized into the cells involved in catabolism by fluid phase endocytosis and that a proportion of the antibody is then bound to intracellular receptors that recognize its Fc region. Receptor-bound IgG molecules are protected from lysosomal degradation and are recycled back into the circulation. In contrast, unbound molecules are degraded. Because the number of receptors is limited, an increase in the concentration of IgG in the circulation results in a shorter $t_{1/2}$ as a result of saturation of the receptors, that is, the proportion of internalized, unbound IgG molecules that are degraded is increased. Conversely a low concentration of IgG results in a longer $t_{1/2}$, as the receptors are not saturated and a smaller proportion of unbound molecules are destroyed. The Brambell hypothesis was proposed in the absence of any knowledge of the nature of the receptor(s) or the origin of the cell(s) involved in IgG catabolism. Subsequently, the receptor was identified as the FcRn [11–13]. FcRn was first recognized as the Fc receptor which delivers maternal IgG across the neonatal intestine and the maternal–fetal barrier [14]. Interestingly, FcRn is a heterodimer of an α-chain (homologous to MHC class I (chain) and β_2-microglobulin [14]. Recent studies indicate that the FcRn is ubiquitously expressed in endothelial cells where it most likely acts to regulate levels of serum IgG [15,16]. Further, studies using transfected [17–19] and nontransfected [20,21] cells have provided evidence that FcRn acts as an IgG transporter.

The role of FcRn in the regulation of the persistence of IgG in the circulation was clearly demonstrated by measuring the $t_{1/2}$ of mouse IgG_1 and IgG_1-derived recombinant Fc fragments in mice that do not express functional FcRn because of homozygous deletion of the gene encoding β_2-microglobulin, a component of FcRn [11]. The $t_{1/2}$s of IgG_1 and of the wild-type Fc fragment are considerably decreased in β_2-microglobulin knockout mice, and serum concentrations of IgG are 30 times lower as a result of the higher rate of IgG catabolism. In this case, the catabolism–concentration effect is absent because of the lack of FcRn. In contrast, IgA or a mutated Fc fragment of IgG, which are unable to bind to FcRn, have the same $t_{1/2}$ in both normal and FcRn-deficient mice (Table 1).

Table 1
$t_{1/2}$s of IgG_1, Fc Fragments, and IgA in Normal and FcRn-Deficient Mice[a]

Mice	IgG_1	Half-life (h) of Fc		IgA
		Recombinant	Mutant	
Normal	97.7	76.9	13.7	25.0
FcRn-deficient	17.6	12.6	14.8	24.0

Data from ref. *11*.

Similar results using different IgG ligands were obtained by other authors *(12,13)*.

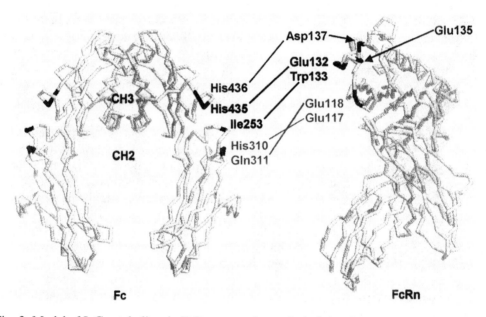

Fig. 2. Model of IgG catabolism in FcRn-expressing endothelial cells *(23)*. IgG is taken up by nonspecific pynocytosis into the endosome containing FcRn. In the acidic environment of the endosomes a proportion of IgG molecules bind to the available FcRn and are recycled to the cell surface by the fusion of endosomes with the plasma membrane. At this level, IgG dissociates from its complex with FcRn owing to the slightly alkaline pH of the environment outside the cell. IgGs that cannot bind to already saturated FcRn or have no affinity for FcRn traffic into lysosomes and are degraded.

The expression of FcRn in almost every tissue analyzed strengthened the hypothesis original proposed by Waldmann and Strober *(22)* that the endothelial cells might be the site of IgG catabolism *(11,15,16)*. Distribution studies of murine IgG_1 and anti-FcRn antibodies indicated that FcRn is expressed in the endothelium of small arterioles and capillaries of the skin and muscle and to a lesser extent in the liver and adipose tissue *(16)*. Functional FcRn is present in both mouse and human endothelial cell lines *(16,21)*. A model of how FcRn functions as an IgG homeostat is illustrated in Fig. 2 *(23)*.

Table 2
Affinity for FcRn and $t_{1/2}$s of Recombinant
Mouse Fc Fragments in Mice

Fc fragment	Relative affinity for mouse FcRn (%)	$t_{1/2}$ (h)
Wild–type	100.0[a]	119.1[b]
Mutants:		
Ile253Ala[c]	18.0	26.2
His310Ala	12.5	16.8
His433Ala	75.0	114.8
Asn434Ala	84.5	110.0
His435Ala	5.0	17.4
His436Ala	20.2	48.7

Data from ref. 27.
[a] Affinity of the wild-type is taken as 100%.
[b] The $t_{1/2}$ of Fc the fragment obtained from IgG$_1$ by papain digestion is 93 h. (Ghetie, *unpublished*).
[c] Nomenclature of mutants is: Ile253Ala = isoleucine mutated to alanine, and so forth.

3. DELINEATION OF THE AMINO ACID RESIDUES INVOLVED IN THE CATABOLISM OF IGG

3.1. Mouse

The identification of the amino acid residues involved in regulating the persistence of IgG was facilitated by the observation that mouse IgG complexed with staphylococcal protein A (SpA) or its 7-kDa fragment B was rapidly eliminated from the circulation *(24)*. Fragment B of SpA binds to the interface of the CH_2–CH_3 domains where the interaction site encompasses three regions comprising amino acid residues 252–254, 308–312, and 433–436 *(25)*. To test the hypothesis that the SpA-binding site overlaps the site of IgG involved in catabolism, amino acid residues from these three regions were altered by in vitro mutagenesis of recombinant Fc fragments *(26,27)*. These mutants were tested for their PK in mice and for their binding affinity for recombinant mouse FcRn. As shown in Table 2, amino acids from both the CH_2 (Ile-253, His-310) and CH_3 (His-435, His-436) domains are essential for the regulation of IgG catabolism. Mutants with short $t_{1/2}$s bind to FcRn with lower affinity *(28)*. The presence of highly conserved histidine residues at positions 310, 435, and, to a lesser extent, 436 provides an explanation for the strict pH dependence (binding at pH 6.0–6.5 and release at pH 7.0–7.5) of the FcRn–IgG (or Fc) interaction that was observed in binding studies *(28,29)*. The pH dependence of the FcRn–IgG interaction explains how IgG salvage might take place in endothelial cells. Hence, it has been hypothesized that IgG molecules are ingested by fluid-phase pinocytosis, traffic into acidic intracellular vesicles (endosomes), and bind to FcRn. The IgG molecules bound to FcRn are recycled back to the membrane, where they are released into the circulation because of the slightly basic pH of the blood (Fig. 2). Conversely, IgG molecules that do not bind to FcRn are destined for lysosomal degradation (reviewed in ref. *23*).

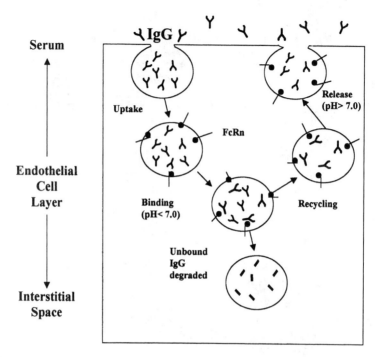

Fig. 3. The structure (α-carbon traces) of human Fc *(25)* and rat FcRn *(47)* with residues predicted to be involved in the interaction shown (based on the structure of the complex rat IgG_{2a} with rat FcRn *[52]*). Glu135 is also involved in mediating interactions with backbone amides of residues 253 and 254. The figure was drawn using RASMOL. (Courtesy of Roger Sayle, Bioinformatics Research Institute, University of Edinburgh, UK.)

The crystal structure of Fc complexed with FcRn is consistent with the results obtained by site-directed mutagenesis, showing that Ile-253, His-310, His-435, and His-436 are involved in the FcRn–IgG interaction *(30,31)*. In addition to these residues, amino acids at positions Thr-256, Pro-257, Pro-307, and Met-309 also play a role in building the FcRn interaction site of IgG in the mouse *(32)*. The good correlation between serum persistence and affinity for FcRn of the Fc fragments (Pearson correlation coefficient = 0.78) (Table 2) suggested that an increase in the affinity of an Fc fragment or IgG would result in a longer $t_{1/2}$ in vivo. Subsequently, a mutated Fc fragment with a 3.5-fold higher affinity for FcRn was obtained from a phage display library. In this fragment, Thr-252, Thr-254, and Thr-256 were mutated to Leu, Ser, and Phe, respectively, and these mutations resulted in an increase in serum $t_{1/2}$ from 93 h to 153 h *(33)*.

The IgG residues that are critical for FcRn binding are located on three spatially proximal loops that are noncontiguous in the primary sequence (Fig. 3). This suggests that the relative positions of the residues might be dependent on the conformation of the β-strands that support them and also on the topology of the CH_2 and CH_3 domains relative to each other. Thus, the detrimental effect of mutating proline to alanine at position 257 *(32)* on the serum half-life is most likely due to perturbation of the conformation of the loop encompassing Ile-253. The removal of the hinge region from the Fc fragment results in a shorter half-life,

Table 3
Affinity for FcRn and $t_{1/2}$s of Recombinant
Human Fc Fragments in Mice

Fc fragment	Relative affinity for mouse FcRn (%)	$t_{1/2}$ (h)
Wild-type[a]	100.0[a]	62.2[b]
Mutants:		
Ile253Ala[c]	21.6	25.3
His310Ala	7.2	19.2
His433Ala	110.2	62.8
His435Ala	7.5	21.7

Data from ref. *39*.
[a]Affinity of the wild-type is taken as 100%.
[b] The $t_{1/2}$ of Fc fragment obtained from IgG_1 by papain digestion is 153 h.
[c]Nomenclature of the mutants is: Ile253Ala = isoleucine mutated to alanine, and so forth.

indicating that the hinge region determines the relative spatial orientation of the CH_2 and CH_3 domains and the configuration at their interface *(34)*. In fact, replacement of the hinge sequence with a synthetic hinge containing a cysteine–cysteine bridge in the context of a different sequence generates an Fc fragment that has a $t_{1/2}$ similar to that of the wild-type fragment *(34)*. The IgG molecule has two CH_2–CH_3 domain interfaces and both are necessary for its normal persistence in the circulation *(35)*. This was demonstrated by using a hybrid recombinant mouse Fc fragment containing one functional and one mutagenized (and hence nonfunctional) FcRn interaction site. The $t_{1/2}$ of the hybrid was decreased by 50% as compared with the wild-type Fc fragment with two functional FcRn binding sites *(35)*. This finding was in agreement with an earlier observation that a rabbit IgG complexed only with one of its CH_2–CH_3 domain interfaces to fragment B of SpA has only 20% of the persistence of the noncomplexed IgG in the circulation of rabbits *(36)*.

The same amino acid residues that are involved in the control of IgG catabolism are also involved in the control of the transfer of IgG from mother to offspring *(27)*, a process also regulated by FcRn *(23)*.

3.2. Human

For the genetic engineering of therapeutic ch and hu MAbs it is important to know whether the amino acid residues critical for FcRn binding in the mouse are equally important for the persistence of human IgG in humans. Ethical reasons precluded the use of humans for PK analyses, but mice provide a suitable model for the study of the catabolism of human IgGs *(37,38)*. The $t_{1/2}$s and the affinities of mutated human Fc fragments for mouse FcRn have shown that Ile-253, His-310, and His-435 are also essential for regulating the $t_{1/2}$ of human IgG in mice (Table 3) *(39)*. These results were confirmed by mapping the binding site for human FcRn on human IgG_1 *(40)*. In addition, it has been shown that other amino acid residues in human IgG_1 are important for its binding to human FcRn.

These include Ser-254 and Lys-288 (both in the CH_2 domain), as well as Ser-415 and His-433 (both in the CH_3 domain) *(40)*. It has also been shown that a change in residue Asn-434 to Ala yielded mutants with an increased affinity for FcRn *(40)*. In the absence of PK, it is, however, difficult to evaluate how these mutants will be handled in vivo. The $t_{1/2}$s of ch IgG antibodies with shuffled constant regions have indicated that, as in the case for mouse IgGs, the conformation of the molecule also contributes to its persistence in the circulation *(41)*. Thus, ch human-mouse IgG containing a γ_4 amino-terminus spliced to a γ_1 carboxy-terminus within the CH_2 domain had a half-life in SCID mice of 282 h, which was greater than either parental IgG (199 h for IgG_1 and 77 h for IgG_4) *(41)*.

3.3. Mouse vs Human

Although the absence of carbohydrates on the Fc region of recombinant IgG has no impact on the persistence of mouse Fc (Table 2), aglycosylated human recombinant Fc has a significantly shorter $t_{1/2}$ than its glycosylated counterpart (Table 3) *(39)*. Thus, there appear to be differences in the requirements for glycosylation between the IgGs from these two species. A comparison of the X-ray crystallographic structures of human and mouse Fc regions has shown that the oligosaccharides attached to the CH_2 domain can form contacts (i.e., a bridge) between the two CH_2 domains in human IgG but not in mouse IgG *(42)*. Thus, the contribution of CH_2 domain-linked carbohydrates to the conformation of CH_2 domains is species related.

The surprisingly short half-life of mouse IgG as compared with human IgG in humans has been explained previously by the assumption that some "natural" anti-galactose antibodies present in human serum can bind to the $Gal\alpha_1$-3Gal residues present *only* on mouse IgG (and IgGs from other mammals), thus shortening its $t_{1/2}$ in the circulation by immune elimination *(43)*. However, therapeutic humanized MAbs produced in murine cells have been reported to have long $t_{1/2}$s, indicating that anti-Gal antibodies are not involved in the rapid removal of murine IgG *(44)*. An alternative explanation for the decreased $t_{1/2}$ of mouse IgG in humans is based on the observation that the mouse IgG isotypes (with the exception of IgG_{2b}) fail to bind to human FcRn, whereas all human isotypes bind to homologous FcRn *(4)* (Ghetie and Ward, *unpublished*). As expected from PK analysis, both human and mouse IgG isotypes bind to mouse FcRn. These results provide a molecular explanation for the short half-lives of therapeutic mouse MAbs in patients as a consequence of their poor affinity for human FcRn. The lack of an interaction between human FcRn and most mouse IgGs indicates that mice cannot be reliably used to extrapolate the $t_{1/2}$s of murine MAbs to humans. Even the PK of humanized MAbs in mice might be different from their PK in humans owing to differences in the fine specificity of FcRn across species. This is suggested by the discrepancy between the half-lives of human IgG isotypes in mice vs humans *(8,37,45)* (Table 4). For example, human IgG_3 has a significantly shorter $t_{1/2}$ than the other isotypes in both humans and mice (owing to the substitution of His by Arg in 435 *[39]*) but the $t_{1/2}$s of IgG_1, IgG_2, and IgG_4 differ considerably in both species (Table 4). Although three isotypes have approximately the same $t_{1/2}$s in humans, in mice, IgG_2 has a much longer $t_{1/2}$ than IgG_1, and IgG_4 (Table 4). To predict the pharmacokinetics of a therapeutic MAb in humans, preclinical studies in mice should therefore be complemented by studies to measure the binding of the MAb to human FcRn.

As in mice, FcRn also plays an essential role in the maternofetal transfer of IgG in humans. The same amino acid residues in human IgG that control the catabolism of IgG are involved in IgG transcytosis across the in vitro perfused placenta *(46)*.

Table 4
$t_{1/2}$ of Human IgG Isotypes
in Mice and Humans

IgG isotype	$t_{1/2}$ (h) in:	
	Mice (37)	Humans (8)
IgG$_1$	162.0	508.8
IgG$_2$	275.3	484.8
IgG$_3$	64.5	170.4
IgG$_4$	71.7	494.4

Table 5
Residues in FcRn Involved in the Binding of IgG

Mouse FcRn	Mouse IgG	Human FcRn	Human IgG
Glu-117	His-310	Glu-117	His-310
Glu-118	Gln-311	Glu-118	Gln-311
Glu-132	His-435[a]	**Asp-132**	His-435[b]
Trp-133	Ile-253	Trp-133	Ile-253
Glu-137	His-436[c]	**Leu-137**	**Tyr-436[d]**

Data from ref. 52.
The amino acid residues in human FcRn and IgG that are different
from their mouse counterparts are in **bold**.
[a] In all mouse isotypes except IgG$_{2b}$ with Tyr at 435.
[b] In all human isotypes except IgG$_3$ allotype with Arg at 435.
[c] In all mouse isotypes except IgG$_{2b}$ with Tyr at 436.
[d] In all human IgG except IgG$_3$ allotype with Phe at 436.

4. LOCALIZATION OF THE INTERACTION SITE FOR IGG ON FCRN

Despite the homology of the α-chain of the FcRn with the major histocompatibility class (MHC) I molecule (14), the "peptide binding groove" of the FcRn is not occupied by peptide owing to close apposition of the α-helical segments that flank this groove (47). The genes encoding both the mouse and human FcRn α-chain have been isolated and characterized (48,49). These two proteins have a high degree of homology in the α_2-domain, which is involved in binding to the Fc region of IgG. The contact amino acid residues at the CH$_2$–CH$_3$ interface of IgG have been determined by both X-ray crystallography of the rat Fc–FcRn complexes (30,31) and by site-directed mutagenesis (50,51). The residues in the α_2-domain that play a direct role in the interactions between IgG and FcRn are conserved in FcRn in both mice and humans with the exception of residues 132 and 137 (Table 5) (Fig. 3). The acidic nature of the four (or three for human) amino acid residues and the role of histidines in the binding of IgG to FcRn suggests that electrostatic forces may play a predominant role in mediating this interaction. Hydrophobic interactions between Trp-133 in FcRn and Ile-253 of IgGs are also involved (31,51). The amino-terminal residue of β_2-microglobulin (Ile), which is conserved in mice and humans, has also been implicated in the binding of IgG to residues Leu-309 and/or Glu-311, but to a lesser extent than the residues in the α_2-domain (31,51).

Differences between mouse and human FcRn occur at residue 132 (Asp in human, Glu in mouse) and 137 (Leu in human, Glu in mouse) (Table 5). Glu-137 (Asp in rat) forms a salt bridge with His-436 of IgG, and this interaction is precluded in the human FcRn owing to the replacement of Glu with Leu (52). Both human IgG and mouse IgG_{2b} have Tyr at position 436, a residue that may establish hydrophobic interactions with Leu-137 in human FcRn. This could explain the lack of binding of mouse IgG_1 and IgG_{2a}, the weak binding of mouse IgG_{2b}, and the strong interactions of human IgGs with human FcRn. However, neither sheep nor bovine IgGs can bind to human FcRn (4) despite the fact that these proteins have Tyr at position 436. This suggests that other differences between human and mouse IgG and/or FcRn might also be responsible for the lack of interactions of some mouse IgG subclasses and human FcRn. Thus, in mouse, as compared with human FcRn, Trp-133 is more exposed to solvent. There is also a two-residue deletion in human FcRn that is located at the carboxy-terminal end of the α_1-domain, in the vicinity of the IgG-binding site. This shortens the α-helix of the α_1-domain and thereby creates a different conformation at the level of the α_1/α_2 platform of these two FcRns. This two-residue deletion also eliminates an Asn residue in human FcRn which is a potential site for glycosylation in mouse FcRn. It has also been suggested that to achieve maximal binding affinity for IgG, dimerization of FcRn is required (52). In the crystal structure of rat FcRn, dimerization is mediated by electrostatic interactions between the carbohydrate residues attached to Asn-225 (53). There can be no such interactions in human FcRn because Asn-225 is replaced by Gln, as demonstrated by the propensity of rat FcRn (highly homologous with mouse) to form dimers in crystals, and by the lack of human dimers in such crystals (52).

5. PK OF MABS AND ITS IN MICE

5.1. Persistence of MAbs in Normal and Tumor-Bearing Mice

The preclinical testing of mouse or ch/hu MAbs in severe combined immunodeficiency (SCID) mice xenografted with various human tumors is usually followed by measuring tumor size (for subcutaneous tumors) or the survival of animals (for disseminated lymphomas and metastatic tumors). The persistence of murine MAbs in normal mice depends on the IgG isotype used (Table 6). Both mouse and rat IgG_{2b} have a short $t_{1/2}$ as compared with the other isotypes. In the case of rat IgG_{2b}, the sequence difference at position 257 (Ala instead of Pro in the other isotypes) is most likely responsible for the short $t_{1/2}$ (32) whereas for mouse IgG_{2b}, the short $t_{1/2}$ is probably due to the substitution of His-435 (in all other isotypes) with Tyr (27). The most frequently used mouse MAbs in clinical trials are of the IgG_1 isotype, which has one of the longest $t_{1/2}$s in mice (45) (Table 6).

In tumor-bearing mice the presence of the tumor acts as a sink for the injected MAb and decreases its $t_{1/2}$. However, if the tumor is saturated with the corresponding MAb, the $t_{1/2}$ is within its normal range. This behavior was demonstrated by using SCID mice xenografted with human Burkitt's Daudi cells and injected with ^{125}I-labeled mouse RFB4 anti-human CD22 previously treated or not with an excess of unlabeled MAbs (Fig. 4) (Ghetie and Vitetta, *unpublished*). The treatment of SCID/Daudi tumor mice with RFB4 prolonged the survival of mice from 30 d (untreated) to 46 d while the same amount of IT constructed with RFB4 and deglycosylated ricin A chain (dgRTA) was more efficient in extending the life of tumor-bearing animals to 73 d (54).

Despite their small size and good tumor penetration, fragments of IgG antibody (Fab, Fv) have very short $t_{1/2}$s and therefore decreased tumor retention. To prolong their persistence in the circulation and increase their therapeutic potential, a site-specific chemical modification of human Fab fragments with polyethyleneglycol (PEG) was performed.

Table 6
$t_{1/2}$ of Murine IgG Isotypes in Mice

Species	IgG isotype	$t_{1/2}$ (h)	Reference
Mouse	1	197	(45)
	2a	207	
	2b	121	
	3	228	
Rat	1	223	(32)
	2a	235	
	2b	57	
	2c	102	

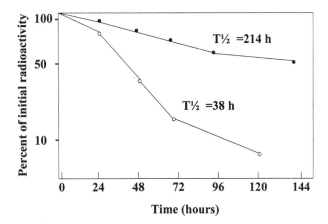

Fig. 4. Elimination curves of ^{125}I-RFB4 in SCID/Daudi mice. Four mice were injected intravenously with 10 µg of radiolabeled RFB4 (○) or intraperitoneally with 10 mg of RFB4 followed 1 h later by 10 µg of radiolabeled RFB4 (●). Radioactivity was measured by whole body counting.

This conferred a longer $t_{1/2}$ and full retention of antigen-binding properties (55). Thus, the $t_{1/2}$ of a Fab–PEG conjugate in rats was prolonged from 0.3 h (nonconjugated Fab) to 4.9 h, which is close to the $t_{1/2}$ of 5.8 h for intact IgG (55). Similar results were obtained using cynomologus monkeys. It was noted that the majority of improvements in the PK were due to a large increase in the α-phase, indicating that less conjugate was lost from the circulation during the equilibration phase. However, the possible use of pegylated IgG fragments instead of the intact IgG in therapy may depend on the ability of such hydrophilic molecules to diffuse through the milieu of the interstitium.

5.2. Persistence of ITs in Normal and Tumor-Bearing Mice

The chemical attachment of toxins or their subunits to MAbs alters their PK. This is at least partially due to nonspecific interactions of the toxin with receptors on cells in a variety

Table 7
Pharmacokinetic Data on MAbs, ITs, and Toxins in Mice

Protein	$t_{1/2}$ (h)		
	(57)	(56)	Ghetie and Vitetta[a]
MAb	114[b]	22[c]	210[d]
IT	10	6	82
Toxin	2[e]	5[f]	26[g]
MAb/IT	11.4	3.7	2.6

[a] Unpublished results.
[b] Anti-Thy 1.1 mouse antibody.
[c] Rat IgG with unknown antibody specificity. In BCL$_1$ tumor-bearing mice a rat IgG anti-IgD antibody has a $t_{1/2}$ of only 12 h.
[d] Anti-human CD22 (RFB4) mouse IgG$_1$ antibody.
[e] RTA.
[f] dgRTA.
[g] Recombinant RTA expressed in *E. coli*.

of tissues. The consequence of this interaction is the much shorter persistence in the circulation of IT vs the MAb used for its preparation (Table 7) (56). The decreased $t_{1/2}$ of ITs vs MAbs is not the result of the modification of the MAb molecule by the crosslinker used for the attachment of the toxin, as indicated by the same half-life of MAbs treated or not treated with N-succinimidyl 3-(2-pyridyldithiopropionate) (SPDP) (57) or N-succinimidyl-oxycarbonyl-α-methyl (2-pyridyldithio)-toluene (SMPT) (Ghetie and Vitetta, *unpublished*) crosslinker. The MAb/IT ratios (Table 7) are inversely proportional to the number of mannose residues on the RTA molecule. Thus, following chemical deglycosylation, 5 of the 18 mannose residues in RTA remain (58). Recombinant RTA expressed in *E. coli* has none. The rapid clearance of the ITs is likely to be mediated through the recognition of mannose-rich oligosaccharides by hepatic Kupfer and sinusoidal endothelial cells (58) which express mannose-binding receptors. The dose-limiting toxicity of ITs constructed with RTA and some other plant and bacterial toxins is vascular leak syndrome (VLS), which is characterized by an increase in vascular permeability resulting in interstitial edema, weight gain, and, in its most severe form, organ failure (59). The nonspecific cytotoxic effect of ITs is thought to be related to their ability to damage the integrity of the endothelial cells of the microvasculature (60). Because the predominant expression site of FcRn is the vascular endothelium, it is possible that treatment with ITs *per se* also alters their persistence in the circulation by altering the "salvaging" function of FcRn in the endothelium. This possibility is supported by results of studies designed to measure the persistence of ^{125}I-labeled mouse MAb in mice treated with an IT. As shown in Fig. 5, the half-life of mouse MAb (RFB4) is considerably shortened after 3 d of consecutive treatment of mice with a dose of RFB4-dgRTA representing 40% of its LD$_{50}$ (Ghetie and Vitetta, *unpublished*). However, the effect of the IT was reversible, as shown by the elimination curves of RFB4, which are similar in normal mice and in mice used 2 wk after treatment with IT (Fig. 5).

Recombinant ITs are molecules containing truncated toxins (e.g., *Pseudomonas exotoxin* [PE] or [PE40]) fused to a recombinant antigen-binding Fv fragment. The Fv fragment comprises the variable regions of the IgG heavy and light chains, which can be linked by either an engineered peptide linker (scFv) or an engineered disulfide bond (dsFv) (61).

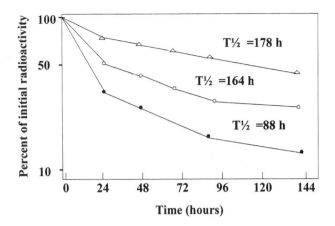

Fig. 5. The effect of IT treatment on the elimination curves of radiolabeled RFB4. Three mice were treated for 3 consecutive days with RFB4-dgRTA followed the next day by intravenous injection of ^{125}I-RFB4 (●) or the same mice were rested 2 wk after completion of pharmacokinetic experiment and injected again with ^{125}I-RFB4 (○). (△), Elimination curve before treatment. Radioactivity was measured in the blood.

These manipulations stabilize the association of VH and VL, which are normally noncovalently bound to each other. Compared to ITs containing intact IgG molecules, both types of recombinant ITs have improved intratumoral penetration in animals (62). However, the rapid blood clearance and monovalency of these small molecules result in significantly decreased tumor retention (63). Thus, the $t_{1/2}$ in mice of a dsFv IT containing a truncated PE was only 15–20 min (64). The very fast elimination is due to the rapid renal clearance of FvITs. This was demonstrated by biodistribution studies of FvIT in nephrectomized mice in which tumor retention of the FvIT was similar to that of IT containing intact IgG (65). Therefore, to achieve antitumor effects in mice, these FvITs should be administered by continuous infusion using miniosmotic pumps (64). Improved $t_{1/2}$s and antitumor activity have been reported for an anti-EpCAM hu MAb fused at the carboxyl-terminal end of the heavy chain to interleukin-2 (IL-2). By introducing single amino acid changes in the junctional sequence between the MAb and IL-2, these fusion proteins showed reduced sensitivity to proteolysis and longer $t_{1/2}$s (66). This work demonstrated that, in addition to its interaction with FcRn, the persistence of these conjugates in the circulation was also dependent on their susceptibility to proteolysis. In support of the implication that the protease sensitivity of IgG affects its persistence in the circulation, human IgG$_3$, which is known to be more susceptible to papain/pepsin proteolysis than IgG$_1$ (67), has the same affinity as IgG$_1$ for human FcRn (52) (Ghetie and Ward, unpublished). However, its $t_{1/2}$ in humans is three times shorter (8). In addition, the shorter $t_{1/2}$ of wild-type recombinant human Fc fragments as compared with Fc fragments generated by papain digestion (Table 3) is not due to a decreased affinity for FcRn, as both fragments bind equally well to FcRn-Sepharose (39). However, analysis of the sensitivities of these two human Fc fragments to pepsin-limited digestion demonstrated that the wild-type Fc fragment is digested about three times more rapidly than the Fc-papain fragment (39).

6. PK OF MABS AND ITS IN CANCER PATIENTS

6.1. Persistence of MAbs in Cancer Patients

The $t_{1/2}$ of any heterologous or homologous IgG antibody infused into a normal recipient does not depend on the amount administered (22). However, this is not the case in tumor-bearing recipients in whom the tumor cells act as a sink. Therefore, it would be predicted that by increasing the dose, or by infusing repeated doses, the tumor will be saturated with the MAbs and the excess will be catabolized at a normal rate. As shown in Fig. 6, this is the case (68,69). Hence, in situations in which tumor cells are present, $t_{1/2}$s are dependent on the dose administered.

PK analyses of the anti-CD20 IgG_1 ch MAb (Rituxan™) have demonstrated that its $t_{1/2}$ in patients with relapsed B-cell lymphoma is 445 ± 361 h (70), a value very close to 500 h for human IgG_1 in normal individuals (8) (Table 4). The half-life of another ch MAb directed against a high molecular weight mucin (TAG-72) expressed on colorectal tumors and constructed with an IgG_4 isotype was only 224 ± 62 h in patients with metastatic colon cancer (71). This value is considerably longer than that of its murine MAb counterpart (24–48 h) (71) but shorter than that of Rituxan™ (70). The shorter half-life could be the result of the different type and burden of the two tumors and not on the isotype, as both IgG_1 and IgG_4 have similar $t_{1/2}$s in humans (8) (Table 4). The $t_{1/2}$ of the anti-TAG-72 ch MAb was considerably shorter (< 24 h) in patients who responded to treatment by eliciting HAMA, indicating that a process of immune elimination and not tumor capture took place (71).

6.2. Persistence of ITs in Cancer Patients

All ITs which have been used to date in clinical trials contain mouse MAbs. Hence, their persistence in the circulation and retention in the body is short irrespective of the toxin used. However, the size of the targeting antibody has an impact on the half life of the IT as shown in Phase I clinical trials using anti-CD22 (RFB4) IT constructed with dgRTA and intact IgG ($t_{1/2}$ = 7.8 h) (72) vs its Fab' fragment ($t_{1/2}$ = 1.5 h) (6). The ITs were administered intravenously in several bolus doses at 48-h intervals but therapeutic concentrations (~1 µg/mL) could be sustained only with ITs constructed with intact IgG (72) (Fig. 7). A high peak concentration of IT in serum and a longer $t_{1/2}$ correlated with both clinical response and toxicity. These results were consistent with those obtained in a murine lymphoma model where a longer $t_{1/2}$ resulted in a better antitumor response (73).

To avoid toxic levels of ITs (> 1 µg/mL) in serum (Fig. 7), and to maintain constant levels of IT in the blood, continuous infusion of anti-CD22 IT was evaluated (74). As compared to bolus infusion, a comparable $t_{1/2}$ (11.4 h), toxicity, immunogenicity, and clinical response were observed. Toxicity depended on the presence or absence of circulating tumor cells (CTCs) with less toxicity observed in patients with CTCs (74). The $t_{1/2}$ of the IT in patients with CTC was shorter (8.8 h) than in patients without CTCs (12.7 h), indicating that in these cases, the CTCs absorbed more IT and thereby reduced its $t_{1/2}$. However, this observation was not confirmed in subsequent clinical studies using combination therapy with a mixture of two ITs (75). In these studies, the $t_{1/2}$ of RFB4 IT was slightly longer for those patients with CTCs (32.1 h and 39.2 h for two dose levels) when compared to those without (24.4 h and 21.6 h for two dose levels). In contrast to the patients lacking these CTCs, patients with even small numbers of CTCs (<50/mm³) tolerated even the highest dose of the combined ITs (30 mg/m²/192 h) (75). The PK of the anti-CD19 (HD37) IT in patients with B-cell lymphomas (76) was similar to that of anti-CD22 IT. Thus, half-lives of 18.2 h and 22.8 h have been reported for anti-CD19 IT administered either by bolus or continuous infusions. In contrast, an anti-CD25 IT administered to patients with Hodgkin's lymphoma had a shorter $t_{1/2}$ (6.1 h), perhaps owing to the bioavailability of tumor cells (77).

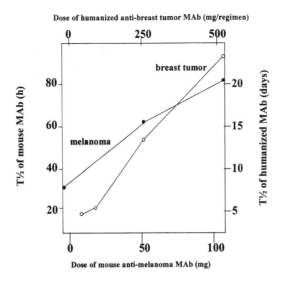

Fig. 6. Variations in pharmacokinetics of MAbs infused in increasing doses in melanoma *(68)* and breast cancer *(69)* patients.

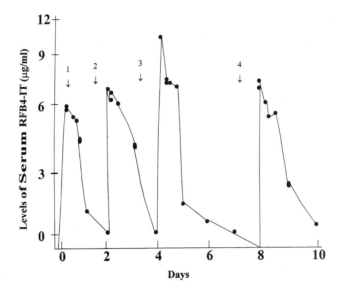

Fig. 7. Pharmacokinetics of RFB4-dgRTA IT *(72)*. The non-Hodgkin's lymphoma patient received four doses of 13.9 mg each. The concentration of IT was measured by radioimmunoassay.

Recombinant ITs constructed with mouse Fv fragments and truncated PE have a very short half-life (<1 h) in patients owing to the low retention of mouse Fv fragments in the circulation and the nonspecific uptake of PE by the liver *(78)*. Despite unfavorable PK, a recombinant IT containing the anti-CD22 (RFB4) dsFv fragment fused to PE38 was efficacious in patients with hairy cell leukemia *(7)*. Thus, in contrast to unconjugated MAbs, ITs may not require a long $t_{1/2}$ if the tumor cells are few in number and accessible to the circulation.

7. PK OF INTRAVENOUS IMMUNOGLOBULIN (IVIG)

IVIG preparations have been used to prevent infection in cancer patients and, in some cases, antitumor effects have been reported. Thus, as compared with untreated patients, mortality in the group of chronic lymphocytic leukemia patients treated with IVIG was lower *(79)*. Similar observations were noted in a study in which regression of a Kaposi sarcoma occurred in human immunodeficiency (HIV) patients treated with IVIG *(80)*. In a study using IVIG-treated SCID mice xenografted with human melanoma or sarcoma, fewer recurrences and prolongation of survival time was observed *(81)*. This was confirmed in SCID mice xenografted with human lymphoma (Daudi) cells (M-A. Ghetie and E. Vitetta, *unpublished*).

The PK of IVIG preparations were obtained by analyzing the plasma elimination curves after infusing IVIG into patients with immunodeficiencies. Alternatively, the elimination of some specific IgG antibodies present in the infused IVIG but not in the serum of the subject has been studied *(82)*. The $t_{1/2}$ of various commercial IVIG preparations in patients with X-linked agammaglobulinemia or with various immunodeficiency syndromes ranged between 26 and 35 d *(82)*. The dose of IVIG recommended for the treatment of patients with humoral immunodeficiencies is approx 0.4 mg/kg/mo, which is somewhat less than the amount of IgG in the intravascular pool of normal subjects but is sufficient to maintain levels above 5 g/L, which is considered to be a critical threshold *(82)*. The $t_{1/2}$s of IgG_1, IgG_2, and IgG_4 isotypes were approx 30 d whereas the $t_{1/2}$ of IgG_3 was 20 d *(83,84)*. This last value is higher than expected based on results from studies with radiolabeled IgG in normal subjects (Table 4) *(8)*, suggesting that the IVIG preparation used in these studies might also contain a proportion of the IgG_3 allotype with His at position 435 *(85)*.

The effect of IVIG in the treatment of some autoimmune diseases may also be due to the concentration–catabolism effect *(22)* in addition to the activation of inhibitory Fc receptors reported by Samuelsson et al. *(86)*. The increased catabolism of endogenous IgG (including autoantibody) by administration of high doses of IVIG (half-life decreased from 20 to 10 d) is the result of the saturation of FcRn in the patients which leads to the destruction of all IgG molecules present in excess *(87,88)*. The contribution of enhanced IgG catabolism to the beneficial effect of IVIG in the treatment of some autoimmune diseases is also supported by the observation that the severity of experimental lupus erythematosus is greatly attenuated in β_2-microglobulin-deficient mice *(89,90)*. The very low levels of IgG and autoantibodies in these mice are the cause of their protection from the disease. Hence, because they lack FcRn, they rapidly catabolize both their normal and their pathogenic IgG autoantibody. Furthermore these FcRn-deficient mice are protected against some other autoantibody-mediated diseases (e.g., bullous pemphigus), as the amount of IgG autoantibody reaching the epidermal target is greatly reduced because of its hypercatabolism *(91)*.

8. ALTERATIONS IN IGG PK IN NON-NEOPLASTIC DISEASES

Alterations in the PK of IgG in individuals with hyper- and hypogammaglobulinemia has been explained by the concentration–catabolism effect *(8,9)* inducing the accelerated or decreased catabolism of IgG in patients with high or low serum IgG concentrations, respectively *(22)*. Hypercatabolism of IgG in diseases involving excessive loss of serum proteins through the kidney (nephrotic syndrome *[92]*), gastrointestinal tract (protein-losing entheropathy *[93]*), or skin (severe burns *[94]*) can be explained by the irreversible loss of IgG in a new catabolic compartment. However, the hypercatabolism of IgG in unrelated diseases such as myotonic dystrophy *(95)*, systemic lupus erythematosus *(96,97)*, rheumatoid arthritis *(96,97)*, Wiskott–Aldrich syndrome *(98)*, and other diseases *(99,100)* remains unexplained. In light of our present knowledge of the mechanism of IgG catabolism *(23)*, the hypercatabolism of IgG in at least some of these diseases might be due to the lack of expression or malfunction of FcRn. With the exception of myotonic dystrophy *(101)* this possibility has not yet been explored.

8.1. Myotonic Dystrophy (DM)

In an early study *(95)* it was demonstrated that the mean survival time of IgG in individuals with DM was 11.4 vs 22.9 d in normal individuals, corresponding to a lower serum concentration (7.5 mg/mL) than in controls (12.1 mg/mL). The rate of IgG synthesis was normal (35.7 mg/kg/d) in patients with DM. Thus, the reduction in the concentration of serum IgG was due solely to the decreased $t_{1/2}$ of IgG. IgG isolated from normal individuals had a similar accelerated rate of catabolism in DM patients, suggesting that the defect is not in the IgG but in the patient's ability to catabolize it. Normal serum concentrations and catabolic rates were measured for albumin, IgM, and IgA, indicating that the alteration is restricted to a single class of serum proteins. One hypothesis to explain IgG hypercatabolism in DM patients is that the genetic alteration in DM suppresses FcRn expression, leading to decreased IgG protection and increased catabolism *(101)*. The gene encoding the FcRn α-chain *(FCGRT)* is localized in the same chromosomal band as DM (19q13.3), 4.1 megabases away *(102)*. This colocalization, however distant, may be compatible with a long range chromosomal effect induced by the DMCTG repeat *(101)*. This hypothesis assumes that a potent *cis*-suppressive mechanism extends even to distant genes such as *FCGRT* inactivating the expression of functional FcRn *(101)*. Because DM is caused by an expanded CTG repeat in the 3'-untranslated region of the DM protein kinase mRNA *(103)*, this mRNA must be transcribed in the vascular endothelial cells where *FCGRT* itself is expressed and mediates IgG protection. The presence of DM protein kinase mRNA was confirmed in FcRn-positive human endothelial cells *(101)*, suggesting that a long range effect of DMCTG expansion on *FCGRT* might explain the hypercatabolism of IgG in DM.

8.2. Systemic Lupus Erythematosus (SLE) and Rheumatoid Arthritis (RA)

In two studies published by different laboratories it was reported that patients with SLE have both higher serum IgG concentrations and higher catabolic rates of IgG than controls *(96,97)*. As shown in Table 8, there is excellent agreement between the data obtained in both laboratories indicating that IgG hypercatabolism is associated with an increased serum concentration. The increase in the concentration of serum IgG in SLE patients is a result of the increase in the synthetic rate, which surpasses the catabolic rate. Because the catabolic rates increase in patients with elevated serum IgG concentration (e.g., myeloma patients) a possible explanation is that hypercatabolism results from the higher concentrations of serum IgG in SLE patients. However, neither study found a correlation between the serum concentration and the fractional catabolic rate in these patients, indicating that the concentration–catabolism effect was not the cause of IgG hypercatabolism *(96,97)*. The accelerated breakdown of IgG could not be explained by any of the factors known to alter IgG catabolism (e.g., loss of protein in urine or gastrointestinal tract) or the treatment with corticosteroids known to induce hypercatabolism of IgG *(104)*. The nature of the phenomenon leading to the hypercatabolism of IgG in these SLE patients may correlate with alterations in the function of FcRn *(23)*. This is supported by the results of experiments using MRL-lpr mice which develop SLE-like disease *(105)*. As in its human counterpart, SLE in mice is characterized by the development of hypergammaglobulinemia and a severe autoimmune syndrome. β$_2$-Microglobulin-deficient mice that do not express FcRn are protected from hypergammaglobulinemia and show a reduction in the titers of autoantibody *(89,90)*.

Table 8
Metabolism of IgG in SLE and RA Patients

Disease	IgG concentration (mg/mL)	$t_{1/2}(h)$ (patients/controls)	Synthetic rate (mg/kg/d)	Reference
SLE	22.8/11.0	14.7/22.7	114.0/30.5	(96)
	18.3/10.7	8.2/18.0	127.5/34.5	(97)
RA	17.6/11.0	13.8/22.7	78.0/30.5	(96)
	16.3/10.7	12.4/18.0	92.6/34.5	(97)

In agreement with these results, treatment of MLR-lpr mice developing SLE with a synthetic peptide that binds to IgG at its FcRn-binding site blocks the development of the disease in the majority of cases *(106)*. These results indicate that modification of the function of FcRn in SLE may interfere with the catabolism of both endogenous IgG and autoantibody *(90)*. If this is the case, mice with SLE should have an accelerated rate of catabolism of IgG. However, in disease-free, SLE-susceptible strains of mice, the $t_{1/2}$s of IgG were indistinguishable from those of resistant strains *(90)*, suggesting that alterations in IgG catabolism take place only after the onset of the disease. In a preliminary experiment using mice with lupus-like disease induced by treatment with pristane *(107)*, the $t_{1/2}$ of mouse IgG_1 was considerably shortened from 208 ± 18 h to 76 ± 8 h 3 mo after treatment (Ghetie and Ward, *unpublished*). However, the serum IgG concentrations in these treated mice was comparable to those of control mice. A possible link between the gene coding FcRn *(FCGRT)* and genes associated with SLE *(Sle3* and *Lrdm1)* was suggested. *FCGRT* has been proposed to be a suitable candidate for an SLE susceptibility locus *(90)*.

Short $t_{1/2}$s have also been reported for patients with RA *(96,97,108)* (Table 8). In patients with SLE or RA, identical $t_{1/2}$s were reported whether the IgG was prepared from the patient or from a normal donor. This demonstrates that hypercatabolism of IgG in RA and SLE patients is a host defect *(96)*. In RA patients the accelerated catabolism of IgG could be due to a defect in the function of FcRn, combined with the presence of rheumatoid factor (RF) which may bind to the administered radiolabeled IgG and remove it from the circulation as an immune complex. It is well known that immune complexes consisting of RF bound to IgG are commonly present in the serum and in the diseased joints *(109)*. Because RFs bind to the FcRn-binding site on IgG *(110)*, they may also accelerate the destruction of IgG by interfering with the protective function of FcRn.

9. FUTURE IMPLICATIONS

The therapeutic efficacy of MAbs in vivo depends on characteristics such as affinity, FcR- and C-binding, serum persistence, and immunogenicity. It also depends on the nature of the disease being treated (primary vs metastatic tumor, early vs late stage).

The characteristics of the MAbs that have been most thoroughly studied are affinity and specificity for the targeted (tumor) antigen. Current technologies now enable us to prepare "custom-made" MAbs with restricted specificities and very high affinities (reviewed in ref. *111*). In contrast, although the amino acid residues involved in the various antigen-dependent effector functions of MAbs have been identified (reviewed in ref. *112*) this knowledge has not yet been applied clinically *(113)*. However, it is likely that a new generation of genetically engineered antibodies with improved effector functions will be available in the near future *(40,113)*.

A major antigen-independent effector function that has an impact on the antitumor activity of MAbs is their ability to bind to FcRn and to persist in the circulation. A long $t_{1/2}$ results in a higher concentration gradient across cellular barriers with better penetration into the targeted tumor. It has been demonstrated in animals as well as in patients that the antitumor activity of MAbs is proportional to their concentration (68,69). The improved PK of ch and hu MAbs vs mouse MAbs is partially responsible for the therapeutic success of these MAbs. The persistence of ch and hu MAbs (which are already similar to "normal" human IgG) can be prolonged further by genetic engineering as suggested by recent experiments using mouse and human Fc fragments or IgG (33,40). To isolate ch and hu MAbs with increased serum $t_{1/2}$s, random mutagenesis and selection could be used to alter amino acid residues in the vicinity of those involved both in FcRn-binding and in modulating the flexibility of the interface angle between the CH_2–CH_3 domains. Mutants should be analyzed for their affinity for human FcRn, the pH dependence of binding, and their persistence in the circulation of mice. Only mutants with favorable features in all three areas should be developed for use in clinical trials. More attention to the PKs of MAbs in Phase I clinical trials should be given, for example, persistence in the circulation, correlations between doses, PKs, maximum tolerated doses (MTDs) and any biological effects.

A decrease in the size of antibody molecules is invariably associated with better tumor penetration. However, this effect is diminished by a much shorter $t_{1/2}$ and a decreased serum concentration due to rapid renal elimination from the circulation. Future goals would be to produce smaller MAbs with longer $t_{1/2}$s. This could be accomplished by attaching Fvs to CH2-CH3 domain interface-like peptides able to bind in a pH-dependent manner to FcRn. The demonstration that an Fc region-derived peptide encompassing residues 308–317 blocks the binding of streptococcal protein G to IgG (114) suggests that peptides encompassing key FcRn-binding residues may be effective (23).

In contrast to MAbs, a decreased $t_{1/2}$ of ITs might be advantageous excess IT (not absorbed by the tumor) is quickly eliminated from the circulation, thus diminishing nonspecific side effects. Therefore the use of ch and hu MAbs instead of mouse MAbs for the construction of ITs would confer longer half-lives, a higher serum concentration, and a better tumor penetration but also an increased toxic side effect. If ch or hu MAbs are used, the portion of the toxin that induces side effects should be identified and altered (Smallshaw et al., submitted).

Finally we must expand our knowledge of how FcRn functions in endothelial cells. This will allow us to control the persistence of MAbs in the circulation not only by altering the structure of MAbs, but also by modulating the function of FcRn. For this purpose, in vitro systems using cells originating from tissues involved in transcytosis of IgG have provided valuable information regarding the mechanisms of intracellular trafficking of IgG and FcRn (19–21). In the future we need to study endothelial cells originating from the vasculature of the tissues involved in IgG catabolism. This could answer the question of how expression of FcRn is regulated in endothelial cells and how fluctuations in the expression of FcRn influence the PKs of MAbs in vivo.

ACKNOWLEDGMENTS

We thank Ms. L. Owens for excellent administrative assistance.

REFERENCES

1. Reichert JM. Monoclonal antibodies in the clinic. Nat Biotechnol 2001; 19:819–822.
2. Kohler G, Milstein C. Continuous cultures of fused cells secreting antibody of predefined specificity. Nature 1975; 256:495–497.
3. Carter P. Improving the efficacy of antibody-based cancer therapies. Nat Rev Cancer 2001; 1:118–129.

4. Ober RJ, Radu CG, Ghetie V, Ward ES. Differences in promiscuity for antibody–FcRn interactions across species: implications for therapeutic antibodies. Int Immunol 2001; 13:1250–1255.

5. Farah RA, Clinchy B, Herrera L, Vitetta ES. The development of monoclonal antibodies for the therapy of cancer. Crit Rev Eukaryot Gene Express 1998; 8:321–356.

6. Vitetta ES, Stone M, Amlot P, et al. A phase I immunotoxin trial in patients with B-cell lymphoma. Cancer Res 1991; 51:4052–4058.

7. Kreitman RJ, Wilson WH, Bergeron K, et al. Efficacy of the anti-CD22 recombinant immunotoxin BL22 in chemotherapy-resistant hairy-cell leukemia. N Engl J Med 2001; 345:241–247.

8. Morell A, Terry WD, Waldman TA. Metabolic properties of IgG subclasses in man. J Clin Invest 1970; 49:673–680.

9. Fahey JL, Robinson AG. Factors controlling serum gamma-globulin concentration. J Exp Med 1963; 118:845–868.

10. Brambell FNR, Hemmings WA, Morris IG. A theoretical model of γ-globulin catabolism. Nature 1964; 203:1352–1355.

11. Ghetie V, Hubbard JG, Kim JK, Ben MF, Lee Y, Ward ES. Abnormally short serum half-lives of IgG in β2-microglobulin-deficient mice. Eur J Immunol 1996; 26:690–696.

12. Junghans RP, Anderson CL. The protection receptor for IgG catabolism is the β_2-microglobulin-containing intestinal transport receptor. Proc Natl Acad Sci USA 1996; 93:5512–5516.

13. Israel EJ, Wilsker DF, Hayes KC, Schoenfield D, Simister NE. Increased clearance of IgG in mice that lack β_2-microglobulin: possible protective role of FcRn. Immunology 1996; 89:573–578.

14. Simister NE, Mostov KE. An Fc receptor structurally related to MHC class I antigen. Nature 1989; 184.

15. Junghans RP. Finally! The Brambel receptor (FcRB) mediator of transmission of immunity and protection from catabolism for IgG. Immunol Res 1997; 16:29–57.

16. Borvak J, Richardson J, Medesan C, et al. Functional expression of the MHC class I-related receptor, FcRn, in the endothelial cells of mice. Int Immunol 1998; 10:1289–1298.

17. Praetor A, Ellinger I, Hunziker W. Intracellular traffic of the MHC class I-like IgG Fc receptor, FcRn, expressed in epithelial MDCK cells. J Cell Sci 1999; 112 (Pt 14):2291–2299.

18. McCarthy KM, Yoong Y, Simister NE. Bidirectional transcytosis of IgG by the rat neonatal Fc receptor expressed in a rat kidney cell line: a system to study protein transport across epithelia. J Cell Sci 2000; 113 (Pt 7):1277–1285.

19. Ramalingam TS, Detmer SA, Martin WL, Bjorkman PJ. IgG transcytosis and recycling by FcRn expressed in MDCK cells reveals ligand-induced redistribution. EMBO J 2002; 21:590–601.

20. Ellinger I, Schwab M, Stefanescu A, Hunziker W, Fuchs R. IgG transport across trophoblast-derived BeWo cells: a model system to study IgG transport in the placenta. Eur J Immunol 1999; 29:733–744.

21. Antohe F, Radulescu L, Gafencu A, Ghetie V, Simionescu M. Expression of functionally active FcRn and the differentiated bidirectional transport of IgG in human placental endothelial cells. Hum Immunol 2001; 62:93–105.

22. Waldmann TA, Strober W. Metabolism of immunoglobulins. Prog Allergy 1969; 13:1–110.

23. Ghetie V, Ward ES. Multiple roles for the major histocompatibility complex class I-related receptor FcRn. Annu Rev Immunol 2000; 18:739–760.

24. Dima S, Medesan C, Mota G, Moraru I, Sjöquist J, Ghetie V. Effect of protein A and its fragment B on the catabolic and Fc receptor sites of IgG. Eur J Immunol 1983; 13:605–614.

25. Deisenhofer J. Crystallographic refinement and atomic models of a human Fc fragment and its complex with fragment B of protein A from *Staplylococcus aureus* at 2.9 and 2.8A resolution. Biochemistry 1981; 20:2361–2370.

26. Kim JK, Tsen M-F, Ghetie V, Ward ES. Identifying amino acid residues that influence plasma clearance of mouse IgG$_1$ fragments by site-directed mutagenesis. Eur J Immunol 1994; 24:542–548.

27. Medesan C, Matesoi D, Radu C, Ghetie V, Ward ES. Delineation of the amino acid residues involved in transcytosis and catabolism of mouse IgG$_1$. J Immunol 1997; 158:2211–2217.

28. Popov S, Hubbard JG, Kim JK, Ober RJ, Ghetie V, Ward ES. The stoichiometry and affinity of the interaction of murine Fc fragments with the MHC class 1-related receptor, FcRn. Mol Immunol 1996; 33:521–530.

29. Raghavan M, Bonagura VR, Morrison SL, Bjorkman PJ. Analysis of the pH dependence of Fc receptor/immunoglobulin G interaction using antibody and receptor variants. Biochemistry 1995; 32:14,649–14,657.

30. Burmeister WP, Huber AH, Bjorkman PJ. Crystal structure of the complex of rat neonatal Fc receptor with Fc. Nature 1994; 372:379–383.

31. Martin WL, West AP, Gan L, Bjorkman PJ. Crystal structure at 2.8A of an FcRn/hererodimeric Fc complex: mechanism of pH-dependent binding. Mol Cell 2001; 7:867–877.
32. Medesan C, Cianga P, Mummert M, Stanescu D, Ghetie V, Ward ES. Comparative studies of rat IgG to further delineate the Fc: FcRn interaction site. Eur J Immunol 1998; 28:2092–2100.
33. Ghetie V, Popov S, Borvak J, et al. Increasing the serum persistence of an IgG fragment by random mutagenesis. Nat Biotechnol 1997; 15:637–640.
34. Kim JK, Tsen MF, Ghetie V, Ward ES. Evidence that the hinge region plays a role in maintaining serum levels of the murine IgG$_1$ molecule. Mol Immunol 1995; 32:467–475.
35. Kim JK, Tsen MF, Ghetie V, Ward, ES. Catabolism of the murine IgG$_1$ molecule: evidence that both CH2-CH3 domain interfaces are required for persistence of IgG$_1$ in the circulation of mice. Scand J Immunol 1994; 40:457–465.
36. Dobre MA, Dima S, Moraru I. Fate of protein A released in circulation after extracorporeal perfusion of plasma over immobilized protein A. Rev Roum Biochem 1985; 22:3–10.
37. Zuckier LS, Georgescu L, Chang CJ, Scharff MD, Morrison SL. The use of severe combined immunodeficiency mice to study the metabolism of human immunoglobulin G. Cancer 1994; 73:794–799.
38. Bazin R, Boucher G, Monier G, et al. Use of hu-IgG-SCID mice to evaluate in vitro stability of human monoclonal IgG antibodies. J Immunol Methods 1994; 172:209–217.
39. Kim JK, Firan M, Radu C, Ghetie V, Ward ES. Mapping the site on human IgG for binding of the MHC class I-related receptor, FcRn. Eur J Immunol 1999; 29:2819–2826.
40. Shields RL, Namenuk AK, Hong K, et al. High resolution mapping of the binding site on human IgG1 for FcγRI, FcγRII, FcγRIII and FcRn and design of IgG1 variants with improved binding to FcγR. J Biol Chem 2001; 276:6591–6604.
41. Zuckier LS, Chang CJ, Scarff MD, Morrison SL. Chimeric human-mouse IgG antibodies with shuffled constant region exons demonstrate that multiple domains contribute to in vitro half-life. Cancer Res 1998; 58:3905–3908.
42. Harris LJ, Larson SB, Hasel KW, McPherson A. Refined structure of an intact IgG$_{2a}$ monoclonal antibody. Biochemistry 1997; 36:1581–1597.
43. Borrebaeck CK, Malmborg AC, Ohlin M. Does endogenous glycosylation prevent the use of monoclonal antibodies as cancer therapeutics? Immunol Today 1993; 14:477–479.
44. Junghans RP. Anti-Gal antibodies—where's the beef? Nat Biotechnol 1999; 17:938.
45. Zuckier LS, Rodriguez LD, Scarff MD. Immunologic and pharmacologic concepts of monoclonal antibodies. Semin Nucl Med 1989; 29:166–186.
46. Firan M, Bawdon R, Radu C, et al. The MHC class I-related receptor, FcRn plays an essential role in the maternofetal transfer of γ-globulin in humans. Int Immunol 2001; 13:993–1002.
47. Burmeister WP, Gastinel LN, Simister NE, Blum ML, Bjorkman PS. Crystal structure at 2.2A resolution of the MHC-related neonatal Fc receptor. Nature 1994; 372:336–343.
48. Ahouse JJ, Hagerman CL, Mittal P, et al. Mouse MHC class I-like Fc receptor encoded outside the MHC. J Immunol 1993; 151:6078–6088.
49. Story CM, Mikulska JE, Simister NE. A major histocompatibility complex class I-like Fc receptor cloned from human placenta: possible role in transfer of immunoglobulin G from mother to fetus. J Exp Med 1994; 180:2377–2381.
50. Raghavan M, Gastinel LN, Chen MY, Bjorkman PJ. Investigation of interaction between the class I MHC-related Fc receptor and its immunoglobulin G ligand. Immunity 1994; 1:303–315.
51. Vaughn DE, Milburn CM, Penny DM, Martin WL, Johnson JL, Bjorkman PJ. Identification of critical IgG binding epitopes on the neonatal Fc receptor. J Mol Biol 1997; 274:597–607.
52. West AP, Bjorkman PJ. Crystal structure and immunoglobulin G binding properties of the major histocompatibility complex-related Fc receptor. Biochemistry 2002; 39:9698–9708.
53. Vaughn DE, Bjorkman PJ. Structural basis of pH-dependent antibody binding by neonatal Fc receptor. Structure 1998; 6:63–73.
54. Ghetie MA, Tucker K, Richardson J, Uhr J, Vitetta E. The antitumor activity of an anti-CD22 immunotoxin in SCID mice with disseminated Daudi lymphoma is enhanced by either an anti-CD19 antibody or an anti-CD19 immunotoxin. Blood 1992; 80:2315–2320.
55. Chapman AP, Antoniw P, Spitali M, West S, Stephens S, King DJ. Therapeutic antibody fragments with prolonged in vivo half-lives. Nat Biotechnol 1999; 17:780–783.
56. Fulton RJ, Tucker TF, Vitetta ES, Uhr JW. Pharmacokinetics of tumor-reactive immunotoxins in tumor-bearing mice: effect of antibody valency and deglycosylation of the ricin A chain on clearance and tumor localization. Cancer Res 1988; 48:2618–2625.

57. Blakely DC, Skilleter DN, Price RJ, et al. Comparison of the pharmacokinetics and hepatotoxic effects of saporin and ricin A-chain immunotoxins on murine liver parenchymal cells. Cancer Res 1988; 48: 7072–7078.

58. Thorpe PE, Detre SI, Foxwell BMJ, et al. Modification of the carbohydrate in ricin with metaperiodate-cyanoborohydride mixtures. Effects on toxicity and in vivo distribution. Eur J Biochem 1985; 147: 197–206.

59. Baluna R, Vitetta ES. Vascular leak syndrome: a side effect of immunotherapy. Immunopharmacology 1997; 37:117–132.

60. Baluna R, Ghetie V, Oppenheimer-Marks N, Vitetta ES. Fibronectin inhibits the cytotoxic effect of ricin A chain on endothelial cells. Int J Immunopharm 1996; 18:355–361.

61. Reiter Y, Brinkmann U, Kreitman RJ, Jung SH, Lee B, Pastan I. Stabilization of the Fv fragments in recombinant immunotoxins by disulfide bonds engineered into conserve framework regions. Biochemistry 1994; 33:5451–5459.

62. Yokota T, Milenic DE, Whitlow M, Schlom J. Rapid tumor penetration of a single-chain Fv and comparison with other immunoglobulin forms. Cancer Res 1992; 52:3402–3408.

63. Milenic DE, Yokota T, Filpula DR, et al. Construction, binding properties, metabolism and targeting of a single-chain Fv derived from pancarcinoma monoclonal antibody CC49. Cancer Res 1991; 51: 6363–6371.

64. Reiter Y, Pastan I. Antibody engineering of recombinant Fv immunotoxins for improved targeting of cancer: disulfide-stabilized Fv immunotoxins. Clin Cancer Res 1996; 2:245–252.

65. Adams GP, Schier R, Marshall K, et al. Increased affinity leads to improved selective tumor delivery of single-chain Fv antibodies. Cancer Res 1998; 58:485–490.

66. Gillies SD, Lo KM, Burger C, Lan Y, Dahl T, Wong WK. Improved circulating half-life and efficacy of an antibody-interleukin 2 immunocytokine based on reduced intracellular proteolysis. Clin Cancer Res 2002; 8:210–216.

67. Michaelsen TE. Fragmentation and conformational changes of IgG subclasses In: Shakib F (ed). The Human IgG Subclasses. Oxford, UK: Pergamon Press, 1990, pp. 31–42.

68. Eger RR, Covell DG, Carrasquillo JA, et al. Kinetic model for the biodistribution of an ^{111}In-labeled monoclonal antibody in humans. Cancer Res 1987; 47:3328–3336.

69. Leyland-Jones B. Administration schedules of Trastuzumab. In: First International Congress on Monoclonal Antibodies in Cancer, Banff, Canada, 2001.

70. Tobinai K, Kobayashi Y, Narabayashi M, et al. Feasibility and pharmacokinetic study of a chimeric anti-CD20 monoclonal antibody (IDEC-C2B8, rituximab) in relapsed B-cell lymphoma. The IDEC–C2B8 study group. Ann Oncol 1998; 9:527–534.

71. Khazaeli MB, Saleh MN, Liu TP, et al. Pharmacokinetics and immune response of ^{131}I-chimeric mouse/human B72.3 (human γ-4) monoclonal antibody in humans. Cancer Res 1991; 51:5461–5466.

72. Amlot PL, Stone MJ, Cunningham D, et al. A phase I study of an anti-CD22-deglycosylated ricin A chain immunotoxin in the treatment of B-cell lymphomas resistant to conventional therapy. Blood 1993; 82:2624–2633.

73. Thorpe PE, Wallace PM, Knowles PP, et al. Improved anti-tumor effects of immunotoxins prepared with deglycosylated ricin A chain and hindered disulfide linkages. Cancer Res 1988; 48:6396–6403.

74. Sausville EA, Headlee D, Stetler-Stevenson M, et al. Continuous infusion of the anti-CD22 immunotoxin IgG-RFB4-SMPT-dgA in patients with B-cell lymphoma: a phase I study. Blood 1995; 85:3457–3465.

75. Messmann RA, Vitetta ES, Headlee D, et al. A phase I study of combination therapy with immunotoxins IgG-HD37-deglycosylated ricin A chain (dgA) and IgG-RFB4-dgA (Combotox) in patients with refractory CD19+, CD22+ B-cell lymphoma. Clin Cancer Res 2000; 6:1302–1313.

76. Stone MJ, Sausville EA, Fay JW, et al. A Phase I study of bolus versus continuous infusion of the anti-CD19 immunotoxin, IgG-HD37-dgA, in patients with B-cell lymphoma. Blood 1996; 88:1188–1197.

77. Engert A, Diehl V, Schnell R, et al. A Phase-I study of an anti-CD25 ricin A-chain immunotoxin (RFT5- SMPT-dgA) in patients with refractory Hodgkin's lymphoma. Blood 1997; 89:403–410.

78. Frankel AE, Kreitman RJ, Sausville EA. Targeted toxins. Clin Cancer Res 2000; 6:326–334.

79. Chapel H, Dicato M, Gamm H, et al. Immunoglobulin replacement in patients with chronic lymphocytic leukemia: a comparison of two dose regimens. Br J Haematol 1994; 88:209–214.

80. Carmeli Y, Mevorach D, Kaminski N, Raz E. Regression of Kaposi's sarcoma after intravenous immunoglobulin treatment for polymyositis. Cancer 1994; 73:2859–2865.

81. Shoenfeld Y, Fishman P. Gamma-globulin inhibits tumor spread in mice. Int Immunol 1999; 11:1247–1251.

82. Morel A. Pharmacokinetics of intravenous immunoglobulin preparations. In: Lee ML, Strand V (eds). Intravenous immunoglobulins in clinical practice. New York, NY: Marcel Dekker, 1997, pp. 1–18.

83. Mankarious S, Lee M, Fisher S, et al. The half-lives of IgG subclasses and specific antibodies in patients with primary immunodeficiency who are receiving intravenously administered immunoglobulin. J Lab Clin. Med 1988; 112:634–640.

84. Lee ML, Mankarious S, Ochs H. The pharmacokinetics of total IgG, IgG subclasses and type specific antibodies in immunodeficient patients. Immunol Invest 1991; 20:193–198.

85. Lefranc MP, Lefranc G. Molecular genetics of immunoglobulin allotype expression. In: Shakib F (ed). The Human IgG Subclasses. Oxford, UK: Pergamon Press, 1990, pp. 43–78.

86. Samuelsson A, Towers TL, Ravetch JV. Anti-inflammatory activity of IVIG mediated through the inhibitory Fc receptor. Science 2001; 291:484–486.

87. Masson PL. Elimination of infectious antigens and increase of IgG catabolism as possible modes of action of IVIG. J Autoimmun 1993; 6:683–689.

88. Yu Z, Lennon VA. Mechanism of intravenous immune globulin therapy in antibody-mediated autoimmune diseases. N Engl J Med 1999; 340:227–228.

89. Mozes E, Kohn LD, Hakim F, Singer DS. Resistance of MHC class I-deficient mice to experimental systemic lupus erythematosus. Science 1993; 261:91–93.

90. Christianson GJ, Brooks W, Vekasi S, et al. β_2-Microglobulin-deficient mice are protected from hypergammaglobulinemia and have defective antibody responses because of increased IgG catabolism. J Immunol 1997; 159:4781–4792.

91. Liu Z, Roopenian DC, Zhou X, et al. β_2-Microglobulin-deficient mice are resistant to bullous penaphigoid. J Exp Med 1997; 186:777–783.

92. Andersen SB, Jarnum S, Jensen H, Rossing N. Metabolism of γ-globulin in the nephrotic syndrome in adults. Scand J Clin Lab Invest 1968; 21:42–47.

93. Mariani G, Strober W. Immunoglobulin metabolism. In: Metzger H (ed). Fc Receptors and the Action of Antibodies: Immunoglobulin Metabolism. Washington, DC: American Society for Microbiology 1990, pp. 94–180.

94. Hansbrough JR, Miller LN, Field TO, Gadd NA. High dose intravenous immunoglobulin therapy in burn patients. Pharmacokinetics and effects on microbial opsonization and phagocytosis. Pediatr Infect Dis J 1988; 7:549–556.

95. Wochner R. D, Drews G, Strober W, Waldman TA. Accelerated breakdown of immunoglobulin G (IgG) in myotomic dystrophy: a hereditary error of immunoglobulin catabolism. J Clin Invest 1966; 45:321–329.

96. Wochner RD. Hypercatabolism of normal IgG; an unexplained immunoglobulin abnormality in the connective tissue diseases. J Clin Invest 1970; 49:454–464.

97. Levy J, Barnett EV, MacDonald NS, Klinenberg JR. Altered immunoglobulin metabolism in systemic lupus erythenatosus and rheumatoid arthritis. J Clin Invest 1970; 49:708–715.

98. Blaese RM, Strober N, Levy AL, Waldmann TA. Hypercatabolism of IgG, IgA, IgM and albumin in the Wiskott–Aldrich syndrome. A unique disorder of serum protein metabolism. J Clin Invest 1971; 50:2331–2338.

99. Waldman TA, Miller EJ, Terry WD. Hypercatabolism of IgG and albumin: a new familiar disorder. Clin Res 1968; 16:45–49.

100. Waldmann TA, Johnson JS, Talal N. Hypogammaglobulinemia associated with accelerated catabolism of IgG secondary to its interaction with an IgG-reactive monoclonal IgM. J Clin Invest 1971; 50:951–959.

101. Junghans RP, Ebralidze A, Tiwari B. Does (CUG)$_n$ repeat in DMPK mRNA "paint" chromosome 19 to supress distant genes to create the diverse phenotype of myotonic dystrophy? A new hypothesis of long-range *cis* autosomal inactivation. Neurogenetics 2001; 3:59–67.

102. Kandil E, Egashira M, Miyoshi O, et al. The human gene encoding the heavy chain of the major histocompatibility complex class I-like Fc receptor (FCGRT) maps to 19q 13.3. Cytogenet Cell Genet 1996; 73:97–98.

103. Seznec H, Lia-Balini AS, Duros C, et al. Transgenic mice carrying large human genomic sequences with expanded CTG repeat mimic closely the DM CTG repeat intergenerational and somatic instability. Hum Mol Genet 2000; 9:1185–1194.

104. Levy AL, Waldmann TA. The effect of hydrocortisone on immunoglobulin metabolism. J Clin Invest 1970; 49:1679–1684.

105. Theofilopoulos AN, Dixon FJ. Murine models of systemic lupus erythematosis. Adv Immunol 1985; 37:269–390.

106. Marino M, Ruvo M, De Falco S, Fassina G. Prevention of systemic lupus erythematosus in MRL/lpr mice by administration of an immunoglobulin-binding peptide. Nat Biotechnol 2000; 18:735–739.

107. Satoh M, Reeves WH. Induction of lupus-associated autoantibodies in BALB/c mice by intraperitoneal injection of pristane. J Exp Med 1994; 180:2341–2346.

108. Catalona MA, Krick EH, De Heer DH, Nakamura RM, Theofilopoulos AN, Vaughan JH. Metabolism of autologous and homologous IgG in rheumatoid arthritis. J Clin Invest 1977; 60:313–322.

109. Jefferis R, Mageed RA. The specificity and reactivity of rheumatoid factors with human IgG In: Shakib F (ed). Autoantibodies to immunoglobulins. Basel, Switzerland: Karger, 1989, pp. 45–60.

110. Corper AL, Sohi MK, Bonagura VR, et al. Structure of human IgM rheumatoid factor Fab bound to its auto antigen IgG Fc reveals a novel topology of antibody-antigen interaction. Nat Struct Biol 1997; 4:374–381.

111. Sensel MG, Coloma MJ, Harvill ET, Shin SU, Smith RI, Morrison SL. Engineering novel antibody molecules. Chem Immunol 1997; 65:129–158.

112. Ward ES, Ghetie V. The effector functions of immunoglobulins: implications for therapy. Ther Immunol 1995; 2:77–94.

113. Idusogie EE, Wong PY, Presta LG, et al. Engineered antibody with increased activity to recruit complement. J Immunol 2001; 166:2571–2575.

114. Frick IM, Wikstrom M, Forsten S, et al. Convergent evolution among immunoglobulin G-binding bacterial protein. Proc Natl Acad Sci USA 1992; 89:8532–8536.

30 Pharmacokinetics of Biologicals

Håkan Mellstedt, MD, PhD, *Jan-Erik Frödin,* MD, PhD, *and Anders Österborg,* MD, PhD

CONTENTS

INTRODUCTION
PHARMACOKINETICS OF CYTOKINES
ANTIGENICITY OF CYTOKINES
PHARMACOKINETICS AND ANTIGENICITY OF THERAPEUTIC MABS
SUMMARY

1. INTRODUCTION

Present therapeutic approaches, including surgery, irradiation, and chemotherapy, will cure up to 50% of all patients with cancer, but many of the remainder will live with chronic disease for many years. There is therefore a need for new therapeutic agents, not only to achieve durable remissions, but also to increase quality of life for patients during and after treatment. This chapter describes the impact and pharmacokinetics of cytokines and monoclonal antibodies (MAbs) in cancer therapy when used as adjuvants to chemotherapy, as therapeutic support, and as anticancer agents in their own right. Such compounds often have a very complex mechanism of action, and multiple effects. The dose–response curve is bell shaped rather than linear, which makes it more difficult to estimate the optimal therapeutic dose (OTD), which is not usually the maximum tolerated dose (MTD) for these compounds. Pharmacokinetic studies provide important data, enabling clinicians to optimize therapeutic strategies.

2. PHARMACOKINETICS OF CYTOKINES

2.1. Interferons

The potential of the interferons as antitumor and antiviral agents has been well established *(1–4)*. The interferon (IFN) protein families, α (produced by leukocytes), β (by fibroblasts and macrophages), and γ (by T cells), all show rapid plasma clearance after intravenous administration *(5)*. Serum concentrations are generally undetectable after 24 h. Terminal elimination half-lives range from 4 to 16 h (α), 1–2 h (β), and 25–35 min (γ). Intramuscular and subcutaneous administration of α and β IFNs results in protracted but reliable absorption: >80% for IFN-α and 30–70% for IFN-γ *(5)*.

Handbook of Anticancer Pharmacokinetics and Pharmacodynamics
Edited by: W. D. Figg and H. L. McLeod © Humana Press Inc., Totowa, NJ

Table 1
Use of IFN in Cancer Treatment in Clinical Studies (1987–2001)

Malignancy	IFN type	Role in therapy
Follicular lymphoma (129,130)	α-2b	Induction[a]
Aggressive follicular lymphoma (131,132)	α-2b	Induction[a]
Multiple myeloma (132)	α-2b	Induction
Multiple myeloma (133,134)	α-2b	Maintenance
Multiple myeloma (135)	β	Induction
Chronic myeloid leukemia (136)	α-2b	Induction
Chronic myeloid leukemia (137)	α-2b	Maintenance
Melanoma (138)	a-2b	Induction[a]
Melanoma (139–142)	α-2b	Maintenance
Melanoma (143)	β, γ	Induction
Renal cell carcinoma (10)	α-2b	Induction
Renal cell carcinoma (144)	β	Induction[b]
Renal cell carcinoma (145)	β	Induction
Renal cell carcinoma (146)	β	Induction[c]

[a] In combination with chemotherapy.
[b] In combination with IL-2.
[c] In combination with GM-CSF and IL-2.

Interferon, in the vast majority of cases IFN-α is used clinically for cancer treatment (see Table 1). Meta-analysis evaluating IFN-α across 24 multiple myeloma (MM) trials involving 4012 patients (6) showed that IFN-α improved progression-free survival by about 6 mo, but the overall survival benefit was small. A meta-analysis of treatment of MM and renal cell carcinoma (RCC) patients, with or without IFN-α, indicated that inclusion of IFN-α in the treatment of 1164 MM patients raised response rates from 17% to 24%; in the 525 RCC patients, IFN-α raised response rates from 8% to 14% (7).

IFN-α can be used in conjunction with IFN-γ and with other biologicals such as interleukin-2 (IL-2) for treatment of advanced RCC (8,9). When compared in a randomized trial, addition of IFN-γ to IFN-α increased the rate (from 12.5% to 20%) and duration of responses (10). IFN-γ may also be used alone (11), or in conjunction with IL-2 (12) or IL-12 (13).

The clinical utility of synthetic interferons has been hampered, however, by rapid clearance from the plasma and degradation by plasma and tissue enzymes. Various modifications have been carried out in an effort to overcome this. The degree and type of glycosylation, for example, has a profound effect on IFN pharmacokinetics: IFN-γ is a dimer containing four glycosylation sites that shows differential clearance due to glycosylation (14). High-mannose glycosylated recombinant IFN molecules expressed in insect cell cultures were taken up by the liver and so eliminated more rapidly from serum than unglycosylated recombinant forms, which in turn were eliminated faster than the natural form (low-mannose glycosylated). Clinical studies, in general, use forms of IFN grown in *Escherichia coli*. These are unglycosylated, which may explain why their clearance is faster than that of natural IFN.

More recently, pegylation has been used to improve pharmacokinetics by addressing the problem of rapid clearance (15,16). Polyethylene glycol (PEG) moieties, inert long-chain

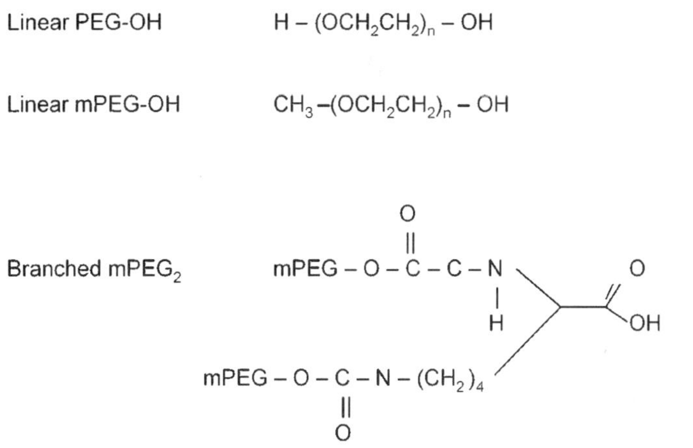

Linear PEG-OH $H - (OCH_2CH_2)_n - OH$

Linear mPEG-OH $CH_3 - (OCH_2CH_2)_n - OH$

Branched mPEG$_2$

$$mPEG - O - \overset{\overset{O}{\|}}{C} - C - \underset{\underset{H}{|}}{N}$$

$$mPEG - O - \underset{\underset{O}{\|}}{C} - N - (CH_2)_4$$

Fig. 1. Structural formulae of poly(ethylene glycol) (PEG) molecules. mPEG and monometho-xypoly(ethylene glycol).

amphiphilic molecules, are linked to any protein of interest, usually via amino groups of lysine residues or the target protein amino-terminus. This decreases antigenicity by steric hindrance of immune recognition, reduces renal clearance, and prolongs the maintenance of serum levels at or near the target dose *(15,17,18)*. As a result, PEG compounds generally have longer serum half-lives and durations of bioactivity than their nonpegylated counterparts *(16)*.

PEG-IFN-α-2a is currently approved for treatment of chronic hepatitis C infection, and pegylated forms of IFN-α and IFN-β are under investigation for use in other conditions. Pegylation has been shown to improve absorption, to increase the elimination half-life ($t_{1/2}\beta$) from 3–8 h to 65 hours, and to decrease systemic clearance (CL) 100-fold *(15)*. There are no significant differences in subcutaneous bioavailability of pegylated forms of IFN.

Effective pegylation may be achieved by attaching a single, large PEG at a single site; a branched-chain PEG at a single site; or multiple small-chain PEGs at several attachment sites (see Fig. 1) *(16)*. PEGs of varying shapes and lengths (5000, 12,000, and 40,000 Da) have been attached to IFN-α-2a and to IFN-α-2b, and although they also extend half-life ($t_{1/2}$) to a similar degree, other pharmacokinetic parameters are affected in a size-dependent manner, with the 5000-Da moiety behaving similarly to unmodified IFN in terms of volume of distribution (V_d) and absorption half-life ($t_{1/2abs}$) *(15)*. Only the 40,000-Da (branched-chain) moiety is associated with a highly decreased V_d and a much more sustained serum concentration *(19)*. This provides for a much more convenient administration schedule, allowing the drug to be given once weekly. This schedule has safety and convenience advantages and can replace the frequently used three-times-weekly schedule *(20)* or the daily schedule required for treatment of melanoma. Using the 40,000-Da PEG forms also allows for higher and more sustained virological responses than those achieved by standard therapy in patients with hepatitis C *(21,22)*. Extensive randomized studies in patients with chronic hepatitis C infection have demonstrated the benefits of pegylated IFN (see Table 2).

An understanding about the distinct pharmacokinetic properties of PEG-IFNs when used as antiviral agents can also be applied to their use as antitumor agents. PEG-IFNs show the same advantages, allowing the intervals between treatments to be reduced from daily or three-times-weekly schedules. The 40,000-Da branched-chain PEG-IFN-α-2b derivative,

Table 2

Randomized Trials of IFN vs PEG-IFN in Chronic Hepatitis C Infection

Study	Schedule	Pharmacokinetic findings	Viral response (at 48 wk)
A (19)	IFN three times weekly (n = 29)	C_{max} declined rapidly	NA
	PEG-IFB once weekly (n = 29)	C_{max} sustained 48–72 h	NA
B (147)	IFN three times weekly (n = 264)	NA	28%
	PEG-IFN once weekly (n = 267)	NA	69%
C (148)	IFN three times weekly + ribavirin (n = 505)	NA	42%
	High-dose PEG-IFN once weekly + ribavirin (n = 511)	NA	54%
	Low-dose PEG-IFN once weekly + ribavirin (n = 514)	NA	47%

NA, Not available.

administered subcutaneously on a weekly basis in RCC, demonstrated antitumor activity and established a dosage (450 µg/wk) suitable for further trials (23). A multicenter Phase II trial conducted in 40 previously untreated patients with advanced RCC using this schedule demonstrated a major response in five patients (four partial and one complete). Median time to progression was 4.8 mo, with 14 patients still under therapy. After 13 mo median follow-up, median survival has not yet been reached, but 72% of patients were alive at 1 yr. The toxicity profile was not appreciably different from that of standard IFN. Serum drug levels were studied in all patients. The mean peak serum concentration (C_{max}) at week 1 was 18 ng/mL, and levels were sustained at close to peak levels over 1 wk. With chronic dosing, drug concentration was increased two- to threefold, and steady state was achieved in about 5 wk. PEG-IFN is currently also under investigation in treatment of chronic myeloid leukemia (24).

These new schedules using PEG-IFNs offer equivalent efficacy and greater convenience and safety than nonpegylated IFNs.

2.2. Erythropoietin

The glycoprotein hormone erythropoietin (EPO) is the primary regulator of erythropoiesis (25). Recombinant forms of human EPO produced in Chinese hamster ovary (CHO) cells (rHuEpo) are used to combat chemotherapy- and cancer-related anemia, either replacing or supplementing red blood cell transfusion, and are highly effective in increasing quality of life (26). Two main recombinant forms of EPO are available, epoetin-α and epoetin-β. These differ slightly in glycosylation, with epoetin-α having more sialic acid residues than epoetin-β, and being more widely used (27).

A study comparing the pharmacokinetics of rHuEpo administered intravenously, intraperitoneally, or subcutaneously, showed that after intravenous infusion, serum rHuEpo levels decayed exponentially from a peak of 3959 mU/mL, with a half-life of 8.2 h. In patients on chronic hemodialysis treatment, bioavailability of ssubcutaneous rHuEpo (21.5%) was seven times greater than that of intraperitoneal rHuEpo. (2.9%) (28). Further work showed bioavailabilities after subcutaneous injection of 31.7% (29), 36% (30), and 20–30% (31), with peak concentrations occurring about 18 h after injection of 5–10% of peak levels obtained after an intravenous dose (31).

Such studies have established the effectiveness, dosage, and optimal route of administration of rHuEpo and have indicated that the high levels reached immediately after intravenous doses are unnecessary either to induce or to sustain erythropoiesis *(32)*. This encourages the use of subcutaneous administration. The constant presence of rHuEPO is critical to erythropoiesis, and although peak plasma values are achieved slowly after subcutaneous administration, rHuEpo levels are then maintained above the critical concentration required. The subcutaneous route sustains rHuEpo levels, prevents death of rHuEpo-dependent cells, and results in more efficient and more sustained erythropoiesis. Subcutaneous administration in 36 healthy adults allowed the pharmacokinetics of once-weekly injection and (fixed dose, 40,000 IU) three-times-weekly injections (weight adjusted 150 IU/kg) to be compared. This study showed that the peak serum concentrations (C_{max}) and the area under plasma concentration–time curve (AUC_{0-168}) for the once-weekly schedule were three times and six times higher than those achieved with the three-times-weekly schedule. Both groups showed similar changes in reticulocytes and red blood cells, and hemoglobin levels from baseline, indicating that these schedules can be considered clinically equivalent. The total weekly dose administered by single injection is greater than that required when three injections are administered.

To improve both pharmacokinetics and effectiveness, further modifications have been made to the glycosylation of rHuEpo. Human physiological EPO has a 40% carbohydrate content and studies have shown that there is a direct relationship between the sialic acid content and the serum half-life and biological activity in vivo *(33)*. Although affinity for the EPO receptor diminishes with increasing sialic acid content, this does not translate to a decrease in activity. The recombinant rHuEpo (Epogen, epoetin-α) used in the majority of cases is a fraction containing molecules with 9–14 sialic acid residues. Isoform 9 has one third of the in vivo activity of isoform 14 owing to the difference in serum half-life.

Hyperglycosylated rHuEpo analogs have altered protein backbones that provide more glycosylation sites. The most active product, novel erythopoiesis stimulating protein (NESP), has five glycosylation sites and can contain up to 22 sialic acid residues. Comparative pharmacokinetic studies were performed in mice that showed that NESP was 3.6 times more potent than rHuEpo when administered three times weekly. Importantly, it also showed that NESP was 13–14 times more potent than rHuEpo when administered once weekly. Studies in dialysis patients *(34,35)* and in pediatric renal disease patients *(36)* also confirmed a longer serum half-life for NESP (see Table 3), and its ability to achieve suitable serum levels by subcutaneous administration in both pediatric and adult patients. Of these studies, the double-blind randomized trial in 11 dialysis patients *(34)* compared the pharmacokinetics of a single dose of rHuEpo with an equivalent mass of NESP, both given by intravenous bolus; in a second comparative study *(35)*, 47 patients were randomized to rHuEpo (three times weekly), NESP three times weekly, or NESP once weekly.

One NESP study of cancer patients used a single injection of NESP given as a single subcutaneous injection prior to the first cycle of chemotherapy, followed by further injections on day 1 of each cycle of subsequent chemotherapy *(37)*. This study indicated that subcutaneous NESP is slowly absorbed, taking about 85 h to reach peak concentration, with a mean $t_{1/2}\beta$ of 32.6 h. Trough serum concentrations of NESP varied within chemotherapy cycles, most likely due to the impact of myelosuppression on pharmacokinetics: within a cycle, the lowest values were found in wk 1 (immediately prior to NESP and chemotherapy), whereas the wk 2 values (1 wk after chemotherapy) were the highest. This may indicate that bone marrow involvement may affect either the clearance or the distribution of NESP. For instance, reduction in erythroid precursors by chemotherapy would allow more NESP to remain in circulation. No antibodies to NESP were detected.

Table 3
Comparative Pharmacokinetics Studies of NESP and rHuEpo

Study population	Schedule	Half-life (h)	Clearance (mL/h/kg)	Bioavailability (%)
Dialysis patients (34) (n = 11)	NESp single dose iv, mean ± SD (n = 11)	25.3 ± 2.2	1.6 ± 0.3	NA
	rHuEpo single dose IV, mean ± SD (n = 10)	8.5 ± 2.4	4.0 ± 0.3	NA
	NESP single dose sc, median (range), (n = 6)	48.8 (33.5–68.0)	NA	37
Dialysis patients (35) (n = 47)	NESP once weekly IV, median (range)	17.8 (15.2–20.4) at wk 1 (n = 11)	2.00 (1.65–2.34) at wk 1 (n = 17)	NA
		23.4 (20.6–26.2) at wk 12 (n = 11)	1.79 (1.42–2.17) at wk 12 (n = 14)	NA
	NESP three times weekly IV, median (range)	13.1 (11.2–14.9) at wk 1 (n = 17)	2.05 (1.51–2.59) at wk 1 (n = 11)	NA
		18.3 (14.4–22.2) at wk 12 (n = 11)	1.90 (1.31–2.49) at wk 12 (n = 11)	NA
	rHuEpo, three times weekly IV, median (range)	6.3 (5.1–7.6) at wk 1 (n = 14)	8.58 (6.72–10.44) at wk 1 (n = 14)	NA
		8.0 (5.7–10.3) at week 12 (n = 14)	NA	NA
Pediatric patients (36) (n = 13)	NESP single dose IV, median (range)	22.1 (12.0–30.0)	2.29 (16.0–86.0)	NA
	NESP single dose SC, median (range)	42.8 (1.60–3.50)	NA	54

NA, Not available

These results demonstrate that the mean elimination half-life of NESP doubles when given sc because this value represents a balance between absorption from the injection site and elimination from the circulation. NESP terminal half-life also appears to be at least twice that achieved with sc rHUEpo (31).

2.3. Granulocyte Colony-Stimulating Factor (G-CSF)

The granulocyte colony-stimulating factor (G-CSF) is used to prevent febrile neutropenia, which is a frequent consequence of high-dose cancer chemotherapy and increases the risk of infectious complications. G-CSF may be given as primary prophylaxis or as support in response to neutropenia (38–40). It also has a role in allogeneic transplantation, as it is effective in mobilizing peripheral blood stem cells (PBSCs) (41).

Like other recombinant cytokines, it can be produced in three ways: using bacterial (E. coli), yeast, or mammalian (usually CHO) cell lines. These recombinant products vary in the amount of posttranslational modification. Bacterial systems do not glycosylate the polypeptide backbone; yeast systems glycosylate to a limited extent; CHO cells glycosylate to a similar extent as the human physiological form of the cytokine (42).

Two main recombinant forms of G-CSF have been produced, the E. coli product, filgrastim (43), and the CHO product, lenograstim (44). In addition, an E. coli derived amino-terminal mutated form (nartograstim, rHuG-CSF-mutein, KW-2228), a pegylated version of nartograstim (Ro-25-8315, PEG-rHuG-CSF-mutein), as well as a pegylated version of filgrastim (PEG-filgrastim, SD-01), are under investigation. Of these, filgrastim has been most extensively investigated in humans.

Filgrastim has consistent and predictable pharmacokinetics when given intravenously or subcutaneously (45). It is rapidly absorbed and peak serum concentrations are achieved 2–8 h after intravenous infusion. The elimination half-life after intravenous or subcutaneous dosing is 2–4 h. After discontinuation of dosing, concentrations decrease to physiological levels within 24 h. In cancer patients, dose-linear clearance can occur during severe neutropenia and after high-dose administration, presumably due to saturation of receptor-mediated clearance. It appears that, in cancer patients, administration of rHuG-CSF increases the number of G-CSF receptors per cell as well as circulating neutrophil counts, resulting in modulation of its own clearance (46). Conversely, dose-dependent clearance is seen after the administration of low doses prior to chemotherapy (45).

Pharmacodynamics and efficacy are directly related to pharmacokinetics, with dose-dependent increases in the numbers of neutrophils and metamyelocytes. Phase I/II trial results from 15 patients given doses ranging from 1 to 60 μg/kg/d demonstrated dose-dependent absolute neutrophil count (ANC) increases, achieving ANCs up to 80×10^9/L (47). Doses > 10 μg/kg/d can also produce dose-dependent increases in monocytes and small increases in lymphocytes.

Like filgrastim, lenograstim achieves higher maximum plasma concentrations after intravenous administration than after subcutaneous administration of the same dose. However, subcutaneous administration resulted in a longer elimination half-life, and a greater and more sustained neutrophil response (48,49). In controlled Phase II dose-ranging studies, which included 66 solid tumor and 121 bone marrow transplantation (BMT) patients, lenograstim doses from 2 μg/kg/d were shown to restore neutrophil counts, and a dose of 5 μg/kg/d was chosen for further clinical trials. Phase III double-blind randomized studies in a further 439 patients with solid tumors or post-BMT confirmed the clinical efficacy of the recommended therapeutic dose of lenograstim (150 μg/m²/d) which is equivalent in efficacy to 5 μg/kg/d (48). Irrespective of route, the most common adverse events were headaches and back/spine pain, and at doses of up to 5 μg kg/d these were mild and generally well tolerated (49).

With regard to myelostimulation (50), low subcutaneous doses of lenograstim (1 μg/kg/d) in 72 healthy volunteers (50) produced ANC increases that did not correlate to C_{max} or the plasma concentration–time curve. This upper limit to the rHuG-CSF transfer rate from subcutaneous tissue to blood may be dependent on the concentration of the G-CSF receptors.

Pharmacokinetics after sc administration of lenogastrim was studied in healthy subjects at doses of 2, 5, and 10 μg/kg/d, given for 5 d to mobilize PBSCs for allogeneic transplantation *(51)*. In this study, peripheral neutrophils increased markedly by up to 13 times from baseline, peaking at about 40×10^9/L on d 5 for both the 5 and 10 μg/kg/d doses. Peak serum concentration (C_{max}) occurred 4 hours after administration and serum G-CSF then declined with time in a log-linear fashion. The C_{max} and 12-h AUC increased dose-dependently, but the minimum drug level increased up to d 2 and then decreased until d 5. Clearance decreased with increasing dosage at the first dose, and increased significantly at the last dose. There was a highly significant correlation between ANC and clearance for each dose. Adverse events most frequently occurred on d 6, with increases of alkaline phosphatase and lactate dehydrogenase, and onset of bone pain. Direct comparisons of the clinical effects of glycosylated and nonglycosylated forms on PBSCs showed that while differences in serum concentrations were observed, this did not influence their ability to mobilize progenitor cells when tested in monkeys *(52)*, in healthy volunteers *(53)*, or in humans with breast cancer *(54)*.

Adverse events appear less frequent with filgrastim than lenograstim *(55)*, although few comparative studies have been carried out.

Nartograstim is a G-CSF mutant produced in *E. coli (56)* in which five amino acids at the terminal region have been replaced. This compound has higher specific activity than the native protein owing to increased serum stability *(57–59)*, although serum concentration–time profiles were found to be very similar to those of filgrastim in monkey studies *(52)*. These pharmacokinetic studies comparing filgrastim, lenograstim, and nartograstim indicated that after intravenous injection, the serum concentration–time profiles of nartograstim were almost identical to those of filgrastim at either 1.5 or 5 μg/kg doses, but that the serum concentration decreased faster after lenograstim administration. After subcutaneous administration, no marked differences were observed between the three forms of rHuG-CSFs, although lenograstim showed lower serum concentrations than both filgrastim and nartograstim. The small differences in pharmacokinetics did not translate into any significant differences in pharmacodynamics, with all compounds having equivalent activity.

As with other cytokines, addition of PEG to G-CSF has great advantages, allowing active serum levels to be sustained over days rather than minutes. Pegylated forms of nartograstim and filgrastim are under investigation. The uninterrupted therapy possible using pegylated G-CSF may also prove more beneficial with regard to ANC recovery after transplant and with regard to efficient mobilization of PBSCs.

Addition of PEG to nartograstim produces a multi-PEG molecule (Ro-25-8315, PEG-rHuG-CSF-mutein) that can further increase serum half-life compared with filgrastim, as first demonstrated in mice *(60)* and monkeys *(61)*, indicating that these compounds can maintain elevated neutrophil doses for extended periods, with the extent of pegylation directly proportional to the increase of in vivo activity. In monkeys receiving subcutaneous injections, peak neutrophil levels could be attained 6 d after a single dose of Ro-25-8315, while similar levels required six daily injections of PEG-rHuG-CSF *(61)*.

In humans, Ro-25-8315 has been compared with filgrastim in 52 healthy male volunteers *(62)*. Part 1 of this study was a double-blind trial in which 40 adults were randomized to receive either placebo or a single subcutaneous dose of Ro-25-8315 at 10, 30, 60, 100, or 150 μg/kg, with eight patients assigned to each dose level in a dose-ascending manner. Part 2 of the trial assigned 12 adults to receive either 5 or 10 μg/kg of filgrastim (using the standard multiple dosing regimen). This consisted of a single subcutaneous dose of filgrastim given on d 1 and then, beginning on d 15, each adult received daily injections of filgrastim for 7 d.

Administration of Ro-25-8315 resulted in substantial increases in ANC, with both ANC_{max} and AUC_{ANC} increasing six- to eight-fold over placebo at the four highest doses tested. These increases were dose-dependent, although over 60 µg/kg the increases were modest. The time to reach maximum plasma concentration was also dose dependent, ranging from 30 h at 10 µg/kg to 104 h at 150 µg/kg. Effects on CD34+ counts showed that mobilization peaked between day 4 and d 5 with Ro-25-8315, earlier than with filgrastim, and that the 60 µg/kg single injection achieved mobilization levels equivalent to daily administration of filgrastim for 1 wk.

Addition of a single chain (20,000 Da) of PEG to filgrastim produces PEG-filgrastim. Studies in rats of this pegylated protein suggest that it has an elimination half-life that is two to four times greater than that of filgrastim (63) and comparative studies in humans have demonstrated its advantages. The first clinical study of PEG-filgrastim in humans was a randomized dose-escalation study carried out in 13 patients with small-cell lung cancer receiving carboplatin and paclitaxel chemotherapy (64). In this study, patients were randomized to receive either daily filgrastim (5 µg/kg/d) or a single injection of PEG-filgrastim at 30, 100, or 300 µg/kg per cycle. The maximum PEG-filgrastim serum concentration and AUC were dose dependent. In cycle 1, maximum values were similar to cycle 0. However, a prolonged plateau of serum concentrations began during cycle 1 and began to decline only with recovery of neutrophil counts. Prechemotherapy median ANCs in patients receiving PEG-filgrastim were increased in a dose dependent fashion, with the duration of this effect also being dose-dependent. After chemotherapy, median ANC nadirs were similar in the filgrastim cohort and the cohort receiving PEG-filgrastim 30 µg/kg; higher nadirs were seen in the cohorts receiving PEG-filgrastim at 100 or 300 µg/kg. No serious adverse events were attributed to G-CSF in any arm, with the most common adverse event in all arms being musculoskeletal pain lasting about 8 d during cycle 1. Mobilization of CD34+ cells was also similar in all arms. Seroreactivity was seen in 4 of 19 samples collected, but no evidence of neutralizing antibodies was found. This work established PEG-filgrastim at 100 µg/kg as effective, with no excessive toxicity associated with prolonged pharmacokinetics.

Mobilization of stem cells by PEG-filgrastim has also been studied in detail in both mice and humans (65). The splenectomized mouse model confirmed that a single-bolus dose of filgrastim could not sustain elevated neutrophil counts beyond 24–48 h irrespective of dose, and that this duration could be extended only by giving multiple injections. A single dose of PEG-filgrastim, however, resulted in increased neutrophil levels for almost 5 d. In a neutropenic setting (induced in mice by chemotherapy with 5-fluorouracil) data indicated that PEG-filgrastim was superior to daily injection of filgrastim. Further, PEG-filgrastim mobilized stem cells in a pattern different from filgrastim. PBSC counts were three times greater after a single injection, and the peak was earlier than could be achieved with multiple-dose filgrastim.

These critical pharmacokinetic observations were confirmed in humans. Healthy subjects were randomized to receive either 30, 60, 100, or 300 µg/kg of PEG-filgrastim. Mobilized CD34+ cells peaked at d 3. At the highest dose, values remained elevated until d 12 or 13, and at other doses, values returned to the normal range at d 9. The duration of this response was longer than that seen with mice. Although direct comparisons with filgrastrim were not made, peak mobilization with PEG-filgrastrim in humans appears to be earlier than the 5.3 d achieved with a 5-d daily regimen of filgrastim (10 µg/kg/d) (66). Overall, results indicate that single-dose PEG-filgrastim is at least as effective as a five-dose schedule of filgrastim in subjects with normal white cell counts, and appears to have advantages in the neutropenic setting when given following myelosupressive therapy, and for mobilization of PBSCs.

One large multicenter trial compared pegylated G-CSF with nonpegylated G-CSF when used once monthly as part of a chemotherapy regimen in 310 breast cancer patients enrolled in 62 centers. A single ssubcutaneous injection of PEG-filgrastim (100 µg/kg per chemotherapy cycle, given on d 2, 24 h after chemotherapy) was demonstrated to be as safe and effective as daily sc injections of filgrastim (5 µg/kg/d, given until ANC recovery with an average of 11 injections per cycle) *(67)*. PEG-filgrastim was given to 154 patients and filgrastim to 156. Incidence of grade IV neutropenia and depth of the ANC nadir was similar in the two arms. In some parameters, such as the duration of grade IV neutropenia between cycles 2 and 4, and the incidence of febrile neutropenia, PEG-filgrastim performed better than filgrastim. Adverse events were similar in the two arms, and no adverse safety patterns or trends were seen with PEG-filgrastim. This work confirms earlier claims for a supportive role for PEG-filgrastim during cancer chemotherapy *(68)*.

2.4. Granulocyte-Macrophage Colony-Stimulating Factor (GM-CSF)

Granulocyte-macrophage colony-stimulating factor (GM-CSF) is the most widely used hematopoietic growth factor used to augment immune responses, usually as an adjuvant to vaccination *(69,70)*. This stimulation of immune effector functions aims to increase the potency of treatment and improve the outcome for patients with various disorders including hematopoeitic and nonhematopoietic malignancies.

Comparative pharmacokinetics studies of glycosylated (produced from CHO cells) and nonglycoslylated (produced from *E. coli*) recombinant GM-CSFs have explored the differences between these forms *(71)*. Twelve patients were randomized to treatment with either bacterial or CHO rHuGM-CSF, first intravenously, then subcutaneously. Both GM-CSF types followed a two-compartment first-order pharmacokinetic model after intravenous administration. The bacterial form showed more rapid absorption, achieved higher peak serum concentrations, and was eliminated faster. The initial rate of clearance ($t_{1/2}\alpha$) of the bacterial form was also higher (7.8 min vs 20 min). After subcutaneous administration, clearance of the *E. coli* form was faster (reversion to pretreatment serum levels took 16–20 h vs > 48 h). However, the more rapid turnover of the bacterial form did not translate into a significantly different effect on neutrophil kinetics. While there was considerable variability between patients, both types of rHuGM-CSF induced an initial fall in ANC immediately after administration, then a sharp increase, passing baseline levels by about 3 h (intravenous) or 3–6 h (subcutaneous) and reaching maximum values after 4.5–9 h (intravenous) and 5–20 h (subcutaneous).

The effects of bacterial and mammalian rHuGM-CSFs on endogenous leukotriene biosynthesis have also been studied, in 21 healthy subjects, linking this marker to the frequency of adverse reactions *(72)*. This study confirmed the more rapid kinetics of the *E. coli* form, linked to faster and larger increases in urinary leukotriene concentrations (2.1- to 44-fold vs 1.4- to 14-fold). Mammalian GM-CSF caused a number of skin reactions; other side effects (flulike symptoms, bone pain, gastrointestinal effects, and dyspnea) predominated in volunteers given bacterial GM-CSF.

Recombinant GM-CSF has potent augmentation effects. In addition to stimulating proliferation of myeloid cells, GM-CSF enhances phagocytosis and killing of invading pathogens and increases chemotaxis of neutrophils and macrophages. It also expands and activates antigen-presenting cells; activates eosinophils; and stimulates monocytes to increase production of IFN-γ, IL-12, and Il-15, so increasing natural killer (NK) cell functions (see review by Mellstedt *[70]*). This has led to its investigation as an adjuvant, used to increase the immune response against tumor-specific antigens.

Tumor vaccines may consist of whole tumor cells, or cell lysates, or purified fractions of specific tumor antigens such as human carcinoembryonic antigen (CEA) or mucins (MUC-1). The cytokinc adjuvant may be administered as soluble protein *(73)*, as protein encapsulated in microsomes *(74)* or by transfer of the cytokine DNA sequence into cells expressing the tumor protein(s) of interest *(75)*. These vaccination protocols are of particular relevance to patients at risk of relapse after surgery has excised solid tumors, as in colorectal cancer (CRC), melanoma, and renal cell carcinoma.

Preclinical models established the importance of prolonged exposure to GM-CSF together with tumor cell proteins, showing that responses in mice were better with low doses of GM-CSF given for 4 d than for 1 d *(73)*, and that good results could be obtained when GM-CSF was encapsulated in slow-release microspheres *(74)*. These preclinical results supported the use of low doses of GM-CSF given for 4 d.

Most CRC cells express CEA, and vaccination using this antigen alone can stimulate antibody production *(76)*. With the addition of GM-CSF these effects are greatly enhanced *(77)*. This latter study treated 18 CRC patients without macroscopic disease, after surgical excision of primary tumor. Local administration of soluble GM-CSF was used, rather than generation of retrovirally GM-CSF-transduced cells. Nine patients received baculovirus-produced rHuCEA alone (100, 300, or 1000 µg), while nine received the same dose plus GM-CSF. All patients in the GM-CSF group developed a strong rHuCEA-dose-dependent IgG antibody response compared with the weak antibody response seen in only one third of the non-GM-CSF patients. All patients in the GM-CSF group also developed a strong rHCEA-specific proliferative T-cell response, and induced IFN-γ production in type 1 T cells. In addition, 45% of GM-CSF patients showed IL-4 production by type 2 T cells.

Further studies are indicated to develop regimens that present the recombinant rHuCEA in such a way as to maximize production of antibodies that can recognize the native protein. After follow-up periods of at least 18 mo from the last vaccination, strong T-cell responses against rHuCEA remained in the GM-CSF group; in the non-GM-CSF group the original weak responses had disappeared *(78)*. This work has demonstrated that local administration of soluble GM-CSF is an inexpensive, simple, and reproducible therapeutic procedure for the successful induction of immunity.

The majority of colorectal carcinomas also express the tumor antigen GA733 (CO 17-1A, KSA, EPCAM) *(79–81)*.

In one study, responses were maintained for the whole observation period of 10 mo after only three injections of GM-CSF with rHuGA773. The responses observed include a strong type 1 T-cell response that seems to be major histocompatibility class (MHC) I as well as class II restricted *(81)*.

The idiotypic immunoglobulins on the surface of myeloma cells can be treated as tumor-restricted antigens, and used in vaccination *(82,83)*. The use of GM-CSF in such protocols appears to be mandatory for frequency and magnitude of the antigen response *(84)*. In five myeloma patients vaccinated with purified M-protein plus low-dose (75 µg/d) GM-CSF at six intervals over a 14-wk period, a transient rise of B cells producing IgM antiidiotypic antibodies was seen in all patients *(85)*. The T-cell response could be characterized as a type 1 response (IFN-γ production), which seemed preferentially to be MHC I restricted. Patients with a low tumor burden are expected to respond most favorably to this kind of therapeutic intervention *(86)*.

GM-CSF-transduced autologous melanoma cells may also be used to treat metastatic melanoma *(87)*. This case history reported a temporary tumor response in a patient who had rapidly progressive disease at the time of vaccination.

RCC may also respond to vaccination strategies, as shown in a Phase I trial in which 16 such patients were treated. Patients were treated in a randomized, double-blind dose-escalation study with equivalent doses of autologous, irradiated RCC vaccine cells with or without ex vivo human GM-CSF gene transfer using a retroviral vector. Patients vaccinated with GM-CSF-transduced vaccines showed histology changes, such as an intense eosinophil infiltrate, while patients who received nontransduced vaccines did not. Treatment was well tolerated, with one patient achieving a partial response *(88)*.

Mixed administration of GM-CSF with other cytokines is under increasing investigation for the treatment of RCC and melanoma. One combination of GM-CSF, IL-2, and IFN-α *(89)*, resulted in considerable expansion and/or activation of various effector cells. In this study, of eight patients with progressive metastatic RCC after nephrectomy, three achieved a complete remission; one out of seven patients with metastatic melanoma achieved a partial remission. MAbs may also be added, such as anti-GA733-3 (anti-CO17A). The use of anti-GA733-3 with GM-CSF and recombinant human IL-2 in 20 CRC patients *(90)* has produced mixed results. Although one patient obtained a partial remission and two patients achieved stable disease for 7 and 4 mo, respectively, the effect of the antibody was less than that anticipated from in vitro studies.

2.5. IL-2

Il-2 is an immune modifier able to activate cytotoxic T lymphocytes (CTL) and NK cells *(91)*. It therefore has potential to treat cancers such as RCC and melanoma. In RCC, RHuIL-2 monotherapy can achieve overall response rates (ORR) of 20% (CR 5%), while in metastatic malignant melanoma, ORRs are about 13% *(92)*. Early studies, reviewed in Anderson and Sorenson *(93)*, indicated that effective treatment of cancer required repetitive long-term high-dose treatment to its very short half-life. Efforts to improve scheduling include pegylation—as for other cytokines that use the kidney as the main site of elimination, pegylation will sustain peak serum levels (see Table 4) *(94)*. Low-dose peritoneal administration also produces longer duration of action *(95)*. Other approaches include administering rHuIL-2 in combination with an anti-IL-2 MAb to enhance targeting and distribution *(96)*, or with other cytokines and MAbs to promote immune modulation *(89,90)*.

2.6. L-12

Like Il-2, IL-12 can stimulate CTL and NK cells, and also has the unique property of promoting development of CD4 T cells, which have a critical role in cell-mediated immunity *(97,98)*. This gives it a role as an antitumor agent also capable of restoring immune function.

Studies in rats and monkeys established that the terminal half-life of rHuIL-12 (produced in *E. coli*) was relatively long ($t_{1/2}\beta$ of up to 14 h) compared with other cytokines such as Il-2. This is likely to be a consequence of its larger molecular weight—Il-12 is a dimer composed of 35,000- and 40,000-Da subunits, compared with the more typical 15,500-Da molecular length of Il-2. It also has a low subcutaneous bioavailability (20-30%).[99] Such pharmacokinetic data led to the adoption of once-weekly single subcutaneous injection for treatment of metastatic melanoma and RCC.

In a pilot study 10 patients with melanoma were given rHuIL-12 (0.5 µg/kg) on d 1, 8, and 15, for two consecutive 28-d cycles. Peak serum levels were reached 8–12 h after the first injection, and became lower with subsequent injections, being undetectable at the end of the second cycle *(100)*. This adaptive response may be due to greater removal of IL-12 from peripheral blood, inhibition of access of injected IL-12 to the bloodstream; or up-regulation of IL-12 receptors. Anti-IL-12 antibodies were not implicated, as assays for such antibodies

Table 4
Pharmacokinetics of rHuIL-2

Patient population	Schedule	Pharmacokinetic findings
Mixed malignancy (149)	IL-2, bolus IV	Median $t_{1/2}\alpha$: 12.9 min Median $t_{1/2}\beta$: 85 min Clearance: 120 mL/min
Mixed malignancy (150) ($n = 20$)	IL= 2 continuous vs bolus IV	Median $t_{1/2}\alpha$: 6.9 min Median $t_{1/2}\beta$: 70–85 min
Pediatric malignancy (151)	IL-2 bolus IV	Median $t_{1/2}\alpha$: 14 min Median $t_{1/2}\beta$: 51.4 min
Ovarian cancer (95) ($n = 14$)	IL IP, for 4 d	Median $t_{1/2}\alpha$: 30 min Median $t_{1/2}\beta$: 9.2 h at d 4 Clearance: 72 mL/h/kg
Renal cell carcinoma (152) ($n = 10$)	IL-2 SC once daily ($n = 7$) vs half-dose twice daily ($n = 3$)	Median $t_{1/2}\beta$: 5.1 h (single dose) Higher AUC found in split dose (vs single dose)
Mixed malignancy (94) ($n = 37$)	IL-2 bolus IV once weekly	Median $t_{1/2}\alpha$: 220 min Median $t_{1/2}\beta$: 942 min Clearance: 4.06 mL/min/m2
Colorectal cancer (113) ($n = 19$)	IL-2 twice daily for 10 d	Single-dose kinetics: Median $t_{1/2}\alpha$: 16 min Median $t_{1/2}\beta$: 10.67 h Clearance: 21.33 mL/min

IP, Intraperitoneal; $t_{1/2}\alpha$, distribution half-life; $t_{1/2}\beta$, elimination half-life (two-compartment model); AUC, area under the concentration–time curve.

proved negative. The attenuation in serum levels was reflected in attenuation of immunomodulation such as stimulation of IFN-α.

A Phase I study in 51 RCC patients randomized them either to three fixed-dose rHuIL-2 injections (0.1, 0.5, and 1.0 µg/kg; $n = 24$) or to an up-titration scheme (lower levels in wk 1, increased to maintenance doses of 0.5, 0.75, 1.0, 1.25, and 1.5 µg/kg in wk 2; $n = 27$) (101). With the up-titration scheme, the maximum tolerated dose was 1.5 µg/kg: at this level, serum IL-12 levels peaked at 706 pg/mL. Peak serum levels were achieved 8–24 h after the first injection, and decreased with a $t_{1/2}\beta$ of 7–21 h. Serum levels after the first maintenance dose in the up-titration scheme were lower than those seen with the equivalent fixed-dose scheme, although half-life and peak time were unchanged. Of the 50 patients evaluable for response, 34 had stable disease, 14 progressed, and 3 were lost to treatment.

In a multicenter Phase II trial, 46 patients with previously untreated advanced RCC were assigned (2:1) to either subcutaneous rHuIL-12 or IFN-α treatment (102). An escalating-dose schedule of rHuIL-12 was used: d 1, 0.1 µg/kg; d 8, 0.5 µg/kg; and d 14, 1.25 µg/kg. Subsequent doses were 1.25 µg/kg. IFN-α was given at 9×10^6 units, three times weekly. Pharmacokinetic studies were carried out in 10 patients. Peak serum concentrations occurred at about 12 h. In contrast to fixed-dose results (13,100), no adaptive response was seen, with C_{max} and AUC remaining constant after repeat dosing. Despite this, low disease responses to rHuIL-12 stopped accrual into this arm after an interim analysis.

This modest clinical activity in RCC and melanoma suggests that the most promising use for IL-12 may be in combination with other cytokines, or as a vaccine adjuvant. One such vaccination study has reported on 48 patients with resected melanoma, vaccinated with two tumor antigen peptides (gp100$_{200-217}$, tyrosinase$_{368-376}$) with or without IL-12 (103). IL-12 augmented cytokine release and enhanced the immune response to the tumor antigens. However, the time to relapse of the IL-12 group was identical to that of the non-IL-12 group (20 mo in the whole cohort). Tumor peptide-reactive CTLs did not increase to a plateau until at least six vaccinations had been given over 3 mo. This suggests that prolonged vaccination schedules may be required for melanoma.

3. ANTIGENICITY OF CYTOKINES

One drawback of using proteins of nonhuman origin for therapeutic purposes is an increase in antigenicity and the risk of triggering an immune response. Detection of such antibodies may predict clinical response and exact information on epitope recognition may also provide information of clinical relevance (104).

The different forms of recombinant interferon show different immunogenicities. Typical incidences of neutralizing antibodies are 17% after IFN-α-2b treatment, and up to 45% (plus 38% binding antibodies) after IFN-α-2a treatment (105). Neutralizing antibodies are associated with treatment failure. Conversely, patients, such as those with multiple myeloma, treated with natural leukocyte interferon do not produce antibodies (106).

Changes in the polypeptide backbone in recombinant proteins can render the protein immunogenic, as has been seen in the case of EPO. Sporadic cases of anti-EPO development have been reported, in some cases causing red-cell aplasia (107–109). Neutralizing antibodies were identified and characterized in 13 patients with red-cell aplasia who had received rHuEpo-α (12 patients) or -β (1 patient) to treat chronic renal failure (110). The antibodies did not target glycosylated moieties. They were shown to be reactive with epitopes specific for folded forms of the protein backbone, except in one case where antibody species reactive with both conformationally folded and linear epitopes were seen. Although, in theory, the additional alterations in the protein backbone of NESP might render this molecule more immunogenic, monitoring of patients treated with NESP has not shown the development of neutralizing antibodies. However, antibodies developed during treatment with rHuEpo-α showed cross-reactivity with other forms of recombinant EPO including NESP (110). NESP therefore is not likely to be able to rescue patients who have already developed red-cell aplasia as a consequence of EPO treatment and the development of neutralizing antibodies.

Binding or neutralizing antibodies have also been seen in response to GM-CSF (75,85,111). The purity of the recombinant product is one factor involved, with some preparations triggering antibodies to contaminant bacterial proteins (104,112). In a study of the significance of binding and neutralizing antibodies in 45 patients, binding antibodies were assayed using solid-phase indirect enzyme-linked immunosorbant assay (ELISA), using the same clinical-grade E. coli-derived recombinant human GM-CSF as was used for therapy (78). Neutralizing antibodies were assayed using the TF-1 cell line which proliferates in response to GM-CSF, using known quantities of GM-CSF used after preincubation with dilutions of patient serum. No patients had antibodies directed against GM-CSF at baseline. However, following therapy, while none of the four MM patients had developed reactivity, 15 of the 41 CRC patients had developed reactive antibodies (37.5%). The incidence was greatest in patients receiving high-dose therapy, and was related to cumulative dose. None of the reactive antibodies were capable of neutralizing GM-CSF activity, and no difference was observed in the stimulation of monocytes or other immune effector cells in patients with or without reactive antibodies.

Table 5
Effect of Antibodies on Pharmacokinetics in Patients with Colorectal Carcinoma (d 10) (113)

	IL-2-antibody negative patients n = 5 (mean ± SD)	IL-2-antibody positive patients n = 3 (mean ± SD)	p
C_{max}	64.00 ± 3.00	12.00 ± 1.7	< 0.0001
T_{max}	3.82 ± 0.29	3.40 ± 0.61	NS
$t_{1/2}$	4.06 ± 1.16	3.66 ± 1.25	NS
AUC (ng · h/mL)	528 ± 71	93 ± 19	< 0.0001
CL/F (L/h)	0.19 ± 0.03	1.08 ± 0.21	< 0.001
V_d/F	1.11 ± 0.18	5.70 ± 1.2	< 0.05

Data from ref. *113*.

C_{max}, Peak serum concentration; T_{max}, time to reach maximum concentration; $t_{1/2}$, serum half-life (one-compartment model); AUC: area under the concentration–time curve; CL/F, total body clearance; V_d/F, distribution volume; NS, not statistically significant.

These results were confirmed in a study of 64 CRC patients *(112)*, in which it was found that only neutralizing antibodies (seen in 9 patients) impaired biological activity, while binding antibodies (seen in 47 patients) did not. These findings indicate that non-neutralizing antibodies to GM-CSF do not reduce an immune response. However, non-neutralizing antibodies to some biologicals may perturb pharmacokinetics by forming aggregates that remove the active molecule from circulation. The effect of binding antibodies has been clearly shown in studies of IL-2 pharmacokinetics in patients with and without anti-IL-2 antibodies *(113)*. Of 19 CRC patients tested for the presence of IL-2 antibodies during therapy with rHuIL-2, rHuGM-CSF, and MAb17-1A, 10 developed antibodies (10 binding, 1 binding/neutralizing). Titers of anti-IL-2 antibodies increased with repeated treatment and reverted to undetectable levels 4–6 mo post-therapy. The presence of antibodies was shown to affect pharmacokinetics significantly, regardless of their neutralization potential (see Table 5). The reduction in serum IL-2 concentration and increased clearance by antibodies also reduced IL-2 impact on lymphocyte counts. These results indicate that non-neutralizing antibodies may be as important clinically as neutralizing antibodies.

4. PHARMACOKINETICS AND ANTIGENICITY OF THERAPEUTIC MABS

Many clinically effective MAbs have now been generated, able to target specific cancers, including CRC *(114–117)*, chronic lymphocytic leukemia (CLL) *(118)*, non-Hodgkin's lymphoma (NHL) *(119)*, melanoma, and breast cancer *(120)*. MAbs directed against cell-surface tumor markers can kill their target cell by a variety of mechanisms including antibody-directed cellular cytotoxity (ADCC), complement-dependent cytotoxicity, (CDC) and apoptosis *(121)*. The exact mechanism of killing varies among unconjugated antibodies: alemtuzumab appears to act primarily by ADCC *(122)* and is less effective in bulky tumors which are poorly supplied with effector cells *(123)*; rituximab cytotoxicity has strong apoptotic and complement-mediated components *(124,125)*; and trastuzumab may act primarily by nonimmune effector mechanisms triggered by signal transduction *(126)*. While all these MAbs are of largely similar molecular weight (about 145,000 Da), their pharmacokinetics vary greatly as a consequence of the different affinities for, and distribution of, the target antigen (see Table 6). However, increasing doses increased AUC *(114)*, which augments the exposure of tumor cells to the MAb.

Table 6
Monoclonal Antibodies in Cancer Treatment

	MAb	Type	Target molecule (cell type)	Pharmacokinetic findings
Colorectal carcinoma (114)	17-1A	Murine	Colon mucosa	Single dose 200 mg: $C_{max\ 2\ h}$: 55 ± 5 μg/mL $t_{1/2}\beta$: 25.9 ± 1.4 h Single dose 500 mg: $C_{max\ 2\ h}$: 132 ± 7 μg/mL $t_{1/2}\beta$: 19.8 ± 1.0 h
Non-Hodgkin's lymphoma (153)	Rituximab	Chimeric	CD20 (B lymphocytes)	$t_{1/2}\alpha$: 1.37 d $t_{1/2}\beta$: 19.9 d CL: 0.0054 L/h/m²
Metastatic melanoma (154)	KM-871	Chimeric	GD-3 (neuroectoderm, melanocytes)	$t_{1/2}\alpha$: 0.40 ± 0.33 d $t_{1/2}\beta$: 7.68 ± 2.94 d
Colorectal carcinoma (155)	anti-A33	Humanized	A33 (GI epithelial cells)	NA
Chronic lymphocytic leukemia /T-cell depletion allograft (156)	Alemtuzumab	Humanized	CD52 (mature lymphocytes)	Detectable in serum 11–23 d post-infusion
Breast cancer (32)	Trastuzumab	Humanized	HER-2 (breast, lung, GI, kidney, and CNS epithelial cells)	$t_{1/2}\alpha$: 9.2 ± 5.3 d C_{max}: 113 ± 35 μg/mL

C_{max}, Peak serum concentration; $t_{1/2}\alpha$, distribution half-life; $t_{1/2}\beta$, elimination half-life; CL, clearance.

As with cytokines, the production of an anti-MAb response may limit efficacy after repeat administration. When rodent antibodies are shown to be immunogenic, this can be addressed by the production of chimeric MAbs, retaining only the rodent variable region, or humanized MAbs, retaining only short sequences of rodent hypervariable regions (see Fig. 2). Although some humanized MAbs show low immunogenicity after repeated dosing (123), others, such as MAb-A33, have triggered responses in a large numbers of patients (in 26 of 41, 63% in one study) (127). The antibodies produced to MAb-A33 included type 1 antibodies (49% of cases: early onset; declined with further treatment), which were associated with accelerated MAb clearance, and type 2 antibodies (17% of cases: late onset, increased with treatment), which were associated with infusion-related adverse reactions. The type 1 response appears to be unique to the A33 system. This persistent immunoreactivity is being addressed by using PEG-Mab-A33, which has shown slowed pharmacokinetics and decreased immunogenicity in xenograft models (128).

5. SUMMARY

Major advances in producing stable and effective therapeutic biological agents have been made in the last decade. Antitumor vaccination programs have been boosted by the use of GM-CSF as an immunomodulator, and further progress is underway as the effects of additional cytokines such as IL-1 and IL-12 are elucidated, individually and in combination.

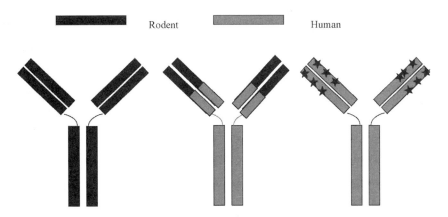

Fig. 2. **(A)** MAb as generated in rodent. **(B)** Chimeric monoclonals: Constant region replaced with human sequence, variable region derived from rodent. **(C)** Humanized monoclonal; hypervariable regions from rodent sequence embedded within fully human framework.

The use of cytokines as chemotherapy support can achieve not only more effective therapy, allowing higher chemotherapy doses to be given, but also a better quality of life, even in patients who are not cured by therapy.

The introduction of more convenient dosing schedules of cytokines such as EPO and G-CSF, made possible by using PEG-cytokines, is also likely to have a beneficial effect on the quality of life of patients with cancer. In the case of EPO, tailoring glycosylation for maximum serum stability has also improved treatment schedules with regard to convenience and efficacy. Pegylation also has the advantage of reducing immunogenicity, which may prove to be of particular value when applied to MAbs with inherent immunogenicity, such as anti-A33.

The large scale production of clinical-grade MAbs achieved in recent years has paved the way to their successful therapeutic use in many conditions, now further enhanced by the synthesis of new humanized and/or pegylated molecules. Significant advances in the treatment of previously intractable forms of cancer have already been made, and these new generations of MAbs, in combination with chemotherapy, have great potential to achieve durable remissions in increasing numbers of patients.

REFERENCES

1. Ahre A, Bjorkholm M, Mellstedt H, et al. Human leukocyte interferon and intermittent high-dose melphalan-prednisone administration in the treatment of multiple myeloma: a randomized clinical trial from the Myeloma Group of Central Sweden. Cancer Treat Rep 1984; 68:1331–1338.
2. Einhorn S, Ahre A, Blomgren H, Johansson B, Mellstedt H, Strander H. Interferon and natural killer activity in multiple myeloma. Lack of correlation between interferon-induced enhancement of natural killer activity and clinical response to human interferon-alpha. Int J Cancer 1982; 30:167–172.
3. Janson CH, Tehrani M, Wigzell H, Mellstedt H. Rational use of biological response modifiers in hematological malignancies—a review of treatment with interferon, cytotoxic cells and antibodies. Leuk Res 1989; 13:1039–1046.
4. Tossing G. New developments in interferon therapy. Eur J Med Res 2001; 6:47–65.
5. Wills RJ, Spiegel HE, Soike KF. Pharmacokinetics of recombinant alpha A interferon following I.V. infusion and bolus, I.M., and P.O. administrations to African green monkeys. J Interferon Res 1984; 4:399–409.

6. Interferon as therapy for multiple myeloma: an individual patient data overview of 24 randomized trials and 4012 patients. Br J Haematol 2001; 113:1020–1034.

7. Hernberg M, Pyrhonen S, Muhonen T. Regimens with or without interferon-alpha as treatment for metastatic melanoma and renal cell carcinoma: an overview of randomized trials. J Immunother 1999; 22:145–154.

8. Krown SE. Interferon treatment of renal cell carcinoma. Current status and future prospects. Cancer 1987; 59:647–651.

9. Locatelli MC, Facendola G, Pizzocaro G, et al. Subcutaneous administration of interleukin-2 and interferon-alpha 2b in advanced renal cell carcinoma: long-term results. Cancer Detect Prev 1999; 23:172–176.

10. Koga S, Nishikido M, Matsuya F, Kanetake H, Saito Y. Subcutaneous administration of interferon alpha and gamma in patients with metastatic renal cell carcinoma. Anticancer Res 1999; 19:5547–5550.

11. Nayak SK, Schiltz PM, Dillman RO. Modulation of renal carcinoma cells in vitro: comparison after transduction with retroviral vector containing a human IFN-gamma gene versus incubation with soluble IFN-gamma. J Interferon Cytokine Res 1999; 19:49–58.

12. Schmidinger M, Steger GG, Wenzel C, et al. Sequential administration of interferon gamma and interleukin-2 in metastatic renal cell carcinoma: results of a phase II trial. Austrian Renal Cell Carcinoma Study Group. Cancer Immunol Immunother 2000; 49:395–400.

13. Rakhit A, Yeon MM, Ferrante J, et al. Down-regulation of the pharmacokinetic-pharmacodynamic response to interleukin-12 during long-term administration to patients with renal cell carcinoma and evaluation of the mechanism of this "adaptive response" in mice. Clin Pharmacol Ther 1999; 65:615–629.

14. Sareneva T, Cantell K, Pyhala L, Pirhonen J, Julkunen I. Effect of carbohydrates on the pharmacokinetics of human interferon-gamma. J Interferon Res 1993; 13:267–269.

15. Harris JM, Martin NE, Modi M. Pegylation: a novel process for modifying pharmacokinetics. Clin Pharmacokinet 2001; 40:539–551.

16. Molineux G. Pegylation: engineering improved pharmaceuticals for enhanced therapy. Cancer Treatment Reviews 2002; 28(Suppl 1):1–4.

17. Kozlowski A, Charles SA, Harris JM. Development of pegylated interferons for the treatment of chronic hepatitis C. BioDrugs 2001; 15:419–429.

18. Kozlowski A, Harris JM. Improvements in protein PEGylation: pegylated interferons for treatment of hepatitis C. J Control Release 2001; 72:217–224.

19. Glue P, Fang JW, Rouzier-Panis R, et al. Pegylated interferon-alpha2b: pharmacokinetics, pharmacodynamics, safety, and preliminary efficacy data. Hepatitis C Intervention Therapy Group. Clin Pharmacol Ther 2000; 68:556–567.

20. Lindsay KL, Trepo C, Heintges T, et al. A randomized, double-blind trial comparing pegylated interferon alfa-2b to interferon alfa-2b as initial treatment for chronic hepatitis C. Hepatology 2001; 34:395–403.

21. Heathcote EJ, Shiffman ML, Cooksley WG, et al. Peginterferon alfa-2a in patients with chronic hepatitis C and cirrhosis. N Engl J Med 2000; 343:1673–1680.

22. Patel K, McHutchison J. Peginterferon alpha-2b: a new approach to improving response in hepatitis C patients. Expert Opin Pharmacother 2001; 2:1307–1315.

23. Motzer RJ, Rakhit A, Ginsberg M, et al. Phase I trial of 40-kd branched pegylated interferon alfa-2a for patients with advanced renal cell carcinoma. J Clin Oncol 2001; 19:1312–1319.

24. Talpaz M. Interferon-alfa-based treatment of chronic myeloid leukemia and implications of signal transduction inhibition. Semin Hematol 2001; 38:22–27.

25. Adamson JW. Erythropoietin: in vitro and in vivo studies of the regulation of erythropoiesis. Schweiz Med Wochenschr 1988; 118:1501–1506.

26. Doweiko JP, Goldberg MA. Erythropoietin therapy in cancer patients. Oncology (Huntingt) 1991; 5:31–7; discussion 38: 43–44.

27. Storring PL, Tiplady RJ, Gaines Das RE, et al. Epoetin alfa and beta differ in their erythropoietin isoform compositions and biological properties. Br J Haematol 1998; 100:79–89.

28. Macdougall IC, Roberts DE, Neubert P, Dharmasena AD, Coles GA, Williams JD. Pharmacokinetics of recombinant human erythropoietin in patients on continuous ambulatory peritoneal dialysis. Lancet 1989; 1:425–427.

29. Nielsen OJ. Pharmacokinetics of recombinant human erythropoietin in chronic haemodialysis patients. Pharmacol Toxicol 1990; 66:83–86.

30. Salmonson T, Danielson BG, Wikstrom B. The pharmacokinetics of recombinant human erythropoietin after intravenous and subcutaneous administration to healthy subjects. Br J Clin Pharmacol 1990; 29:709–713.

31. Macdougall IC, Roberts DE, Coles GA, Williams JD. Clinical pharmacokinetics of epoetin (recombinant human erythropoietin). Clin Pharmacokinet 1991; 20:99–113.

32. Besarab A. Physiological and pharmacodynamic considerations for route of EPO administration. Semin Nephrol 2000; 20:364–374.

33. Egrie JC, Browne JK. Development and characterization of novel erythropoiesis stimulating protein (NESP). Br J Cancer 2001; 84(Suppl 1):3–10.

34. Macdougall IC, Gray SJ, Elston O, et al. Pharmacokinetics of novel erythropoiesis stimulating protein compared with epoetin alfa in dialysis patients. J Am Soc Nephrol 1999; 10:2392–2395.

35. Allon M, Kleinman K, Walczyk M, et al. The pharmacokinetics of novel erythropoeisis stimulating protein (NESP) following chronic intravenous administration is time- and dose-linear. JASN 2000; 11: 248A.

36. Lerner R, Kale AS, Warady BA, et al. The pharmacokinetics of novel erythropoeisis stimulating protein (NESP) in pediatric patients with chronic renal failure or end stage renal disease. JASN 2000; 11:282A.

37. Heatherington AC, Schuller J, Mercer AJ. Pharmacokinetics of novel erythropoiesis stimulating protein (NESP) in cancer patients: preliminary report. Br J Cancer 2001; 84(Suppl 1):11–16.

38. Carral A, Sanz GF, Sanz MA. Filgrastim for the treatment of leukemia relapse after bone marrow transplantation. Bone Marrow Transplant 1996; 18:817–819.

39. Flinn IW, Byrd JC, Morrison C, et al. Fludarabine and cyclophosphamide with filgrastim support in patients with previously untreated indolent lymphoid malignancies. Blood 2000; 96:71–75.

40. Steinmetz HT, Schulz A, Staib P, et al. Phase-II trial of idarubicin, fludarabine, cytosine arabinoside, and filgrastim (Ida-FLAG) for treatment of refractory, relapsed, and secondary AML. Ann Hematol 1999; 78:418–425.

41. Leyvraz S, Ketterer N, Perey L, et al. Intensification of chemotherapy for the treatment of solid tumours: feasibility of a 3-fold increase in dose intensity with peripheral blood progenitor cells and granulocyte colony-stimulating factor. Br J Cancer 1995; 72:178–182.

42. Petros WP. Pharmacokinetics and administration of colony-stimulating factors. Pharmacotherapy 1992; 12:32S–38S.

43. Osslund T, Boone T. Biochemistry and structure of filgrastim. In: Morstyn G, Dexter T, Foote M, (eds). Filgrastim in Medical Practice. New York, NY: Marcel Dekker, 1998, pp. 41–49.

44. Dunn CJ, Goa KL. Lenograstim: an update of its pharmacological properties and use in chemotherapy-induced neutropenia and related clinical settings. Drugs 2000; 59:681–717.

45. Roskos LK, Cheung E, Vincent ME, Foote M, Morstyn G. Pharmacology of filgrastim (r-metHuG-CSF). In: Morstyn G, Dexter T, Foote M, (eds). Filgrastim in Medical Practice. New York, NY: Marcel Dekker, 1998, pp. 49–71.

46. Terashi K, Oka M, Ohdo S, et al. Close association between clearance of recombinant human granulocyte colony-stimulating factor (G-CSF) and G-CSF receptor on neutrophils in cancer patients. Antimicrob Agents Chemother 1999; 43:21–24.

47. Morstyn G, Campbell L, Souza LM, et al. Effect of granulocyte colony stimulating factor on neutropenia induced by cytotoxic chemotherapy. Lancet 1988; 1:667–672.

48. Marty M. The optimal dose of glycosylated recombinant human granulocyte colony stimulating factor for use in clinical practice: a review. Eur J Cancer 1994; 30A(Suppl 3):S20–S25.

49. Houston AC, Stevens LA, Cour V. Pharmacokinetics of glycosylated recombinant human granulocyte colony-stimulating factor (lenograstim) in healthy male volunteers. Br J Clin Pharmacol 1999; 47:279–284.

50. Hayashi N, Kinoshita H, Yukawa E, Higuchi S. Pharmacokinetic and pharmacodynamic analysis of subcutaneous recombinant human granulocyte colony stimulating factor (lenograstim) administration. J Clin Pharmacol 1999; 39:583–592.

51. Akizuki S, Mizorogi F, Inoue T, Sudo K, Ohnishi A. Pharmacokinetics and adverse events following 5-day repeated administration of lenograstim, a recombinant human granulocyte colony-stimulating factor, in healthy subjects. Bone Marrow Transplant 2000; 26:939–946.

52. Tanaka H, Tanaka Y, Shinagawa K, Yamagishi Y, Ohtaki K, Asano K. Three types of recombinant human granulocyte colony-stimulating factor have equivalent biological activities in monkeys. Cytokine 1997; 9:360–369.

53. Watts MJ, Addison I, Long SG, et al. Crossover study of the haematological effects and pharmacokinetics of glycosylated and non-glycosylated G-CSF in healthy volunteers. Br J Haematol 1997; 98:474–479.

54. de Arriba F, Lozano ML, Ortuno F, Heras I, Moraleda JM, Vicente V. Prospective randomized study comparing the efficacy of bioequivalent doses of glycosylated and nonglycosylated rG-CSF for mobilizing peripheral blood progenitor cells. Br J Haematol 1997; 96:418–420.

55. Milkovich G, Moleski RJ, Reitan JF, et al. Comparative safety of filgrastim versus sargramostim in patients receiving myelosuppressive chemotherapy. Pharmacotherapy 2000; 20:1432–1440.

56. Kuwabara T, Kato Y, Kobayashi S, Suzuki H, Sugiyama Y. Nonlinear pharmacokinetics of a recombinant human granulocyte colony-stimulating factor derivative (nartograstim): species differences among rats, monkeys and humans. J Pharmacol Exp Ther 1994; 271:1535–1543.

57. Suzuki T, Tohda S, Nagata K, Imai Y, Murohashi I, Nara N. Enhanced effect of mutant granulocyte-colony-stimulating factor (KW-2228) on the growth of normal and leukemic hemopoietic progenitor cells in comparison with recombinant human granulocyte-colony-stimulating factor (G-CSF). Acta Haematol 1992; 87:181–189.

58. Fujii I, Nagahara Y, Yamasaki M, Yokoo Y, Itoh S, Hirayama N. Structure of KW-2228, a tailored human granulocyte colony-stimulating factor with enhanced biological activity and stability. FEBS Lett 1997; 410:131–135.

59. Yamasaki M, Konishi N, Yamaguchi K, Itoh S, Yokoo Y. Purification and characterization of recombinant human granulocyte colony-stimulating factor (rhG-CSF) derivatives: KW-2228 and other derivatives. Biosci Biotechnol Biochem 1998; 62:1528–1534.

60. Bowen S, Tare N, Inoue T, et al. Relationship between molecular mass and duration of activity of polyethylene glycol conjugated granulocyte colony-stimulating factor mutein. Exp Hematol 1999; 27: 425–432.

61. Eliason JF, Greway A, Tare N, et al. Extended activity in cynomolgus monkeys of a granulocyte colony-stimulating factor mutein conjugated with high molecular weight polyethylene glycol. Stem Cells 2000; 18:40–45.

62. van Der Auwera P, Platzer E, Xu ZX, et al. Pharmacodynamics and pharmacokinetics of single doses of subcutaneous pegylated human G-CSF mutant (Ro 25-8315) in healthy volunteers: comparison with single and multiple daily doses of filgrastim. Am J Hematol 2001; 66:245–551.

63. Tanaka H, Satake-Ishikawa R, Ishikawa M, Matsuki S, Asano K. Pharmacokinetics of recombinant human granulocyte colony-stimulating factor conjugated to polyethylene glycol in rats. Cancer Res 1991; 51:3710–3714.

64. Johnston E, Crawford J, Blackwell S, et al. Randomized, dose-escalation study of SD/01 compared with daily filgrastim in patients receiving chemotherapy. J Clin Oncol 2000; 18:2522–2528.

65. Molineux G, Kinstler O, Briddell B, et al. A new form of Filgrastim with sustained duration in vivo and enhanced ability to mobilize PBSC in both mice and humans. Exp Hematol 1999; 27:1724–1734.

66. Lane TA, Ho AD, Bashey A, Peterson S, Young D, Law P. Mobilization of blood-derived stem and progenitor cells in normal subjects by granulocyte-macrophage- and granulocyte-colony-stimulating factors. Transfusion 1999; 39:39–47.

67. Holmes FA, O'Shaughnessy JA, Vukelja S, et al. Blinded, randomized, multicenter study to evaluate single administration pegfilgrastim once per cycle versus daily filgrastim as an adjunct to chemotherapy in patients with high-risk stage II or stage III/IV breast cancer. J Clin Oncol 2002; 20:727–731.

68. Morstyn G, Foote MA, Walker T, Molineux G. Filgrastim (r-metHuG-CSF) in the 21st century: SD/01. Acta Haematol 2001; 105:151–155.

69. Masucci G, Wersall P, Ragnhammar P, Mellstedt H. Granulocyte-monocyte-colony-stimulating factor augments the cytotoxic capacity of lymphocytes and monocytes in antibody-dependent cellular cytotoxicity. Cancer Immunol Immunother 1989; 29:288–292.

70. Mellstedt H, Fagerberg J, Frodin JE, et al. Augmentation of the immune response with granulocyte-macrophage colony-stimulating factor and other hematopoietic growth factors. Curr Opin Hematol 1999; 6:169–175.

71. Hovgaard D, Schifter S, Rabol A, Mortensen BT, Nissen NI. In vivo kinetics of 111indium-labelled autologous granulocytes following i.v. administration of granulocyte-macrophage colony-stimulating factor (GM-CSF). Eur J Haematol 1992; 48:202–207.

72. Denzlinger C, Tetzloff W, Gerhartz HH, et al. Differential activation of the endogenous leukotriene biosynthesis by two different preparations of granulocyte-macrophage colony-stimulating factor in healthy volunteers. Blood 1993; 81:2007–2013.

73. Kwak LW, Young HA, Pennington RW, Weeks SD. Vaccination with syngeneic, lymphoma-derived immunoglobulin idiotype combined with granulocyte/macrophage colony-stimulating factor primes mice for a protective T-cell response. Proc Natl Acad Sci USA 1996; 93:10,972–10,977.

74. Golumbek PT, Azhari R, Jaffee EM, et al. Controlled release, biodegradable cytokine depots: a new approach in cancer vaccine design. Cancer Res 1993; 53:5841–5844.

75. Abe J, Wakimoto H, Yoshida Y, Aoyagi M, Hirakawa K, Hamada H. Antitumor effect induced by granulocyte/macrophage-colony-stimulating factor gene-modified tumor vaccination: comparison of adenovirus- and retrovirus-mediated genetic transduction. J Cancer Res Clin Oncol 1995; 121:587–592.

76. Kantor J, Irvine K, Abrams S, Kaufman H, DiPietro J, Schlom J. Antitumor activity and immune responses induced by a recombinant carcinoembryonic antigen-vaccinia virus vaccine. J Natl Cancer Inst 1992; 84:1084–1091.

77. Samanci A, Yi Q, Fagerberg J, et al. Pharmacological administration of granulocyte/macrophage-colony-stimulating factor is of significant importance for the induction of a strong humoral and cellular response in patients immunized with recombinant carcinoembryonic antigen. Cancer Immunol Immunother 1998; 47:131–142.

78. Mellstedt H, Fagerberg J, Osterborg A. Local low-dose of soluble GM-CSF significantly augments an immune response against tumour antigens in man. Eur J Cancer 1999; 35(Suppl 3):S29–S32.

79. Shetye JD, Rubio CA, Harmenberg U, Ware J, Duvander A, Mellstedt HT. Tumor-associated antigens common to humans and chemically induced colonic tumors of the rat. Cancer Res 1990; 50:6358–6363.

80. Mosolits S, Harmenberg U, Ruden U, et al. Autoantibodies against the tumour-associated antigen GA733-2 in patients with colorectal carcinoma. Cancer Immunol Immunother 1999; 47:315–320.

81. Mellstedt H, Fagerberg J, Frodin JE, et al. Ga733/EpCAM as a target for passive and active specific immunotherapy in patients with colorectal carcinoma. Ann NY Acad Sci 2000; 910:254–261.

82. Bergenbrant S, Yi Q, Osterborg A, et al. Modulation of anti-idiotypic immune response by immunization with the autologous M-component protein in multiple myeloma patients. Br J Haematol 1996; 92:840–846.

83. Fagerberg J, Ragnhammar P, Mellstedt H. Idiotypic network responses and anti-idiotypes in cancer therapy. In: Shoenfeld Y, Kennedy RC, Ferrone S, (eds). Idiotypes in Medicine: Autoimmunity, Infection, and Cancer. Amsterdam, The Netherlands: Elsevier Science, 1997, pp. 491–498.

84. Osterborg A, Henriksson L, Mellstedt H. Idiotype immunity (natural and vaccine-induced) in early stage multiple myeloma. Acta Oncol 2000; 39:797–800.

85. Osterborg A, Yi Q, Henriksson L, et al. Idiotype immunization combined with granulocyte-macrophage colony-stimulating factor in myeloma patients induced type I, major histocompatibility complex-restricted, CD8- and CD4-specific T-cell responses. Blood 1998; 91:2459–2466.

86. Mellstedt H, Osterborg A. Active idiotype vaccination in multiple myeloma. GM-CSF may be an important adjuvant cytokine. Pathol Biol (Paris) 1999; 47:211–215.

87. Ellem KA, O'Rourke MG, Johnson GR, et al. A case report: immune responses and clinical course of the first human use of granulocyte/macrophage colony-stimulating-factor-transduced autologous melanoma cells for immunotherapy. Cancer Immunol Immunother 1997; 44:10–20.

88. Simons JW, Jaffee EM, Weber CE, et al. Bioactivity of autologous irradiated renal cell carcinoma vaccines generated by ex vivo granulocyte-macrophage colony-stimulating factor gene transfer. Cancer Res 1997; 57:1537–1546.

89. de Gast GC, Klumpen HJ, Vyth-Dreese FA, et al. Phase I trial of combined immunotherapy with subcutaneous granulocyte macrophage colony-stimulating factor, low-dose interleukin 2, and interferon alpha in progressive metastatic melanoma and renal cell carcinoma. Clin Cancer Res 2000; 6: 1267–1272.

90. HjelmSkog A, Ragnhammar P, Fagerberg J, et al. Clinical effects of monoclonal antibody 17-1A combined with granulocyte/macrophage colony-stimulating factor and interleukin-2 for treatment of patients with advanced colorectal carcinoma. Cancer Immunol Immunother 1999; 48:463–470.

91. Kintzel PE, Calis KA. Recombinant interleukin-2: a biological response modifier. Clin Pharm 1991; 10:110–128.

92. Whittington R, Faulds D. Interleukin-2. A review of its pharmacological properties and therapeutic use in patients with cancer. Drugs 1993; 46:446–514.

93. Anderson PM, Sorenson MA. Effects of route and formulation on clinical pharmacokinetics of interleukin-2. Clin Pharmacokinet 1994; 27:19–31.

94. Meyers FJ, Paradise C, Scudder SA, Goodman G, Konrad M. A phase I study including pharmacokinetics of polyethylene glycol conjugated interleukin-2. Clin Pharmacol Ther 1991; 49:307–313.

95. Freedman RS, Gibbons JA, Giedlin M, et al. Immunopharmacology and cytokine production of a low-dose schedule of intraperitoneally administered human recombinant interleukin-2 in patients with advanced epithelial ovarian carcinoma. J Immunother Emphasis Tumor Immunol 1996; 19:443–451.

96. Oya M, Marumo K, Murai M, Tazaki H. Pharmacokinetics and antitumor effects of an interleukin-2 immunocomplexing agent in murine renal cell carcinoma. Int J Urol 1996; 3:141–144.

97. Gately MK, Gubler U, Brunda MJ, et al. Interleukin-12: a cytokine with therapeutic potential in oncology and infectious diseases. Ther Immunol 1994; 1:187–196.

98. Brunda MJ, Gately MK. Interleukin-12: potential role in cancer therapy. Important Adv Oncol 1995;3–18.

99. Nadeau RR, Ostrowski C, Ni-Wu G, Liberato DJ. Pharmacokinetics and pharmacodynamics of recombinant human interleukin-12 in male rhesus monkeys. J Pharmacol Exp Ther 1995; 274:78–83.

100. Bajetta E, Del Vecchio M, Mortarini R, et al. Pilot study of subcutaneous recombinant human interleukin-12 in metastatic melanoma. Clin Cancer Res 1998; 4:75–85.

101. Motzer RJ, Rakhit A, Schwartz LH, et al. Phase I trial of subcutaneous recombinant human interleukin-12 in patients with advanced renal cell carcinoma. Clin Cancer Res 1998; 4:1183–1191.

102. Motzer RJ, Rakhit A, Thompson JA, et al. Randomized multicenter phase II trial of subcutaneous recombinant human interleukin-12 versus interferon-alpha 2a for patients with advanced renal cell carcinoma. J Interferon Cytokine Res 2001; 21:257–263.

103. Lee P, Wang F, Kuniyoshi J, et al. Effects of interleukin-12 on the immune response to a multipeptide vaccine for resected metastatic melanoma. J Clin Oncol 2001; 19:3836–3847.

104. Wadhwa M, Ragnhammar P, Mellstedt H, Gallo P, Thorpe R. Immunogenicity of therapeutic cytokines. Pharmeuropa Special Issue; Proceedings Biologicals Beyond 2000; 177–189.

105. Oberg K, Alm G. The incidence and clinical significance of antibodies to interferon-a in patients with solid tumors. Biotherapy 1997; 10:1–5.

106. Osterborg A, Engman K, Bjoreman M, et al. Patients treated with natural (leukocyte-derived) interferon (IFN)-alpha do not develop IFN antibodies. Eur J Haematol 1991; 47:234–235.

107. Casadevall N, Dupuy E, Molho-Sabatier P, Tobelem G, Varet B, Mayeux P. Autoantibodies against erythropoietin in a patient with pure red-cell aplasia. N Engl J Med 1996; 334:630–633.

108. Prabhakar SS, Muhlfelder T. Antibodies to recombinant human erythropoietin causing pure red cell aplasia. Clin Nephrol 1997; 47:331–335.

109. Peces R, de la Torre M, Alcazar R, Urra JM. Antibodies against recombinant human erythropoietin in a patient with erythropoietin-resistant anemia. N Engl J Med 1996; 335:523–524.

110. Casadevall N, Nataf J, Viron B, et al. Pure red-cell aplasia and antierythropoietin antibodies in patients treated with recombinant erythropoietin. N Engl J Med 2002; 346:469–475.

111. Ullenhag G, Bird C, Ragnhammar P, et al. Incidence of GM-CSF antibodies in cancer patients receiving GM-CSF for immunostimulation. Clin Immunol 2001; 99:65–74.

112. Wadhwa M, Hjelm Skog AL, Bird C, et al. Immunogenicity of granulocyte-macrophage colony-stimulating factor (GM-CSF) products in patients undergoing combination therapy with GM-CSF. Clin Cancer Res 1999; 5:1353–1361.

113. Hjelm Skog AL, Wadhwa M, Hassan M, et al. Alteration of interleukin 2 (IL-2) pharmacokinetics and function by IL-2 antibodies induced after treatment of colorectal carcinoma patients with a combination of monoclonal antibody 17-1A, granulocyte macrophage colony-stimulating factor, and IL-2. Clin Cancer Res 2001; 7:1163–1170.

114. Frodin JE, Lefvert AK, Mellstedt H. Pharmacokinetics of the mouse monoclonal antibody 17-1A in cancer patients receiving various treatment schedules. Cancer Res 1990; 50:4866–4871.

115. Ragnhammar P, Fagerberg J, Frodin JE, et al. Effect of monoclonal antibody 17-1A and GM-CSF in patients with advanced colorectal carcinoma-long-lasting, complete remissions can be induced. Int J Cancer 1993; 53:751–758.

116. Mellstedt H, Frodin JE, Masucci G, et al. The therapeutic use of monoclonal antibodies in colorectal carcinoma. Semin Oncol 1991; 18:462–477.

117. Shetye J, Ragnhammar P, Liljefors M, et al. Immunopathology of metastases in patients of colorectal carcinoma treated with monoclonal antibody 17-1A and granulocyte macrophage colony-stimulating factor. Clin Cancer Res 1998; 4:1921–1929.

118. Osterborg A, Dyer MJ, Bunjes D, et al. Phase II multicenter study of human CD52 antibody in previously treated chronic lymphocytic leukemia. European Study Group of CAMPATH-1H Treatment in Chronic Lymphocytic Leukemia. J Clin Oncol 1997; 15:1567–1574.

119. Anderson DR, Grillo Lopez A, Varns C, Chambers KS, Hanna N. Targeted anti-cancer therapy using rituximab, a chimeric anti-CD20 antibody (IDEC-C2B8) in the treatment of non-Hodgkin's B-cell lymphoma. Biochem Soc Trans 1997; 25:705–708.

120. McKeage K, Perry CM. Trastuzumab: a review of its use in the treatment of metastatic breast cancer overexpressing HER2. Drugs 2002; 62:209–243.

121. Mellstedt H. Passive and active specific immunotherapy in colorectal carcinoma. In: Jacombsen A (ed). Colorectal Cancer. Current Status and Future Persepctives. Copenhagen, Denmark: Bøhm Offset 1999, pp. 157–164.

122. Dyer MJ, Hale G, Hayhoe FG, Waldmann H. Effects of CAMPATH-1 antibodies in vivo in patients with lymphoid malignancies: influence of antibody isotype. Blood 1989; 73:1431–1439.

123. Keating MJ, Flinn I, Jain V, et al. Therapeutic role of alemtuzumab (Campath-1H) in patients who have failed fludarabine: results of a large international study. Blood 2002; 99:3554–3561.

124. Maloney DG. Mechanism of action of rituximab. Anticancer Drugs 2001; 12(Suppl 2):S1–S4.

125. Byrd JC, Kitada S, Flinn IW, et al. The mechanism of tumor cell clearance by rituximab in vivo in patients with B-cell chronic lymphocytic leukemia: evidence of caspase activation and apoptosis induction. Blood 2002; 99:1038–1043.

126. Pegram M, Slamon D. Biological rationale for HER2/neu (c-erbB2) as a target for monoclonal antibody therapy. Semin Oncol 2000; 27:13–19.

127. Ritter G, Cohen LS, Williams C, Jr., Richards EC, Old LJ, Welt S. Serological analysis of human anti-human antibody responses in colon cancer patients treated with repeated doses of humanized monoclonal antibody A33. Cancer Res 2001; 61:6851–6859.

128. Deckert PM, Jungbluth A, Montalto N, et al. Pharmacokinetics and microdistribution of polyethylene glycol-modified humanized A33 antibody targeting colon cancer xenografts. Int J Cancer 2000; 87:382–390.

129. Arranz R, Garcia-Alfonso P, Sobrino P, et al. Role of interferon alfa-2b in the induction and maintenance treatment of low-grade non-Hodgkin's lymphoma: results from a prospective, multicenter trial with double randomization. J Clin Oncol 1998;–16:1538–1546.

130. Haase-Statz S, Smalley RV. Role of interferon-alfa in NHL: still controversial? Oncology (Huntingt) 1999; 13:1147–1163.

131. Soubeyran P, Debled M, Tchen N, et al. Follicular lymphomas—a review of treatment modalities. Crit Rev Oncol Hematol 2000; 35:13–32.

132. Cooper MR. A review of the clinical studies of alpha-interferon in the management of multiple myeloma. Semin Oncol 1991; 18:18–29.

133. Westin J. Interferon therapy during the plateau phase of multiple myeloma: an update of a Swedish multicenter study. Semin Oncol 1991; 18:37–40.

134. Mandelli F, Avvisati G, Amadori S, et al. Maintenance treatment with recombinant interferon alfa-2b in patients with multiple myeloma responding to conventional induction chemotherapy. N Engl J Med 1990; 322:1430–1434.

135. Liberati AM, Cinieri S, Senatore MG, et al. Phase I-II trial on natural beta interferon in chemoresistant and relapsing multiple myeloma. Haematologica 1990; 75:436–442.

136. Giles FJ, Kantarjian H, O'Brien S, et al. Results of therapy with interferon alpha and cyclic combination chemotherapy in patients with Philadelphia chromosome-positive chronic myelogenous leukemia in early chronic phase. Leuk Lymphoma 2001; 41:309–319.

137. Goldman JM, Druker BJ. Chronic myeloid leukemia: current treatment options. Blood 2001; 98:2039–2042.

138. Legha SS. The role of interferon alfa in the treatment of metastatic melanoma. Semin Oncol 1997; 24:S24–S31.

139. Cascinelli N, Belli F, MacKie RM, Santinami M, Bufalino R, Morabito A. Effect of long-term adjuvant therapy with interferon alpha-2a in patients with regional node metastases from cutaneous melanoma: a randomised trial. Lancet 2001; 358:866–869.

140. Dubois RW, Swetter SM, Atkins M, et al. Developing indications for the use of sentinel lymph node biopsy and adjuvant high-dose interferon alfa-2b in melanoma. Arch Dermatol 2001; 137:1217–1224.

141. Reintgen D, Balch CM, Kirkwood J, Ross M. Recent advances in the care of the patient with malignant melanoma. Ann Surg 1997; 225:1–14.

142. Grob JJ, Dreno B, de la Salmoniere P, et al. Randomised trial of interferon alpha-2a as adjuvant therapy in resected primary melanoma thicker than 1.5 mm without clinically detectable node metastases. French Cooperative Group on Melanoma. Lancet 1998; 351:1905–1910.

143. Schiller JH, Storer B, Bittner G, Willson JK, Borden EC. Phase II trial of a combination of interferon-beta ser and interferon-gamma in patients with advanced malignant melanoma. J Interferon Res 1988; 8:581–589.

144. Krigel RL, Padavic-Shaller KA, Rudolph AR, Konrad M, Bradley EC, Comis RL. Renal cell carcinoma: treatment with recombinant interleukin-2 plus beta-interferon. J Clin Oncol 1990; 8:460–467.

145. Rinehart JJ, Young D, Laforge J, Colborn D, Neidhart JA. Phase I/II trial of interferon-beta-serine in patients with renal cell carcinoma: immunological and biological effects. Cancer Res 1987; 47: 2481–2485.

146. Schmidinger M, Steger G, Wenzel C, et al. Sequential administration of interferon-gamma, GM-CSF, and interleukin-2 in patients with metastatic renal cell carcinoma: results of a phase II trial. J Immunother 2001; 24:257–262.

147. Zeuzem S, Feinman SV, Rasenack J, et al. Peginterferon alfa-2a in patients with chronic hepatitis C. N Engl J Med 2000; 343:1666–1672.

148. Manns MP, McHutchison JG, Gordon SC, et al. Peginterferon alfa-2b plus ribavirin compared with interferon alfa-2b plus ribavirin for initial treatment of chronic hepatitis C: a randomised trial. Lancet 2001; 358:958–965.

149. Konrad MW, Hemstreet G, Hersh EM, et al. Pharmacokinetics of recombinant interleukin 2 in humans. Cancer Res 1990; 50:2009–2017.

150. Lotze MT, Matory YL, Ettinghausen SE, et al. In vivo administration of purified human interleukin 2. II. Half life, immunologic effects, and expansion of peripheral lymphoid cells in vivo with recombinant IL 2. J Immunol 1985; 135:2865–2875.

151. Pais RC, Ingrim NB, Garcia ML, et al. Pharmacokinetics of recombinant interleukin-2 in children with malignancies: a Pediatric Oncology Group study. J Biol Response Mod 1990; 9:517–521.

152. Kirchner GI, Franzke A, Buer J, et al. Pharmacokinetics of recombinant human interleukin-2 in advanced renal cell carcinoma patients following subcutaneous application. Br J Clin Pharmacol 1998; 46:5–10.

153. Iacona I, Lazzarino M, Avanzini MA, et al. Rituximab (IDEC-C2B8): validation of a sensitive enzyme-linked immunoassay applied to a clinical pharmacokinetic study. Ther Drug Monit 2000; 22:295–301.

154. Scott AM, Lee FT, Hopkins W, et al. Specific targeting, biodistribution, and lack of immunogenicity of chimeric anti-GD3 monoclonal antibody KM871 in patients with metastatic melanoma: results of a phase I trial. J Clin Oncol 2001; 19:3976–3987.

155. Welt S, Divgi CR, Real FX, et al. Quantitative analysis of antibody localization in human metastatic colon cancer: a phase I study of monoclonal antibody A33. J Clin Oncol 1990; 8:1894–1906.

156. Rebello P, Cwynarski K, Varughese M, Eades A, Apperley JF, Hale G. Phamacokinetics of Campath-1H in bone marrow transplant patients. Cytotherapy 2001; 3:261–267.

31 Exposure–Response Relationship of Anticancer Agents

A Clinical Pharmacology and Biopharmaceutics Regulatory Perspective

Atiqur Rahman, PhD

CONTENTS

1. INTRODUCTION

The exposure–response evaluation in drug development supports the efficacy and safety evaluation of drugs for marketing approval and for dose modifications in special populations *(1,2)*. In the past, the US Food and Drug Administration (FDA) received limited pharmacokinetic and pharmacodynamic information for the evaluation and approval of an anticancer drug and subsequently for the labeling of an approved drug. Cytotoxic agents such as antimetabolites, anthracyclines, alkylating agents, and platinum drugs were developed based on the maximum tolerated dose (MTD) concept. The dose/exposure and response (efficacy or toxicity) relationships of these cytotoxic agents were very steep and the therapeutic ranges of these agents were usually narrow. The dose and dosing regimens of most of the drugs were modified and optimized post-drug approval through research by the cancer research groups such as the National Cancer Institute, the Pediatric Oncology Group, the South West Oncology Group, and so forth, or by the recognized cancer treatment centers. The results of these dose-finding clinical trials were published in journals and later included in the prescription label of the drug. The major goal of the cancer therapy has been to obtain clinical response at the expense of tolerable toxicity. As a result, exposure response assessments through prospective clinical trial have been rare and when they have been performed the trials have mostly focused on the determination of exposure associated toxicity of the drugs *(3–7)*.

Handbook of Anticancer Pharmacokinetics and Pharmacodynamics
Edited by: W. D. Figg and H. L. McLeod © Humana Press Inc., Totowa, NJ

The FDA faces the challenge to balance the benefit and risks of medicine use by patients through rational drug development and through the post-marketing surveillance (MEDWATCH) and research. Exposure–response relationships contribute significantly in the assessment of benefit and risks of a medicine use by a patient. The importance and value of understanding the exposure–response relationships of cancer drugs during drug development have become well recognized, especially in light of the new targets for cancer treatments (8–16). The FDA and the pharmaceutical companies have become proactive in generating important exposure–response information in drug development and drug labeling to enhance the safe use of the drugs by cancer patients.

Current cancer treatment involves various approaches, modalities such as surgery, radiation therapy, neo-adjuvant and adjuvant treatment, site-specific treatments, and so forth. Cytotoxic agents are intended to kill tumor cells and have a risk-to-benefit profile that is quite different from that of the therapy developed for a particular cellular target such as a receptor or a biomarker. The development of the cytotoxic agent focuses on achieving the MTD in patients with a good performance status to increase the probability of therapeutic benefit; mostly desired is the improved survival. As a result, the relationship between exposure and the onset of drug response, the maximum response, and the response profile is not well characterized and understood. Tumor response and increased survival in this situation are considered pharmacodynamic effects with no defined relationship to the exposure in the responding population, and the reasons for the absence of response in the nonresponding patients remain unexplained. Therefore, the safe use of these agents involves complex patient factors that can tip the outcome of the therapy from the desired therapeutic benefit to an undesirable serious toxicity. On the other hand, hormonal therapy for breast cancer or prostate cancer involves drugs intended to interact with receptors, targets, or enzymes at the cellular level and produce the desired effects. These therapies are better tolerated and the toxicity profiles of these agents are quite different from the toxicity profiles of the cytotoxic agents (17–20). The exposure–response profiles of these agents are mostly shallow and the therapeutic range is large. The optimum therapeutic dose or exposure may be well below the MTD or tolerated exposure. Dose selection of these agents is based on target interactions such as enzyme inhibition, receptor occupancy, biomarker inhibition, and so forth.

The dose–toxicity evaluation of anticancer agents was routinely performed in clinical studies. However, the exposure–response evaluations most of the time failed to demonstrate a correlation between the exposure and response mainly because of the following reasons:

1. Inadequate understanding of the interpatient pharmacokinetic variability.
2. Inadequate understanding of drug's mechanism of actions.
3. Selection of inappropriate biomarker or response endpoints.
4. Selection and measurement of inappropriate moiety (inactive entity) in the biological matrix used as the exposure variable.
5. Selection of inappropriate sampling time.
6. Selection of inappropriate exposure variable.
7. Absence of evaluation of placebo or low dose drug effect in exposure–response studies.

Therefore, to assess any exposure–response relationship we have to understand the pharmacokinetic variability of a drug, select appropriate response variables associated with disease progression and drug response, and characterize the appropriate moiety in the biological matrix that is associated with the pharmacologic or adverse effect of the drug (21). Also, the trials should include treatment arms to evaluate the placebo effect or low dose drug effect on response variables.

2. MEASURES OF EXPOSURE AND RESPONSE

The exposure variables are usually determined from the concentration–time profiles of the parent drug and/or any of its appropriate active or toxic metabolites. In oncology, exposure variables are better defined and established than the response variables. Various exposure variables of a drug may be associated with different response effects. Anthracycline-induced cardiomyopathy is considered to be associated with the maximum concentration, whereas exposure as measured by the area under the curve seems to be related to leucopenia *(22)*. Sometimes the moiety responsible for the pharmacologic effect of a drug may be different from the moiety associated with the toxicity of the drug. For example, the active metabolites, fluorouridine triphosphate generated in the cells from 5-fluorouracil disrupt RNA synthesis and fluorodeoxyuridine monophosphate inhibits the thymidylate synthase enzyme, interrupting DNA synthesis of the proliferative cells and producing tumor cell death *(23–25)*. On the other hand, the urinary catabolite, α-fluoro-β-alanine (FBAL) is likely associated with the neurotoxic effects of the drug *(26–28)*. Therefore, the two moieties influences the risk–benefit associated with the exposure to the two moieties after 5-fluorouracil therapy. In oncology, the evaluation of the exposure–response relationship mostly correlates exposure with hematological (neutropenia, leucopenia thrombocytopenia, hemoglobin, etc.) and nonhematological (diarrhea, liver enzymes, edema, nausea, vomiting, etc.) toxicities *(29–31)*.

In the assessment of the exposure variables, all the active moieties associated with either the pharmacologic effects or the toxic effects of the drug should be measured. Mostly total drug concentration in a biological fluid is measured; however, when drugs are highly protein bound, and when protein binding varies significantly among patients, unbound drug concentration as an exposure variable may show a better correlation with drug's response *(32)*.

Association of a response variable with disease progression and with the response to a drug therapy is the key in the evaluation of exposure response relationship, which is rare in oncology *(33)*. The importance of response variable measurements depends on the pharmacokinetics of the drug and the exposure range studied. When the pharmacokinetics of a drug is highly variable or a wide exposure range is studied in a patient population the measured response variable may be able to identify a threshold for a response *(1)*.

2.1. Exposure Variables

Exposure variables are assessed from the concentration–time profiles of drugs in blood or plasma. Rarely, cerebrospinal fluid or other biological matrix may be sampled and drug concentration measured. Exposure variables may be divided into two main categories; concentration measurements and area under the concentration–time curve measurements (AUC). The concentration measurements are usually maximum concentration (C_{max}), steady-state concentration (C_{ss}), and threshold concentration associated with the safety or effectiveness of a drug or any of its active metabolite. Cytotoxic agents are usually administered once during a 3- or 4-wk cycle. In such a dosing regimen, the exposure variable is the maximum concentration measured from the concentration–time profile after the first dose in cycle 1 or subsequent cycles. When treatment involves daily dosing on a continuous basis or weekly treatment (daily $\times$ 5) with a rest period or a long-term continuous infusion, the C_{ss} of a drug is usually the exposure variable that is correlated with the effectiveness or toxicity of a drug *(7,30)*. In case of daily dosing, obtaining the blood sample prior to administering a dose assesses the steady-state concentration, after the drug concentration has achieved steady state. This measurement represents the minimum plasma or blood concentration at steady state. When a drug is infused over a long period (48– 96 h), C_{ss} is assessed towards the end of the infusion duration after the steady state is achieved.

Sometimes the drug concentrations may be determined in the second or subsequent cycles of therapy to understand the relationship between drug concentration and the long-term toxicity or the cycle specific toxicity of a drug. Preclinical studies are often conducted to identify a target concentration that achieves a desired or undesired effect. For example, hematologic toxicity is sometime associated with a threshold concentration that is maintained for a certain duration following drug administration. Neutropenia associated with paclitaxel therapy is related to the duration of time that plasma concentrations are at or above 0.05 μM value *(34,35)*. Therefore, threshold concentration sometime represents the exposure variable for exposure–response assessment.

The AUC measurement is another pharmacokinetic parameter that represents an exposure variable in the assessment of exposure response relationship of a drug. Carboplatin is dosed to achieve a target AUC based on renal function and desired platelet nadir for maximum therapeutic benefit *(31,36)*. The AUC measurements are usually considered for exposure–response relationship for drugs that are taken on a chronic basis such as hormonal agents, some targeted therapy, and palliative therapy. There are three types of AUC measurements: AUC from time zero to infinity ($AUC_{0-\infty}$), AUC from time zero to last measured concentration time (AUC_{0-t}), and AUC at the steady state (AUC_{ss}).

For cytotoxic agents administered once every 3–4 wk, the AUC is determined using the trapezoidal rule from time zero to the last measured concentration and then the residual area is calculated from the last measured concentration and the elimination rate constant *(37)*. The area under the plasma concentration–time curve from time zero to last determine concentration time is used after the first dose or at the steady-state level. After the steady state is achieved, AUC measurements may be for a particular dosing interval, that is, 6 h, 8 h, or 12 h, depending on how frequently the drug is taken at steady state. A list of exposure variables is presented in Table 1. Rarely, drug clearance values may be associated with the toxicity parameters in exposure response evaluation. The changes in the clearance of a drug because of organ impairment are usually associated with the toxicity of the drug in such a patient population.

The concentration–time profiles should be long enough to cover five elimination half-lives of the drug for a reliable exposure measurement. Also, when the steady-state measurements are obtained the samples should be collected after the subjects have been dosed for at least five elimination half-lives of the drug *(37)*.

2.2. Response Variables

Response variables can be of two types: efficacy variables and safety variables. Hematological measurements may represent both efficacy and safety variables depending on the purpose of the therapy and the degree of inhibition associated with the entity measured *(38–41)*. There are three major categories of response variables: biomarkers, surrogate endpoints, and the clinical endpoints. A limited list of response variables in oncology is presented in Table 1. Sometimes more than one response variable may be assessed for the exposure response relationship evaluation.

2.2.1. BIOMARKERS

A number of biological markers are currently assessed in various types of cancer to understand the role of these markers with diagnosis, disease progression, and drug response *(42–46)*. Some of the biomarkers are associated with the diagnosis and disease progression, whereas others are associated with the therapeutic intervention and disease palliation. A biomarker such as prostate-specific antigen (PSA) is related to the early detection and disease progression for prostate cancer *(47–50)*. Sometime course of therapy is dictated by

Table 1
Measures of Exposure and Response in Oncology

Exposure variables	Response variables
Area under the curve $AUC_{(0-\infty)}$, $AUC_{(0-t)}$, AUC_{ss}	Biomarkers EGFR, VGEF, proteosome, CA-125, etc.
Concentrations C_{max}, C_{ss}, threshold concentrations	Surrogate endpoints Tumor response, time to tumor response, hematologic response, cytogenetic response, etc.
Parameters Clearance	Clinical endpoints Survival, quality of life measures

the PSA status of a patient. The expression of human epidermal growth factor (HER2-Neu) is associated with therapeutic response to herceptin and paclitaxel therapy in advanced breast cancer *(51,52)*. However, PSA and HER2-Neu are not directly related to the therapeutic intervention or the therapeutic outcome. Some of the biomarkers, such as tyrosine kinases, vascular endothelial growth factors, epidermal growth factor receptors, cyclooxygenase, and so forth. are associated with the drug's mechanism of action with uncertain relationship to the clinical outcome. In the past, CD4 cell counts were considered a reliable biomarker in the assessment of anti-acquired immune deficiency syndrome (AIDS) drugs. However, in oncology a reliable marker such as CD4 cell counts for drug evaluation is yet to be established.

2.2.2. Surrogate Endpoints

Tumor shrinkage and time to tumor progression are acceptable surrogates to predict clinical benefit for solid tumors in cancer drug development. Hematologic and cytogenetic responses are also considered surrogates to predict clinical benefit for hematologic malignancies. Cancer drugs have received accelerated approval for serious life-threatening illnesses with no approved therapy based on surrogate response. In relapsed and refractory settings, surrogates are expected to reasonably likely predict clinical benefit. Accelerated approval allows marketing of promising drugs prior to establishing clinical benefit of the drug. At the time of approval, the FDA requires a commitment from the pharmaceutical company to conduct clinical trial(s) to establish clinical benefit, post-approval. Oxaliplatin with 5-fluorouracil for the treatment of first-line colorectal cancer patients received accelerated approval based on tumor response and time to tumor progression *(53)*. The initial approvals of docetaxel, capecitabine, irinotecan, temozolomide, gemtuzumab ozogamycin, and imatinib were based on surrogate response. In cancer drug development, dose selection for efficacy trials sometimes use surrogate associated exposure–response relationship information. For example, selection of a 400-mg dose of imatinib for treating chronic myeloid leukemia (CML) patients was based on 98% complete hematologic response at or above 300 mg dose tested in the Phase 1 trials *(54)*. Human immunodeficiency virus (HIV) viral load for the AIDS drugs or cholesterol levels and blood pressure measurements for cardiovascular drugs are considered surrogates that have direct association with drug response and clinical benefit. Drugs have received FDA approval based on these surrogate endpoints. However, similar surrogate endpoints that directly correlate with the clinical benefit of a drug are not present in oncology.

2.2.3. CLINICAL ENDPOINTS

In cancer, survival and "quality of life" assessment are usually considered the endpoints associated with the direct clinical benefit of a therapy. Survival is usually considered the credible endpoint for clinical benefit in both early and advanced stages of cancer. Approval of drugs for the first-line treatment of solid tumors are mostly based on survival. Gemcitabine approval for advanced or metastatic pancreatic cancer was based on clinical benefit response, survival, and time to disease progression *(55)*, whereas, mitoxantrone was approved based on palliative response associated with pain for patients with hormone-refractory prostrate cancer *(56)*. In certain situations, dose–response studies using survival as the response variable have been conducted *(57,58)*.

3. EXPOSURE–RESPONSE RELATIONSHIPS IN ONCOLOGY DRUG DEVELOPMENT

Prospectively developed exposure–response relationships for oncology drugs are rare; however, recent drug development included exploratory exposure–response assessment mostly focusing on exposure–toxicity relationship. Several pharmacokinetic and pharmacodynamic factors including cellular efflux, topoisomerase I and II modulation, lactone stability, and alteration of metabolism influence the antitumor response and toxicity of camptothecins *(59)*. Intravenous busulfan is approved in combination with cyclophosphamide for bone marrow ablation prior to allogeneic stem cell transplantation for the CML patients. A target exposure to busulfan balances both effectiveness and toxicity from its treatment. Exposure (AUC) of < 900 μM·min has been associated with failure of bone marrow ablation whereas hepatic venoocclusive disease is associated with AUC of 1300–1500 μM·min *(60)*. Therefore, busulfan therapy is targeted to achieve an AUC within 900–1300 μM·min for optimum benefit from the treatment. Modeling and simulations of data obtained from a pediatric study indicated that only 60% of the patients achieve a target AUC of 900–1350 μM·min with the first dose of busulfan *(61)*. Therefore, based on the modeling of the exposure data from the pediatric study, the labeling recommends therapeutic drug monitoring to obtain a safe exposure for bone marrow ablation with minimum toxicity. After the first dose of busulfan, a dose adjustment method based on body weight to modify the subsequent doses of busulfan to achieve the target exposure is included in the label *(61)*.

Zolendronic acid is indicted for the treatment of patients with multiple myeloma and patients with documented bone metastases from solid tumors, in conjunction with standard antineoplastic therapy *(62)*. The drug is also indicated for the treatment of hypercalcemia of malignancies. The pharmacokinetics of zolendronic acid and markers of bone metabolism were assessed in a Phase 1 study of advanced cancer patients with osteolytic bone metastases *(63)*. Various urinary markers of bone resorption, such as *N*-telopeptide, pyridinoline, deoxypyridinoline, hydroxyproline, calcium, and creatinine were measured and an attempt was made to correlate the bone markers with the pharmacokinetics of the drug. Urinary *N*-telopeptide levels decreased 40–60% in the 0.1- to 0.4-mg dose groups compared to 70–80% reduction in the 0.8- to 4.0-mg dose groups. In the 8-mg dose group, > 80% reduction in *N*-telopeptide was noted *(63)*. Pyridinoline and deoxypyridinoline levels decreased at doses > 1.5 mg dose. Urinary excretion plays a major role in zolendronic acid disposition. Zolendronic acid clearance significantly correlated with the creatinine clearance. The exposure–response modeling predicted association between risk of renal deterioration and AUC as shown in Fig. 1 *(64)*, and the FDA recommended in the label a dose adjustment of zolendronic acid based on the creatinine clearance of a patient *(62)*.

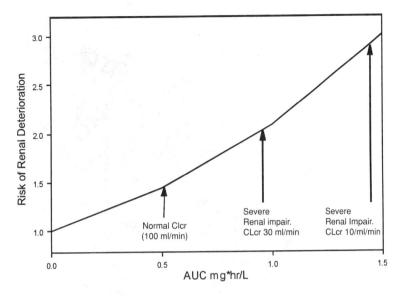

Fig. 1. The risk of renal deterioration vs zolandronic acid AUC.

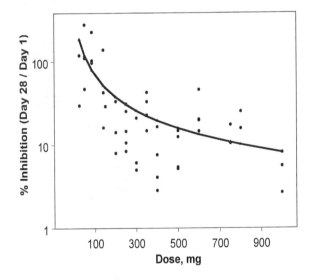

Fig. 2. Relationship between imatinib dose and the inhibition of WBC count in CML patients.

Imatinib is indicated for the treatment of CML and for the treatment of gastrointestinal stromal tumors. The drug is a potent Bcr-Abl tyrosine kinase inhibitor. Imatinib administration decreased the white blood cell (WBC) counts over time in a dose-dependent manner as shown in Fig. 2 *(65)*. Nonlinear mixed effects pharmacokinetic modeling suggested that body weight and age are important covariates governing the exposure of imatinib and the probability of edema as shown in Fig. 3 *(65)*. The probability of grade 3 edema in blast crisis CML patients as a function of steady-state drug concentration and age is shown in Fig. 4 *(65)*.

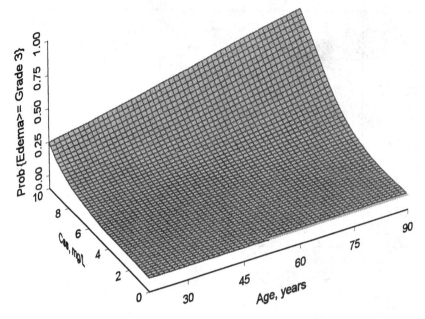

Fig. 3. Probability of a grade 3 or greater edema occurrence in blast crisis CML patients as a function of plasma steady-state concentration and age after administration of imatinib.

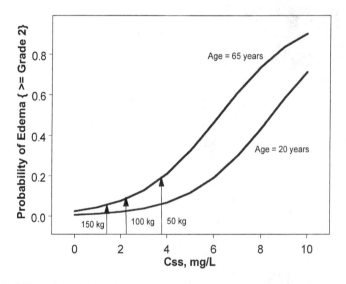

Fig. 4. The probability of grade 2 or greater edema occurrence in blast crisis CML patients as a function of steady-state drug concentration. The *arrow* indicates the probability of edema in a 65-yr-old patient increases with decreased body weight.

Older CML patients are identified as a subpopulation that is highly susceptible to grade 3 or higher edema based on the exposure–toxicity relationship of the drug.

Taxotere is indicated for the treatment of advanced or metastatic breast and non-small-cell lung cancer. Docetaxel clearance decreased and AUC increased in patients with mild to moderate liver function impairment (SGOT and/or SGPT > 1.5 times ULN) (66). Patients with higher bilirubin, SGOT and/or SGPT, or alkaline phosphatase are at increased risk for developing grade 4 neutropenia, febrile neutropenia, infections, severe thrombocytopenia, severe stomatitis, severe skin toxicity, as well as death due to toxicity (66). The recommendation to obtain bilirubin, SGOT or SGPT, and alkaline phosphatase values prior to each cycle of therapy and to discontinue therapy in case of hepatic impairment is stated in the package insert of docetaxel (66).

Carboplatin is indicated in the treatment of advanced ovarian cancer. Dosing of this drug is based on the relationship between carboplatin exposure and hematologic toxicity in pretreated patients a target exposure based on AUC for single agent carboplatin balances the risk between developing toxicity (thrombocytopenia and leukopenia) and achieving an effective treatment (36). The dose of the drug is based on the target AUC to achieve and the renal status of the patient.

The discovery of various targets associated with the tumor growth and proliferation is expected to lead the pharmaceuticals to explore exposure–response relationship of the new cancer agents in drug development. Because the utility of exposure–toxicity relationship in oncology is well established, research should focus on investigations on relationships between exposure and activity of an agent. The establishment of reliable markers associated with the disease and disease progression will be helpful in this regard.

4. GUIDANCES ON EXPOSURE–RESPONSE RELATIONSHIPS

The FDA guidance on exposure–response relationships elaborates on the regulatory applications, study design, and data analysis aspects of the clinical trials to be conducted during drug development to assess the exposure–response relationship of a drug (1). The purpose of the guidance is to encourage prospective collection of exposure–response data in the clinical trials to support the safety and efficacy evaluation of a drug. The guidance describes under what circumstances an exposure response study provides (1) primary evidence of safety and effectiveness of a drug, (2) supportive evidence for the primary efficacy studies, (3) evidence to support new target population or an altered dosage forms or an altered doses/dosing regimens, or routes of administration. The guidance discusses integrating exposure–response relationship assessment in all phases of drug development. The guidance also elaborates on the format and content for reports of exposure–response studies in a regulatory submission. The exposure–response study designs are described in the guidance with emphasis on prospective collection of information to support regulatory decisions. The guidance provides a pediatric decision tree integrating pharmacokinetic and pharmacodynamic in drug development for pediatric population (1).

The International Conference on Harmonization (ICH) also published guidance, ICH E4 on dose–response information to support drug registration (2). The guideline describes the usefulness of dose or concentration–response relationship assessment from the global drug development perspectives. The dose–response information is expected to allow multiple regulatory agencies making approval decisions from a common database. The guidance emphasizes the importance of evaluating exposure response data throughout all phases of drug development. The guidance highlights the strengths and limitations of various study designs and the limitations associated with conducting dose–response studies for drugs for life-threatening diseases, such as cancer. ICH has also published guidance on ethnic factors in the acceptability of foreign clinical data (67). The guidance describes pharmacokinetic and pharmacodynamic studies and pharmacodynamic endpoints. The guidance elaborates on bridging studies to support drug approval in a region based on the clinical data generated in another region. The exposure–response study using an established pharmacodynamic effect that is related to a clinical endpoint may be acceptable as a bridging study.

Table 2
Guidances Providing General and Specific Statements
Regarding Exposure–Response Relationship

1. Guidances providing general statements

   Providing clinical evidence of effectiveness for human drugs and biological products

   Guideline for the format and content of the clinical and statistical sections of an application

   ICH E4, dose response information to support drug registration

   ICH E5, ethnic factors in the acceptability of foreign clinical data

2. Guidances providing specific statements

   ICH E7, studies in support of special populations: geriatrics

   Study of evaluation of gender differences in the clinical evaluation of drugs

   Pharmacokinetics in patients with impaired renal function: study design, data analysis, and impact on dosing and labeling

   Pharmacokinetics in patients with impaired hepatic function: study design, data analysis, and impact on dosing and labeling

   In vivo metabolism/drug interactions studies: study design, data analysis, and recommendations for dosing and labeling

   Population pharmacokinetics

Source: FDA Guidance, Exposure–Response Relationships—Study Design, Data Analysis, and Regulatory Applications.

Various regulatory guidances that mention the values of understanding exposure-response relationship in drug development and drug use are presented in Table 2 *(1)*. These guidances are expected to promote evaluation of exposure–response relationships during drug development and provide an understanding of regulatory decision making based on exposure–response relationship of a drug.

5. EXPOSURE–RESPONSE INFORMATION IN LABELING

The exposure–response information is included in the Clinical Pharmacology section of the label and in certain situations in the Warnings and Precautions sections of a label. Information about the effects of antiestrogenic agents on estrogen suppression, on the levels of corticosteroids, and on other endocrine effects is included in the label of these hormonal agents. The dose-related pharmacodynamic effect of exemestane on estrogen suppression is included in the Clinical Pharmacology section of the label *(68)* as follows:

Pharmacodynamics

Effect on Estrogens: Multiple doses of exemestane ranging from 0.5 to 600 mg/day were administered to postmenopausal women with advanced breast cancer. Plasma estrogen (estradiol, estrone, and estrone sulfate) suppression was seen starting at a 5-mg daily dose of exemestane, with a maximum suppression of at least 85% to 95% achieved at a 25-mg dose. Exemestane 25 mg daily reduced whole body aromatization (as measured by injecting radiolabeled androstenedione) by 98% in postmenopausal women with breast cancer. After a single dose of exemestane 25 mg, the maximal suppression of circulating estrogens occurred 2 to 3 days after dosing and persisted for 4 to 5 days.

The label also mentions that exemestane did not affect cortisol or aldosterone secretion at baseline or in response to adrenocorticotropic hormone (ACTH). Arimidex package insert includes dose-related serum estradiol suppression by anastrozole *(69)*. Similar information about the pharmacodynamic effects of letrozole is also included in the label of Femara *(70)*.

In the Platinol label, a box warning *(71)* states, "Cumulative renal toxicity with Platinol-AQ is severe. Other major dose-related toxicities are myelosuppression, nausea, and vomiting." Although this statement is derived from clinical experience in the absence of a thoroughly investigated exposure–response evaluation, the statement indicates the importance of exposure–response evaluation for cytotoxic agents. The Warning section of the label states that there is an association between severe neuropathies in patients and higher doses or greater frequencies of cisplatin administration than those recommended *(71)*. Similarly in the Box warning section of the docetaxel label, an association between liver dysfunction and increased risk for the development of grade 4 neutropenia, febrile neutropenia, infections, severe thrombocytopenia, severe stomatitis, severe skin toxicity, and death due to toxicity is stated *(66)*.

In the label of Zometa *(62)*, the pharmacodynamics of zolendronic acid is mentioned in the Clinical Pharmacology section as follows:

Pharmacodynamics: Clinical studies in patients with hypercalcemia of malignancy (HCM) showed that single-dose infusions of Zometa are associated with decreases in serum calcium and phosphorus and increases in urinary calcium and phosphorus excretion.

In the "Renal Insufficiency" subsection of the Clinical Pharmacology section of Zometa, there is a warning about increased risk of renal deterioration with increased AUC based on pharmacokinetic–pharmacodynamic modeling *(62)*.

The exposure–response relationship constitutes the basis for dose modifications, particularly in special populations, such as geriatric and pediatric populations, different ethnic groups, renal or hepatic impaired patients, and patients on other concomitant medications. Although exposure–toxicity relationships of oncology drugs are evaluated in clinical trials and dose modifications are recommended in the label, the relationship between exposure and effectiveness information of cancer drugs is seldom found in the label.

6. CONCLUSIONS

Aggressive cancer therapy to obtain a cure or to increase survival has to be balanced with knowledge of exposure–response relationship of a drug for optimal drug use and possible individualized therapy. In oncology, dose adjustment based on toxicity is a traditional practice, especially for cytotoxic agents *(36,53,72,73)* and under certain circumstances when severe toxicity is manifested, subsequent doses or cycles of therapy are withheld until the toxicity is resolved. However, these adjustments are done empirically in the absence of any exposure–response information and may not provide optimum benefit from the therapy. New targets are being discovered and drugs are developed against these targets. Understanding the exposure-associated target response in early development will allow selection of optimum dose and/or dosing regimen for pivotal efficacy and safety studies. In the pivotal trials, exposure–response assessment can validate the hypothesis generated in the early drug development and provide a dosing algorithm or prediction for special populations. In the clinical trial protocols dose modifications are proposed based on toxicity; the dose is either withdrawn until the severity of the toxicity reduces to an acceptable level or the dose is reduced by a certain fraction for the next cycle. The inherent assumption is that the toxicity at least in part is associated with the exposure to the drug. However, the relationship between the exposure levels from the modified dosing and the clinical response is not usually defined in these trials.

The exposure–response relationship is the principle that forms the basis on which rational dose adjustment can be made for patients who are excluded from the registration clinical trials. Inclusion and exclusion criteria for pivotal clinical trials for registration include patients with good performance status and adequate organ (renal and hepatic) function. Patients on various concomitant medications are excluded from the trial. However, in the community practice physicians treat patients who have compromised performance status, are on concomitant medications, and have impaired organ function. Rational dose adjustment in such special populations is possible if the exposure–response relationship of the drug is well defined. Death due to drug toxicity is not uncommon in cancer treatment and dose adjustment based on toxicity is expensive. Therapeutic drug monitoring helps to avoid toxicity and optimize drug therapy. The concept of therapeutic drug monitoring is mostly based on exposure–toxicity relationship.

From the regulatory perspectives, exposure–response information not only helps in drug development, but under certain circumstances may provide supportive evidence for approval of a drug (1). The FDA promotes evaluation of exposure–response relationship during drug development as well after a drug is approved (74,75). Although exposure–response evaluation of cancer drugs has been rare in the past, recognition of the utility of exposure–response relationship in drug development and targeted therapy in oncology relying on various safety and efficacy markers are expected to promote exposure response evaluation and optimal and individualized therapy in the future.

REFERENCES

1. Guidance for Industry. Clinical Pharmacology. Exposure–response relationships: study design, data analysis, and regulatory applications. United States Food and Drug Administration. Center for Drug Evaluation and Research. Website: (http://www.fda.gov/cder/guidance/index.htm).
2. International Conference on Harmonisation. Guidance on dose response information to support drug registration. Fed Reg 1994; 59:55,972–55,976.
3. Egorin MJ, Van Echo DA, Olman EA. Whitacre MY, Forrest A, Aisner J. Prospective validation of a pharmacologically based dosing scheme for the cis-diammine-dichloroplatinum(II) analogue diammine-cyclobutane-dicarboxylatoplatinum. Cancer Res 1985; 45:6502–0506.
4. O'Dwyer PJ, LaCreta F, Engstrom PF, et al. Phase I/pharmacokinetic reevaluation of thioTEPA. Cancer Res 1991; 51:3171–3176.
5. Fanucci MP, Walsh TD, Fleisher M, et al. Phase I and clinical pharmacology study of trimetrexate administered weekly for three weeks. Cancer Res 1987; 47:3303–3308.
6. Noe DA, Rowinsky EK, Shen HS, et al. Phase I and pharmacokinetic study of brequinar sodium (NSC 368390). Cancer Res 1990; 50:4595–4599.
7. Clark PI. Clinical pharmacology and schedule dependency of the podophyllotoxin derivatives. Semin Oncol 1992; 19:20–27.
8. Hehlmann R. Current CML therapy: progress and dilemma. Leukemia 2003; 17:1010–1012.
9. O'Brian SG, Guilhot F, Larson RA, et al. Imatinib compared with interferon and low-dose cytarabine for newly diagnosed chronis-phase chronic myeloid leukemia. N Engl J Med 2003; 348:994–1004.
10. Huang J, Frischer JS, Serur AS, et al. Regression of established tumors and metastases by potent vascular endothelial growth factor blockade. Proc Natl Acad Sci USA 2003; 100:7785–7790.
11. Xiong B, Sun TJ, Yuan HY, Hu MB, Hu WD, Cheng FL. Cyclooxygenase-2 expression and angiogenesis in colorectal cancer. World J Gastroenterol 2003; 9:1237–1240.
12. Kausch I, Lingnau A, Endl E, et al. Antisense treatment against Ki-67 mRNA inhibits proliferation and tumor growth in vitro and in vivo. Int J Cancer 2003; 105:710–716.
13. Thiagalingam S, Cheng K, Lee HJ, Mineva N, Thiagalingam A, Ponte JF. Histone deacetylases: unique players in shaping the epigenetic histone code. Ann NY Acad Sci 2003; 983:84–100.

14. Frankel SR. Oblimersen sodium (G3139 Bcl-2 antisense oligonucleotide) therapy in Waldenstrom's macroglobulinemia: a targeted approach to enhance apoptosis. Semin Oncol 2003; 30:300–304.

15. Uren A, Merchant MS, Sun CJ, et al. Beta-platelet-derived growth factor receptor mediates motility and growth of Ewing's sarcoma cells. Oncogene 2003; 22:2334–2342.

16. Mitchell BS. The proteasome—an emerging therapeutic target in cancer. N Engl J Med 2003; 348: 2597–2598.

17. Crucitta E, Locopo, N, Silvestris N, De Lena M, Lorusso V. The role of letrozole (Femara®) in breast cancer therapy: a clinical review. Drugs Today (Barc) 2001; 37:639–644.

18. Druker BJ, Moshe T, Debra JR, et al. Efficacy and safety of a specific inhibitor of the BCR-ABL tyrosine kinase in chronic myeloid leukemia. N Engl J Med 2003; 344:1031–1037.

19. Berenson JR, Vescio RA, Rosen LS, et al. A Phase I dose-ranging trial of monthly infusions of zoledronic acid for the treatment of osteolytic bone metastases. Clin Cancer Res 2001; 7:478–485.

20. Pallis AG, Mavroudis D, Androulakis N, et al. ZD-1839, a novel, oral epidermal growth factor receptor-tyrosine kinase inhibitor, as salvage treatment in patients with advanced non-small-cell lung cancer. Experience from a single center participating in a compassionate use program. Lung Cancer 2003; 40:301–307.

21. Evans WE. Clinical pharmacodynamics of anticancer drugs: a basis for extending the concept of dose-intensity. Blut 1988; 56:241–248.

22. Danesi R, Fogli S, Gennari A, Conte P, Del Tacca M. Pharmacokinetic-pharmacodynamic relationships of the anthracycline anticancer drugs. Clin Pharmacokinetic 2002; 41:431–444.

23. Longley DB, Harkin DP, Johnston PG. 5-Fluorouracil: mechanisms of action and clinical strategies. Nat Rev Cancer 2003; 3:330–338

24. Grem JL. Fluorinated pyrimidines. In: Chabner B, Collins J (eds). Cancer Chemotherapy: Principles and Practice, Chapter 7. Philadelphia PA: JB Lippincott, 1990, pp. 180–224.

25. Tsukamoto Y, Kato Y, Ura M, Horii I, Ishitsuka H, Kusuhara H, Sugiyama T. A physiologically based pharmacokinetic analysis of capecitabine, a triple prodrug of 5-FU, in humans: the mechanism for tumor-selective accumulation of 5-FU. Pharm Res 2001; 18:1190–1202.

26. Koenig H, Patel A. Biochemical basis for fluorouracil neurotoxicity. The role of Krebs cycle inhibition by fluoroacetate. Arch Neurol 1970; 23:155–160.

27. Akiba T, Okeda R, Tajima T. Metabolites of 5-fluorouracil, alpha-fluro-beta-alanine and fluoroacetic acid, directly injure myelinated fibers in tissue culture. Acta Neuropathol (Berl) 1996; 92:8–13.

28. Cao S, Baccanari DP, Rustum YM, et al. Alpha-fluro-beta-alanine: effects on the antitumor acticity and toxicity of 5-fluorouracil. Biochem Pharmacol 2000; 59:953–960.

29. Grochow LB, Jones RJ, Brundrett RB, et al. Pharmacokinetics of busulfan: correlation with veno-occlusive disease in patients undergoing bone marrow transplantation. Cancer Chemother Pharmacol 1989; 25:55–61.

30. Trump DL, Egorin MJ, Forrest A, Willson JK, Remick S, Tutsch KD. Pharmacokinetic and pharmacodynamic analysis of fluorouracil during 72-hour continuous infusion with and without dipyridamole. J Clin Oncol 1991; 9:2027–2037.

31. Jodrell DI, Egorin MJ, Canetta RM, et al. Relationship between carboplatin exposure and tumor response and toxicity inpatients with ovarian cancer. J Clin Oncol 1992; 10:520–524.

32. Sparreboom A, Nooter K, Loos WJ, Verweij J. The (ir)relevance of plasma protein binding of anticancer drugs. Neth J Med 2001; 59:196–207.

33. van den Bongard HJ, Mathot RA, Beijnen JH, Schellens JH. Pharmacokinetically guided administration of chemotherapeutic agents. Clin Pharmacokinet 2000; 39:345–367.

34. Kearns CM, Gianni L, Egorin MJ. Paclitaxel pharmacokinetics and pharmacodynamics. Semin Oncol 1995; 22:16–23.

35. Belani CP, Kearns CM, Zuhowski EG, et al. Phase I trial, Including pharmacokinetic and pharmacodynamic correlations, of combination paclitaxel and carboplatin in patients with metastatic non-small-cell lung cancer. J Clin Oncol 1999; 17:676–684.

36. Physicians' Desk Reference, 57th Edit. Paraplatin (carboplatin for injection). Medical Economics/Thomson PDR, 2003, pp. 1126–1129.

37. Gibaldi M, Perrier D. Drugs and the Pharmaceutical Sciences, Vol. 15: Pharmacokinetics, 2nd Edit. New York, NY: Marcel Dekker, 1982, pp. 1–198.

38. Roboz GJ, Knovich MA, Bayer RL, et al. Efficacy and safety of gemtuzumab ozogamicin in patients with poor-prognosis acute myeloid leukemia. Leuk Lymphoma 2002; 43:1951–1955.

39. Garcia-Manero G, Talpaz M, Giles FJ, et al. Treatment of Philadelphia chromosome-positive chronic myelogenous leukemia with weekly polyethylene glycol formulation of interferon-alpha-2b and low-dose cytosine arabinoside. Cancer 2003; 97:3010–3016.

40. Kantarjian HM, Gandhi V, Cortes J, et al. Phase II clinical and pharmacology study of clofarabine in patients with refractory or relapsed acute leukemia. Blood First Edition Paper, prepublished online June 5, 2003; DOI 10.1182/blood-2003-03-0925.

41. Van Den Bent MJ, Taphoorn MJ, Brandes AA, et al. Phase II study of first-line chemotherapy with temozolomide in recurrent oligodendroglial tumors: The European Organization for Research and Treatment of Cancer brain tumor group study 26971. J Clin Oncol 2003; 21:2525–2528.

42. Garcea G, Sharma RA, Dennison A, Steward WP, Gescher A, Berry DP. Molecular biomarkers of colorectal carcinogenesis and their role in surveillance and early intervention. Eur J Cancer 2003; 39: 1041–1052.

43. Hedman M, Arnberg H, Wernlund J, Riska H, Brodin O. Tissue polypeptide antigen (TPA), hyaluronan and CA 125 as serum markers in malignant mesothelioma. Anticancer Res 2003; 23:531–536.

44. Glas AS, Roos D, Deutekom M, Zwinderman AH, Bossuyt PM, Kurth KH. Tumor markers in the diagnosis of primary bladder cancer. A systematic review. J Urol 2003; 169:1975–1982.

45. Berenson JR, Vescio R, Henick K, et al. A Phase I, open label, dose ranging trial of intravenous bolus zolandronic acid, a novel bisphosphonate, in cancer patients with metastatic bone disease. Cancer 2001; 91:144–154.

46. Zheng L, Li S, Boyer TG, Lee W-H. Lessons learned from *BRCA1* and *BRCA2*. Oncogene 2000; 19:6159–6175.

47. Catalona WJ, Smith DS, Ratliff TL, et al. Measurement of prostate-specific antigen in serum as a screening test for prostate cancer. N Engl J Med 1991; 324:1156–1161.

48. Woolf SH. Screening for prostate cancer with prostate-specific antigen. N Engl J Med 1995; 333:1401–1405.

49. Roach M 3rd. The role of PSA in the radiotherapy of prostate cancer. Oncology (Huntingt) 1996; 10: 1143–1153.

50. Khan MA, Partin AW. Management of high-risk populations with locally advanced prostate cancer. Oncologist 2003; 8:259–269.

51. Luftner D, Luke C, Possinger K. Serum HER-2/*neu* in the management of breast cancer patients. Clin Biochem 2003; 36:233–240.

52. Lipton A, Ali SM, Leitzel K, et al. Serum HER-2/*neu* and response to the aromatase inhibitor letrozole versus tamoxifen. J Clin Oncol 2003; 21:1967–1972.

53. Physicians' Desk Reference, 57th Edit. Eloxatin (oxaliplatin for injection). Medical Economics/Thomson PDR, 2003, pp. 2999–3003.

54. Mauro MJ, Druker BJ. STI571: targeting BCR-ABL as therapy for CML. Oncologist 2001; 6:233–238.

55. Physicians' Desk Reference, 57th Edit. Gemzar (gemcitabine HCl for injection). Medical Ecomonics/Thomson PDR, 2003, pp. 1837–1842.

56. Physicians' Desk Reference, 57th Edit. Novantrone (mitoxantrone for injection concentrate). Medical Economics/Thomson PDR, 2003, pp. 1747–1752.

57. Diehl V, Frankllin J, Pfreundschuh M, et al., German Hodgkin's Lymphoma Study Group. Standard and increased-dose BEACOPP chemotherapy compared with COPP-ABVD for advanced Hodgkin's disease. N Engl J Med 2003; 348:2386–2395.

58. Therasse P, Mauriac L, Welnicka-Jaskiewicz M, et al. Final results of a randomized Phase III trial comparing cyclophosphamide, epirubicin, and fluorouracil with a dose-intensified epirubicin and cyclophosphamide + filgrastim as neoadjuvant treatment in locally advanced breast cancer: an EORTC-NCIC-SAKK multicenter study. J Clin Oncol 2003; 21:843–850.

59. Jung LL, Zamboni WC. Cellular, pharmacokinetic, and pharmacodynamic aspects of response to camptothecins: can we improve it? 2001; 4:273–288.

60. Grochow LB, Jones RJ, Brundrett RB, et al. Pharmacokinetics of busulfan: correlation with veno-occulusive disease in patients undergoing bone marrow transplantation. Can Chemother Pharmacol 1989; 25:55–61.

61. Busulfex (busulfan) injection label. Website: (www.fda.gov/cder/foi/label/2003/20954se2-2004_busulfex_lbl.pdf).

62. Physicians' Desk Reference, 57th Edit. Zometa (zolandronic acid for injection). Medical Economics/Thomson PDR, 2003, pp. 2341–2345.

63. Berenson JR, Vescio RA, Rosen LS, et al. A Phase I dose-ranging trial of monthly infusions of zolendronic acid for the treatment of osteolytic bone metastases. Clin Can Res 2001; 7:478–485.

64. NDA Review. NDA 21-386. Zometa (zoledronic acid) injection. EFOI. Website: (www.fda.gov/cder/approval/index.htm).
65. NDA Review. NDA 21-335. Gleevec (imatinib mesylate) capsules. EFOI. Website: www.fda.gov/cder/approval/index.htm).
66. Physicians' Desk Reference, 57th Edit. Taxotere (docetaxel for injection). Medical Economics/Thomson PDR, 2003, pp. 773–779.
67. International Conference on Harmonisation. Guidance on ethnic factors in the acceptability of foreign clinical data; availability. Fed Reg 1998; 63:31,790–31,796.
68. Physicians' Desk Reference, 57th Edit. Aromasin (exemestane tablets). Medical Economics/Thomson PDR, 2003, pp. 2692–2695.
69. Physicians' Desk Reference, 57th Edit. Arimidex (anastrazole tablets). Medical Economics/Thomson PDR, 2003, pp. 653–656.
70. Physicians' Desk Reference, 57th Edit. Femara (Letrazole tablets). Medical Economics/Thomson PDR, 2003, pp. 2269–2272.
71. Physicians' Desk Reference, 52nd Edit. Platinol (cisplatin for injection). Medical Economics/Thomson PDR, 1998, pp. 756–758.
72. Physicians' Desk Reference, 57th Edit. Xeloda (capecitabine tablets). Medical Economics/Thomson PDR, 2003, pp. 2952–2959.
73. Physicians' Desk Reference, 57th Edit. Temodar (temozolamide capsules). Medical Economics/Thomson PDR, 2003, pp. 3081–3083.
74. Peck CC, Barr WH, Benet LZ, et al. Opportunities for integration of pharmacokinetics, pharmacodynamics, and toxicokinetics in rational drug development. J Clin Pharmacol 1994; 34:111–119.
75. Lesko LJ, Rowland M, Peck CC, Blaschke TF. Optimizing the science of drug development: opportunities for better candidate selection and accelerated evaluation in humans. J Clin Pharmacol 2000; 40:803–814.

32   Identifying Agents to Test in Phase III Trials

Thomas G. Roberts Jr., MD, Thomas J. Lynch Jr., MD, and Bruce A. Chabner, MD

CONTENTS

1. INTRODUCTION

The greatest thing in this world is not so much where we are, but what direction we are moving.

—*Oliver Wendell Holmes (1809–1894)*

The revolution of molecular medicine, to a considerable degree the result of investment in the understanding of cancer biology, has produced a dynamic time for the development of cancer drugs. This scientific revolution, coupled with the increasing prominence of the biotechnology industry, has led to an unprecedented proliferation of cancer drugs under investigation. According to a recent survey by the Pharmaceutical Researchers and Manufacturers of America, the number of anticancer drugs in the clinical pipeline rose 87% from 1995 to 2001 *(1)*. A major driver has also been the unmet need of patients with cancers; cancer is the second leading cause of death in the United States *(2)* and is estimated to eclipse cardiovascular disease within this century. As of 2001, there were an estimated 1345 antineoplastic drugs in development, with 837 in the preclinical stage and 196, 219, and 67 in clinical Phases I, II, and III, respectively (Fig. 1; *3*) This diverse group includes novel agents that target cell cycle regulation, signal transduction, angiogenesis, and drug resistance reversal, to name a few. To place these numbers in perspective, the total number of antineoplastic drugs in development is greater than the total of the next two most represented therapeutic classes (antiinfective and cardiovascular system drugs) combined *(3)*.

Handbook of Anticancer Pharmacokinetics and Pharmacodynamics
Edited by: W. D. Figg and H. L. McLeod © Humana Press Inc., Totowa, NJ

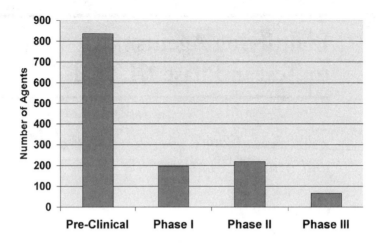

Fig. 1. Estimated number of cancer drugs in development by phase. (Data from Parexel's Phar-maceutical R&D Statistical Sourcebook 2001.)

At the same time that cancer drugs under investigation have multiplied, clinical trials in oncology have become increasingly regulated *(4)*, expensive *(5)*, and time consuming *(6)*. Oncology trials are not only resource intensive, but often they also yield disappointing results, making the clinical development phase risky from a sponsor's perspective *(7)*. For example, of the 280 antineoplastic agents brought into clinical trials from 1975 to 1994, only 29 ultimately advanced to receive marketing approval from the Food and Drug Administration (FDA) *(8)*. More recent data on success rates for the development of new anticancer drugs are only slightly more encouraging and show that oncology drugs have the second lowest approval rate of all therapeutic drug classes *(7)*.

Taken together, these figures herald a new phase in the history of cancer treatment. Two issues define the time. First, the emergence of targeted therapy necessitates new strategies for clinical drug development. The same rules that have been used for cytotoxic drugs are unlikely to be useful for targeted agents. Second, there are now many more potential drug targets and more new chemical entities (NCEs) in the clinic. The resources of government and industry are sufficient to test only a fraction of the NCEs in large clinical trials. Choices must therefore be made about which agents to introduce into and advance through the clinical development phase for new drugs. Of all the possible choices that must be made during the development of a cancer drug (see Fig. 2), none is more important or more involved than deciding which agents to advance to Phase III testing. This chapter focuses on this high-stakes decision point and offers a decision model to guide the process, both for standard cytotoxics and molecularly targeted agents (MTAs). An overview of the clinical trials process in oncology and the salient issues surrounding Phase III cancer trials also provided.

1.1. Prevalence of Clinical Trials in Oncology

Ever since Sidney Farber published in 1948 his findings that the administration of ami-nopterin could induce temporary remissions in children with leukemia *(9)*, a complex process of clinical testing has evolved to evaluate rigorously new cancer treatments. The subsequent application of this process by clinical investigators has produced curative treatments in leukemias, lymphomas, and germ-cell tumors and has led to significant improvements in survival for many patients with solid tumors such as breast *(10)* and colorectal cancer *(11)*.

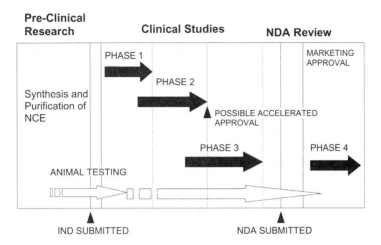

Fig. 2. The new drug development process. NCE, New chemical entity; IND, investigational new drug; NDA, new drug application.

Despite these successes, the prognosis of most patients diagnosed with advanced epithelial cancers is grim; and overall clinical progress has been slow, particularly when compared to progress in other areas in medicine *(12)*. To be sure, cancer has been a formidable opponent. Fueled by the promise of better treatments and the recent emergence of targeted therapy *(13)*, clinical research in oncology is now flourishing. As of March 2002 the Physicians Data Query (PDQ) database maintained by the National Cancer Institute (NCI) showed that in the United States alone, 497 Phase I, 931 Phase II, and 376 Phase III clinical trials were open *(14)*. With a swelling interest in a vast spectrum of MTAs directed at specific differences between host and tumor, these numbers are likely to continue to burgeon *(15)*.

1.2. Overview of the Clinical Trials Process

Before a new antineoplastic agent or NCE can advance from in vitro and animal testing to be given to human subjects in a clinical trial, the FDA must approve an investigational new drug (IND) application. In year 2000, oncology-related IND applications comprised 12.5% of all active commercial INDs *(3)*, making antineoplastics the most numerous of any therapeutic class. Once IND approval has been granted, the drug classically enters into three sequential phases of clinical trials, each representing a distinct set of goals and challenges. If the results from these clinical trials yield particularly promising results, the sponsor may choose to submit a new drug application (NDA) to the FDA to seek marketing approval for a specific indication. A schematic representation of this process is shown in Fig. 2. With the advent of MTAs, which will likely be first approved for use in combination with cytotoxic agents, the classic, sequential order of the clinical trials process may require modification (see Subheading 4.).

1.2.1. Phase I Trials

Phase I trials represent the first experience with the agent, regimen, or dosing schedules in humans. For cytotoxic drug, the major objectives of Phase I trials are to (1) determine maximum tolerated dose (MTD) that is appropriate to use for Phase II trials; (2) characterize the toxicity profile, focusing in particular on dose limiting toxities (DLTs); and (3) collect relevant pharmacokinetic (PK) and pharmacodynamic (PD) data *(16)*. An appropriate schedule and starting dose for Phase I is chosen based on PK and efficacy data from animal experiments. In the Phase I trials, dose escalation in humans continues in successive cohorts of patients until the DLT is reached, at which point additional patients are treated at the dose just below the DLT level to confirm its safety.

For targeted therapies, which may have biological activity well below the MTD, the standard end point for Phase I trials (toxicity) may not be appropriate *(17)*. Important endpoints for these agents may be the demonstration of in vivo target engagement and the achievement of satisfactory PKs (i.e., inhibitory concentration for a given period of time), as the goal for targeted agents is to determine the optimal biological dose rather than the MTD. Because the target in tumor tissue may be inaccessible and because repeat biopsies before and during treatment may not be possible, surrogate markers of biological effect, such as imaging studies or target measurement in accessible normal tissues, may provide useful information. Changes in Phase I trial designs to evaluate both the biological as well as toxic and pharmacologic properties of these MTAs, alone and in combination with cytotoxic agents, are now being offered *(18,19)*.

Whereas Phase I trials are typically performed in small numbers of *normal* subjects in most other areas of medicine, Phase I trials of antineoplastics typically enroll cancer patients with advanced disease who are resistant to all standard treatments, yet have preserved performance status and organ function. Because toxicity rather than response is the primary endpoint, these trials do not need to be performed separately for each tumor type. That said, recognition of therapeutic benefit *is* sought during this phase, but the combination of small numbers of patients; low starting doses of the investigational drugs; and the drug-resistant, advanced disease of the study participants all compromise the chance of demonstrating clinical benefit *(20)*. A relatively recent review of a 3-yr Phase I experience at M.D. Anderson Cancer Center showed an overall response rate of 3% *(21)*. This low response rate was similar to the 4% overall response rate reported earlier in an analysis of Phase I trials sponsored by the NCI *(22)*. When responses are seen, they help direct which diseases to test in the Phase II efforts. For both standard cytotoxic and MTAs, a successful Phase I trial will (1) determine a dose and schedule to test in later phases and (2) demonstrate that further testing will not be compromised by prohibitive toxicity.

1.2.2. PHASE II TRIALS

The primary focus of Phase II trials is to determine efficacy in different tumor types. They also provide additional opportunities to refine and expand PK data, broaden the experience with toxicity through larger populations treated with multiple cycles of drug, and perform biological and imaging studies that enhance the understanding of the drug's action *(16)*. Phase II trials have been typically performed as single-arm, single-institution studies *(23)* and have taken 1–3 yr to complete, with the data held by the primary investigator. Now, many Phase II trials are multicentered, take only 4–6 mo to complete, with the aggregate data held only by the industry sponsor. When successful, these trials often demonstrate the first evidence of efficacy in humans. The typical Phase II endpoint for standard cytotoxic drugs is tumor regression (i.e., complete, partial, or minor responses). Trials of MTAs, which may be cytostatic, may incorporate additional end points such as target inhibition and time to progression (TTP), although an accurate assessment of TTP may be difficult in a small, nonrandomized Phase II study.

Phase II trials are designed to maximize the chance of detecting a clinical response or biological activity and thus avoid erroneously concluding that an agent is inactive (type II error). These mutual goals are met by selecting patients who have maximum performance status and minimal prior chemotherapy. In a typical, two-stage design, 10–25 patients will be entered to evaluate response. Optimized designs for Phase II trials have been offered depending on the target response rate and chosen error limits *(16)*. Under one such design, if there are no responses in the first 12 evaluable patients, there is only a 10% chance of rejecting a drug that has a true response rate of 20% *(16)*, and the trial is suspended. If one or more of the patients respond, an additional 20–30 patients are entered in order to refine the estimate of response rate. Although these trials are typically directed at patients who have received prior therapy, "window of opportunity" designs in which a Phase II drug is given prior to a standard treatment are sometimes employed in previously untreated patients who have excellent performance status. Even when the Phase II drug was ineffective, this type of approach did not have a negative impact on subsequent response to established drugs, or on overall survival in breast cancer *(24)*. The reliability of data from Phase II trials is compromised by their small size, patient selection bias, and lack of a concurrent control group. Taken together, Phase I and II trials are referred to as *developmental* or learning trials that help inform decisions regarding which agents to advance to confirmatory testing in Phase III trials.

1.2.3. PHASE III TRIALS

Phase III trials are large, usually randomized, multiinstitutional, resource-intensive efforts that seek to determine if the investigational treatment shows clinically important benefit over a widely accepted standard of care. The hallmarks of Phase III trials include (1) a control group receiving standard therapy, (2) a broad selection of patients so that results can be applied in the community, and (3) the measurement of endpoints that have direct relevance to patients such as TTP, survival, or relief of symptoms *(25)*. Compared to Phase I and II trials, Phase III trials require hundreds of patients or more and are considerably more difficult to execute. As such, they are much more expensive to complete. Despite their substantial challenges, Phase III trials provide the most reliable source of efficacy data, and their results are the most important criteria for approval by the FDA. Of the more than 85 approved oncology drugs in the United States for almost 150 indications, approximately two-thirds of the approved indications were based on data from Phase III trials *(26)*.

The reliability of Phase III trials derives from the elimination of selection bias, broad eligibility criteria, and multiinstitutional participation, all of which allow the collection of accurate and generalizable results. The large numbers of patients enrolled in Phase III trials also provide data on infrequent or delayed toxicities that may not manifest in a smaller group of selected patients. For example, the cardiotoxicity associated with the monoclonal antibody trastuzumab (Herceptin), particularly when combined with an anthracycline, became clearly evident only during the course of a Phase III trial *(27)*. Phase III trials are therefore the primary vehicle for establishing that a candidate treatment offers overall benefit over the standard and are often referred to as *registration* or *pivotal trials* because of their traditionally preeminent role in the approval process. Selected characteristics of Phase I, II, and III trials are shown in Table 1.

1.2.4. PHASE IV TRIALS

Phase IV trials are performed in the postmarketing period and are often undertaken by a sponsoring organization or firm in order to seek additional marketing indications. Phase IV trials may also be required as a part of qualifications set forth under accelerated marketing approval to collect addition safety data and provide evidence of clinical benefit.

Table 1
Selected Characteristics of Clinical Trials of Cancer Drugs

	Cancer treatment trials		
	Phase I	Phase II	Phase III
Number of patients	20–30	30–100	200–thousands
Primary endpoints	MTD, DLT	RR, TTP	Survival, TTP, QOL
Mean duration (mo) [a]	26	43	54
Indexed mean cost per patient (Phase I = 100) [a,b]	100	75	64
Indexed mean cost per phase (Phase III = 100) [a–c]	10	22	100
Randomization	No	Varies	Yes
Typical no. of institutions	One	One	Multiple

MTD, Maximum safe dose; DLT, dose-limiting toxicity; RR, response rate; TTP, time to progression; QOL, quality of life.

[a] Data derived from ref. *1*.

[b] Based on aggregate trial data from all therapeutic classes and not limited to cancer trials.

[c] Calculations were performed using 25, 75, and 400 patients for Phases I, II, and III, respectively.

The FDA is increasingly granting these qualified approvals under the accelerated approval and expanded access effort begun in 1996 *(28)*, an issue that is discussed in detail later in the chapter.

2. THE ROLE OF PHASE III TRIALS IN ONCOLOGY

Phase III comparative trials yield the highest quality data in oncology.

—*James Cox, M.D., The Janeway Lecture 2000 (29)*

2.1. The Advantages of Randomization

As alluded to in the preceeding, Phase III trials represent the definitive method to determine whether an investigational therapeutic regimen offers clinically meaningful benefit compared to an existing standard *(30)*. The power of these trials relates in large part to their application of randomization. Randomization offers two major advantages compared to any other control technique. First, it eliminates selection bias with respect to assignment of treatments. Because oncologists can often select which patients are likely to have a good outcome based on their performance status and the underlying disease biology, the elimination of selection bias with respect to assignment of treatments is critical. Second, randomization inherently balances over time all covariates (prognostic factors), both known and unknown, between the treatment arm(s) and the control arm, thus allowing the groups to be truly comparable. Importantly, randomization minimizes variation in the groups with respect to both known and unknown prognostic factors, whereas adjustment techniques used in nonrandomized designs can control only for *known* prognostic factors *(31)*. The randomization process can be made even more powerful if factors known to be strongly related to outcome (e.g., cytogenetic abnormalities in acute myelogenous leukemia) are used to stratify patients prior to randomization. This stratification process ensures that these factors will be adequately balanced.

The power of the Phase III trial is well illustrated in the history of chemotherapy for melanoma *(32,33)*. The standard of care for metastatic melanoma had been single-agent dacarbazine (DTIC), producing response rates between 10% and 20%. A single-institution Phase II trial, published in 1984, demonstrated a significantly higher response rate of 55% with combination therapy (dacarbazine, cisplatin, carmustine, and tamoxifen; later referred to as the Dartmouth regimen). Additional Phase II trials with the Dartmouth regimen were performed with confirmatory results *(34,35)*. When a randomized Phase III trial, involving 240 patients (121 in the DTIC arm and in the 119 Dartmouth arm), was then undertaken based on the Phase II data, there was no demonstrated statistically significant difference in survival or response between the two arms *(36)*. Response rates for both arms were similar to the original data from single-agent DTIC. Similar examples can be found within all areas of oncology *(37,38)*. While adjustment techniques to control for patient selection in Phase II trials are increasingly being suggested *(33)*, this example demonstrates how potentially misleading conclusions obtained from patient selection in Phase II trials can be mitigated by an adequately powered, randomized Phase III effort.

2.2. Historical Perspective of Randomized Trials in Oncology

The first randomized clinical trials in cancer, comparing various radiation therapy techniques and doses, can be traced back to the late 1940s in the United Kingdom *(39)*. Randomized trials in medical oncology followed later with the first randomized trial comparing two regimens for the treatment of acute leukemia *(40)* published in 1958. The first randomized study in solid tumors *(41)* was published shortly thereafter. Almost from their inception, randomized Phase III trials in oncology have been controversial and have led to contention within the field, based mostly on ethical considerations and difficulties with their execution. One observer even remarked that "Phase III trials are essentially worthless for determining anything except the talent of the medical experts who design the trials" *(42)*.

In part because of these views, randomized trials in oncology grew slowly, and by 1972, only about one in five clinical cancer trials had any control group at all, let alone a randomized one *(43)*. Chalmers' articulation of the sentiment that "just as controls were not necessary to demonstrate the efficacy of penicillin....controls will not be necessary to recognize the cure for cancer" *(43)* represented a widely held optimistic notion that dramatically effective treatment advances would make controlled trials unnecessary. This mindset, which has been characterized by Cox as *res ipsa loquitur* or "the thing speaks for itself," was undoubtedly reinforced by the early successes of chemotherapy *(39)*, such as the ability of methotrexate to eradicate gestational choriocarcinoma in the 1950s and cyclophosphamide to cure African children with Burkitt's lymphoma in the 1960s.

Over the last 30 yr, there has been a growing appreciation for the importance of Phase III trials in oncology and a movement away from the mindset of *res ipsa loquitur*. Both the disappointments and progress of clinical cancer research have influenced this sea change. In terms of the disappointments, the fruits of the early optimism have not been realized. While there have been dramatic instances when an incurable disease has been transformed into an easily controlled or curable disease by a new treatment, as for example, cisplatin for germ cell tumors of the testis, cladribine for hairy cell leukemia, or imatinib mesylate (Gleevec) for chronic myelogenous leukemia (CML), these successes have been infrequent. Most advances in oncology over the last 30 yr have instead been incremental, and have required Phase III trials. When chemotherapy was first given to children with Burkitt's lymphoma, there was no need to compare to a standard. Because of the progress derived from clinical research, there now exist some effective therapies for most forms of cancer. Because most new drugs are only incrementally better than the standard, if at all, randomized trials of sufficient power have been required to provide evidence of significant benefit.

2.3. Alternatives to a Randomized Phase III Trial

2.3.1. Historical Controls

For various reasons, including the expense and the logistic hurdles of Phase III trials, alternatives have been proposed. One alternative is to compare response or survival rates in a treatment group to those of a historical control group. Clinical trials that employ historical controls require fewer patients, are much less expensive, and are completed more rapidly compared to trials using a randomized concurrent control group *(44)*. These trials also invoke fewer ethical concerns because all the patients receive the investigational treatment. There are two major problems that limit the utility of trials that employ historical controls. First, these trials rely on the tenuous assumption that the survival rate in historical controls is sufficiently similar to randomized control groups to allow for valid comparisons. Unfortunately, subtle differences in patient selection or pretreatment staging, and differences in methods of evaluation of response for the same disease, can lead to outcome differences between the treatment group and the historical control group that may be difficult or even impossible to interpret. A second and related problem is that relevant historical databases may not be available for the disease and particular stage in question. Technological and demographic changes can invalidate existing historical databases. For example, the widespread application of mammography led to a sharp rise in the recognition of ductal carcinoma *in situ* (DCIS), a condition for which adequate historical databases did not exist. Similarly, appropriate historical databases were lacking for the malignancies associated with the acquired immunodeficiency syndrome. As treatment standards evolve and new screening and staging tools emerge (e.g., positron emission tomography), historical databases lose their applicability.

The utility of historical controls in oncology was tested formally in an analysis of 118 major treatment studies in six types of malignancies (breast cancer, colon cancer, gastric cancer, lung cancer, melanoma, and soft tissue sarcoma). Of these studies, 43 concurrent randomized control groups and historical control groups were identified that matched exactly for (1) disease, (2) stage, (3) major prognostic factor, (4) outcome parameter reported, and (5) follow-up time. The overall results showed that 18 of 43 (42%) matched control groups had median survival that differed by > 10%, with a significant proportion of the matched controls (21%) differing by > 20%. For unclear reasons, studies in gastric cancer and breast cancer showed better agreement between historical control groups and randomized control groups than the other four malignancies studied. Remarkably, among the groups where survival differed significantly between the historical and concurrent randomized control groups, almost all (94%) of the randomized control groups had survival superior to that of the historical controls *(44)*.

The fact that historical control groups tend to do worse than randomized controls may explain why so many treatments look promising in Phase II trials (using historical controls) only to fail to show comparative benefit in their subsequent Phase III experience (using concurrent controls). This reality was demonstrated in an analysis of Phase II trials that were followed by a corresponding Phase III experience in extensive-stage small-cell lung cancer. Even though 44 out of 56 (79%) historically controlled trials found the investigational therapy to be more effective, only 10 out of the 50 (20%) corresponding randomized-controlled trials confirmed such a benefit *(45)*. Taken together these data provide a compelling argument against drawing indiscriminate conclusions regarding the utility of investigational treatments based solely on comparisons with historical controls.

Despite the need for caution in the use of historical controls, there are two major circumstances in which it may be necessary or preferable to use them. In the first case, there may be such small numbers of patients with a disease that randomization would be unfeasible or impossible even in the cooperative group setting (e.g., sarcomas, anaplastic thyroid cancer, phyloides tumor of the breast). In the second case, concurrent controls may not be required if there is a dramatic improvement in response a disease with a uniformly poor outcome (e.g., imatinib mesylate in interferon-resistant CML).

2.3.2. ADJUSTMENT TECHNIQUES

Adjustment techniques can be used in historically controlled trials as an attempt to mitigate the effect of selection bias on Phase II trials. Any control group that is employed other than one using randomization requires either that (1) the control and treatment groups are identical in every important prognostic factor with the exception of the treatment under study (which is unlikely) or that (2) it is possible to adjust for all relevant differences *(31)*. Efforts to adjust for differences in nonrandomized groups represent an area of intense biostatistical research, whose yield has not yet translated into widespread application. Of particular interest are Bayesian approaches that incorporate quantification of variability derived from changes over time and between institutions *(46)* and other models that attempt to standardize the effect of patient selection in nonrandomized trials by creating risk categories *(33)*. Efforts to validate these approaches and to decide when, if ever, they may truly substitute for a Phase III trial are underway.

2.3.2. SEQUENTIAL TECHNIQUES

Another alternative to a randomized controlled trial is to use the patients as their own controls. In this approach, one compares endpoints such as RR and TTP with an approved therapy, and subsequent RR or TTP in the same patients with a new therapy. In one recent and well publicized instance *(47)*, colon cancer patients who progressed while on irinotecan had the monoclonal antibody IMC-C225 (C225, Erbitux), an inhibitor of the epidermal growth factor receptor, added to irinotecan when they progressed. Because responses were found *(48)*, the claim was made that these responses were evidence of reversal of irinotecan resistance. The drug was submitted to the FDA for consideration under accelerated approval. The FDA responded with a "refusal-to-file" (RTF) letter, which means that the agency determined it was not possible to evaluate the drug's efficacy from the data presented. According to the FDA's RTF letter summarized in *The Cancer Letter*, the study design was deemed "not adequate and well-controlled." Specifically the FDA cited, in addition to protocol violations, that the sequential study design created uncertainty regarding (1) the refractoriness of patients to further irinotecan treatment and (2) the potential contribution of C225's single-agent activity to the regimen. The FDA stated that additional trials directly comparing single-agent irinotecan and single-agent C225 to a combination of irinotecan and C225 would be required for NDA consideration *(49)*. While sequential approaches using the patient as their own control may provide early evidence of efficacy, the experience with C225 demonstrates the risk inherent in submitting an NDA that relies on a pivotal trial that is not adequately controlled.

2.4. Ethical Considerations of Randomization and the Concept of Equipoise

Phase III trials have undergone the most intense ethical scrutiny of any aspect of the clinical cancer research *(50,51)*. The goals of Phase III trials are universally lauded, but the methodology, particularly the application of randomizing cancer patients to receive either an investigation treatment or the standard of care, has been the subject of considerable and still unresolved debate *(52)*. The ethical basis of Phase III trials is predicated on the requirement of *equipoise*. This term was originally defined by Fried *(53)* as a state of genuine uncertainty on the part of the clinical investigator as to the whether the treatment or control arm is likely to offer greater benefit for the patient in question. It follows that since the moral responsibility of the physician as healer is greater than his or her responsibility as investigator, the ethical basis to enroll a patient into a Phase III trial is eroded as soon as the physician is no longer in equipoise.

The problem with requiring equipoise for the individual oncologist enrolling patients on randomized trials is that it is likely to be present the minority of time *(54)*. Because oncologists tend to have strong views regarding the promise of greater efficacy or less toxicity for the treatments under consideration *(35)*, the ethical basis of randomized research has been drawn into sharp question. Equipoise may also be eroded as interim results become available, narrowing the "window of opportunity" to perform many Phase III trials *(55)*. These ethical considerations, particularly with respect to the absence of equipoise, have been sufficiently bothersome that some prominent observers have argued for the abandonment of the randomized clinical trials in cancer altogether *(52,56)*. Despite these strong views, most clinical investigators and ethicists now accept a broader view of equipoise, requiring that it need be present only within the *medical community* and not necessarily for the individual oncologist enrolling the patient into a trial *(57)*. For each institution, an institutional review board (IRB), often including lay personnel, ultimately decides the ethical merits of a new trial.

The informed consent document has also become a major focus of the debate. Most oncologists feel comfortable enrolling patients onto randomized trials if the informed consent document accurately portrays the randomization process and the alternatives to the trial. Since many patients agree to participate in a clinical trial because it is the only way to get access to a potential drug, many trials will also allow those patients who were randomized to standard treatment to cross over to the investigational arm at the time of relapse.

Much of the impetus for the establishment of the informed consent process and ethically sound research grew out of the publication of Henry Beecher's article in the *New England Journal of Medicine* in 1966 *(58)*. Beecher detailed in this article many disturbing examples of peer-reviewed research that contained egregious violations of established ethical principles. In one example that involved a young woman with advanced melanoma, a metastatic lesion was excised and implanted into her mother in the hopes of later using the mother's serum to establish an immune-mediated treatment response. Sadly, the therapy failed and the patient died. Even more disturbing was that fact that the mother soon died of metastatic melanoma herself. The public spotlight in response to this publication led to a rapid increase in the public scrutiny of cancer research that continues to the present day *(50)*.

2.5. Effect on the Physician–Patient Relationship

Entering a patient into a randomized trial may have an effect on the physician–patient relationship. Sociological research has shown that physician authority derives from the patient's perception of the physician's expert knowledge and individualized decision-making power. By entering a patient into a randomized trial, physicians *de facto* admit uncertainty and relinquish some autonomy in the eyes of their patients *(59)*. This real or perceived effect appears to be more prominent in the community setting (which represents 60% of clinical trial activity) where the oncologists may not have played a role in the overall trial design and may not garner the prestige associated with authorship or credit *(60)*.

This concern of oncologists—that randomized trials influence relationships with their patients—appears to be particularly acute when the treatment arms under question are vastly different (e.g., consolidation chemotherapy vs bone marrow transplant in acute myelogenous leukemia). One important trial in breast cancer, which randomized women to lumpectomy without radiation, lumpectomy with radiation, or total mastectomy, had difficulty accruing patients. One study explored the reasons for the disappointing accrual; it was found that an overwhelming majority of physicians (73%) who failed to enter patients into the trial expressed as their primary concern the possible negative effect on the physician–patient relationship *(61)*. Trials that compare relatively similar treatments appear to have fewer problems with accrual. As an example, the ATAC trial, which randomized women with newly diagnosed breast cancer to receive adjuvant therapy with either tamoxifen, an aromatase inhibitor, or both, accrued more than 9000 patients in 3 yr *(62)*.

Compared to research on oncologists' views on randomization, less is known about patients' concerns. What is increasingly clear, however, is that patients empower themselves with information, often through the Internet, and come armed with information and with strong preferences about treatment. These preferences may have the effect of inducing patient dropout once enrollment occurs if the randomized treatment is not the one they desired, unless patients are blinded with respect to their treatment or crossover is permitted. Taken together, these issues may affect accrual on and integrity of Phase III trials, thus limiting their power to detect small but significant differences.

2.6. Cost of Phase III Trials

The cost of developing new antineoplastic drugs is remarkably high. While data specific to the cost of developing cancer drugs in unavailable, the most recent estimate of the average total cost (i.e., preclinical plus clinical costs) of developing a representative new drug from concept to FDA approval is $802 million *(63)*. Although this figure includes in the calculation the cost of developing other drugs that fail, the total is still staggering. A substantial proportion of this cost is spent on clinical development, with Phase III trials representing by far the majority (72%) of clinical drug development costs *(64)*. The expense of Phase III trials in oncology has likely restricted their growth over the past 10 yr. While developmental trials (Phases I and II) in solid tumors increased by 9–15% per year from 1990 to 2000, the annual increase in Phase III trials lagged considerably. In fact, the annual increases in Phase III trials during that time exceeded 5% for in only three tumor types (breast, prostate, and colorectal). For leukemia, urologic cancers, and brain tumors, the number of Phase III trials actually decreased *(65)*. The disproportionate cost of Phase III trials in oncology may change as the expense of earlier trials increase for MTAs, which may require elaborate "proof of principle" studies in Phases I and II.

The expense of Phase III trials in general relates to their large numbers of patients, the need for coordination over many institutions, and requirements for detailed and long-term data collection. Because their high costs and requirements for coordination, Phase III trials are generally sponsored only by pharmaceutical firms or by the cooperative groups of the NCI. Much of the industry data on development costs is proprietary and not available. Extrapolating from available data, it is possible to estimate that these trials can run into the tens of millions of dollars, making them the single largest investment of time and resources in the drug development process. The amount of effort involved in this process and the need for coordination between centers have led to the growth of the contract research organization (CRO). In the past, management of Phase III trials was done "in house" by the industry sponsor. Now most Phase III trials and many multicenter Phase II trials are managed by the CRO.

2.7. Financial Effects on the Health Care System

Because the costs of Phase III trials are so high, reimbursement by third-party payers has been a contentious issue and one deserving of brief discussion. There are three important areas of costs in clinical cancer trials. The first is the administrative costs of the study. This cost is usually wholly covered by the sponsoring organization or firm. The second area is the "usual and customary care" cost for the treatment of the patient that occurs irrespective of whether the patient participates in a clinical trial. This cost has historically been reimbursed by third-party payers such as private insurance or Medicare, but in the late 1980s and early 1990s cost constraints led to a trend of third party payers to refuse to reimburse for the clinical costs incurred for cancer patients on clinical trials. This trend created great fear among clinical researchers (66) and a debate as to who should cover these "usual and customary care" costs. Several recently published studies have demonstrated that the incremental clinical costs of enrolling cancer patients onto clinical trials are either modestly higher (67) or in some cases even lower (68). Fueled in part by these data, President Clinton issued an executive memorandum in year 2000 directing Medicare to reimburse health care providers for the routine costs of patient care associated with participation in clinical trials (69). Many private insurers have voluntarily followed in line, and a growing number of states require such coverage. The third area of cost from a reimbursement view is *extra* costs to patient care generated specifically by the patient's participation in a clinical trial. Of these extra costs, the sponsor generally pays for additional diagnostic tests that are anticipated, while insurers typically cover additional supportive care and hospitalizations attendant with the trial (70).

2.8. Duration of Phase III Trials

Closely tied to the cost of Phase III trials is the time that they take to complete. By one estimate, using data supplied by pharmaceutical companies and maintained in the Tufts Center for the Study of Drug Development NCE database, the mean length of Phase III trials in oncology from 1990 to 1997 was an impressive 53.9 mo (4.5 yr) (3). The time interval is determined by multiple factors: (1) time to complete accrual, (2) time for 80% of "events" such as progression or death to take place, and (3) collection and analysis of the data. The companies did not specify if this 4.5 yr included time to conceive the trial, write the protocol, and get through the IRB approval process. Even if this "startup" time is included in the estimate, Phase III trials in oncology remain time consuming. In fact they are the most time consuming among all therapeutic categories of drugs under development and all types of cancer trials (3). To place the estimate into perspective, the mean duration of Phase III trials for antiinfective agents during the same period was almost half as long at 28.7 mo (2.4 yr). Likewise, the mean length of Phase I and II trials in oncology during the same time were considerably shorter.

The length of Phase III trials contributes to the overall long duration of antineoplastic drug development and at the same time cuts into the patent life of the drug, and the expected return on investment once approval is granted. Based on a study from the Tufts Center for the Study of Drug Development, the mean time from synthesis to FDA approval for antineoplastics approved between 1990 and 1999 was 16.2 yr, making them by far the most time consuming drugs to develop of any therapeutic class (6). Of this 16.2 yr, 4.4 was spent in preclinical development, 10.4 in clinical development, and 1.4 under FDA evaluation. These times can be compared to 13.7 yr of total development time for cardiovascular drugs, with 2.6, 8.8, and 2.3 yr spend in preclinical development, clinical development, and FDA review, respectively. Because of an agreement of the Tuft's authors to publish their proprietary data in aggregate form only, it is not possible to provide development times for individual oncology drugs that have been approved.

2.9. Approval Times and Regulatory Issues

Despite the fact that FDA approval times for cancer drugs have shortened, an increasingly stringent regulatory environment requires more demanding, expensive, and time-consuming trials *(71)*. Specifically, requirements by institutional review boards (IRBs) and the FDA have led to growing complexity in the design, administration, and monitoring of cancer trials in addition to heightened scrutiny of the resultant data. This environment has created shorter approval phases but much longer clinical phases. For example, whereas the average total time of development (from IND filing to FDA marketing approval) increased from 5.0 yr for the seven drugs approved in the 1960s to 10.8 yr for the 20 drugs approved from 1990 to 1996, the FDA approval phase fell from 2.0 yr in the 1960s to approx 1.6 yr in the 1990s *(72)*.

The regulatory aspect of drug development is a moving target, as it is impacted by statutory changes as well as by the political environment. New developments in the approval process promise to accelerate and/or encourage drug development in oncology, and include *fast track designation, priority review, orphan drug approval*, and *accelerated approval*. *Fast track* refers to a formal mechanism of interacting with the FDA during the drug development process to seek regulatory input through scheduled meetings during development. The fast track designation is intended for agents that address an unmet need and allow for the submission of NDA applications in sections rather than all components simultaneously. *Priority review*, which also is intended for agents addressing an unmet medical need, refers to the shortened time frame that the FDA targets for reviewing a completed application. As compared to the standard 10-mo target for FDA action from time of submission of a completed application, priority status resets the target date for FDA action at 6 mo. *Orphan drug approvals* are available for drugs intended to treat diseases affecting fewer than 200,000 people in the United States. These approvals have the same approval standards and time frames as the other reviews but allow for a longer period of marketing exclusivity. Lastly, *accelerated approval* (also known as Subpart H) is an FDA program that is intended to make promising products for life-threatening diseases available on the basis of preliminary evidence such as surrogate markers (e.g., response rates) prior to formal demonstration of patient benefit (e.g., survival advantage). By FDA mandate, accelerated approvals are qualified, and require postmarketing trials that have survival or quality of life endpoints. Of the 11 drugs approved to date using the accelerated approval mechanism, only 3 (capecitabine, docetaxel, and irinotecan) have fulfilled the obligation to provide follow-up studies demonstrating survival benefit for full approval *(26)*. Table 2 provides a compilation of the endpoints underlying FDA approval, the registration strategy employed by the sponsor, and the 2001 sales revenues for the major anticancer drug approved from 1996 through 2001.

3.SUCCESS RATES AND GOALS OF PHASE III CANCER TRIALS

A problem well-stated is a problem half solved.

—*Charles Kettering*

3.1. Clinical Phase Attrition Rates

Before discussing the specific criteria for entry into a Phase III trial, it is helpful to offer perspective on the historical attrition rates of novel agents in each phase of clinical development. Given the impressive cost, duration, and commitment that Phase III trials require, it is not surprising that clinical research on the vast majority of new agents is terminated prior to their evaluation in a pivotal Phase III trial. Success rates for all new chemical entities that entered clinical trials (in all therapeutic classes) from 1981 to 1992 have been reviewed *(7)*.

Table 2
Recent Approval Characteristics of Selected Antineoplastic

Generic name (trade name; distributor)	Treatment indication	Approval date	Highest phase on which approval was originally based [a]	Major endpoint(s)	Accelerated approval for original indication?	Randomized Phase IV studies required?	Priority review? (approx FDA approval time)	Additional indications?	Estimated market size for yr 2001 [b] (millions)
Docetaxel (Taxotere; Aventis)	Locally advanced or metastatic breast cancer that has progressed during anthracycline-base treatment.	05/1996	Phase II	Tumor response	Yes	Yes	Yes (21 mo)	Yes, metastatic NSCLC	$689
Gemcitabine (Gemzar; Eli Lilly)	First-line treatment of locally advanced or metastatic pancreatic cancer and second-line treatment for pancreatic cancer patients previously treated with 5-FU	05/1996	Phase III	Clinical benefit; survival	No	No	Yes (12 mo)	Yes, advanced lung cancer	$723
Topotecan (Hycamtin; Glaxo Smith Kline)	Treatment of metastatic ovarian cancer after failure of first-line chemotherapy	05/1996	Phase III	Tumor response; survival	No	Yes	Yes (5 mo)	Yes, second-line SCLC	Not available from primary sources
Irinotecan (Camptosar; Pharmacia & Upjohn)	Metastatic carcinoma of the colon or rectum that has progressed/recurred after treatment with 5-FU	06/1996	Phase II	Tumor Response	Yes	Yes	Yes (6 mo)	Yes, first-line in metastatic colon in combination	$613
Letrozole (Femara; Novartis)	Advanced breast cancer in postmenopausal women	07/1997	Phase III	TTP, TTTF, tumor response	No	No	No (12 mo)	Yes, first-line in metastatic ER/PR+ positive breast	Not available from primary sources

Drug (Trade name; Company)	Indication	Date	Phase	Endpoint				Price
Rituximab (Rituxan; Genentech)	Relapsed or refractory low-grade or follicular, B-cell non-Hodgkin's lymphoma	11/1997	Phase II	Tumor response	No	No	No	No	$779
Capecitabine (Xeloda; Roche)	Metastatic breast cancer resistant to both paclitaxel and an anthracycline regimen or for whom further anthracycline therapy may be contraindicated	04/1998	Phase II	Tumor response	Yes	Yes	Yes (6 mo) colon cancer	Yes, metastatic currency	$170 Required conversion from CHF[b]
Trastuzumab (Herceptin; Genentech)	Certain breast cancer patients who have tried chemotherapy with little success or as a first-line treatment for metastatic disease when used in combination with paclitaxel	09/1998	Phase III	Tumor response; survival	No	No	No	No	$346
Temozolomide (Temodar; Schering-Plough)	Refractory anaplastic astrocytoma (i.e., patients who have progressed on regimen containing nitrosourea and procarbazine)	08/1999	Phase II	Tumor response	Yes	Yes	Yes (6 mo)	No	$180
Epirubicin (Ellence; Pharmacia & Upjohn)	Component of adjuvant therapy in patients with evidence of axillary node tumor involvement following resection of primary breast cancer	09/1999	Phase III	Survival	No	No	Yes (9 mo)	No	$261
Exemestane (Aromasin; Pharmacia & Upjohn)	Advanced breast cancer in postmenopausal women whose disease has progressed following tamoxifen therapy	10/1999	Phase III	Survival	No	No	Yes (10 mo)	No	$47

Continued on next page

Table 2 (Continued)
Recent Approval Characteristics of Selected Antineoplastic

Generic name (trade name; distributor)	Treatment indication	Approval date	Highest phase on which approval was originally based [a]	Major endpoint(s)	Accelerated approval for original indication?	Randomized Phase IV studies required?	Priority review? (approx FDA approval time)	Additional indications?	Estimated market size for yr 2001 [b] (millions)
Gemtuzumab (Mylotarg; Wyeth-Ayerst)	Patients with CD33 positive acute myeloid leukemia in first relapse who are 60 yr or older and who are not considered candidates for cytotoxic chemotherapy	05/2000	Phase II	Complete remission rates	Yes	Yes	Yes (6 mo)	No	Not available from primary sources but available from less than $50
Aresenic trioxide (Trisenox; Cell Therapeutics)	Induction of remission and consolidation in patients with acute promyelocytic leukemia who are refractory to, or have relapsed from, retinoid and anthracycline chemotherapy	10/2000	Phase II	Complete remission rates	No	No	Yes (6 mo) Approval granted 3 yr from first human testing[a]	No	Less than $10
Alemtuzumab (Campath; Millennium)	Treatment of B-cell chronic lymphocytic leukemia who have treated with alkylating agents and who have failed fludarabine therapy	05/2001	Phase II	Tumor response rates	Yes	Yes	No	No	NA
Imatinib (Gleevec; Novartis)	Treatment of chronic myeloid leukemia in blast crisis, accelerated phase, or in chronic phase failure of interferon-α therapy	05/2001	Phase I	Hematologic and cytogenetic response	Yes	Yes	Yes (2.5 mo) Approval granted 3 yr and 3 mo from first human testing[a]	Yes, gastrointestinal stromal tumors	$152 Required currency conversion from CHF[b]

[a] Aproval criteria were taken from the "Oncology Tools" section of the FDA website (available at http://www.fda.gov).
[b] All revenue data were gathered from annual reports. Where indicated, currency conversions were required using the prevailing exchange rate during 3/2002.

Of the drugs that did not receive marketing approval in this interval, terminations occurred during or immediately after Phase II trials for slightly more than 50%. Another 30–40% of the terminations occurred during or immediately after Phase I trials. The remaining terminations (approx 10%) occurred during Phase III trials or during a failed FDA review. These data establish that clinical development on the great majority of drugs entering clinical testing will terminate prior to a their entering a Phase III trial.

3.2. Success Rates of Phase III Trials

3.2.1. INDUSTRY-SPONSORED TRIALS

The selectivity used to choose the agents that are tested in Phase III trials enriches for success during Phase III trials and subsequent NDA submission. Because of this selectivity, the majority (78%) of all industry-sponsored drugs (in all therapeutic categories) that enter these trials will ultimately go on to receive FDA marketing approval for at least one indication (7). Success rates for Phase III industry-sponsored trials specific to oncology have not been reviewed, but their success rate is likely to be somewhat less than the 78% figure calculated for the aggregate. This prediction is based on two facts. First, antineoplastic drugs have had among the lowest overall success rates of marketing approval, with only 16% of antineoplastics entering industry-sponsored Phase I trials from 1981 to 1992 ultimately receiving FDA approval (7). Second, FDA data show that since 1995, only 75–80% of oncology-related NDAs *submitted to the FDA* ultimately received marking approval (73). Therefore unless every oncology-related NCE that entered a Phase III trial was submitted for FDA review, the percentage of antineoplastics that enter Phase III trials and then go on to obtain FDA approval is less than the 78% figure calculated for NCEs in all therapeutic classes. The current rate of antineoplastic development translates into approximately three to five oncology-related NCE approvals per year (12). It will be interesting to monitor the success rates of antineoplastics over the nest several years to see if the number of oncology-related approvals will increase in proportion to the increasingly sophisticated and targeted nature of drug discovery for cancer.

3.2.2. TRIALS SPONSORED PRIMARILY BY INSTITUTIONS AND COOPERATIVE GROUPS

Several recent studies have evaluated the success of Phase III trials sponsored primarily by non-industry groups. A recent analysis examining 33 Phase III trials in advanced stage-non-small-cell lung cancer sponsored by North American Cooperative Groups or institutions over a 22-yr period revealed that only 5 (15%) of the 33 trials found a statistically significant prolongation in survival for one of the treatment arms (74). A similar study in small-cell lung cancer trials found that only 5 (24%) of 21 phase III studies from 1972 to 1990 identified a treatment arm with survival benefit. For the aggregate, the success rate of Phase III trials in oncology appears somewhat better. Of the 529 Phase III trials with more than 200 patients published between 1989 and 1998 in the *Proceeding of the American Society of Clinical Oncology* (of which only 18% identified an industry sponsor), the treatment arm showed a statistically significant ($p < 0.05$) improvement over the control arm in the trial's primary endpoint (usually survival or TTP) in slightly less than half (44%) of the trials (75,76). Reassuringly, there have been remarkably few trials in which the outcome in the investigational arm(s) has been inferior. Overall, these relatively disappointing results have prompted questioning of the process by which industry and non-industry sponsors choose agents to be tested in Phase III trials, and suggestions to improve the choices of these agents are now being offered (77; see Subheading 4.).

3.3. Goals of Phase III Trials

3.3.1. INDUSTRY SPONSORS

It is critical that the goals are clearly defined before a Phase III trial is undertaken. It is only through defining specific goals and asking definitive questions that the ultimate result of a Phase III trial can be assessed. For industry sponsors, the intent of a Phase III trial is almost always to achieve one of three goals: (1) to gain marketing approval for an agent's first treatment indication; (2) to change physician use for an already approved drug, independent of marketing approval; or (3) to achieve an additional marketing indication for an approved drug. Although off-label drug use (i.e., using drugs for indications other than those approved by the FDA) of chemotherapy is prevalent in oncology (78), pharmaceutical representatives are prohibited from commenting on unapproved indications of their drugs. Because of these marketing restrictions, pharmaceutical companies weigh the costs of trying to achieve additional marketing indications against the expected additional revenue from being able to market actively for those indications.

3.3.2. NON-INDUSTRY SPONSORS

For non-industry sponsors (e.g., cooperative groups), the goals of Phase III trials are not financially driven because the sponsors do not have a financial stake in the trials. Rather, the investigators seek to improve the standard of care for a particular disease, often by comparing combinations of already approved drugs and/or treatment modalities. It is imperative that these cooperative group trials begin by asking an important question. If the most interesting anticipated outcome is not particularly helpful to the field, then the trial is not likely to be worth the effort (79). The usual endpoint of these trials is improvement in survival, although other goals such as reduction in toxicity, quality of life, sparing of surgical removal of an organ, or "clinical benefit" may be used as primary or secondary endpoints. The recently published randomized trial run by the Eastern Cooperative Oncology Group comparing four doublet chemotherapy regimens for advanced non-small-cell lung cancer (38) is a good example of a cooperative group sponsored trial.

4. CRITERIA FOR ENTERING INTO A PHASE III TRIAL: A DECISION MODEL

Destiny...is not a matter of chance, it is a matter of choice; it is not a thing to be Waited for, it is a thing to be achieved.

—Williams Jennings Bryan

The previous sections have described in general terms the benefits and drawbacks of Phase III trials, emphasizing on one hand their power through size and randomization and on the other hand their costs, ethical concerns, and complexity (Table 3). Even more fundamental, and at times more perplexing than the design and execution of a Phase III trial, is the selection of experimental treatments to be tested. There are limited resources to support the huge commitment of time, effort, and money required of these trials. Because only 2–3% of cancer patients in the United States participate in clinical trials (80), access to eligible patients can also be limiting. For these reasons, usually no more than a few Phase III studies are conducted for a given disease at any one time (81). If an important question is not asked or an agent with little promise tested, a Phase III trial, even if expertly executed, will not move the field forward and will only detract from the opportunity to ask other questions. The yield from Phase III trials can be increased from thoughtful and rigorous choices of which agents to test in them.

Table 3
Benefits and Drawbacks of Phase III Trials in Oncology

Benefits	Drawbacks
• Eliminates selection bias	• Very high cost
• Allows generalization to broad population	• Difficult to coordinate and execute
• Produces data on delayed or infrequent toxicities	• May involve ethical considerations and effect doctor–patient relationship
• May be best suited to evaluate molecularly targeted agents	• May introduce delays in drug approval
• Allows for pivotal trial design suitable for determination of eventualmarketing approval	• Has an historically high rate of failure in showing comparative benefit of new agents

Table 4
Critical Factors for Advancing to Phase III

• Unique and compelling target—not sufficient in absence of preclinical and clinical activity
• Favorable pharmacokinetics—good bioavailability if oral, long half-life, drug levels that exceed the (inhibitory) threshold by several multiples with trough levels above the threshold
• Acceptable toxicity—the less the better, especially if the drug is to be used in chronic therapy
• Evidence of strong activity—including some evidence of antitumor response in Phase II
• Potential role in treating a disease and the need for new treatments in that disease

These choices are difficult, because each agent in question is unique in its pharmacological characteristics, treatment potential, toxicity profile, and strategic role in the sponsor's portfolio. The underlying cancer biology on which the treatments are based is often incompletely understood. Making the decision even more challenging is the fact that several predictions about the future need to be made, including regulatory trends and changes in the standard of care for the disease the agent is intended to treat. Although difficult, making thoughtful decisions about which agents to test in Phase III trials is critical to our field. The skills and creativity that clinical investigators bring to this decision, in conjunction with the scientific advances, will ultimately determine the rate and quality of improvements in cancer care.

It is increasingly clear that there is no standardized or "cookie cutter" formula for making the critical Phase III "go/no go" decision. The varied properties of many of the newer MTAs, along with varied, disease-specific approval thresholds, demand an increasingly individualized developmental and registration strategy *(24,82)*. Because the decision is so complex, the Phase III "go/no go" question can be approached best by using a decision model. Our conceptual model is presented below and is intended to be applicable to any anticancer agent under development. The critical components of the model are listed in Table 4.

In the broadest sense, the question that must be answered by a decision model is whether the expected benefit from a Phase III trial exceeds the large investment in time and resources required for its design, execution, and follow-up. The criteria with which to answer this question can be grouped into five important considerations unique to each agent in question.

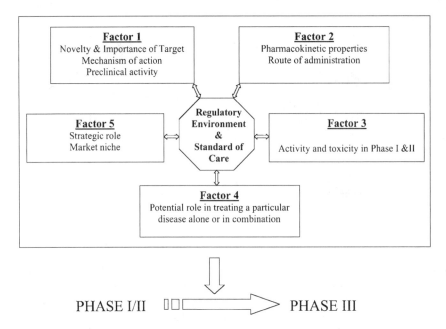

Fig. 3. Schematic view of the Phase III decision model. (From ref. *128*, with permission.)

These include the agent's (1) novelty of mechanism of action and preclinical evidence for activity; (2) pharmacokinetic properties in developmental (Phase I and II) trials; (3) activity and toxicity in developmental trials; (4) potential role in treating a disease either alone or in combination; and (5) strategic value to the sponsor and potential market niche. For each agent, certain factors will take precedence in the "go/no go" decision, but none should be considered in isolation. Agents or treatments that rank highly in all of these critical areas should be preferentially chosen for testing in Phase III trials. Those agents with poor rankings in one or more of the above criteria should not be advanced to Phase III testing, or done so with due circumspection. For those drugs under consideration for testing in Phase III registration trials, their merits must be further judged against the backdrop of the evolving standard of care and prevailing regulatory environment (Fig. 3). The individual components of the model are discussed in detail below.

4.1. The Five Factors of the Phase III Decision Model

4.1.1. FACTOR I: THE MECHANISM OF ACTION AND PRECLINICAL ACTIVITY

4.1.1.1. The Mechanism of Action

Because most cancer drug development is now focused on modulating molecular targets, the importance of the agent's intended molecular target and how well it is engaged are critical components of the Phase III decision model. Targeted therapy represents a departure from the classical, empirical paradigm of cancer drug discovery. Under the old paradigm, cytotoxic drugs typically were discovered through screening thousands of molecules to find those that had activity against tumor cells growing in tissue culture or in animals. Once a lead compound was identified, its structure was optimized and the best schedule of administration established. The major preclinical endpoint was evidence of tumor regression in animal models, which inconsistently correlated with tumor response in humans.

Subsequent decisions regarding which cytotoxic agents to test in Phase III trials were based on whether a threshold of activity was achieved in Phase II trials with an agent that had an acceptable toxicity profile and satisfactory PKs. The agent's mechanism of action and preclinical activity also influenced these decisions, as testing drugs with unique or new mechanisms of action (e.g., topoisomerase inhibitor) were favored over those with established or less specific mechanisms (e.g., alkylator). Likewise, the primary way to generate interest in a second-in-a-class drug was to show a lack of cross-resistance with the first agent in preclinical models. Yet, because the drugs were cytotoxic and their activity could be evaluated in Phase II trials, these factors were often less influential in deciding whether to test an agent in Phase III compared to the actual results of the Phase II experience.

The remarkable gains in knowledge in the understanding of molecular biology over the last 20 yr have led to the ability to move away from the empirical paradigm and toward specific molecular targets. An inflection point may have already been reached with respect to deriving additional utility from cytotoxic chemotherapy in the treatment of the most cancers (83). For these reasons, the majority of potential cancer drugs under development have novel mechanisms of action and are targeted to specific molecules thought to be germane to the pathogenesis of cancer (84). With the emergence of this approach, the perceived importance of the target has become distinctly more influential to the "go/no go" decision and in some cases provides a major impetus to proceed to a pivotal Phase III trial.

Prioritizing which agents to test in Phase III trials on the basis of the perceived importance of the molecular target is a daunting task. Few targets have been adequately validated in human systems. The presence of redundant and compensatory cellular pathways, innate and acquired drug resistance, and heterogeneous and genetically unstable tumors can all decrease the clinical utility of a particular drug target (85). The sheer number and classes of potential drug targets can overwhelm the scientist and the clinical investigator alike.

Defining what makes a target "important" and offering a framework to classify mechanism of action can clarify the process of selecting targets. For the purposes of the Phase III decision model, a target is considered "important" if it is (1) uniquely or markedly overexpressed in specific type of cancer (i.e., tumor specific); (2) physiologically active in the given clinical setting (i.e., active at a time when treatment can be initiated); and (3) essential for the survival of the cancer in question (i.e., rate limiting), but not essential for the survival of normal tissues. Applying these criteria can help limit the number of targets on which to concentrate. Whereas the number of genetic mutations that are present in an average tumors is thought to exceed 10,000 (86), the number of "important" mutations that are required for tumorigenesis and that meet the criteria presented above is likely to be much lower (in the range of 5–10) for each individual tumor (87,88). Therefore, with all other factors being equal, an agent should be prioritized for Phase III testing to the extent that its target fulfills the three criteria listed above.

No target exists in isolation. Because the effective treatment of most advanced cancers will likely require engaging multiple targets at various times, it is useful to categorize the large number of targets into a mechanistic framework. One approach is to collate molecular targets around the acquired capabilities likely shared by most (if not all) cancer cells (89). These include (1) self-sufficiency in growth signals, (2) evasion of apoptosis, (3) limitless replicative potential, (4) sustained angiogenesis, and (5) tissue invasion and metastasis. Each of these acquired capabilities contains its own growing set of cellular pathways and potential drug targets. Some of the more prominent targets and their corresponding drugs under development are shown in Table 5. Targeting each of these capabilities will likely be important to a greater or lesser degree for each tumor type and disease stage. For example, early in the course of a myeloproliferative disorder, targeting growth signal autonomy or

Table 5
Examples of Drug Targets Under Investigation

Acquired capability	Potential drug targets	Drugs under investigation
Self-sufficiency in growth signals	Upregulated EGFR Tumor production of PDGF	Tarceva, Iressa, Gleevec
Evasion of apoptosis	Bcl-2 IGF-1	Genasense
Limitless replicative potential	Telomerase	None yet in clinical trials
Susatained angiogenesis	VEGF and its receptor	Many
Tissue invasion and metastasis	MMPs	Many

EGFR, Epidermal growth factor receptor; PDGF, platelet derived growth factor; IGF-1, insulin-like growth factor-1; VEGF, vascular endothelial growth factor; MMP, matrix metalloproteinase.

evasion of apoptosis may have the greatest treatment utility. It follows that agents that inhibit targets that contribute to these capabilities should therefore be preferentially chosen for Phase III testing for individuals with early disease. In contrast, the greatest clinical utility in the treatment of advanced pancreatic cancer may be derived from targeting angiogenesis or metastasis, as these capabilities may become rate limiting for disease progression late in the disease course. Effective control of some tumors such as advanced non-small cell lung cancer may require simultaneous modulation of multiple targets within several (or even all) of these acquired capabilities.

It is important to be clear about whether the target is "important" before proceeding to Phase III testing, especially for the MTAs. Sometimes the target can be so tantalizing that an enormous amount of clinical development is undertaken before adequate validation of the target and mechanism of action has been accomplished, as was the case with matrix metalloproteinase (MMP) inhibitors (90). At least five MMP inhibitors advanced to late stages of development before the precise role of various MMPs in cancer progression was known. Of the 15 Phase III trials undertaken with these agents, none has shown a significant survival benefit, and two of them have shown poorer survival as compared to placebo (90). The MMP experience can be contrasted with the development of imatinib mesylate for CML. The role of bcr–abl kinase, imatinib mesylate's target in CML, was rigorously characterized prior to the drug's clinical development. The bcr–abl kinase is an activated oncogene product that can be detected in virtually all patients with the CML. It is sufficient to cause the disease and absolutely required to sustain it. Its normal counterpart, the abl kinase, is found in nonmalignant tissues, but it is not critical to normal physiology. When this target is inhibited in tissue culture experiments, the malignant cells die but normal bone marrow cells do not. Thus the target fulfills all three of the above criteria and is therefore deemed important. The importance of the target coupled with imatinib mesylate's own pharmacological merits contributed to the fact that it was approved for marketing on the basis of Phase I/II data in just over 3 yr from its initial testing in humans, requiring < 3 mo under FDA review. Although it is uncertain whether other targets as important as the bcr–abl kinase will be identified in most cancers, its properties make it a standard against which other molecular targets can be measured, as they are considered for preferential testing in pivotal trials.

After determining the importance of a target and placing it in the mechanistic framework described in the preceding, the next issue that should be addressed is whether the agent effectively engages the target. Because it is vastly easier to inhibit an aberrantly overexpressed function than it is to restore a deleted or underexpressed function, most targets under investigation represent dominant or overexpressed functions within cancer cells *(91)*. The basic strategy for most MTAs involves inhibiting these aberrantly expressed functions. For example, the production of platelet-derived growth factor (PDGF) by glioblastomas represents an acquired property that may be exploited in a drug development strategy. Imatinib mesylate, a small-molecule inhibitor of the PDGF receptor as well as of the bcr–abl kinase, is now being evaluated in clinical trials for patients with glioblastomas. Advances in gene therapy technology may some day allow for the restoration of deleted function (e.g., tumor suppressor genes such as *p53*), but these approaches have thus far been disappointing. Classes of drugs that have been used for inhibitory purposes include small molecules, monoclonal antibodies, antisense oligonucleotides, and natural products, to name a few. Each type of specific targeting agent has it particular advantages and limitations that must be considered throughout the development process. These issues are beyond the scope of this chapter but are discussed in detail throughout the rest of this volume.

With regard to inhibitors, the two specific issues that must be addressed are the agent's potency and selectivity. Agents that do not engage their targets at sufficiently low concentrations (i.e., IC_{50} in the low nanomolar range for most inhibitors) typically should not be chosen for late-stage clinical testing. Rather, attempts should be made to identify more potent inhibitors. The agent's specificity is equally important in the decision model, but its role is not as straightforward. Greater target specificity is generally favored, as it broadly correlates with decreased toxicity. The epidermal growth factor (EGFR) inhibitor OSI-774 (Tarceva) is a example of an potent and selective inhibitor with an IC_{50} of 20 n*M* and an approx 1000-fold greater specificity for its receptor compared to other kinases. These properties allow for almost complete inhibition of OSI-774's target at drug levels that are associated with minimal toxicity *(92)*. In some cases, however, some lack of target specificity can be exploited in the development of a drug, as long as it does not lead to unacceptable toxicity. Agents that inhibit multiple targets may either be more effective in treating a particular tumor or may be used to treat multiple tumor types. Imatinib mesylate, for example, inhibits three targets: bcr–abl, c-kit, and the PDGF receptor. Different targets provide the mechanism of action for its established role in CML (bcr–abl) and gastrointestinal stromal tumors (c-kit) but also the rationale for clinical investigation in several other tumor types such as prostate cancer and glioblastoma, which are thought to be driven by overexpression of PDGF.

The number of potential targets will undoubtedly grow in number and quality as genomics and proteomics research defines additional pathways of tumorigenesis and tumor progression *(93,94)*. The exciting recent report of somatic missense mutations of the *BRAF* gene (an *RAF* gene), which are present in 66% of malignant melanomas and at lower frequency in several other human cancers *(95)*, illustrates the point. In this work, genomic DNA from cancer cell lines and from corresponding matched lymphoblastoid cell lines from the same individuals was screened for sequence variants of the *BRAF* gene between the individual's tumor cells and the normal tissues. A single-base substitution on exon 15 was found in the melenoma cell lines that led to elevated kinase activity of the mutated BRAF protein. Remarkably, this mutated protein was capable of transforming NIH3T3 cells. For those individuals with the mutation, these data define the mutant BRAF protein as a potential target, although its role in promoting proliferation of human tumor cells in vivo has not been established. Not surprisingly, these data have already prompted efforts to develop small molecule inhibitors of the mutated protein.

4.1.1.2. Preclinical Activity

The next component in the Phase III Decision Model involves evaluating the agent's preclinical activity. Cytotoxic and molecularly targeted agents require separate strategies for this purpose. For cytotoxic agents, the first evidence of preclinical activity is typically sought through incubation of agents with established tumor cell lines. Testing agents in combination is performed routinely to determine whether they display antagonism, additivity, or synergy. Tests of activity and toxicity of the new agent in rodent tumor models (alone or in combination with other agents) then follow. Two of the most commonly used rodent models include the hollow fiber (HF) assay and the human tumor xenograft model. The HF model is utilized mainly for screening purposes, in which 12 different tumor cell lines from tissue culture are introduced into hollow glass or plastic chambers in the intraperitoneal or subcutaneous space of mice and are then exposed to test agents at two doses. Antiproliferative activity is then determined by retrieving the fibers and assaying cell mass. A complex scoring system for agents tested in this model has been created, with the basis being that its application to the selected cell lines would have resulted in the detection of 95% of the currently available cytotoxics *(84)*.

Agents that show activity in the HF model are usually advanced to testing in the human xenograft models, as increasing intraperitoneal hollow fiber activity has been shown to correlate with subsequent activity in the human xenograft models *(96)*. These xenograft models are created by injecting or transplanting human cancer cells into immunocompromised (nude) mice and then using the mice to test the agent's activity. The tissue can be introduced intravenously, subcutaneously, or even orthotopically at a common site of metastasis. The important limitation of these nude mice models is that they do not recapitulate host–tumor interactions because of the immunocompromised state of the mice. To model these host–tumor interactions, transgenic mice that develop *de novo* cancers are being developed to test cytotoxic agents, but their ability to predict clinical efficacy has yet to be established *(97)*.

Unfortunately, a strong correlation has not been found between cytotoxic activity in a particular histology in the tumor models and subsequent efficacy in clinical trials of the same human cancer histology. However, for agents with activity in at least one third of the xenograft models, there does seem to be a correlation with at least some subsequent clinical efficacy *(96)*. The comparative preclinical activity of the oral fluoropyrimidines capecitabine (Xeloda) and UFT is illustrative. Capecitabine, which ultimately showed equivalence to intravenous flourouracil plus leucovorin in two Phase III trials, was effective (defined as > 50% growth inhibition) in 18 of 24 xenograft models (75%) and achieved FDA approval for first-line treatment of colorectal cancer. In comparison, UFT, another orally active fluoropyrimidine, showed activity in only 5 of 24 models (21%) and subsequently did not meet FDA standards for equivalence to flourouracil plus leucovorin in its pivotal trials. There are clearly exceptions to these rules, and the preclinical assessment of activity for cytotoxic agents should be used predominantly to guide *early* development.

MTAs that are not cytotoxic require an alternative strategy to define their preclinical activity. Most MTAs that have proceeded to clinical trials have inhibited tumor growth in mouse models designed to provide proof of concept regarding the putative mechanism of action. The preclinical goals of the MTAs include establishing the importance of the target to tumorigensesis and demonstrating in vivo target engagement and downstream biological and molecular effects. This information can be very useful in helping to make the decision to test an agent in a Phase III trial particularly if the agent is cytostatic and not clearly effective in Phase II testing. Preclinical evidence of anti-tumor activity is critical to the go-ahead decision. At present, evaluation of many targeted agents can not be met by using the standard preclinical models designed for cytotoxic agents. Instead, each new agent may require unique genetically engineered mouse (GEM) models. The technological progress in this field has been astonishing *(97)*. For example, GEM models now exist in which tetracycline-based inducible systems can be used to turn on or off the expression of almost any target of interest. Somatic mutations can also be engineered to be preferentially expressed in specific tissues. This approach was used to express activated k-*ras* in lung epithelium of mice, leading to the predisposition of those mice to develop non-small-cell lung cancer *(98)*. This model is ideally suited to for the preclinical testing of k-*ras* inhibitors to determine if they can prevent or delay the development or progression of the endogenous lung cancer. While these models are largely unvalidated in terms of their ability to subsequently predict clinical response, they will undoubtedly provide the basis for most preclinical testing of the MTAs. As an indication of their perceived importance, the NCI established the mouse models of human cancer consorium (MMHCC; http://emice.nci.nih.gov/) in 1999 to fund research and maintain comprehensive databases on these GEM models.

The preclinical activity of a standard cytotoxic agent typically holds less influence regarding whether to take it to Phase III testing as compared to its activity in Phase II trials. For the MTAs, in contrast, preclinical activity may hold as much or greater influence in decisions about late-stage testing for three reasons. First, the preclinical activity can provide the most powerful validation of the target and mechanism of action. Second, because some MTAs are not cytotoxic when used alone, response in Phase II may not be an appropriate endpoint, and the decision to advance to Phase III trials may need to be based on the knowledge that when satisfactory pharmacokinetics are achieved in animal models, the drug exerts its intended biological effect *(17)*. Some evidence of biological effects in humans, and particularly a low level of clinical tumor response, have supported most but not all decisions to proceed to Phase III. This was the case with ZD1839 (Iressa) and trastuzumab (Herceptin), in which the decisions to undergo Phase III testing were based primarily on the novelty of the mechanism, importance of the target, established preclinical activity, and favorable PKs in the setting of limited single-agent activity (10–20%) in developmental trials. Third, decisions regarding which agents to use in combination for late-stage development can often be worked out most efficiently in the preclinical setting. Most MTAs will be used in combination with standard cytotoxics, as many of them lower the apoptotic threshold of standard cytotoxics. This concept is illustrated by the pro-apoptotic agent Bcl-2 antisense (Genasence), which has been shown to increase substantially the activity of standard chemotherapy in multiple tumor cell line and rodent models *(99,100)*, and is now being tested in Phase III combination trials with these agents.

4.1.2. Factor II: Pharmacokinetic Properties in Phase I and II Trials

The PK of oncology drugs under investigation act as a bridge integrating data from preclinical testing through the early clinical trials *(101)*. PK properties (e.g., bioavailability, peak and trough concentrations, area under the curve, clearance, half-life) determine the appropriate route of administration, treatment schedule, and dose to be used in later trials *(84)*. As such, these properties represent a critical component of the Phase III Decision Model. Favorable PK properties include (1) high percentage and consistent bioavailabilty, if oral; (2) a long half-life (i.e., > 8 h, which allows for once per day dosing of oral agents); and (3) drug levels at a trough that exceeds the threshold dose needed to inhibit the target in preclinical experiments. These properties are necessary but not sufficient in deciding to test an agent in a Phase III trial. All things being equal, however, favorable PKs in Phase I and II testing are essential to the decision to proceed with Phase III testing.

For most MTAs, prolonged and continuous target inhibition will likely be required to inhibit tumor progression. Because of the inconvenience of using intravenous infusion pumps, these agents will be administered orally. While oral chemotherapy appears to be preferred by patients *(102,103)* and may be associated with pharmacoeconomic *(104)* and quality-of-life advantages, its large-scale application raises issues of drug compliance *(105)*, variability in bioavailability, and drug–drug interactions. Many oral chemotherapy agents display small intrapatient and interpatient variability in drug levels at low drug doses but substantially more when higher doses are employed. This variability may be dangerous when the therapeutic window is narrow, as is the case with oral etoposide *(106)*, but may be less threatening for an MTA such as ZD1839 (Iressa), which has a wider therapeutic window.

During the preclinical and early clinical development periods, it is critical to find dosing schedules that produce drug levels that sustain activity during trough periods and maintain selectivity during peak periods. The PK properties of OSI-774 (Tarceva) demonstrate the principle. Based on the pharmacodynamic studies in animals (corrected for interspecies differences in protein binding), OSI-774 plasma concentrations of 0.5 μg/m: were estimated to be the threshold required to inhibit tumor proliferation sufficiently. In the Phase I trial, on a daily dosing regimen, all but one patient achieved steady-state minimum plasma concentrations at the MTD that exceeded the 0.5 μg/mL threshold; and, the average steady-state plasma concentration at the MTD was more than twice the threshold value *(92)*. These data, together with the drug's toxicity profile, demonstrated that the agent could be given on a daily, uninterrupted dose schedule that was well tolerated and that achieved and sustained biologically relevant drug concentrations. Based on the importance of the target, favorable PKs, and modest evidence of antitumor activity in non-small-cell lung cancer, OSI-774 was chosen for Phase III testing.

4.1.3. Factor III: Activity and Toxicity in Phase I and II Trials

The activity and toxicity seen in the Phase I and II experiences represent the third component of the Phase III Decision Model. Most agents that have an acceptable toxicity and favorable PK profile in Phase I trials will undergo further efficacy testing in Phase II. For the MTAs, simultaneous Phase I/II trials in combination with selected cytotoxic agents may be initiated in parallel with single-agent Phase II to take advantage of synergy observed in preclinical studies. Among their several advantages, Phase II trials allow verification of dose and schedule before advancing to a definitive Phase III effort and provide concrete evidence of target inhibition and hopefully antitumor activity. The results from these early efficacy trials, even among MTAs, still exert a great influence in terms of choosing which agents to advance to Phase III.

When overwhelming activity is noted during the Phase II trial in an otherwise untreatable disease (e.g., imatinib mesylate in gastrointestinal stromal tumor), Phase III trials are unnecessary for approval. When this situation is not present, the decision to advance to Phase III rests at least in part on whether an agent's activity (alone or in combination) in Phase I and II trials exceeds a threshold as compared to the standard treatments. There are several measurements of activity that can be employed for this purpose.

4.1.3.1. Pharmacodynamic and Therapeutic Effects in Phase I and II Trials

Increasingly, attempts are made to demonstrate target engagement in humans by measuring biochemical markers in tissues during early clinical development. This approach was used during the Phase I trial of the small molecule farnesyltransferase inhibitor (FTI) SCH66336. In this study, buccal mucosal cells were sampled during treatment and assayed for the presence of prelamin A, a polypeptide whose processing is dependent on farnesylation.

Before treatment with the FTI, prelamin A was not detected in buccal mucosal cells because of its farnesylation and subsequent cellular processing. With increasing doses of the FTI, a dose-dependent increase in the percentage of patients with detectable levels of non-farncsylated prelamin A was found, with five out of five patients having detectable levels of the nonfarnesylated protein at the second highest dose of 350 mg of SCH6636 *(107)*. This work represented the first demonstration of in vivo inhibition of farnesyl protein transferase in human.

In another example of evaluating in vivo target engagement, skin biopsies were obtained from cancer patients undergoing treatment with the EGFR inhibitor ZD1839 (Iressa). The investigators demonstrated during a Phase I trial that ZD1839 could thin the stratum corneum, suppress EGFR phosphorylation in all EGFR-expressing cells, and increase expression of markers of maturation and apoptotis *(108)*. Importantly, these changes occurred even at doses several times lower than the MTD of 850–1000 mg/d. In both of these case, these data helped the sponsoring companies choose the dose to use in later-stage testing and added assurance that large investments in Phase III trials were justifiable in terms of safety *(82,107,108)*.

Unfortunately, several issues currently limit the widespread application of these pharmacodynamic approaches to assess biological activity. First, the target tissue in question is often not readily available except through repeated, invasive biopsies. To avert this problem, efforts are currently underway to collect circulating tumor cells that have derived from the tumor using genetic and immunologic probes. Second, if the drug has activity mediated through a target other than the one hypothesized, the molecular test will not provide useful information. Third, there has generally not been adequate clinical validation in regard to whether target engagement assessed through these approaches will correlate with clinically relevant endpoints such as survival or quality of life. Whereas these issues represent an area under active investigation, standard criteria with which to gauge activity such as response rates can still be very useful.

4.1.3.2. Response Rates

Response rates are relevant for cytotoxic drugs and for MTAs that are either used in combination with standard cytotoxics or that are pro-apoptotic. Response rates are usually not helpful in evaluating agents that have growth inhibition as their primary mechanism of action as (i.e., cytostatic agents). That said, there has yet to be an oncology drug approved in the Untied States, excluding supportive and facilitating agents (e.g., leucovorin), that did not show at least some single-agent antitumor response in a developmental trial *(109)*. Evaluating antineoplastic drugs by response rates as a surrogate to clinical benefit relies on the prediction that tumor shrinkage will lead to either lengthened survival, the unambiguous measure of efficacy, or improved quality of life *(110)*. Although this prediction appears to hold true for hematological malignancies, the correlation of response rates in Phase II trials to survival in Phase III in solid tumors is unpredictable and appears to vary by tumor. If the duration of response is brief or if the percentage of response is low, there may not be any increase in median survival in a Phase III trial. Even with the consistent application of prospective response criteria, such as the RECIST criteria defined by the NCI, response rates can be misleading. Because patient selection and clinician bias can affect response rates, response rates should be interpreted cautiously when deciding whether to test an agent in Phase III *(26,111,112)*.

The reason for the historical failure of many drugs in late-stage testing is that Phase III trials are often initiated on agents based on positive Phase II trials (compared to historical controls) performed in highly selected patients *(77,111)*. This point is well illustrated in an

Table 6
Drugs and Indications Approved Using Accelerated Approval Based on Response Rates

Drug	Indications
Amifostine (Ethyol)	Reduction in platinum toxicity in non-small-cell lung cancer
Capecitabine (Xeloda)	Refractory metastatic breast cancer
Celecoxib (Celebrex)	Reduction of polyp number in familial adenomatous polyposis
Liposomal cytarabine (DepoCyt)	Lymphomatous meningitis
Dexrazoxane (Zinecard)	Cardioprotection during anthracycline treatment
Docetaxel (Taxotere)	Second-line metastatic breast cancer
Liposomal doxorubicin (Doxil)	AIDS related Kaposi's sarcoma and refractory ovarian cancer
Gemtuzumab (Mylotarg)	Acute myelogenous leukemia
Imatinib mesylate (Gleevec)	Chronic myelogenous leukemia and GIST
Irinotecan (Camptosar)	Second-line metastatic colon cancer
Temozolamide (Temodar)	Second-line anaplastic astrocytoma

analysis of 21 Phase III trials of extensive-stage small-cell lung cancer initiated from 1972 through 1990. Most of the treatment regimens were chosen for Phase III testing based on an apparently positive Phase II result, but very few of the chosen treatments demonstrated a survival advantage in Phase III. Response rates in the Phase II trials were compared to median survival in the corresponding Phase III trials. Interestingly, no significant correlation between the two was found (77). In fact the only predictor of a Phase III survival benefit for the treatment arm over the control arm was the overall survival time in the preceding Phase II trial.

Even within Phase III trials, there may be little correlation between response rates and survival. A recent meta-analysis of 25 randomized trials in advanced colorectal cancer treated with fluoropyrimidine-based regimens showed that in the aggregate there was a very weak (although significant) correlation between response rates and survival (113). To improve the predictive ability of response rates, some investigators attempted compare survival of responders to that of nonresponders to make inferences regarding efficacy. This is a flawed approach, however, because patients who live long enough to have a response are likely to live longer irrespective of whether the treatment is effective or not (114).

In recent years, the FDA has devoted attention to whether approval can be based on surrogate markers such as response rate. In 1996 the FDA's accelerated approval program for investigational cancer treatments stated that, for many cancer therapies, the use of objective evidence of tumor shrinkage is an appropriate basis for accelerated approval (72). To make the approval full, however, the company must perform additional trials with "due diligence" to show evidence of survival advantage and improved quality of life in the postmarketing setting (28). The opportunity for accelerated approval is limited to specific malignancies for which no effective treatment currently exists. Agents such as irinotecan in colon cancer and docetaxel in breast cancer originally received accelerated approval by demonstrating meaningful response rates as second-line therapies (26). Postapproval trials subsequently demonstrated an improvement in survival. To date, 11 new drugs for 13 indications have been approved using this accelerated approval mechanism (Table 6).

As more effective treatments accumulate, gaining approval based solely on response is likely to become more difficult. This appears to have been the case for oxaliplatin subsequent to the approval of irinotecan. In the pivotal Phase III trial of oxaliplatin plus 5-fluorouracil

(5-FU)/leucovorin vs 5-FU/leucovorin as first-line treatment for advanced colorectal cancer, the overall response rate was significantly higher for the oxaliplatin arm (50% vs 22%; $p < 0.001$), but there was not a statistically significant overall survival difference *(115)*. The FDA concluded from this data that oxaliplatin should not receive marketing rights for first-line treatment of colorectal cancer because survival has become the efficacy standard in the United States for metastatic colorectal cancer. Regulatory agencies in other countries have disagreed with this action, as oxaliplatin has been approved in Europe for at least 3 yr. While the positive result is of great interest to the academic community, particularly in view of the fact that no other platinum analogue has proven activity in this disease, marketing approval for a first-line indication was not achieved. Additional testing of this agent in combination with other agents and in various schedules is now underway with promising results *(116)*. Based in part on these data, the FDA recently granted second-line approval for oxaliplatin in combination with 5-FU/leucovorin for patients with metastatic colorectal cancer who have recurred or progressed on 5-FU/leucovorin and irinotecan.

The FDA assesses not only overall response rates but also the number of complete responses, duration of responses, the reproducibility of response rates in other trials, and the history of using the response rate surrogate for the disease and class of drug in question *(111)*. In most cases, two well-conducted, positive Phase III trials are necessary to gain full marketing approval *(26)*. However, in selected cases (drug-refractory patients, rare diseases) *bona fide* complete responses in a small number of patients in Phase II trials may be sufficient for approval. For example, a small number of complete responses was the basis for approval of cladribine in hairy cell leukemia and ifosfamide for third-line testis cancer *(111)*. The question of whether to advance an agent into Phase III testing based on response rates in Phase II trials is therefore complex. The answer depends on the disease and the clinical setting in question, whether a response threshold has been eclipsed relative to the standard of care, and most important whether the agent has demonstrated a favorable therapeutic ratio (activity/toxicity).

4.1.3.3. Balancing Activity with Toxicity: The Therapeutic Ratio

For all cancer treatments under development, activity in developmental trials must be assessed in the context of toxicity. In fact, the FDA's major criterion for efficacy is evidence of patient benefit with a favorable risk–benefit profile *(26)*. To make this tradeoff visually accessible, two developmental matrices are offered to show how activity and toxicity combine to inform decisions about whether to test an agent in Phase III *(128)*. A matrix for novel cytotoxic agents is presented in Fig. 4, and an analogous one for novel MTAs is presented in Fig 5. Before providing examples of how an agent's placement on the matrix influences the Phase III "go/no go" decision, a general orientation is helpful.

Investigational treatments are placed on the matrix based on their biologic activity in developmental trials on the x-axis and relative toxicity on the y-axis. Those treatments with strong evidence of activity and modest toxicity compared to the standard of care are located toward the Southwest corner and are termed *Superstars*. Agents with less evidence of activity but still with relatively modest toxicity are located toward the southeast (Fig 4) or south (Fig. 5) and are referred to as *Incrementalists*. Those potential treatments with strong evidence of activity but with significant toxicity are termed *Trade-offs* and are located in toward the northwest corner. Lastly, the treatments that are unfortunate enough to have both little evidence of biologic activity and significant toxicity are located toward the northeast and are termed Castaways, because they are unlikely to enter further clinical testing. The matrix is useful, because the designations given to treatments under review help to determine the need for a Phase III trial.

	Large	Small
Toxicity		
Significant	**TRADE-OFFS** Attempt to circumvent toxicity Phase III usually required	**CASTAWAY** Discontinue development
Modest	**SUPERSTAR** Phase III may not be required May be approved after Phase II	**INCREMENTALIST** Consider for Phase III based on Treatment void to be filled

Fig. 4. Proposed classification matrix for novel cyotoxics.

Toxicity	Strong Evidence of Tumor Regression	Modest Evidence of Tumor Regression Good PKs Target Inhibition in Man	Only Target Inhibition	No Biological Activity
Significant	**TRADE-OFFS** Attempt to circumvent toxicity Phase III usually required	**? CASTAWAY** Consider going back to Phase I-II	**CASTAWAY** Consider going back to Phase I-II	**CASTAWAY** Discontinue development
Modest	**SUPERSTAR** Phase III may not be required May be approved after Phase II	**INCREMENTALIST** Consider for Phase III	**? INCREMENTALIST** Consider for Phase III based on Treatment void to be filled	**CASTAWAY** Discontinue development

Fig. 5. Proposed classification matrix for novel MTAs. (From ref. *128*, with permission.)

For different reasons, the *Superstar* and *Castaway* treatments tend not to enter Phase III trials. The *Superstar* classification typically refers to novel treatments with vastly improved response rates, acceptable therapeutic ratios, and little competition in the disease under investigation. Because of their impressive characteristics, these treatments may require Phase III testing for FDA approval, as they become approved (or become the standard of care) on the merits of their earlier-phase clinical testing. Examples of "Superstar" treatments among the cytotoxics include paclitaxel for platinum-resistant ovarian cancer, cladribine for hairy cell leukemia, and MOPP (merchlorethamine, vincristine, procarbazine, and prednisone) for Hodgkin's disease (HD). Because of their favorable activity and toxicity profile compared to available treatments at the time, none of these examples required a Phase III trial for FDA approval or widespread acceptance. The paradigmatic and most recent "Superstar" among the MTAs is imatinib mesylate (Gleevec) for CML and gas-trointestinal stromal tumor. As mentioned ealier, imatinib mesylate was approved by the FDA for treatment of CML in less than 3 mo without the need for Phase III data. Another example of *Superstar* MTA is the differentiating agent ATRA (Vesanoid) in the treatment of acute promyelocytic leukemia, an agent whose favorable activity and toxicity profile also allowed it to be approved without the need for a Phase III trial. The only problem with *Superstars* in the drug development process is their rarity.

In contrast to the *Superstars*, the *Castaway* treatments show little evidence of improved biologic activity for the diseases they are intended to treat and have relatively poor toxicity profiles. An example of a cytotoxic *Castaway* treatment is mitoguazone, which has a unique mechanism of action (as an inhibitor of *S*-adenosylmethionine decarboxylase) and modest activity against acute myelogenous leukemia and lymphomas *(117)*. Because its activity was not an improvement over the standard treatments at the time of development and because of unacceptable mucositis associated with its use, development was terminated *(8)*. While development on this agent was attempted to be revived for the treatment of AIDS-related non-Hodgkin lymphoma, its relatively poor activity to toxicity profile continued to limit developmental progress. For the MTAs, the MMP inhibitors mentioned above (such as Tanomastat) provide examples of *Castaways (90)*. Novel cytotoxics or MTAs that fall into the "Castaways" category are unlikely to warrant later-stage testing unless the following two conditions are met: (1) there is large market potential with little competition within that market and (2) less toxic schedules can be identified.

The other two treatment classifications, the *Incrementalists* and *Trade-offs*, typically require Phase III testing. As much as the *Superstars* are rarified, *Incrementalist* treatments represent the typical characterization of a cytotoxic agent (or an MTA in combination with cytotoxics) at the completion of Phase II testing. These treatments show promise in Phase II by both demonstrating modest biological activity with acceptable toxicity, but to a lesser extent than the *Superstars*. Because it is usually impossible to determine how much patient selection bias creates the promise demonstrated in Phase II trials, the *Incrementalists* typically require Phase III testing if FDA approval is to be sought or if clinical benefit is to be confirmed. Examples of cytotoxic *Incrementalists* include gemcitabine (Gemzar) in the treatment of pancreatic cancer, vinorelbine (Navelbine) in the treatment of non-small-cell lung cancer, and paclitaxel in the adjuvant treatment of node-positive breast cancer. All of these agents required Phase III testing for FDA approval for their respective indication. For the MTAs, an example of and *Incrementalists* is trastuzumab (Herceptin) for HER2-overexpressing breast cancers. For its first-line indication in breast cancer, trastuzumab was tested in a large, Phase III trial to show that the combination with paclitaxel had greater efficacy when compared to paclitaxel alone. Another example of an *Incrementalist* MTA is ZD1839 Iressa, whose favorable toxicity profile in the setting of modest activity may provide the basis for it approval in advanced, previously treated NSCLC. It should be noted that whenever a *Superstar* therapy has been established in a disease, subsequent treatments, even if very promising, will often be considered *Incrementalists* and require Phase III testing to confirm relative benefit or noninferiority. An example of this phenomenon is the fact that the acceptance of doxorubicin, bleomycin, vinblastine, and dacarbazine (ABVD) over MOPP as the standard treatment for Hodgkin's disease occurred after many years of availability for ABVD and only after a large, Phase III trial showed equal survival (compared to MOPP) but improved toxicity for the ABVD arm *(118)*.

The *Trade-off* designation is the last of the four. These treatments have substantial evidence of biological activity but at the price of significant toxicity. Examples of "Trade-off" treatments (and their major toxicity) early in their development included doxorubicin for treatment of advanced breast cancer (congestive heart failure), vincrisitine for lymphomas (neurotoxicity), and cisplatin for germ cell tumors (renal toxicity). In each of these cases, attempts were successfully made to minimize toxicity by modifying dose or schedule or by applying supportive medication *(8)*. If, on the other hand, the toxicity of a novel *Trade-off* agent with promising activity cannot be circumvented, the agent will usually require Phase III testing for definitive demonstration of overall clinical benefit.

4.1.3.4. Randomized Phase II Trials

Randomized Phase II trials are now increasingly being used to screen promising new agents. These trials allow evaluation of several treatments on a common patient population. An increasingly popular design is to test a standard regimen plus a novel MTA against the standard regimen alone. A recent example of this design is the randomized Phase II trial of a recombinant monoclonal antibody to vascular endothelial cell growth factor (VEGF) (rhuMAB VEGF) in which 99 patients with advanced non-small-cell lung cancer (NSCLC) were randomized to receive either the standard regimen (carboplatin plus paclitaxel) or the standard regiment plus rhuMAB VEGF *(119)*. Another design is to simultaneously test several doses or schedules of a new agent to choose the best one for Phase III testing. This approach was employed in the recent Phase II trial of ZD1839 (Iressa) in advanced non-small-cell lung cancer (IDEAL-2) where patients were randomized to receive either 250 or 500 mg/d of ZD1839 *(120,121)*. Randomized Phase II trials have the major benefit of providing some assurance that a positive result is meaningful or that a dose or schedule chosen for Phase III testing is optimal *(122)*. As such, they should be considered screening trials to help justify continued development. It is important that they not be confused with Phase III trials *(16)*. Compared to Phase III trials, randomized Phase II trials are smaller, are not typically powered to allow for stratification, contain more narrow eligibility requirements, and are not designed to provide a definitive answer to the question at hand.

4.1.3.5. Time-to-Progression in Phase II

Whereas response rates have been the most useful surrogate for cytotoxic drugs, time-to-progression (TTP) has been the one most often proposed for assessing cytostatic agents in Phase II trials. TTP is typically defined as the time from enrollment to documented progression of tumor size based on imaging tests (and not on biochemical tumor markers). This endpoint was used for the approval basis of letrozole (Femara) for first-line therapy for estrogen-receptor-positive metastatic breast cancer *(26)*. When this end point is used to approve a drug claim, it is always followed by a commitment to provide follow up survival data to the FDA.

The two major benefits of using TTP include the need for smaller sample size and shorter follow-up time *(26)*. Unfortunately, even in Phase III trials, the use of TTP as a surrogate marker is suspect. The trouble mainly derives from the difficulty in standardization across treatment centers because of the limitation imposed by the frequency of obtaining imaging studies especially in comparison with historical controls. There have been recent calls for more uniform methods of evaluating TTP in clinical trials. One proposed method is to measure the proportion of nonprogressors at fixed time points such as 3- or 6-mo intervals *(123)*. Even is the problem with standardization were resolved, there are other limitations. When effective blinding is not performed, investigator bias may be present in interpreting clinical data such as radiology films. There is also scarcity of historical control databases with TTP as an endpoint. Because of these issues, TTP has generally not been an acceptable registration end point for the FDA. Several presentation before the FDA's Oncology Drug Advisory Committee (ODAC) discussing TTP as an end point in a first-line setting have not resulted in Committee support for it to be used as a basis for recommending approval *(26)*.

Because of these limitations, TTP should not typically be used in isolation to decide whether to enter a Phase III trial.

4.1.3.6. Clinical Benefit

The FDA has placed increasing importance on quality-of-life (QOL) endpoints for assessing approval of new anticancer drugs *(124)*. Although global QOL data have not yet formed a basis for oncology drug approval, specific symptom control has been used as important component of the approval for pamidronate (Aredia) in multiple myeloma and breast cancer and for topotecan (Hycamptin) for second line therapy for limited stage small-cell lung cancer *(111)*. As such, symptom control data are increasingly collected in Phase II trials and used to help make decisions about whether to enter Phase III testing. This strategy was employed in the case of gemcitabine (Gemzar). After patients receiving gemcitabine reported having a benefit in disease-related symptoms during the Phase II trial *(125)*, a randomized Phase III effort was designed to target clinical benefit*(126)*. This "clinical benefit response," based on consumption of analgesic medications, pain intensity, performance status, and weight change, was predefined with the FDA and later proven in the Phase III trial of gemcitabine in pancreatic cancer. The clinical benefit response ultimately provided a substantial portion of the FDA's basis for marketing approval. QOL data are compromised by the fact that the patients and investigators are often not blinded, end points are subjective, and there is inconsistent correlation with other changes in patient status such as tumor response or toxicity *(111)*. As was the case with gemcitabine, clinical benefit should be influential in the decision for trial advancement or approval when few effective treatments exist for a highly symptomatic patient population.

4.1.4. FACTOR IV:
POTENTIAL ROLE EITHER ALONE OR IN COMBINATION IN TREATING A DISEASE

Most novel agents that show promise in the preclinical and Phase I periods will advance to efficacy testing in several Phase II trials designed to measure activity in a specific tumor type. If a threshold of activity is reached for the agent under development in at least one of these efficacy trials (with acceptable toxicity and pharmacological properties) an approval strategy will then be considered. In most cases, the approval strategy will employ at least one and most likely two Phase III trials. The major question that must be addressed prior to pursuing an expensive registration trial is: For what disease and which line of treatment will marketing approval be sought? This question is critical because it can affect the likelihood and speed of achieving marketing approval as well as the ultimate market size and treatment niche of the agent if approved. In general, a first-line approval strategy is riskier (because the agent is compared to the most active treatment) but the potential return is greater because of a larger market size. Depending on the activity of the agent in early efficacy trials, the risk may be warranted by the potential for return. It is generally true that most agents approved for second- and third-line indications are eventually approved as single agents (e.g., paclitaxel for second-line ovarian cancer, ifosfamide for third line testis cancer). Conversely, most agents with first-line indications are approved for use in combination (e.g., irinotecan plus fluorouracil and leucovorin for first-line colon cancer).

For targeted therapy, the choice of disease for Phase III testing is based on the perceived importance of the agent's target in the disease in question as well as the activity displayed in that disease in preclinical phase and in developmental trials. The progression for most MTAs through clinical development will likely be Phase I (assessing for target inhibition and satisfactory PKs without major toxicity) to Phase II (confirming target inhibition and lack of toxicity while assessing biological activity) to Phase I/II in combination with cytotoxics (looking for drug interactions, toxicity, PKs, and response). If the combination of the MTA with the reference regimen is at least as good as the reference regimen alone in terms of response in Phase I/II, has no significant or problematic toxicity, and has satisfactory PKs, the combination may then be considered for Phase III trial with survival as the primary endpoint. At least initially, most MTAs will have their major role as acting in synergy with cytotoxics or radiation to lower the apoptotic threshold to therapy *(123)*. It seems likely that cytotoxics will still provide the foundation for most cancer chemotherapy for the foreseeable future. The choice of which cytotoxics to test in combination with the MTA should be made on the basis of (1) non-overlapping toxicity and favorable PKs between the MTA and the cytotoxics in question, (2) the currently approved or widely accepted cytotoxic regimen, and (3) preclinical evidence of additivity or synergy.

4.1.5. FACTOR V:
POTENTIAL FOR MARKET NICHE AND STRATEGIC ROLE FOR THE SPONSOR

Regardless of how promising an agent appears with respect to the other four factors, a drug is less likely to advance to Phase III testing if the market size is insufficient to support a positive return on investment or if the agent does not play a strategic role in the sponsor's portfolio. In most cases, the decision to continue to development a drug at any stage depends on whether the drug's estimated present value of future revenues exceeds the anticipated total development, distribution, and marketing costs. When revenues exceed costs, profits can be made. As Phase III trials represent the single largest clinical development cost, it is obviously prudent to evaluate the likely demand for the drug before investing tens of millions of dollars on a Phase III effort. These demand estimates must take into account "off-label" usage, additional potential indications, changes in reimbursement schedules, and alterations in the standard of care for the disease in question during the several years of Phase III development. This demand must then be balanced against the likelihood of achieving marketing approval and a market niche if a Phase III registration trial is executed and successful. It is estimated that more than 30% of drugs entering clinical trials are abandoned primarily on the basis of these economic considerations *(7)*. If a compound's efficacy appears promising, but its predicted return on investment appears unfavorable, it can be offered to the NCI or the cooperative groups to develop under their sponsorship and at their expense.

The last of the factors that sponsors, both industrial and nonindustrial, consider prior to moving a drug to Phase III is the strategic value of the agent or treatment under question. For an industrial sponsor, the short-term value of their shares may be closely linked to whether or not they decide to take an agent to a Phase III trial. This is especially true for biotechnology firms, for whom market capitalization can change dramatically simply by the announcement of a beginning or premature termination of a Phase III trial. In addition to the effect on stock value, the Phase III decision is heavily influenced by concern over speed to market. If approval can be based on Phase II data alone and thus avert a time-consuming Phase III trial, several additional years of exclusive marketing rights may be realized amounting to hundreds of millions or even billions of dollars. This enticement must be balanced against the risk of submitting an NDA to the FDA without convincing Phase III data, leading to a failure to achieve approval (or even be considered for NDA review as was the case with C225 in irinotecan-refractory colon cancer). Finally, industrial sponsors may make decisions regarding Phase III development based on the composition of their drug portfolio and overarching priorities of the company *(127)*. A presence in the cancer drug market may in itself be valuable, apart from expectations of significant short-term profit. For the nonindustrial sponsor such as the NCI, these strategic considerations are based more on the novelty of the agent, the perceived importance of the question to be answered, and the treatment void to be filled. As an example of how the Phase III Decision Model can be applied, an evaluation of two selected agents that have recently advanced to Phase III trials is presented in Table 7.

Table 7
Factor Analysis for Selected Agents in Phase III Trials

Agent	OSI-774 (Tarceva)	Bcl-2 antisense oligo (Genasense)
Sponsor	Genentec	Genta
Trial design	Randomized to carboplatin (C) plus paclitaxel (P) with OSI-774 or placebo in previously untreated patients with advanced non-small-cell lung cancer	Randomized to fludarabine (F) plus cyclophosphamide (Cy) with or without Genasense in patients with relapsed chronic lymphocytic leukemia (CLL)
	Factor 1	
Target	EGFR receptor	Bcl-2 mRNA
Mechanism of action	Receptor inhibition leading to cell-cycle arrest and apoptosis in EGFR-dependent cell	Selective reduction in protein levels of Bcl-2 by using an 18-mer phosphorothioate oligonucleotide against Bcl-2 mRNA
Potency (IC-50 in tumor cells)	Excellent (20 nm)	Good (170 nm)
Selectivity	Excellent (1000-fold greater selectivity for EGFR compared to other kinases)	Good (The oligos polyanionic properties may produce nonspecific binding)
Target engagement	Intratumural EGFR inhibition with 50% effective doses of 9 mg/kg	Demonstrated in Phase I trial by PBMCs and biopsies
Preclinical activity	Growth inhibition of human tumor xenografts in athymic mice with 50% effective dose of 9 mg/kg/d	Induction of apoptosis in multiple cell lines and activity in human tumor xenograft models
Preclinical toxicity	Negligible up to 15 mg/kg/d; Corneal perforations with protracted perforations > 50 mg/kg/d for 7 d	Negligible at doses up to 10 mg/kg/d
Required concentration for antitumor effect	0.5 µg/mL	1 µg/mL
Activity in combination	Additive effects with cisplatin, paclitaxel, and gemcitabine	Synergistic effects with multiple standard cytotoxics and antimetabolites
	Factor 2	
Route	Oral	IV continuous infusion
Bioavailability	70–90%	100%
Intersubject PK variability	Moderate	Moderate
Elimination $t_{1/2}$	24 h	2–7 h, depending on route of administration
Elimination mechanism	Hepatic metabolism	Renal excretion
MTD	150 mg/d	4.1 mg/kg/d
Average steady-state plasma concentration at MTD	1.2 µg/mL	3.2 µg/mL
DLT(s)	Diarrhea	Fatigue, thrombocytopenia, fever
	Factor 3	
Phase I activity	One complete response, two minor responses, and several patients with stable disease	1 complete response, 2 minor response, and several patients with stable disease
Phase II activity	Objective RR of 10–15% in 3 Phase II trials. Objective RR of 14% in Phase II trial of NSCLC	No Phase II trial in CLL
Phase II Toxicity	Acceptable (skin rash and diarrhea)	NA
	Factor 4	
Basis for disease choice	RR in Phase II; perceived importance of target in disease progression	Responses in Phase I. Perceived importance of target in low-grade, non-Hodgkin's lymphoma
Choice of combination	In vitro additivity with carboplatin (C) and paclitaxel (P); C + P is current reference standard for metastatic NSCLC; nonoverlapping toxicity	Cy + F is accepted salvage regimen; nonoverlapping toxicity
	Factor 5	
Market size	Very large market size for NSCLC	Small to moderate market size for CLL
Phase III trials in other Cancers	None	Yes. Muliple myeloma, melanoma, others

5.CONCLUSION

The real voyage of discovery consists not in seeking new landscapes, but in having new eyes.

—Marcel Proust

If it is ever true that success lies within the journey, it is so for the clinical development of anticancer drugs. Clinical trials in oncology in general, and Phase III trials in particular, have become dramatically more complex, expensive, and time consuming. These challenges have coincided with the emergence of a large new cohort of diverse, molecularly based antineoplastic agents whose evaluation and approval depends on the successful employment of Phase III trials, often with limited evidence that the agent will add benefit. "Picking the winners from a sea of plenty" *(81)* will become increasing complex and will continue to be as much art as science. To the extent possible, however, these decisions should be made individually, based on the fundamental criteria and factors set forth in this chapter.

REFERENCES

1. Pharmaceuticals Research and Manufacturers of America. New medicines in development for cancer. Washington, DC: PhRMA 2001, pp. 1–56.
2. American Cancer Society. Cancer Facts and Figures 2001. Atlanta, GA: American Cancer Society, 2001.
3. Parexel's Pharmaceutical R&D Statistical Sourcebook 2001. Boston, MA: Parexel International Corporation, 2002.
4. Lasagna L, Frei E III. The impact of regulations, tradition, and experimental design on clinical cancer trials: report and recommendations resulting from Washington Cancer Trials Conference. Am J Clin Oncol 1996; 19:325–329.
5. DiMasi JA, Bryant NR, Lasagna L. New drug development in the United States from 1963 to 1990. Clin Pharmacol Ther 1991; 50:471–486.
6. DiMasi JA. New drug development in the United States from 1963 to 1999. Clin Pharmacol Ther 2001; 69:286–296.
7. DiMasi JA. Risks in new drug development: approval success rates for investigational drugs. Clin Pharmacol Ther 2001; 69:297–307.
8. Von Hoff DD. There are no bad anticancer agents, only bad clinical trial designs—twenty-first Richard and Hinda Rosenthal Foundation Award Lecture. Clin Cancer Res 1998; 4:1079–1086.
9. Farber S, Diamond LK, Mercer RD, Sylvester RF, Wolff JA. Temporary remissions in acue leukemia in children produced by folic acid antagonist, 4-aminopteroyl-glutamic (aminopterin). N Engl J Med 1948; 238:787–793.
10. NIH Consensus Conference. Treatment of early-stage breast cancer. JAMA 1991; 265(3):391–395.
11. NIH Consensus Conference. Adjuvant therapy for patients with colon and rectal cancer. JAMA 1990; 264:1444–1450.
12. Schein PS. The case for a new national program for the development of cancer therapeutics. J Clin Oncol 2001; 19:3142–3153.
13. Chabner BA. The oncologic four-minute mile. Oncologist 2001; 6:230–232.
14. PDQ. March, 2002 (available at Website: http://www.cancer.gov/cancer_information/pdq/)
15. Chabner BA, Boral AL, Multani P. Translational research: walking the bridge between idea and cure—seventeenth Bruce F. Cain Memorial Award lecture. Cancer Res 1998; 58:4211–4216.
16. Simon R. Clinical trials in cancer. In: DeVita VT Jr, Hellman S, Rosenberg SA, editors. Cancer: Principle & Practice of Oncology. Philadelphia, PA: Lippincott Williams & Wilkins, 2001, pp. 521–538.
17. Newell DR. Pharmacologically based Phase I trials in cancer chemotherapy. Hematol Oncol Clin North Am 1994; 8:257–275.
18. Eisenhauer EA. Phase I and II trials of novel anti-cancer agents: endpoints, efficacy and existentialism. The Michel Clavel Lecture, held at the 10th NCI- EORTC Conference on New Drugs in Cancer Therapy, Amsterdam, 16–19 June 1998. Ann Oncol 1998; 9:1047–1052.
19. Gelmon KA, Eisenhauer EA, Harris AL, Ratain MJ, Workman P. Anticancer agents targeting signaling molecules and cancer cell environment: challenges for drug development? J Natl Cancer Inst 1999; 91:1281–1287.

20. Von Hoff DD, Turner J. Response rates, duration of response, and dose response effects in phase I studies of antineoplastics. Invest New Drugs 1991; 9:115–122.
21. Smith TL, Lee JJ, Kantarjian HM, Legha SS, Raber MN. Design and results of Phase I cancer clinical trials: three-year experience at M.D. Anderson Cancer Center. J Clin Oncol 1996; 14:287–295.
22. Estey E, Hoth D, Simon R, Marsoni S, Leyland-Jones B, Wittes R. Therapeutic response in Phase I trials of antineoplastic agents. Cancer Treat Rep 1986; 70:1105–1115.
23. Mariani L, Marubini E. Content and quality of currently published Phase II cancer trials. J Clin Oncol 2000; 18:429–436.
24. Frei E, III. Clinical trials of antitumor agents: experimental design and timeline considerations. Cancer J Sci Am 1997; 3:127–136.
25. Simon R. Randomized clinical trials in oncology. Principles and obstacles. Cancer 1994; 74(9 Suppl): 2614–2619.
26. Hirschfeld S, Pazdur R. Oncology drug development: United States Food and Drug Administration perspective. Crit Rev Oncol Hematol 2002; 42:137–143.
27. Gianni L. Tolerability in patients receiving trastuzumab with or without chemotherapy. Ann Oncol 2001; 12(Suppl 1):S63–S68.
28. Food and Drug Administration. Reinventing the regulation of cancer drugs: accelerating approval and expanding access. 1996.
29. Cox JD. Evidence in oncology. The Janeway lecture 2000. Cancer J 2000; 6:351–357.
30. Green SB. Patient heterogeneity and the need for randomized clinical trials. Control Clin Trials 1982; 3:189–198.
31. Byar DP, Simon RM, Friedewald WT, et al. Randomized clinical trials. Perspectives on some recent ideas. N Engl J Med 1976; 295:74–80.
32. Fazzari M, Heller G, Scher HI. The Phase II/III transition. Toward the proof of efficacy in cancer clinical trials. Control Clin Trials 2000; 21:360–368.
33. Mazumdar M, Fazzari M, Panageas KS. A standardization method to adjust for the effect of patient selection in Phase II clinical trials. Stat Med 2001; 20:883–892.
34. McClay EF, Mastrangelo MJ, Berd D, Bellet RE. Effective combination chemo/hormonal therapy for malignant melanoma: experience with three consecutive trials. Int J Cancer 1992; 50:553–556.
35. Hellman S. Editorial: Randomized clinical trials and the doctor–patient relationship. Cancer Clin Trials 1979; 2:189–193.
36. Chapman PB, Einhorn LH, Meyers ML, et al. Phase III multicenter randomized trial of the Dartmouth regimen versus dacarbazine in patients with metastatic melanoma. J Clin Oncol 1999; 17:2745–2751.
37. Fisher RI, Gaynor ER, Dahlberg S, et al. Comparison of a standard regimen (CHOP) with three intensive chemotherapy regimens for advanced non-Hodgkin's lymphoma. N Engl J Med 1993; 328: 1002–1006.
38. Schiller JH, Harrington D, Belani CP, et al. Comparison of four chemotherapy regimens for advanced non-small-cell lung cancer. N Engl J Med 2002; 346:92–98.
39. Cox JD. Evolution and accomplishments of the Radiation Therapy Oncology Group. Int J Radiat Oncol Biol Phys 1995; 33:747–754.
40. Frei E 3rd, Holland JF, Schneiderman MA, et al. A comparitive study of two regimens of combination chemotherapy in acute leukemia. Blood 1958; 13(12):1126–1147.
41. Zubrod CG, Schneiderman M, Frei E III, et al. Appraisal of methods for the study of chemotherapy of cancer in man: comparative therapeutic trial of thiophosphoramide. J Chron Dis 1960; 11:7–23.
42. Jones TC. How can clinical research and regulatory processes meet the challenge of rapid drug discovery? Curr Drug Discov 2001; 17–19.
43. Chalmers TC, Block JB, Lee S. Controlled studies in clinical cancer research. N Engl J Med 1972; 287:75–78.
44. Diehl LF, Perry DJ. A comparison of randomized concurrent control groups with matched historical control groups: are historical controls valid? J Clin Oncol 1986; 4:1114–1120.
45. Buyse M, Thirion P, Carlson RW, Burzykowski T, Molenberghs G, Piedbois P. Re: A model to select chemotherapy regimens for phase III trials for extensive-stage small-cell lung cancer. J Natl Cancer Inst 2001; 93:399–401.
46. Simon R, Thall PF, Ellenberg SS. New designs for the selection of treatments to be tested in randomized clinical trials. Stat Med 1994; 13:417–429.
47. Reynolds T. Biotech firm faces challenges from FDA, falling stock prices. J Natl Cancer Inst 2002; 94:326–328.

48. Saltz L, Rubin M, Hochster H, et al. Cetuximab (IMC-C225) plus irinotecan (CPT-11) is active in CPT-11-refractory colorectal cancer (CRC) that expresses epidermal growth factor receptor (EGFR). Proc ASCO 20: abstract 7.2001.

49. FDA says ImClone data insufficient to evaluate colorectal cancer drug C225. The Cancer Letter. 2002; 28:1–5.

50. Daugherty CK. Impact of therapeutic research on informed consent and the ethics of clinical trials: a medical oncology perspective. J Clin Oncol 1999; 17:1601–1617.

51. Rosner F. The ethics of randomized clinical trials. Am J Med 1987; 82:283–290.

52. Hellman S, Hellman DS. Of mice but not men. Problems of the randomized clinical trial. N Engl J Med 1991; 324:1585–1589.

53. Fried C. Medical Experimentation: Personal Integrity and Social Policy. Amsterdam, Oxford: North Holland Publishing Company, 1974.

54. Antman K, Amato D, Wood W, et al. Selection bias in clinical trials. J Clin Oncol 1985; 3:1142–1147.

55. Piantadosi S. Clinical Trials: A Methodological Perspective. New York, NY: John Wiley & Sons, 1997.

56. Gehan EA, Freireich EJ. Non-randomized controls in cancer clinical trials. N Engl J Med 1974; 290:198–203.

57. Freedman B. Equipoise and the ethics of clinical research. N Engl J Med 1987; 317:141–145.

58. Beecher HK. Ethics and clinical research. N Engl J Med 1966; 274:1354–1360.

59. Kodish E, Lantos JD, Siegler M. Ethical considerations in randomized controlled clinical trials. Cancer 1990; 65(10 Suppl):2400–2404.

60. Coltman C. Southwest Oncology Group workshop on clinical trials. Cancer 1990; 65:2385–2390.

61. Taylor KM, Margolese RG, Soskolne CL. Physicians' reasons for not entering eligible patients in a randomized clinical trial of surgery for breast cancer. N Engl J Med 1984; 310:1363–1367.

62. Tobias JS, Baum M, Thornton H. Clinical trials in cancer: what makes for a successful study? Ann Oncol 2000; 11:1371–1373.

63. Tufts Center for the Study of Drug Development . November, 2001 (available at Website: http://www.tufts.edu/med/csdd/nov30coststudy/pressrelease.html)

64. DiMasi JA, Hansen RW, Grabowski HG, Lasagna L. Cost of innovation in the pharmaceutical industry. J Health Econ 1991; 10:107–142.

65. Hillner BE. Trends in published cancer clinical trial reports 1990–2000. Proc ASCO 21: abstract 974.2002.

66. Antman K, Schnipper LE, Frei E III. The crisis in clinical cancer research. Third-party insurance and investigational therapy. N Engl J Med 1988; 319(1):46–48.

67. Wagner JL, Alberts SR, Sloan JA, et al. Incremental costs of enrolling cancer patients in clinical trials: a population-based study. J Natl Cancer Inst 1999; 91:847–853.

68. Bennett CL, Stinson TJ, Vogel V, et al. Evaluating the financial impact of clinical trials in oncology: results from a pilot study from the Association of American Cancer Institutes/Northwestern University clinical trials costs and charges project. J Clin Oncol 2000; 18:2805–2810.

69. Arnold K, Vastag B. Medicare to cover routine care costs in clinical trials. J Natl Cancer Inst 2000; 92:1032.

70. Fleming ID. Barriers to clinical trials. Part I: Reimbursement problems. Cancer 1994; 74(9 Suppl): 2662–2665.

71. Roche K, Paul N, Smuck B, et al. Factors affecting workload of cancer clinical trials: results of a multicenter study of the National Cancer Institute of Canada Clinical Trials Group. J Clin Oncol 2002; 20:545–556.

72. Shulman SR, Wood-Armany MJ. Accelerating access to cancer drugs. J Biolaw Business 1999; 2:38–44.

73. Hirschfeld S. Personal communication. Division of Oncology Drug Products, Center for Drug Evaluation and Research, Food and Drug Administration. July, 2002.

74. Breathnach OS, Freidlin B, Conley B, et al. Twenty-two years of Phase III trials for patients with advanced non-small-cell lung cancer: sobering results. J Clin Oncol 2001; 19:1734–1742.

75. Krzyzanowska MK, Pintilie M, Tannock I. Burying of unwanted results: a survey of more than 500 large randomized clinical tirals presented at ASCO meetings to determine the probabililty and causes of failure to publish. Proc ASCO 21: abstract 973.2002.

76. Krzyzanowska M. Personal communication. Center for Outcomes and Policy Research. Dana Farber Cancer Institute, June 2002.

77. Chen TT, Chute JP, Feigal E, Johnson BE, Simon R. A model to select chemotherapy regimens for phase III trials for extensive-stage small-cell lung cancer. J Natl Cancer Inst 2000; 92:1601–1607.

78. Laetz T, Silberman G. Reimbursement policies constrain the practice of oncology. JAMA 1991; 266:2996–2999.

79. Kaufman D. Cancer therapy and the randomized clinical trial: good medicine? CA Cancer J Clin 1994; 44:109–114.

80. The March: Coming Together to Conquer Cancer: Report from The March Task Force. 2002. 1998.

81. Scher HI, Heller G. Picking the winners in a sea of plenty. Clin Cancer Res 2002; 8:400–404.

82. Averbuch S. Personal communication. AstraZeneca Pharmaceutical, Wilmington, DE, March, 2002.

83. Carney DN. Lung cancer—time to move on from chemotherapy. N Engl J Med 2002; 346:126–128.

84. Johnson J, Monks A, Hollingshead M, Sausville E. Preclinical aspects of cancer drug discovery and development. In: Chabner B, Longo D (eds). Cancer Chemotherapy & Biotherapy. Philadephia, PA: Lippincott Williams & Wilkins, 2001, pp. 17–36.

85. Reddy A, Kaelin WG. Using cancer genetics to guide the selection of anticancer drug targets. Curr Opin Pharmacol 2002; 2:366–373.

86. Stoler DL, Chen N, Basik M, et al. The onset and extent of genomic instability in sporadic colorectal tumor progression. Proc Natl Acad Sci USA 1999; 96:15,121–15,126.

87. Renan MJ. How many mutations are required for tumorigenesis? Implications from human cancer data. Mol Carcinogen 1993; 7:139–146.

88. Fearon ER, Vogelstein B. A genetic model for colorectal tumorigenesis. Cell 1990; 61:759–767.

89. Hanahan D, Weinberg RA. The hallmarks of cancer. Cell 2000; 100:57–70.

90. Coussens LM, Fingleton B, Matrisian LM. Matrix metalloproteinase inhibitors and cancer: trials and tribulations. Science 2002; 295:2387–2392.

91. Clark JW. Targeted therapy. In: Chabner BA, Longo D (eds). Cancer Chemotherapy & Biotherapy. Philadephia. PA: Lippincott Williams & Wilkins, 2001, pp. 891–910.

92. Hidalgo M, Siu LL, Nemunaitis J, et al. Phase I and pharmacologic study of OSI-774, an epidermal growth factor receptor tyrosine kinase inhibitor, in patients with advanced solid malignancies. J Clin Oncol 2001; 19:3267–3279.

93. Ramaswamy S, Golub TR. DNA microarrays in clinical oncology. J Clin Oncol 2002; 20:1932–1941.

94. Bichsel VE, Liotta LA, Petricoin EF, III. Cancer proteomics: from biomarker discovery to signal pathway profiling. Cancer J 2001; 7:69–78.

95. Davies H, Bignell G, Cox C, et al. Mutations of the BRAF gene in human cancer. Nature 2002; 417:949–954.

96. Johnson JI, Decker S, Zaharevitz D, et al. Relationships between drug activity in NCI preclinical in vitro and in vivo models and early clinical trials. Br J Cancer 2001; 84:1424–1431.

97. Van Dyke T, Jacks T. Cancer modeling in the modern era: progress and challenges. Cell 2002; 108: 135–144.

98. Fisher GH, Wellen SL, Klimstra D, et al. Induction and apoptotic regression of lung adenocarcinomas by regulation of a K-Ras transgene in the presence and absence of tumor suppressor genes. Genes Dev 2001; 15:3249–3262.

99. Kitada S, Takayama S, De Riel K, Tanaka S, Reed JC. Reversal of chemoresistance of lymphoma cells by antisense-mediated reduction of bcl-2 gene expression. Antisense Res Dev 1994; 4:71–79.

100. Jansen B, Schlagbauer-Wadl H, Brown BD, Bryan RN, van Elsas A, Muller M et al. bcl-2 antisense therapy chemosensitizes human melanoma in SCID mice. Nat Med 1998; 4:232–234.

101. Collins JM. Pharmacology and drug development. J Natl Cancer Inst 1988; 80:790–792.

102. Liu G, Franssen E, Fitch MI, Warner E. Patient preferences for oral versus intravenous palliative chemotherapy. J Clin Oncol 1997; 15:110–115.

103. Borner MM, Schoffski P, de Wit R, et al. Patient preference and pharmacokinetics of oral modulated UFT versus intravenous fluorouracil and leucovorin: a randomised crossover trial in advanced colorectal cancer. Eur J Cancer 2002; 38:349–358.

104. Twelves C, Boyer M, Findlay M, et al. Capecitabine (Xeloda) improves medical resource use compared with 5- fluorouracil plus leucovorin in a Phase III trial conducted in patients with advanced colorectal carcinoma. Eur J Cancer 2001; 37:597–604.

105. Partridge AH, Avorn J, Wang PS, Winer EP. Adherence to therapy with oral antineoplastic agents. J Natl Cancer Inst 2002; 94:652–661.

106. Wurthwein G, Krumpelmann S, Tillmann B, et al. Population pharmacokinetic approach to compare oral and i.v. administration of etoposide. Anticancer Drugs 1999; 10:807–814.

107. Adjei AA, Erlichman C, Davis JN, et al. A Phase I trial of the farnesyl transferase inhibitor SCH66336: evidence for biological and clinical activity. Cancer Res 2000; 60:1871–1877.

108. Albanell J, Rojo F, Averbuch S, et al. Pharmacodynamic studies of the epidermal growth factor receptor inhibitor ZD1839 in skin from cancer patients: histopathologic and molecular consequences of receptor inhibition. J Clin Oncol 2002; 20:110–124.

109. One of the authors (TGR) confirmed single agent response rates in at least one developmental trial for all of the currently approved oncology drugs listed in the Oncology Tools section of the FDA website. Also confirmed this statement with Steven Hirschfeld, M.D. Division of Oncology Drug Products, Center for Drug Evaluation and Research, Food and Drug Administration. July, 2002.

110. Korn EL, Arbuck SG, Pluda JM, Simon R, Kaplan RS, Christian MC. Clinical trial designs for cytostatic agents: are new approaches needed? J Clin Oncol 2001; 19:265–272.

110. Pazdur R. Response rates, survival, and chemotherapy trials. J Natl Cancer Inst 2000; 92:1552–1553.

112. Therasse P, Arbuck SG, Eisenhauer EA, et al. New guidelines to evaluate the response to treatment in solid tumors. European Organization for Research and Treatment of Cancer, National Cancer Institute of the United States, National Cancer Institute of Canada. J Natl Cancer Inst 2000; 92:205–216.

113. Buyse M, Thirion P, Carlson RW, Burzykowski T, Molenberghs G, Piedbois P. Relation between tumour response to first-line chemotherapy and survival in advanced colorectal cancer: a meta-analysis. Meta-Analysis Group in Cancer. Lancet 2000; 356:373–378.

114. Weiss GB, Bunce H III, Hokanson JA. Comparing survival of responders and nonresponders after treatment: a potential source of confusion in interpreting cancer clinical trials. Control Clin Trials 1983; 4:43–52.

115. de Gramont A, Figer A, Seymour M, et al. Leucovorin and fluorouracil with or without oxaliplatin as first-line treatment in advanced colorectal cancer. J Clin Oncol 2000; 18:2938–2947.

116. Goldberg RM, Morton RF, Sargent DJ, et al. N9741: Oxaliplatin (Oxal) or CPT-11 + 5-fluorouracil (5FU)/Leucovorin (LV) or OXAL + CPT-11 in advanced colorectal cancer (CRC). Initial toxicity and response data from a GI intergroup study. Proc ASCO 21: abstract 511.2002.

117. Warrell RP Jr, Burchenal JH. Methylglyoxal-bis(guanylhydrazone) (Methyl-GAG): current status and future prospects. J Clin Oncol 1983; 1:52–65.

118. Canellos GP. New treatments for advanced Hodgkin's disease: an uphill fight beginning close to the top. J Clin Oncol 2002; 20:607–609.

119. DeVore R, Fehrenbacher L, Herbst RS, Langer CJ, Kelly K, Gaudreault J et al. A randomized Phase II trial comparing Rhumab VEGF (recombinant humanized monoclonal antibody to vascular endothelial cell growth factor) plus carboplatin/placitaxel (CP) to CP alone in patients with stage IIIB/IV NSCLC. Proc ASCO 2000.

120. Kris MG, Natale RB, Herbst R, et al. Efficacy of gefitinib, an inhibitor of the epidermal growth factor receptor tyrosine kinase, in symptomatic patients with non-small cell lung cancer: a randomized trial. JAMA. 2003; 290:2149-58.

121. Ranson M, Hammond LA, Ferry D, et al. ZD1839, a selective oral epidermal growth factor receptor-tyrosine kinase inhibitor, is well tolerated and active in patients with solid, malignant tumors: results of a phase I trial. J Clin Oncol 2002; 20:2240–2250.

122. Simon R, Wittes RE, Ellenberg SS. Randomized Phase II clinical trials. Cancer Treat Rep 1985; 69:1375–1381.

123. Dy GK, Adjei AA. Novel targets for lung cancer therapy: part II. J Clin Oncol 2002; 20:3016–3028.

124. Beitz J, Gnecco C, Justice R. Quality-of-life end points in cancer clinical trials: the U.S. Food and Drug Administration perspective. J Natl Cancer Inst Monogr 1996; 7–9.

125. Casper ES, Green MR, Kelsen DP, et al. Phase II trial of gemcitabine (2,2'-difluorodeoxycytidine) in patients with adenocarcinoma of the pancreas. Invest New Drugs 1994; 12:29–34.

126. Burris HA, III, Moore MJ, Andersen J, et al. Improvements in survival and clinical benefit with gemcitabine as first- line therapy for patients with advanced pancreas cancer: a randomized trial. J Clin Oncol 1997; 15:2403–2413.

127. Lawson W, Risk L. Portfolio management: improving the process. Curr Drug Discov 2001; 34–36.

128. Roberts Jr T G, Lynch Jr TJ, Chabner BA. The Phase III trial in the era of targeted therapy: unraveling the "go or no go" decision. J Clin Oncol 2003; 21:3683–3695.

33 Clinical Trial Designs for Approval of New Anticancer Agents

A Clinical Science

Daniel D. Von Hoff, MD

CONTENTS

INTRODUCTION
METHODS TO SELECT AGENTS THAT WILL BE ACTIVE IN THE CLINIC
GENERAL ASPECTS OF CLINICAL TRIAL DESIGN FOR APPROVAL
SPECIAL TRIAL DESIGNS, PARTICULARLY SUITED
    FOR CYTOSTATIC AGENTS
A UNIQUE ENDPOINT FOR APPROVAL
SPECIAL CHALLENGES IN CLINICAL TRIAL DESIGN FOR APPROVAL
OTHER COMMENTS ON CLINICAL TRIALS FOR APPROVAL

1. INTRODUCTION

Development of new anticancer and cancer prevention agents presents significant challenges to clinical trialists. The correct design of all phases of clinical trials is essential to ensure as rapid and as successful a development as possible. One must have a plan that will give the new agent the best chance of matching its preclinical activity. Because there have been problems with this in the past, it is virtually certain that many promising new agents were dismissed as being inactive because of flaws in clinical trial design. This chapter provides information on multiple types of clinical trial designs that can and have been used for approval of new anticancer (and prevention) agents. Multiple and unique types of endpoints are also included in the chapter.

2. METHODS TO SELECT AGENTS THAT WILL BE ACTIVE IN THE CLINIC

Of course, if people knew for certain how to select agents that would definitely work in the clinic it is likely we would be much further along in our treatment of patients with cancer. However, there are some techniques that have been reported in the literature and that our drug development teams in San Antonio and in Tucson have used to increase the chances of bringing agents into clinical trials that will eventually be approved for clinical use (see Table 1).

Handbook of Anticancer Pharmacokinetics and Pharmacodynamics
Edited by: W. D. Figg and H. L. McLeod © Humana Press Inc., Totowa, NJ

Table 1

Chronology of Methods Used by a Drug Development Team to Try to Increase
the Percentage of Agents That Will Eventually Be Approved for Clinical Use

5-yr period	Method used for selection to take into Phase I trial	No. approved/ no. taken into trial	Percent approved
1978–1983	"Next agent to come along"	3/26	12%
1984–1989	Staquet [a] data on animal models	8/26	31%
1990–1995	Staquet data + any new mechanism of action	11/24	46%
1996–2001	Staquet data + any new mechanism of action + targeted monoclonal antibodies	8[b]/26	TE [c]

[a]Staquet MJ, et al. Cancer Treat Rep 1983; 67:753.
[b]Likely that many more than five will be approved.
[c]Estimate 67% of all agents taken into Phase I trials will be approved.

As can be seen in Table 1, in the period of 1978–1983 our team just took the "next agent to come along" into the Phase I clinical trials. Unfortunately, only 3 of the 26 agents (12%) we took into Phase I trials during that time period were subsequently approved by the Food and Drug Administration (FDA). Clearly, we needed to do better than that. In 1983, a significant publication by Staquet and colleagues (1) reviewed the success of the various murine or human tumor cell lines that were being utilized as in vivo systems by the National Cancer Institute to evaluate all of the potential antineoplastic agents. In that study they noted that murine leukemias L1210 and P388, the murine B16 melanoma, and the MX-1 mammary human tumor xenograft were the most predictive for antitumor activity in the clinic. These models were even more predictive if one used tumor regression or percent cure (≥ 45-d survivors) as an endpoint.

Models that were not predictive included the murine colon cancers Co26 and Co38, the CX-1 and LX-1, human tumor xenografts, and the Lewis lung model. As can be seen in Table 1, when we utilized the Staquet suggested models to select agents for Phase I trials, the success rate for our program (as judged by the percent of new agents that were eventually approved by the FDA divided by all of the agents that we took into Phase I trials during that period) increased to 31%. In 1990 our team had the clinical impression that every time we took a new agent with a new mechanism of action into a Phase I clinical trial (e.g., tubulin inhibitors, such as docetaxel or paclitaxel, topoisomerase I inhibitors such as topotecan or CPT11, or a chain terminator such as gemcitabine) it was very likely that the drug would eventually be approved (if the pivotal trial were designed correctly; see below). As can be seen in Table 1, using the additional parameter of a new mechanism of action, the success rate again appeared to improve.

The introduction of targeted monoclonal antibodies (MAbs) has also appeared to increase success rates. As is noted in Table 1, by using the Staquet criteria plus the new mechanisms of action criteria, plus MAbs, it is estimated that nearly 67% of all new agents brought into Phase I trials will eventually demonstrate antitumor activity significant enough for approval by the FDA (provided that the appropriate pivotal trials are designed for the agent).

The point of MAbs is worth emphasizing. Table 2 details the MAbs that have been approved or are demonstrating enough activity that it is anticipated that they will be approved. If one has a MAb specific to a particular cell surface antigen or receptor, it appears to be an excellent prognostic factor for activity and for approval.

In summary, with some rather simplistic approaches, we believe some of the risk of development of new anticancer agents can be taken out of the process. In fact the likelihood of success can be very high.

Table 2
Example of New Mechanisms of Action Against Specific Targets:
Monoclonal Antibodies Against Specific Targets

Target	Monoclonal antibody(s)	Clinical activity
CD20	Rituximab (Rituxan®)	Lymphoma
Her2/neu	Trastuzumab (Herceptin®)	Breast, others
CD33	Gentazimab zogomycin (Mylotarg®)	Acute leukemia
CD52	Alemtuzumab (CAMPATH®)	CLL
CD20	Radiolabeled ibritumomab (Tiuxetan; Zevalin®)	Lymphoma
CD20	Radiolabeled tositumomab (Bexxar®)	Lymphoma
EGFR	IMC-225 [a]; ABX-EGF [a]	Colorectal
17-1A	Edrecolomab (Panorex [a,b]	Colorectal cancer
VEGF	Bevacizumab (Avastin) [a]	Colorectal cancer, renal cell, lung
Others	Many others	Others

[a] Not yet approved by the FDA.
[b] Approved in Germany.

3. GENERAL ASPECTS OF CLINICAL TRIAL DESIGN FOR APPROVAL

It was stated above that agents with new mechanisms of action had a high probability of success—if the pivotal trials with the agent were designed correctly. To achieve that high probability of success some important aspects of clinical trial design include:

1. Try to select a clinical situation that closely mimics what was found in the preclinical data package. For example, if the new agent demonstrated only growth delays in an animal system, one should probably not design pivotal trials with response rate (e.g., tumor shrinkage) as a primary endpoint. Rather, one should utilize median survival or time to tumor progression (TTP) or time to treatment failure (TTF) as primary endpoints. The TTP or TTF endpoints are usually acceptable to regulatory agencies only if the trial is double-blinded. This is because clinicians caring for patients, and patients themselves, are most anxious to get off of a control arm and on to the new agent arm. This frequently will lead to a declaration that the control arm is not working so the patient can be crossed over to the new agent arm of the study. Thus, double-blinding is very helpful if it is at all possible. Another, more cumbersome method is to use an outside, independent, blinded review panel to assess tumor progression.

2. Make sure the sample size is large enough to give the new agent a real chance. For example, a sample size that allows one to detect only a 50% improvement in survival is too small of a sample size because that hurdle for any new agent is almost certainly too high (50% improvement). This is a setup for failure. Sample size must be large enough to give the new agent a chance e.g., a 25% improvement.

3. It is clear that if you are expecting an agent to be used to change the upfront treatment for patients with a specific type of tumor, two well controlled (and randomized) Phase III trials will need to be performed. Normally two *well controlled* trials does not necessarily mean they have to be randomized trials. For example, well controlled could mean a well monitored study, or a study in which patients serve as their own controls (see Subheading 4.1.). However, in the upfront situation, where the new agent is planned to change standard treatment, it is very likely that two *randomized* Phase III trials will be a necessity. There may be one exception to the two well controlled randomized Phase III trials requirement. It might be possible to obtain approval for the new agent to be used in an "upfront" situation if the level of significance for the primary endpoint

of the Phase III trial is $p < 0.001$. As many experienced investigators can attest, a p value of that magnitude is indeed unusual in most Phase III trials.

4. It is frequently said that one must have an improvement in survival for a new agent to be approved. That is, of course, desirable. However, survival has not always been required. Table 3 details the new agents brought to the FDA Oncology Advisory Board for approval, the type of study(ies) that lead to approval, and the parameters used for that approval. As can be seen in that Table 3, there were 69 approvals and 16 disapprovals (note that some agents were brought multiple times for approval in different indications). As can be seen in that table there were 25 approvals based primarily on response, 16 on survival, 10 on TTP, and 18 based on other primary endpoints. There were 27 approvals based on Phase II trials and 42 approvals based on Phase III trials. One can also note from Table 3 that a variety of other endpoints have been used as primary parameters for approval (e.g., control of pleural effusion, reduction in dysplasia, etc.).

   It is this investigator's personal experience that regulatory agencies will entertain endpoints other than survival (see below) if that new endpoint is discussed prospectively with and in detail with the regulatory agencies. They, like us, like challenges.

5. As is noted above, the FDA and other world regulatory agencies have approved new agents based on response (as a surrogate for survival or for benefit for the patient). The landmark publication that really codified response rate as a surrogate was the article by O'Shaugnhessy and colleagues (2) in which the general guidelines were put forth for approval based on Phase II results. There are many FDA observers who feel that response is no longer an approvable strategy, but Table 3 does document that it still can be a strategy for approval under the right circumstances, including:

   a. a very high response rate or a substantial/complete response rate (where the responses are durable) which is something unexpected for a new agent. The best example of this is the high response rates noted with arsenic trioxide for patients with refractory acute promyelocytic leukemia.

   b. a lower response rate but a low incidence of side effects. An excellent example of this is the Phase II experience with Herceptin® for patients with refractory breast cancer (with response rates of 11% but with no significant side effects).

If you plan to use a Phase II strategy for approval, in general it is better to utilize a Phase II trial design with a reference arm. Otherwise there is a concern about patient selection (e.g., selection of long-term survivors regardless of treatment). Two possible strategies to give most reviewers confidence that it is indeed your new agent that is making a difference include trial designs such as:

a.   Patients with a refractory malignancy ⟨ High dose of the new agent / Lower dose of the new agent

Endpoints: response rate or time to tumor progression (if the arms are blinded).

b.   Patients with a refractory malignancy ⟨ New agent / Clinician's choice

Endpoint: response rate—as it is more difficult to blind the trial.
(*Note*: this could be a 2:1 randomized of new agent vs clinician's choice.)

Table 3
Anticancer Agents Considered by the Oncology Advisory Committee and Biologics
Committee of the U.S. Food and Drug Administration, September 1993–June 2002[a]

Agent (disease)	Type of trial(s) performed	Approved/ disapproved	Primary parameter for approval
Bleomycin (malignant pleural effusions)	Randomized Phase III	Approved	Treatment and prevention of recurrent pleural effusions
Paclitaxel (breast cancer)	Phase II	Approved	Response rate
Vinorelbine (non-small-cell lung cancer)	Phase III	Approved	Survival
Vinorelbine (breast)	Phase III	Disapproved 6/7/94	—
Tamoxifen (breast cancer)	Phase III	Approved	Bioavailability of different dose sizes
Porfimer (esophageal)	Phase II	Approved	Reduction of obstruction and palliation of dysphagia
Pegaspargase (patients who require but are allergic to asparaginase)	Phase III	Approved	Fewer toxicities
Tretinoin (acute promyelocytic leukemia)	Phase II	Approved	Response
Docetaxel (breast)	Phase II	Disapproved 12/18/94	—
Doxorubicin—liposomal (Doxil) (AIDS-related KS)	Phase II	Approved	Response
Nilutamide (prostate)	Phase III	Approved	Time to progression
Interferon α-2a (CML)	Phase III	Approved	Response
Daunorubicin (AIDS related KS) —liposomal (DaunoXome)	Phase III	Approved	Response
Gemcitabine (pancreatic cancer)	Phase III	Approved	Clinical benefit
Interferon α-2b (melanoma postoperative adjuvant)	Phase III	Approved	Time to recurrence
Anastrozole	Phase III	Approved	Time to progression
Toremifene	Phase II	Approved	Response
Docetaxel (breast)	Phase II	Approved	Response
Bicalutamid (prostate)	Phase III	Approved	Time to progression
Talc (pleural effusion sclerosing agent)	Phase II	Approved	Recurrence of pleural effusions
Goserelin acetate (breast)	Phase III	Approved	Time to tumor progression
Topotecan (ovarian cancer)	Phase II	Approved	Response
Irinotecan (colorectal cancer)	Phase II	Approved	Response
Pamidronate (bone metastases)	Phase II	Approved	No. of bone events
Carmustine implant (Gliadel wafer) (glioblastoma multiforme)	Phase III	Approved	Survival
Mitoxantrone (prostate)	Phase III	Approved	Time to progression
Bropiramine (bladder cancer in situ)	Phase III	Disapproved 9/11/96	—
BCG vaccine (prophylaxis of papillary bladder)	Phase III	Approved	Decreased recurrence of papillary carcinoma
Letrozole (breast)	Phase III	Approved	Time to progression
Idarubicin (with other drugs for leukemia)	Phase III	Approved	Survival, less toxicity
Mitoguazone (AIDS-related lymphoma)	Phase II	Disapproved 6/23/97	—
Anegrelide (thrombocytothemia)	Phase II	Approved	Reduction in number of platelets
Paclitaxel (AIDS-related KS)	Phase II	Approved	Response
Liarozole (prostate)	Phase III	Disapproved 6/24/97	—
Vorozole (breast)	Phase III	Disapproved 9/15/97	—
Porfimer sodium (for reduction of obstruction and palliation of non-small-cell lung cancer)	Phase II	Disapproved 9/18/97	—

Continued

Table 3 (Continued)
Anticancer Agents Considered by the Oncology Advisory Committee and Biologics
Committee of the U.S. Food and Drug Administration, September 1993–June 2002[a]

Agent (disease)	Type of trial(s) performed	Approved/ disapproved	Primary parameter for approval
Porfimer sodium (for treatment of endobronchial carcinoma)	Phase II	Approved	Response
Paclitaxel (paxene) (AIDS-related KS)	Phase II	Approved	Response
DepoCyt (cytarabine foam) (carcinomatous meningitis)	Phase II	Disapproved 12/18/97	—
Proleukin (recombinant human interleukin 2)	Phase II	Approved	Response
Rituximab (low-grade lymphoma)	Phase II	Approved	Response
Etoposide phosphate (lung cancer in combination with other drugs)	Phase III	Approved	Comparative kinetics
Capecitabine (breast cancer after failure on paclitaxel and anthracylines)	Phase II	Approved	Response
Gemcitabine (non-small-cell lung)	Phase III	Approved	Survival
Paclitaxel (non-small-cell lung)	Phase III	Approved	Survival
Paclitaxel (ovarian first line)	Phase III	Approved	Survival
Docetaxel (breast cancer locally advanced or metastatic)	Phase III	Approved	Survival
Valrubicin	Phase II	Disapproved 6/11/98	—
Topotecan (small cell)	Phase III	Approved	Survival
Denileukin diftitox-Ontak (cutaneous T-cell lymphoma)	Phase II	Approved	Response
Valrubicin (treatment of patients with BCG refractory carcinoma in situ of the bladder)	Phase II	Approved	Time to recurrence
Suramin hexasodium (prostate)	Phase III	Disapproved 9/1/98	—
Trastuzumab (Herceptin®) (breast)	Phase II	Approved	Response
Tamoxifen (breast cancer risk reduction)	Phase III	Approved	Reduction in breast cancer in high-risk cancer
Porfimer sodium (non-small-cell)	Phase III	Approved	Reduction of obstruction and palliation of symptoms in patients with completely or partially obstructing non-small-cell lung cancer.
Irinotecan (colorectal)	Phase III	Approved	Survival
Cytarabine (DepoCyt) (lymphomatous meningitis)	Phase II	Approved	Response
Alitretinoin (panretin gel) for AIDS-related KS	Phase II	Approved	Response
Temozolomide (anaplastic astrocytoma)	Phase II	Approved	Response
Busulfan (transplant)	Phase II	Approved	Conditioning regimen for bone marrow transplant in combination with other chemotherapy agents and for radiotherapy
Temozolomide (melanoma)	Phase III	Disapproved 3/23/90	—
Epirubicin (breast)	Phase III	Approved	Survival
Liposomal doxorubicin (Doxil)—ovary	Phase III	Approved	Time to progression
Liposomal doxorubicin (breast)	Phase III	Disapproved 9/16/99	—
Tegafur and uracil (UFT)	Phase III	Disapproved 9/16/99	—

Continued

Table 3 (Continued)
Anticancer Agents Considered by the Oncology Advisory Committee and Biologics Committee of the U.S. Food and Drug Administration, September 1993–June 2002[a]

Agent (disease)	Type of trial(s) performed	Approved/ disapproved	Primary parameter for approval
Interferon (Roferon-A) Adjuvant for melanoma	Phase III	Approved	Survival Time to recurrence
Paclitaxel (node positive breast)	Phase III	Approved	Diminished recurrence
Docetaxel (lung cancer)	Phase II and III	Approved	Survival
Bexarotene (Targretin) (cutaneous lymphoma)	Phase II	Approved	Response
Celecoxib (familial polyposis)	Phase III	Approved	Reduction and regression of adenomatous colorectal polyps in familial polyposis in patients
Aminolevulimic (actinic keratoses)	Phase III	Approved	Prevent recurrence
Irinotecan (first-line colorectal)	Phase III	Approved	Survival
Oxaliplatin (colorectal)	Phase III	Disapproved 3/16/00	—
Gemtuzimab zogomycin (Mylotarg®) (acute leukemia)	Phase II	Approved	Response
Anastrozole (first-line breast)	Phase III	Approved	Time to progression
Histamine dihydrochloride (melanoma)	Phase III	Disapproved 12/13/00	—
Campath (CLL)	Phase II	Approved	Response
Intradose (cisplatin–epinephrine gel) (head and neck cancer)	Phase III	Disapproved 4/15/01	—
Diclofenac (actinic keratoses)	Phase III	Approved	Decrease in number of actinic keratoses
Imatinib mesylate (CML)	Phase III	Approved	Response
Tamoxifen (breast)	Phase III	Approved	To reduce risk of invasive breast cancer
Capecitabine (colorectal)	Phase III	Approved	Equivalence in survival—less toxicity
Capecitabine (breast in combination with docetaxel)	Phase III	Approved	Survival
Faslodex (breast cancer)	Phase III	Approved	Time to progression
Ibritumomab tiuxetan	Phase III	Approved	Survival

Note: This table does not include chemoprotective and other supportive care agents.

[a] The source for much of this information is: http://www.accessdata.fda.gov/scripts/cder/onctools/odacmeeting.cfm and http://www.accessdata.fda.gov/scripts/cder/onctools/druglist.cfm.

Note added in final editorial review: Since this chapter was prepared a paper by Johnson and colleagues (J Clin Oncol 21:1403–1411, 2003) was published. That paper described the endpoints for approval for all new cancer agents from January 1990 to November 2002. They documented that endpoints *other than survival* were the basis for approval for 39 of 57 (68%) of the oncology drug marketing applications for regular approval and for all 14 applications granted accelerated approval.

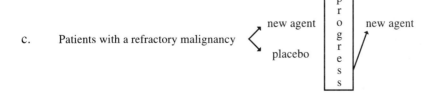

Endpoint: Time to tumor progression with a crossover allowed.

These types of randomized Phase II trials help (page 587) ensure everyone that there is no super-selection of your study population to select for patients who would have a favorable outcome irrespective of which treatment they were given.

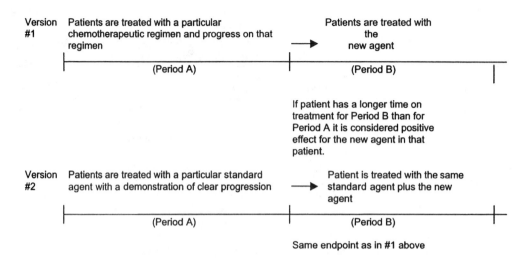

Fig. 1. Two versions of patients as their own control type of trial design.

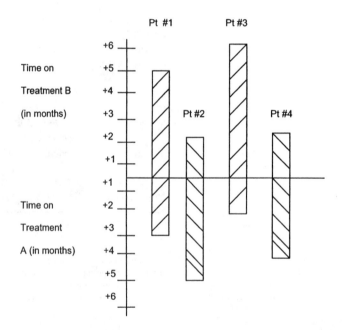

Fig. 2. Suggested manner for plotting time on treatment for period B vs time on treatment for period A. As an example, patient 1 was on treatment B for 5 mo vs on treatment A for 3 mo (which is a positive result). Patient 2 was on new agent B for 2 mo but on the prior regimen A for 5 mo—a negative result.

4. SPECIAL TRIAL DESIGNS, PARTICULARLY SUITED FOR CYTOSTATIC AGENTS

4.1. Patients as Their Own Controls

This is a trial design that, until recently, was all but forgotten. There are at least two versions of this trial design, detailed in Fig. 1. As can be seen in Fig. 1, version 1, any patient who has a longer time on treatment on regimen B than on regimen A is considered a positive

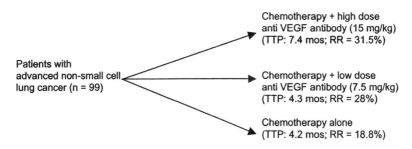

Fig. 3. Randomized Phase II trial of a monoclonal anitbody to VEGF.

result (it is usually not an expected result for a patient to remain on treatment with a second-line regimen for a longer time than on a first-line regimen). This is certainly an inexact situation, as time on treatment is not the same as time to progression, but it is easier to measure when one does not have scans and X-ray films at regular intervals for the first regimen, as one usually has for the second regimen. Even though this is an inexact clinical trial situation, this trial design might offer some insight on whether or not the agent is having an effect on the natural history of the patient's disease. Figure 2 details how the data for such a comparison can be plotted. Based on past experience (3), if ≥30% of patients have a longer time on the new agent than on the regimen they received just prior to the new agent, that is a promising result that should be pursued.

Version 2 of patients as their own control is also detailed in Fig. 1. To try this version of patients as their own controls one must have some preclinical information demonstrating that there is some synergy between the new cytostatic agent and the agent the patient is currently receiving. It is also critical in this design to make *very certain* that the patient is progressing on regimen A (best ascertained by an independent committee). Once again, the endpoint is the same as it is for version 1 and the data can also be plotted as noted in Fig. 2. It needs to be emphasized again that this type of trial is only an *exploratory trial*— but a trial that may again give hints of the agent changing the natural history of the disease. It is not a definitive trial design. This latter (version 2) design has already had a checkered start in that it was utilized for the design for the initial filing of the anti-epidermal growth factor receptor monoclonal antibody C225 *(4)*. The problem with that filing, however, was that it appears that there was unclear documentation as to whether or not the patient progressed on the initial regimen of CPT 11 (period A) to which the C225 was added (during period B). That particular situation should not discourage the clinical investigator from trying version 2 (Fig. 1) of patients as their own controls *if* the new cytostatic agent demonstrates synergy with the standard cytotoxic agent (or other cytostatic agents for that matter).

The reader is referred to an excellent analysis by Mick and colleagues *(5)* on the sequentially measured paired failure time (i.e., patients as their own controls) trial design. That analysis details the important statistical considerations when one is evaluating the patients as their own controls approach.

4.2. The Randomized Phase II Trial

This type of trial design was mentioned above. With some clever additional variations it can yield a great deal of information. Figure 3 details perhaps one interesting randomized Phase II trial, done by DeVore and colleagues *(6)* with a cytostatic agent. As noted in Fig.

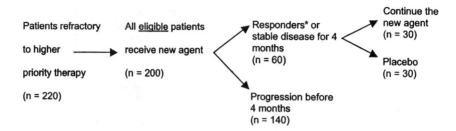

Fig. 4. Randomized discontinued design. *Note: some versions of this design have all of the responders continue to receive the study drug (e.g., they are not randomized to continue the agent versus to receive a placebo).

3, the study was a three-arm study of chemotherapy vs chemotherapy plus a low dose of a MAb to VGEF vs chemotherapy plus a high dose of a MAb to VGEF.

As can be seen in Fig. 3, one of the endpoints for the study, in addition to toxicities, was the TTP. Once again, TTP can be a somewhat inexact endpoint and one that is not usually acceptable to a regulatory agency (except if the arms of the study are blinded—and this study was not). However, the above study design can provide information as to what sample sizes may be needed for an new drug application (NDA)-directed study. Such a study design can also provide information as to whether patients will participate in such a study, accrual rates, and so forth. Such a study design also yields valuable information on the safety of the various arms of the study.

An important option for the study outlined in Fig. 3 is to continue with the study in a randomized fashion, selecting only one of the MAb-containing arms for comparison with the chemotherapy alone arm. This approach can save significant activation time for a new protocol (e.g., continue the randomized Phase II trial and power it up to be large enough for a Phase III trial rather than writing and activating a whole new Phase III trial).

Another randomized Phase II trial that yielded very important information and which serves as an excellent model for solving drug development issues is a trial performed with the agent capecitabine (Xeloda®). After results became available from the Phase I clinical trials with several different schedules of the agent, there was uncertainty as to just which schedule was the best. Therefore a randomized Phase II trial was conducted to determine which schedule (and dose) of capecitabine would be best to take into expanded Phase II and Phase III clinical trials (7). Patients were randomized to receive either: (a) 1331 mg/m^2/d continually; (b) 2510 mg/m^2/d intermittently, or (c) 1657 mg/m^2/d plus leucovorin 60 mg/d p.o. intermittently. The specific aims were to evaluate the safety and efficacy of each schedule. Cleverly, one of the efficacy endpoints utilized (in addition to response rate) was TTP. Utilizing TTP as a parameter of efficacy allowed a finer tuning because it allowed for a continuous assessment (in days) vs the dichotomous variable of response (response or no response). This clever randomized Phase II design showed that schedule "b" was the best schedule in terms of toxicities and efficacy. That schedule was then taken on into successful Phase II and Phase III trials, which led to the very rapid approval of capecitabine.

4.3. Randomized Discontinuation Trial Designs

This is a unique trial design for the development of cytostatic agents that has several very desirable features and yet seems as though it might be a very very difficult trial to complete (8,9). In reality, our team at the Arizona Cancer Center just participated in placing patients on a clinical trial utilizing this randomized discontinuation design and we have found excellent patient participation in the study. The trial design is as outlined in Fig. 4. The design is particularly well suited for a new cytostatic agent that everyone wants to receive (just as the new agent endostatin was).

As noted in Fig. 4, all eligible patients initially received the new agent. Those who progress before 4 mo of treatment are completed are removed from the study. Those patients who do have a response or have stable disease for 4 mo are then randomized to continue the therapy or receive a placebo. The patients are carefully observed and if they have progressive disease (and are receiving placebo), they are placed back on the new agent. The endpoint for the study is the TTP for patients who continue on the therapy vs the TTP for patients who receive placebo.

The randomized discontinuation trial design has been used for testing new agents against the AIDS virus but it is just beginning to be used to evaluate new anticancer agents. Obviously when used in the situation with a new AIDs drug(s) one has viral titers to follow (vs computed axial tomography [CAT] scans and other imaging techniques for oncologists to follow a patient's tumor). The viral titers are more sensitive than our scans are. Also, some investigators question the ethics of randomizing patients who are responding to the new agent to continue, or discontinue that therapy. This problem can be addressed by randomizing only the patients with stable disease (and not the responders). Very carefully administered informed consent is obviously a necessity. One other potential problem with the randomized discontinuation design is that there is a theoretical problem in comparing the patients continued on therapy vs those on placebo if there is a carryover effect of the agent (i.e., it could still be having an effect on the placebo group).

Regardless of its downsides, the randomized discontinuation trial design is one that should be considered for a new cytostatic agent. It does allow for a greater number of patients to have access to a potentially exciting new agent.

5. A UNIQUE ENDPOINT FOR APPROVAL

5.1. Clinical Benefit

In the early development of the chain terminator gemcitabine there were some patients with pancreatic cancer who demonstrated a decrease in their tumor-related pain and an increase in their appetite and weight (10). Gemcitabine had a new mechanism of action. It did not cause regression of pancreatic cancer growing in nude mice but rather it caused a slowing of growth of the pancreatic cancer xenografts growing in nude mice (MIA Pa Ca, PANC-1 and PAN C02) (11,12). Therefore, it was likely that one would not see a complete or partial response in patients. In conversations with Dr. Bob Temple at the FDA (still at the FDA) and Dr. Gregory Burke (now at Novartis) our team was alerted to the fact that one endpoint they could accept in a trial was "fixing what bothers the patient." The term clinical benefit was derived from that conversation. Clinical benefit was not necessarily a quality of life parameter but it was an attempt to measure "fixing what bothers the patient." Because the three most common problems experienced by patients with pancreatic cancer included pain, weight loss, and a deterioration in performance status, Dr. John Anderson at Eli Lilly devised an algorithm to measure clinical benefit (13). This algorithm utilized pain (measured by the Memorial Pain Assessment Card) performance status (measured by the Karnofsky scale because it had a broader range of 0–100 in increments of 10 rather than the ECOG or SWOG scales which have a range of only 0–5), and a direct measurement of weight (with clear cut definitions of what constituted weight gain or weight loss) (13). The pivotal trial design for gemcitabine was as follows:

Table 4
Results of Randomized Trial of Gemcitabine vs 5-FU

Parameter	5-FU arm (n = 63)	Gemcitabine arm (n = 63)	p Value
Clinical benefit (% of patients)	4.8%	23.8%	0.0022
Response rate	0	5.4%	
Time to progression (mo)	1.0	3.2	0.0002
Survival			
Median (mo)	4.41	5.65	0.0025
1 yr	2%	18%	

Data from ref. *14*.

Patients with advanced, symptomatic pancreatic cancer ⟨ Weekly gemcitabine / Weekly 5–FU

The primary endpoint for the study was an improvement in clinical benefit, with the secondary endpoints including response rate, median survival, and percentage of patients alive at 1 yr *(14)*. Table 4 details the results of the study.

As can be seen in Table 4, the study was positive for clinical benefit as well as for the other parameters. Gemcitabine was approved for use for treatment of patients with locally advanced or metastatic pancreatic cancer by the Oncology Drug Advisory Committee (ODAC) and by the FDA on the basis of this one study. In addition, there was a Phase II trial that was uncontrolled but demonstrated a similar survival (and response) to that found in the randomized phase III study *(15)*. Gemcitabine was approved for treatment of patients with locally advanced or metastatic pancreatic cancer. Many observers who were present at the ODAC felt that gemcitabine would not have been approved if clinical benefit were the only parameter that was improved by gemcitabine. The other item of note is that gemcitabine was approved for frontline treatment of patients with advanced pancreatic cancer based on only one randomized trial. Observers at the ODAC felt that was because there were very few options for patients (and no prior controlled trials ever demonstrated an improvement in survival for any single agent) with advanced pancreatic cancer that gemcitabine was approved.

It is of note that no other attempts have been made to bring a new agent to the FDA using the clinical benefit parameter as the primary endpoint of the study. However, this investigator believes that with the proper algorithm it could be a solid primary endpoint for other pivotal trials with a new agent.

6. SPECIAL CHALLENGES IN CLINICAL TRIAL DESIGNS FOR APPROVAL

6.1. Analogs

Unfortunately in anticancer drug development we are still in the sulfonamide era—meaning that it is probably more productive to find agents with new mechanisms of action (for greater progress) than to work on analogs. However, there have been many commercial successes with analogs, largely based on less (or different) toxicities rather than on improved efficacy *(16–19)*. The types of trials for approval for an analog program could be:

a. Patients whose tumors are progressing on the parent compound (with very clear documentation of that progress) → Patient is treated with the analog
Endpoint: Response rate

Endpoint: Response rate

Issues with this design include a very refractory patient population. However, if the analog has activity in that setting, it will certainly have a substantial chance for approval (20).

b. Treat patients with the new analog who have a tumor type that is not responsive to the parent compound → Patient is treated with the analog
Endpoint: Response rate

Endpoint: Response rate

The issue here is that it is unlikely the analog will work in this situation. However, if it does work in this situation it also will have an excellent chance for eventual approval.

c. Patients with a disease usually responsive to the parent compound ↗ New analog
↘ Parent compound

Endpoints: Survival, response rate, TTP toxicities

This is the best way to evaluate a new analog and the most likely way for an analog to be approved by regulatory agencies. Of course, superiority in one of the endpoints (not equivalence) is usually more convincing for approval.

7. OTHER COMMENTS ON CLINICAL TRIALS FOR APPROVAL

Given the difficulty of treating patients with cancer, this author (as do many others in the field) believes that we should do everything we can to gain approval for new agents so patients have options. There are frequently numerous criticisms passing back and forth between investigators, regulators, educators, survivors, and others. At times their criticisms are valid—that perhaps we are asking for so much proof that an agent works (e.g., an improvement in survival) that it is discouraging to all involved and actually dampens any enthusiasm for development of new agents. It is this author's belief that the more these different constituencies communicate and work together (without assigning blame), the better chance we will have to develop innovative endpoints and trial designs for more rapid approval. Our job, together, is to obtain more options for clinical trial designs that allow development of new agents that work for our patients.

ACKNOWLEDGMENTS

This work was supported by the National Foundation for Cancer Research, Center for New Therapies Development at the Arizona Cancer Center. Dr. Von Hoff is a fellow of the National Foundation for Cancer Research.

REFERENCES

1. Staquet MJ, Byar DP, Green SB, Rozencweig M. Clinical predictivity of transplantable tumor systems in the selection of new drugs for solid tumors: rationale for a three-stage strategy. Can Treat Rep 1983; 67:753–765.
2. O'Shaughnessy JA, Wittes RE, Burke G, et al. Commentary concerning demonstration of safety and efficacy of investigational anticancer agents in clinical trials. J Clin Oncol 1991; 9:2225–2232.
3. Von Hoff DD. There are no bad anticancer agents. Only bad clinical trial designs—Twenty-first Richard and Hinda Rosenthal Foundation Award Lecture. Clin Cancer Res 1998; 4:1079–1086.

4. Saltz L, Rubin M, Hochster H, et al. Cetuximab (IMC-C225) plus irinotecan (CPT-11) is active in CPT-11-refractoy colorectal cancer (CRC) that expresses epidermal growth factor receptor (EGFR). Proc Annu Meet Am Soc Clin Oncol 2001; 20:3a: abstract 7.

5. Mick R, Crowley JJ, Carroll RJ. Phase II clinical trial design for noncytotoxic anticancer agents for which time to disease progression is the primary endpoint. Control Clin Trials 2000; 21:343–359.

6. DeVore RF, Fehrenbacher L, Herbst R, et al. A randomized Phase II trial comparing rhumab VEGF (recombinant humanized monoclonal antibody to vascular endothelial cell growth factor) plus carboplatin/paclitaxel (CP) to CP alone in patients with stage IIB/IV NSCLS. Proc Annu Meet Am Soc Clin Oncol 2000; 19:485a: abstract 1896.

7. Findlay M, Van Cutsem E, Kocha W, et al. A randomised phase II study of Xeloda™ (capecitabine) in patients with advanced colorectal cancer. Proc Annu Meet Am Soc Clin Oncol 1997; 16:227a: abstract 798.

8. Ratain MJ. Development of target-based antineoplastic agents. In: Perry MC (ed). American Society of Clinical Oncology Educational Book. Alexandria, VA: American Society of Clinical Oncology, 1999, pp. 71–75.

9. Kopec JA, Abrahamowicz M, Esdaile JM. Randomized discontinuation trials: utility and efficiency. J Clin Epidemiol 1993; 46:959–971.

10. Casper ES, Green MR, Kelsen DP. Phase II trial of gemcitabine (2′,2′-difflurodeoxycytidine) in patients with adenocarcinoma of the pancreas. Invest New Drugs 1994; 12:29–34.

11. Schultz RM, Merriman RL, Toth JE, et al. Evaluation of new anticancer agents agains the MIA PaCa-2 and PANC-1 human pancreatic carcinoma xenografts. Oncol Res 1993; 3:223–228.

12. Merriman RL, Hertel LW, Schultz R, et al. Comparison of the antitumor activity of gemcitabine and ara-C in a panel of human breast, colon, lung and pancreatic xenograft models. Investig New Drugs 1996; 14:243–247.

13. Anderson JS, Burris HA, Casper E. Development of a new system for assessing clinical benefit for patients with advanced pancreatic cancer. Proc Annu Meet Am Soc Clin Oncol 1994; 13:461: abstract 1600.

14. Burris H, Moore M, Anderson J, et al. Improvements in survival and clinical benefit with gemcitabine as first-line therapy for patients with advanced pancreas cancer: a randomized trial. J Clin Oncol 1997; 15:2403–2413.

15. Rothenberg ML, Moore MJ, Cripps MC, et al. A Phase II trial of gemcitabine in patients with 5-FU-refractory pancreas cancer. Ann Oncol 1996; 7:347–353.

16. Bontenbal M, Andersson M, Wildiers J, et al. Doxorubicin vs epirubicin, report of a second-line randomized phase II/III study in advanced breast cancer. Br J Cancer 1998; 77:2257–2263.

17. Gasparini G, Dal Fior S, Panizzoni GA, Favretto S, Pozza F. Weekly epirubicin versus doxorubicin as second line therapy in advanced breast cancer. A randomized clinical trial. Am J Clin Oncol 1991; 14: 38–44.

18. Jain KK, Casper ES, Geller NL, et al. A prospective randomized comparison of epirubicin and doxo-rubicin in patients with advanced breast cancer. J Clin Oncol 1985; 3:818–826.

19. Alberts DS, Green S, Hannigan EV, et al. Improved therapeutic index of carboplatin plus cyclophos-phamide versus cisplatin plus cyclophohshphamide: Final report by the Southwest Oncology Group of a phase III randomized trial in stages III and IV ovarian cancer. J Clin Oncol 1992; 10:706–717.

20. Valero V, Jones SE, Von Hoff DD, et al. A Phase II study of docetaxel in patients with paclitaxel-resistant metastatic breast cancer. J Clin Oncol 1998; 16:3362–3368.

34 Pharmacogenetic Counseling

Jill M. Kolesar, Pharm D

1. INTRODUCTION

Originally identified as early as 500 BCE by Pythagoras, who connected "sallowness" to ingestion of fava beans, now understood as hemolytic anemia caused by eating fava beans by individuals with glucose-6-dehydrogenase deficiency (G6DP) deficiency, the field of pharmacogenetics emerged as a scientific discipline with the landmark discoveries of Werner Kalow in the 1950s. Kalow was the first to identify the genetic basis for differences in affinity of plasma cholinesterases for the anesthetic succinylcholine and that those individuals with reduced affinity for succinylcholine experienced prolonged paralysis, apnea, and sometimes death.

Important advances in molecular biology, genetics, and biotechnology, culminating in the human genome project brings us today to "genetic medicine" of which pharmacogenetics is an integral part. With the advance of genetic medicine into everyday practice the importance of understanding and appropriately using pharamcogenetic information and communicating that information to patients is a priority.

The role of genetics in predicting and diagnosing disease is well established, while the field of clinical pharmacogenetics is still emerging. In most cases, the inherited disease predisposition genes are important in diagnosing a disease and as a potential target for gene therapy; however, a disease predisposition gene usually does not influence how an individual responds to a given medication.

Oncology is unique in two respects: first that there are both inherited genetic traits, such as the thiopurine methyltransferase (TPMT) deficiency associated with drug response and acquired genetic traits or mutations such as *p53* mutations that influence response to therapy and second, the disease causing genetic traits and the drug response traits are exceedingly difficult to separate. In many cases, such as that with imitinab (Gleevec), the genetic mutation causes the disease, is used to diagnose the disease, and predicts who will respond to the

Handbook of Anticancer Pharmacokinetics and Pharmacodynamics
Edited by: W. D. Figg and H. L. McLeod © Humana Press Inc., Totowa, NJ

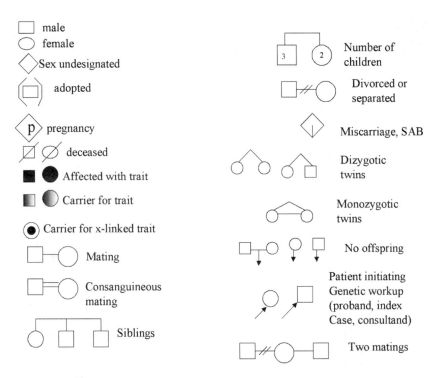

Fig. 1. Standard figures for constructing a pedigree.

therapy. Therefore the genetics of the disease as well as the therapy must be considered in the clinical use of pharmacogenetic information and in pharmacogenetic counseling.

2. OVERVIEW OF CLINICAL GENETICS

Understanding the terminology and principles of basic clinical genetics are essential for health professional engaged in pharmacogenetic counseling (1,2). Construction of a pedigree is the basic documentation used in taking a genetic history and certain conventions, as diagrammed in Fig. 1, exist. First, females are always represented as circles and males as squares, with a horizontal line between the two signifying mating. Individuals with a particular trait are represented with a filled-in circle or square, carriers with a half-filled-in circle or square. Offspring from a mating are designated by a vertical line perpendicular to the horizontal line signifying the mating and are ordered with the firstborn from left to right.

Other important definitions include: An *allele* is one alternative form of a given allelic pair; more than two alleles can exist for any specific gene, but only two of them will be found within any individual. An *allelic pair* is defined as the combination of two alleles that comprise the gene pair. A *homozygote* is an individual containing only one allele at the allelic pair; for example, *DD* is homozygous dominant and *dd* is homozygous recessive. A *heterozygote* is an individual with one of each member of the gene pair, for example, the *Dd* heterozygote The *genotype* is the specific allelic combination for a certain gene or set of genes and the *phenotype* is the outward manifestation of the trait (3).

2.1. Mendelian Genetics

2.1.1. DOMINANT INHERITANCE

As initially identified by the Augustinian monk Gregor Mendel in 1865, from the study of purple and white pea flowers, dominance is defined as the allele that expresses itself at the expense of an alternate allele. In conditions that are inherited in an autosomal dominant fashion, affected individuals are heterozygous for an autosomal dominant disease gene and a normal gene. In such cases, the presence of the abnormal gene results in the clinical expression or phenotype of a disease or a condition. All individuals with a dominant trait must carry the abnormal gene with a 50% chance that they will pass this gene on to their offspring *(3)*.

In human cancers, *BRCA1* is inherited in an autosomal dominant fashion, therefore, as outlined in Fig. 2A, a parent with the *BRCA1* gene will pass the gene on to 50% of her children. If the gene were 100% *penetrant*, defined as the frequency with which individuals carrying a given locus (or genotype) exhibit the phenotype, all of the gene carriers would exhibit the disease. The penetrance of *BRCA1* is still under debate, but is estimated to be between 38% and 67%. If it were 50% penetrant, as diagrammed in Fig. 2B, 50% of the children would have the gene, but only half of those would develop the disease. However, individuals who carry the gene who do not develop disease will still have a 50% chance of passing that gene to their children, and again assuming 50% penetrance, 50% of the children who receive the gene will develop disease. See Fig. 2C *(1–3)*.

2.1.2. RECESSIVE INHERITANCE

In *recessive* inheritance, an allele's expression is suppressed in the presence of a dominant allele. The parents have the gene for a particular disease, such as cystic fibrosis, but because they are phenotypically normal, they are unaware of it. Their offspring have a 25% chance of inheriting the disease-causing allele from both of their parents and having the phenotype and a 50% chance of inheriting one allele from one of their parents and becoming carriers of the trait. See Fig. 3.

An interesting exception is that of retinoblastoma, the first example of a tumor suppressor gene, showing that cancer could be caused not only by activation of a protooncogene, but also by mutation or loss of a tumor suppressor gene. In the United States, Europe, and Japan retinoblastoma occurs in approx 1 per 20,000 births. Approximately 60% of all cases are unilateral and not heritable; about 10% are unilateral and heritable (with or without positive family history); 5% are bilateral, with family history; and 25% are bilateral new germline mutants that are inheritable in subsequent generations.

Therefore approx 40% of retinoblastomas are hereditary, and require one germline mutation and one somatic mutation, as described by the classic two-hit model proposed by Knudesen. A simple explanation of two mutational hits is that they occur in the two copies of the same gene; that is, although predisposition or susceptibility to disease is dominantly inherited, oncogenesis or the expression of the tumor is recessive. The second hit may be a new intragenic mutation, gene deletion, chromosomal loss, or somatic recombination. This concept of *multihit somatic mutations* (in local tissue or organs) on top of a *constitutional mutation* (present in the germline) forms the basic concept for the heritable forms of cancers including colon cancer and breast cancer *(1–4)*.

2.1.3. SEX-LINKED DISORDERS

Sex-linked disorders, such as hemophilia, are recessive alleles, but are carried on the X chromosome. Therefore in females, with two X chromosomes, two alleles are required to

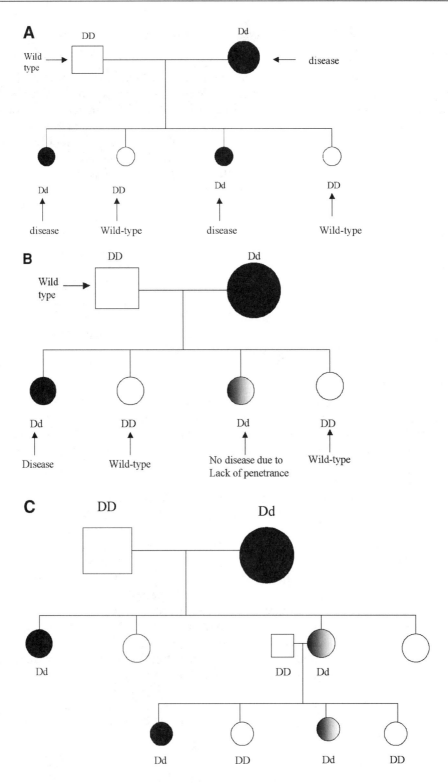

Fig. 2. **(A)** Dominant inheritance, 100% penetrance. **(B)** Dominant inheritance, 50% penetrance. **(C)** Dominant inheritance, 50% penetrance, third generation.

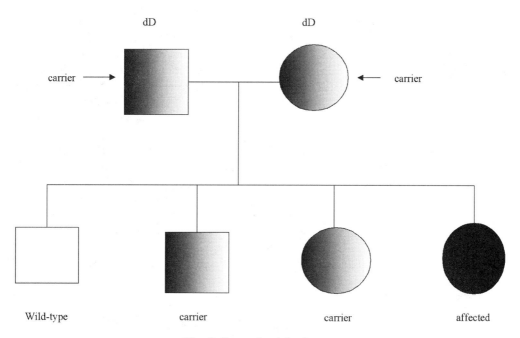

Fig. 3. Recessive inheritance.

express a phenotype, whereas in males, with only one X chromosome, only one copy is required to express the phenotype. Because men inherit their X chromosome from their mother, sex-linked traits are always transmitted from mother to son. Despite some cancers occurring exclusively in males (e.g., prostate cancer) or females (e.g., ovarian cancer) there is currently no evidence to suggest that any cancers are X-linked or carried on the X chromosome, but are related to other differences between the sexes *(1–3)*.

2.1.4. SNPs AND HAPLOTYPES

Single nucleotide polymorphisms (SNPs) are single basepair variations in DNA sequence. Because SNPs are mutations that have occurred in a prior generation, SNPs represent our genetic evolutionary history, and individuals with the same SNP likely share a common ancestor.

Even more interesting is the enormous number of SNPs. There are currently 1.42 million known SNPs that are found at a density of one SNP per 1.91 kilobases, with the density even higher in regions containing genes *(5)*. The International SNP Map Working Group estimates that they have identified 60,000 SNPs within genes ("coding" SNPs), or one coding SNP per 1.08 kilobases of gene sequence. In addition, 93% of genes contain a SNP, and 98% are within five kilobases of a SNP *(5)*.

Genome-wide linkage analysis and positional cloning have already identified hundreds of genes associated with human disease *(6)*. However, for the most part the identified diseases are rare disorders, where a single gene mutation is sufficient to cause the disease(6). Identifying the gene that predisposes for common disorders has proven much more difficult and suggests that a haplotype, or combination of genes at a closely linked site, may in fact be responsible for common diseases and that a single genotype may contribute but not solely determine a phenotype *(7–9)*.

There is increasing support for the "common variant–common disease hypothesis," which proposes that most of the genetic contributions to disease susceptibility arise from variants that are relatively common in the susceptible population *(10)*. Testing this hypothesis would entail a systematic case-control analysis of all common variants in the human genome to identify the major causative genetic contributions to a disease *(6)*. However, the major limitation to this approach is that technology is not sufficiently advanced to support this large-scale (1.42 million SNPs must be sequenced per case) project.

Haplotyping may be one method to accomplish this goal with existing or developing technology. The haplotyping proposal is based on the observation that SNPs are not inherited independently; rather, sets of adjacent SNPs are inherited in blocks and each block has only a few common haplotypes *(8)*. This means that although a block may contain many SNPs, it takes only a few SNPs to uniquely identify or "tag" each of the haplotypes in the block *(8)*.

The National Institute of Health (NIH) has recently launched an initiative to develop a haplotype map, the so-called HapMap, which will be a description of the set of haplotype blocks and the SNPs that tag them. The HapMap is expected to be valuable by reducing the number of SNPs required to examine the entire genome for association with a phenotype from 10 million SNPs to roughly 300,000 tag SNPs.

2.2. Acquired Variability

2.2.1. Chromosomal Rearrangements and the Leukemias

Chromosomal rearrangements are seen in 70–80% of leukemias with many occurring in a nonrandom fashion and certain translocations associated regularly with the various leukemia subtypes. The clonality of leukemias and consistency of rearrangements suggest that chromosomal aberrations are essential to the development of different leukemia subtypes *(11)*.

Chromosomal aberrations may be in number or structure. Chromosomal losses due to deletions, unbalanced translocations, or complete loss of chromosomes are usually negative prognostic indicators. There may also be a net gain in chromosomal material, including trisomy or polysomy, which has a better prognosis when compared to chromosomal loss. The structural changes in chromosomes generally involve translocations, in which genetic material is exchanged between two different chromosomes *(11)*.

This exchange can lead to oncogenesis by two general pathways: first, two new chimeric or combination genes may be generated by the translocations (see Fig. 4A), and second a new or strong promoter may be translocated just upstream from a protooncogene (see Fig. 4B).

The majority of leukemia-causing aberrations are translocations that fuse two genes and generate a chimeric protein; these are described in Table 1 *(11)*. Clinically all patients undergo cytogenetic analysis for categorization of their leukemia. In addition to disease categorization, cytogenetics are used for selecting therapy in two specific examples: the t(15:17) characteristic of M3 variant of acute myelogenous leukemia (AML) *(12,13)* and the t(9:22) *(14)*, also known as the Philadephia chromosome, characteristic of chronic myelogenous leukemia (CML).

Prior to 1988, the natural history of M3 AML was that approx 40% of individuals had essentially benign disease and excellent long-term survival, regardless of therapy, and another 40% with early mortality occurring within 1 yr. The natural history of M3 AML was changed forever by the discovery of t(15:17) by Rowley in 1977 *(15)*. Work in subsequent years concentrated on understanding the function of the fusion protein PML-RAR-α.

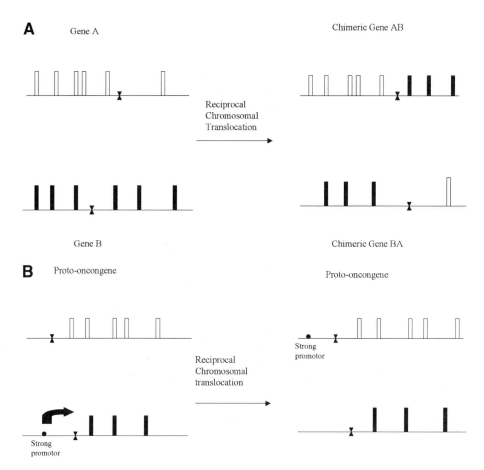

Fig. 4. (**A**) Generation of novel fusion genes by chromsomal translocation. (**B**) Activation of cellular protooncogenes.

Table 1
Frequent Chromosomal Abnormalities in Leukemias

Chromosomal rearrangement	Leukemia	Clinical implications
t(8;21)(q22;q22)	AML–M2 (20%)	Improved prognosis
t(12;21)(p13;q22)	Childhood ALL (20%)	Improved prognosis
t(15;17)(q22;q12)	AML–M3 (95%)	Excellent prognosis. Induction with all-*trans*-retinoic acid.
t (9;22)(q34;q11) The Philadelphia chromosome	CML (>95%) Adult ALL (25%)	Excellent prognosis for those with CML and an indication for imitinab. Poor prognostic factor for ALL
t(1;19)(p23;p13)	Childhood ALL (2–5%)	Intermediate prognosis
t(6;9)(p23;q24)	AML preceded by MDS	Unfavorable prognosis
Inv (16)(p13;22) or t(16;16)(p13q22)	AML–M4 with eosinophilia	Favorable prognosis

The physiological function of PML is still unknown; however, RAR-α is a retinoic acid receptor, its function central to differentiation of myeloid cells by binding to DNA response elements in combination with either steroid or thyroid receptors with a net result of regulation of adjacent genes. The PML-RAR-α fusion protein is unable to perform this regulatory function and M3-AML results *(13)*. Administration of all-trans retinoic acid corrects this defect and allows cells to differentiate. Clinically, administration of 45 mg/m^2/d of all-*trans*-retinoic acid for 90 d prior to daunarubicin and ara-c results in elimination of early mortality and improves the long-term survival from 40% to 80%. This is probably the first example in oncology in which genetics was used to select drug therapy, certainly with impressive results.

Recently, a small molecule directed toward the Philadelphia chromosome, t(9:22) has shown excellent response rates in CML *(16)*. Imitinab was approved after one of the shortest evaluation periods in history for an antineoplastic and achieves single-agent response rates of > 70% when compared to interferon-α with response rates of approx 30%. In addition to CML, imitinab was recently approved for gastrointestinal stromal tumors (GIST) tumors that are positive for an additional tyrosine kinase, c-kit.

2.2.2. POINT MUTATIONS AND THE SOLID TUMORS

The development of solid tumors is now seen as a complex, multistep process that depends on both external carcinogenic influences and subcellular genetic defects *(17)*. This is in contrast to hematological malignancies, where one mutation, usually a translocation, results in clonal growth *(11)*. The genetic defects common to solid tumors may be caused by a variety of mechanisms—directly by mutagenic carcinogens or inherited, or may occur sporadically *(18)*.

The first types of genes important in carcinogenesis are the susceptibility genes, which are generally inherited and are usually drug and xenobiotic metabolizing enzymes and are discussed in Subheading 3. In addition, mutations in mismatch repair genes, clinically associated with the hereditary nonpolyposis colon cancer (HNPCC) may occur. The normal function of mismatch repair genes is to repair damaged DNA; therefore individuals with deficiencies in these enzymes are more likely to accumulate mutations in cancer causing genes *(18)*.

The genes that are associated with the development of malignancy, rather than the predisposition when dysfunctional, are broadly categorized as oncogenes or tumor suppressor genes *(18)*.

2.2.2.1. Oncogenes

Oncogenes are normal genes (known as protooncogenes prior to mutation) that may become oncogenes either by incorporation of a retrovirus into the genetic material or, more commonly, by mutation *(19)*.

Oncogenes, by definition, confer malignant properties onto a cell, resulting in gain of function; that may occur by amplification where the affected gene overproduces a protein that drives cell proliferation or enhances survival, or it may occur by production of a mutant protein that escapes control mechanisms that normally constrain its proliferative activity. Oncogenes generally encode proteins that stimulate cellular growth or survival, including growth factors, growth factor receptors, intracellular signal transducers, and transcription factors.

An oncogene typically acts as a dominant gene, with a mutation in one allele sufficient to cause the phenotype. However, with few exceptions, oncogenes are not inherited and usually contribute to the pathogenesis of cancer by somatic mutations within the cells of the target tissues *(17,18)*.

There has been much debate over the role of *p53*, as an oncogene, a tumor suppressor gene, or a DNA repair gene, however; whatever its classification, *p53* is one of the most clinically significant mutations and is used as a diagnostic test for Li–Fraumeni syndrome, is under evaluation for predicting prognosis in various solid tumors, and is in clinical trials as gene therapy to enhance chemosensitivity *(17,18)*.

2.2.2.2. Tumour Suppressor Genes

In contrast to oncogenes, tumor suppressor genes, in their normal state, encode proteins that inhibit proliferation or promote loss. These genes contribute to carcinogenesis when they develop mutations resulting in a loss of function. In this case the normal gene tends to act in a dominant fashion and only when both alleles are damaged will the effect of the mutant gene be apparent. Because of this, mutations in single alleles of tumor suppressor genes may be inherited *(17,18)*.

Tumor suppressor genes that are routinely screened as art of clinical management and diagnosis of disease include *APC*, *RB*, *MEN1*, and *VHL* all of which are thought to play important roles in slowing cellular growth.

3. PHARMACOGENETICS AND CANCER PREDISPOSITION
3.1. Xenobiotics

Xenobiotic drug-metabolizing enzymes, including the cytochrome P450s, are essential not only in metabolizing clinically useful drugs, but also in detoxifying environmental carcinogens. Therefore, a long-standing yet largely still unproven hypothesis for carcinogenesis is that polymorphisms *(20,21)* in these metabolizing enzymes lead to altered metabolism, either increased activation or decreased inactivation of environmental carcinogens, prolonged exposure to genotoxic compounds, and hence cancer. Numerous case control and epidemiological studies have been reported and have been reviewed recently by Bartsch *(22)* as well as Guengerich *(23)*.

What is well known is that cytochrome P450 enzymes are involved in the activations of numerous carcinogens *(24,25)*. The role of cyp 1A1 in benzopyrene metabolism; 1A2 in toluene and the heterocyclic amines found in broiled meat; 1B1 in nitropyrenes; 2E1 in benzene, butadiene, chloroform, vinyl chloride; and 3A4 in aflatoxin metabolism are well established *(20,21)*.

There is substantial evidence from animal models that susceptibility to cancer induced by chemical carcinogens is greatly influenced by variations in P450 enzymes. Although not as conclusive as the animal studies, population epidemiologic evidence supports 1A1 inducibility, potentially related to the *2B* genotype, with susceptibility to tobacco-induced cancers, including lung and head and neck, in Japanese populations *(25–28)*, but not in Caucasian or other populations *(22–24,29)*, and an association of the *1A2 *2F* genotype with an increased risk of colon cancer and bladder cancer. See Table 2.

NADP(H)quinone: oxidoreductase (NQO1) is a two-electron reductase with a characteristic polymorphism, the *2 that has been associated with both benzene toxicity and the development of leukemia *(30)*. In a case-control study conducted in Shanghai China, subjects homozygous for the *2 allele had a 7.6-fold (95% confidence interval, 1.8–31.2) increased risk of benzene poisoning compared to subjects who carried one or two wild-type *NQO1* alleles *(31)*. In a series of infant leukemias with *MLL* rearrangements versus unselected cord blood controls, *MLL*-rearranged leukemias were more likely to have genotypes with low *NQO1* function (heterozygous CT or homozygous TT at nucleotide 609) than controls (odds ratio, 2.5; $p = 0.015$) *(32)*. In addition, Caucasian non-small-cell lung

---

Table 2
Human Drug Metabolizing Enzymes Potentially Important in Carcinogenesis

Allele	Variant	Population	Cancer risk	Strength of association
1A1	M1, M2	Caucasians	Lung	Controversial
1A1/GST	GST/M1	Japanese smokers	Lung	Strong consistent association in multiple studies
NQO1	*2	Benzene exposed	Aplastic anemia, leukemia	Strong association in one large population study
NQO1	*2	Prior chemotherapy	MDS, AML	Consistent effect in multiple studies

cancer patients homozygous for the *2 allele have much poorer survival than those who are wild-types or heterozygotes (33).

Overall there is no polymorphism that is commonly accepted to predispose an individual to cancer or to cause cancer, and there are no clinically used screening tests. Therefore, the current in vitro and epidemiological data appear to support another long held notion that carcinogenesis is multifactorial and suggest that haplotypes, most likely in combination with environmental exposures, will have better predictive power. It appears likely that we may be discussing a "chemoprevention haplotype" with our patients to develop a tailored cancer prevention plan.

3.2. American Society of Clinical Oncology (ASCO) Guidelines (34)

The American Society of Clinical Oncology's Policy Statement for Genetic Testing of Cancer Susceptibility was approved on March 2003 and is available on-line at www.asco.org. It is a policy written for genetic testing related to cancer predisposition, rather than pharmacogenetics. However, because this policy contains important information for DNA testing that can be easily applied to pharmacogenetics and because in the field of oncology today's disease-causing genes are tomorrow's targets, the guidelines are briefly reviewed. See Table 3.

3.2.1. CRITERIA FOR A GENETIC TEST

First, ASCO recommends that genetic testing be performed only when the following criteria are met:

1. Individual has personal family history suggestive of a genetic cancer susceptibility condition.
2. The test can be adequately interpreted.
3. The results will affect the management of the patient or his or her family.

While a strong family history may not be as important to pharmacogenetic testing, criteria 2 and 3 can be easily extrapolated and criterion 1 may be changed to individuals expected to receive the drug in question.

4. PHARMACOGENETICS AND CANCER

4.1. Genotypes that Predict Toxicity

4.1.1. THIOPURINE METHYLTRANSFERASE

TPMT deficiency is inherited as an autosomal recessive trait, with 89–94% of Caucasians having high activity, 6–11% with intermediate activity and 0.3% with very low or

Table 3
Clinically Important Polymorphism in Predicting Toxicity in Cancer Patients

Gene	Variant	Phenotype	Drug	Clinical use
TPMT	*2, *3A, *3C	Increased toxicity	6-MP, pediatric ALL	Routine screening. Homozygous variants receive empiric dose reduction of 90%.
DPD	*2A	Increased toxicity	5-FU	Not clinically useful, low sensitivity
UGT1A1	*28	Increased toxicity	Irinotecan	Under investigation
MTHFR	C677T	Severe myelosuppression	CMF[a] regimen	Under investigation

[a] Cyclophosphamide, methotrexate, and 5-FU.

no activity. This deficiency is largely explained by three polymorphisms in the *TPMT* gene (*2, *3A, *3C) which also have a profound influence on 6-MP tolerance and dose intensity in children with ALL. While these polymorphisms are rare, they are certainly important, with cases reports of toxic deaths attributed to 6-MP dating back several decades *(36,37)*. In a recent clinical trial, children who were homozygous for one of the alleles required 6-MP dose reductions of 91%, while heterozygotes require a dose reduction of approx 50%. Children with dose reductions had equivalent overall survival when compared with children receiving full dose of 6-MP, suggesting that TPMT polymorphisms are important for drug metabolism and toxicity, but play no role in the pathogenesis of ALL *(38)*.

TPMT screening is recommended for children starting therapy with 6-MP with empiric dose reductions for those with genotypes associated with a deficiency. See Table 3.

4.1.2. DIHYDROPYRIMIDINE DEHYDROGENASE (DPD)

DPD is the first and rate-limiting enzyme in the three-step catabolic pathway for the endogenous pyrimidine bases uracil and thymine and is the enzyme primarily responsible for converting 5-fluorouracil (5-FU) to its inactive form, DHFU. DPD is widely expressed in both normal and tumor tissue, including the liver, gastrointestinal mucosa, and peripheral blood mononuclear cells *(39,40)*.

Familial DPD deficiency is an inborn error of metabolism inherited in an autosomal recessive manner with widely variable penetrance. Affected children present with a variety of neurological syndromes. DPD deficiency is reported in approx 3–5% of Caucasians and results from one of more than 20 reported polymorphisms in the *DPD* gene, although the *2A appears to be one of the most significant *(41,42)*. Diasio et al., *(43)* have documented more than 350 cases of DPD deficiency in patients receiving 5-FU and seven toxic deaths. However, other investigators have shown that only 33–66% of individuals with severe myelotoxicity related to 5-FU administration actually have a known polymorphism, underscoring the complexity of this phenotype *(44)*. Therefore, routine clinical screening for DPD is not currently recommended.

4.1.3. UDP-GLUCURONOSYLTRANSFERASE (UGT)

Irinotecan's active metabolite, SN-38, is glucuronidated by the 1A1 isoform of UGT. The *28 variant is best studied and occurs in 3–10% of the population. Several groups have shown both prospectively and retrospectively that the *28 variant is a risk factor for both severe neutropenia and diarrhea in patients receiving irinotecan, most likely due to a decreased capacity to glucuronidate SN-38, associated with a longer $t_{1/2}$ and area under the concentration–time curve (AUC) of the active component SN-38 *(45,46)*. However, like DPD, not all individuals with severe toxicity have the genotype, indicating that other factors in addition to this genotype are important in determining irinotecan toxicity. Ongoing clinical trials are investigating many aspects of irinotecan disposition, including, mdr, mrp, and carboxyesterases *(45)*. Currently, routine clinical assessment of UGT polymorphisms is not recommended.

4.1.4. METHYLENETETRAHYDROFOLATE REDUCTASE (MHFR)

A common polymorphism, occurring as a homozygous variant in up to 10% of Caucasians, occurs as a C677T in the *MHFR* gene. The normal function of *MHFR* is to regulate the intracellular folate pool used in DNA and protein synthesis. Individuals homozygous for the *MHFR* gene have only 35% of normal enzyme capacity and accumulate 5,10-methylenetetrahydrofolate (CH_2THF) in purine and pyrimidine synthesis *(47)*.

Severe toxicity, primarily myelosuppression, was reported in breast cancer patients with this polymorphism receiving cyclophosphamide, methotrexate, and 5-FU (CMF). The authors suggest that an excess of CH_2THF increases the ability of 5-FU to inhibit thymidylate synthetase (TS) and therefore increased myelosuppression. The relationship between this polymorphism and TS appears convincing, as a recent Phase 1 trial with the TS inhibitor raletrexid, reported that individuals with the polymorphism had no toxicities associated with raletrexid *(47)*. Although interesting, *MHFR* polymorphisms are not ready for routine clinical use.

4.2. Genotypes that Predict Efficacy

4.2.1. THYMIDYLATE SYNTHETASE

TS is the intracellular target of 5-FU and several studies have demonstrated that TS induction is associated with resistance to 5-FU and that decreases in tumor TS is associated with improved sensitivity to 5-FU *(48)*. The endogenous level of *TS* expression is controlled by polymorphic variation in the enhancer region of the TS gene. The variants contain two, three, four, and nine copies of 28-basepair tandem repeated sequences (*TSER*2*, *TSER*3*, *TSER*4*, *TSER*9*). When compared to the *TSER*2* allele, in vitro assays demonstrate that *TS* expression of the *TSER*3* is 2.6 times that of the *TSER*2* allele. Marsh and colleagues *(49)* analyzed genomic DNA from patients with colon cancer and found that 29% of patients were homozygous for *TSER*3*, 16% were homozygous for *TSER*2*, and 55% were heterozygous. In 24 patients who received 5-FU, 40% of responders were homozygous for the *TSER*2*, compared to 20% of nonresponders, and those with the *TSER*2* polymorphism had an improvement in median survival of 16 mo when compared to the *TSER*3* groups, with a 12-mo survival. See Table 4.

4.2.2. CYTOCHROME P450 2D6

While 5-hydroxytryptamine$_3$ (5-HT$_3$) receptor antagonists represent a major advance in the treatment of chemotherapy-induced nausea and vomiting, there is still a substantial minority of individuals who do not respond to antiemetic therapy, up to 30%. A number of reasons for poor response to antiemetics have been identified, including female sex, young age, and no prior history of alcohol consumption. Kaiser and colleagues *(50)* recently reported that variations in CYP2D6 metabolism may be responsible for some anitemetic nonresponders receiving the CYP2D6 substrates tropisetron and ondansetron.

Table 4
Clinically Important Pharmacogenetics in Predicting Efficacy in Cancer Patients

Gene	Variant	Phenotype	Drug	Clinical use
TS	*2, *3 tandem repeat	*3 with increased expression, *2 with improved survival	5-FU	Under investigation
2D6	UM, EM, PM	UM with increased emesis, PM with no emesis	Ondansetron Tropisetron	Under investigation
2D6	UM, EM, PM	Nonresponder	Codeine	Under investigation
TI	Induction	Improved response	Irinotecan	Under investigation

Of the 270 patients evaluated, 7.8% were categorized as poor metabolizers, 32.6% had one active allele, 58.1% had two active alleles and were extensive metabolizers, and 1.5% were ultraextensive metabolizers. Individuals who were ultraextensive metabolizers experienced significantly more episodes of vomiting and those who were poor metabolizers had no episodes of vomiting. These results suggest that the ultraextensive metabolizers may require other approaches to emesis control or higher doses of ondansetron and tropisetron. However, before these results may be applied routinely, further studies should evaluate them prospectively.

In addition to 5-HT receptor antagonists, the CYP2d6 polymorphism is important in activation of the prodrug codeine to its active form, morphine. Individuals with a poor metabolizer genotype (PM), up to 6–10% of Caucasian populations, have been identified as nonresponders to codeine (51,52).

4.2.3. Topoisomerase I (TI)

Numerous in vitro evaluations suggest that increased TI predicts a better response to irinotecan and that mitomycin-c (MMC) can induce TI expression. A recent Phase I trial (53) tested the hypothesis that MMC could induce TI in vivo and that TI induction would predict response to therapy. Forty subjects were enrolled in this Phase 1, where MMC was given as a 6 mg/m^2 dose on the day prior to irinotecan with escalating doses every 21 d. The maximum tolerated dose (MTD) of irinotecan was 125 mg/m^2 and responders had an eight times higher induction in *TI* gene expression in peripheral blood lymphocytes when compared to nonresponders.

This regimen is currently under evaluation in a Phase II trials for breast and esophageal cancer.

5. PHARMACOGENETIC COUNSELING IN CLINICAL PRACTICE

The discipline of genetic counseling has arisen from an arena of medicine where a genetic test could diagnose disease (often in a fetus) but there was no accepted medical management. The options to the parent were to continue or to terminate the pregnancy. In a situation such as this, in which there is no medically correct answer, it is primarily an individual choice of the patient. Therefore one of the hallmarks of genetic counseling was that it was nondirective. The genetic counselor provides information about the genetic risk and explains the available options, but does not recommend the one "right" action. The goal of genetic counseling in this instance is to provide the information necessary to individuals to allow them to select a course of action consistent with their own personal beliefs and preferences (54).

In the era of pharmacogenomics, genetic testing for disease predispostion, diagnosis of cancer, and drug response have arisen. In these cases there is almost always a medically "correct" answer. In fact, genetic testing in these circumstances may be viewed as nothing more than a basic laboratory test, where the information is used to direct or target a therapy (55–57). This realization has prompted Burke and colleagues (58)to propose a categorization scheme of genetic tests based on their ethical, legal, and social implications.

The first question that should be answered with regard to a genetic test is: Is there effective, acceptable treatment available? If this is the case, then the test will improve health and should be recommended to patients. Examples of this include newborn screenings for inborn errors of metabolism, in which identification and dietary therapy prevent mental retardation; the MEN2, hereditary thyroid cancers, and other genetic tests, in which identification and surgery prevent a fatal cancer and TMPT deficiency, in which screening and dose adjustment will prevent extreme toxicity. On the other hand, where there is no acceptable medical management but the information may help in reproductive or other planning the focus should be on providing the information and focusing on the individual's personal choice. Examples of this include Huntington's disease (HD), a neurological disorder with 100% penetrance that does not develop until the mid-50s and prenatal testing, where the only option is pregnancy termination.

The second consideration is the clinical validity of the test. In a test that is highly clinically valid, the mutation or polymorphism has high penetrance and its presence routinely predicts high risk of disease. Both MEN2 and HD testing have high clinical validity, although they differ in availability of treatment.

What of the situation in which the test is not a good predictor of risk, in the case of low or uncertain penetrance? One example of this is DPD deficiency, in which at least one half of subjects with unusual toxicity do not have the DPD variant. If an individual is tested for DPD and found to be deficient, there are no data available to guide us in an appropriate dose reduction. Alternatively, if he or she tests negative, he or she still has an approximately 50% likelihood of unusual toxicity.

5.1. Who is Tested?

There are several methods for categorizing candidates for genetic testing; however, because children represent a special situation, we shall consider them first. With regard to children and their protection, the Institute of Medicine (IOM) (59) has made firm recommendations as to the appropriate use of genetic testing:

1. Newborn screening should not be mandatory without evidence of its necessity for detection and effective treatment of specific disorders.
2. Children should only be tested for disorders for which a curative or preventive treatment exists and is needed.

Therefore, it appears that it is universally agreed that genetic testing for TPMT deficiency in children who will receive 6-MP is an appropriate preventive strategy to avoid excessive toxicity, while incorporating this into the newborn screenings is unnecessary.

With regard to adults, the ASCO (34) recommendations should be followed, namely, that the patient should have a high risk of cancer before being tested for a cancer predisposition gene or about to receive a drug with a given metabolic profile for a pharmacogenetic test, the test should be adequately interpreted; and the results will influence the medical management of the patient.

5.2. Nature of the Test and Testing Conditions

An important consideration in selecting a genetic test is the nature of the test itself. The parameters of the test, including the sensitivity, specificity, false-positive and false-negative rates should be understood prior to ordering the test, as this information is essential in communicating the meaning of test results to the patient.

The laboratory itself must be able to provide accurate, state-of-the-art genetic predisposition testing to at-risk families. In addition to basic Clinical Laboratory Improvement Act (CLIA) requirements, available measures of laboratory competence include successful participation in inspection and survey programs, appropriate state licensing, and credentialing of laboratory directors and staff by the American Board of Medical Genetics (ABMG) *(60)*.

5.3. Mode of Inheritance

Cancer may be caused by both germline and somatic mutations. The difference, in particular the risk that it poses for progeny generations, must be clearly communicated to patients *(34)*.

5.4. Benefits

The primary benefits of genetic and pharmacogenetic testing are to diagnose disease earlier, where specific interventions can be employed, as in the case of *BRCA1* testing; to prevent toxicity, as in the case of TPMT; or to select the therapy most likely to benefit the patient, as in the case of TI induction. In all cases the benefits of testing should clearly outweigh the risks prior to initiating testing *(34,59)*.

5.5. Risks

The physical risks of genetic testing are really quite minor, and are the risks associated with phlebotomy, including bruising, bleeding, and infection. However, the psychological and social risks may in actuality be quite severe. A number of studies suggest genetic test results may increase anxiety, and may actually increase high-risk behaviors in a subset of individuals. However, a recent meta-analysis of women counseled for *BRCA1*, showed a decline in anxiety *(61)*.

Results of genetic testing may lead to discrimination by insurance companies and in the workplace. Another concern is that because DNA may be stored for an extended period of time, it may be used in the future for other purposes. There is currently no federal legislation regulating genetic tests; most states have enacted some form of legislation, although this is highly variable among different states. For the most recent information on health care legislation visit the Human Genome website at http://www.ornl.gov/hgmis/elsi/legislat.html#II.

5.6. Informed Consent (34)

All patients undergoing genetic testing should provide informed consent, both within a clinical trial and if the test is used to direct routine clinical management. The basic elements of informed consent include information about the specific test, implications of a positive and a negative test, the possibility that the test may not be informative, options for risk estimation without genetic testing, risk of passing the mutation to children, technical accuracy of the test, fees involved, risk of psychological distress, risk of employer or insurance discrimination, confidentiality, and options for surveillance after testing.

5.7. Ownership and Inheritability

As genetic testing offers unique opportunities, it also offers unique challenges. Because genetic information is inherited according to specific rules, if you know the genetic history of one family member it is often a simple matter to surmise accurately genetic information of other family members. For example, a 56-yr-old Ashkenazi Jewish woman with breast cancer who has four unmarried daughters is secretly tested for *BRCA1*. She tests positive but does not want to disclose the results to her children. She also does not tell them she has breast cancer because she thinks this will hurt their chances for marriage. Thinking about the genetics of *BRCA1*, inherited in an autosomal dominant manner, and with a penetrance of approx 50%, we can easily surmise that statistically, two daughters will have the genotype, one will have the phenotype, and two will unaffected. So who owns the genetic information? We can look to an IOM recommendation *(59)* that states:

> *Confidentiality may be breached in disclosure to relatives only when attempts to elicit voluntary disclosure fail and there is high probability of irreversible or fatal harm to the relative without disclosure* (59).

In this case there is a good probability that at least one daughter's health may be improved by the knowledge of her mother's *BRCA1* status.

Consider the same family. You contact all four daughters, and they all decide on testing When the results come back, two have the genotype and two are unaffected. One week later you receive a phone call from the fiancé of one of the tested daughters. He wants to know the results of the test before going through with the wedding. Again we can consult the IOM report for guidance.

> *Genetic information about a patient's carrier status should not be revealed to the patient's spouse without the patient's permission* (59).

In this case it would be inappropriate to reveal your patient's genetic information to her fiancé. It will not change anyone's medical management and should be considered the confidential information of that patient.

6. CONCLUSION

Genetic testing in cancer is important for screening for disease susceptibility, diagnosing disease, and for selecting and adjusting therapy. Although there are still relatively few examples of clinically routine genetic tests, the number of available tests is likely to rise dramatically in the ensuing years. As new genetic tests are introduced health care professionals must carefully evaluate them for their clinical utility and work with patients to manage their health care appropriately.

REFERENCES

1. Khabele D, Runowicz CD. Genetic counseling, testing, and screening for breast and ovarian cancer: practical and social considerations. Curr Women Health Rep 2002; 2:163–169.

2. Loud JT, Peters JA, Fraser M, Jenkins J. Applications of advances in molecular biology and genomics to clinical cancer care. Cancer Nurs 2002; 25:110–122.
3. Jenkins J, Blitzer M, Boehm K, et al., the Core Competency Working Group of the National Coalition for Health Professional Education in Genetics. Recommendations of core competencies in genetics essential for all health professionals. Genetics in Medicine, 2001; 3:155–158.
4. Burke W, Emery J. Genetics education for primary-care providers. Nat Rev Genet 2002; 3:561–566.
5. International Human Genome Sequencing Consortium. Initial sequencing and analysis of the human genome. Nature 2001; 409:860–921.
6. Lazzeroni LC, Karlovich CA. Genotype to phenotype: associations, errors and complexity. Trends Genet 2002; 18:283–284.
7. Ardlie KG, Kruglyak L, Seielstad M. Patterns of linkage disequilibrium in the human genome. Nat Rev Genet 2002; 3:299–309.
8. Gabriel SB, Schaffner SF, Nguyen H, et al. The structure of haplotype blocks in the human genome. Science 2002; 296:2225–2229.
9. Stoneking M. From the Evolutionary Past. Nature 2001; 409:821–823.
10. Judson R, Stephens JC, Windemuth A. The predictive power of haplotypes in clinical response. Pharmacogenomics 2000; 1:15–26.
11. Rowley JD. The critical role of chromosome translocations in human leukemias. Annu Rev Genet 1998; 32:495–519.
12. Gao J, Erickson P, Gardiner K, et al. Isolation of a yeast artificial chromosome spanning the 8;21 translocation breakpoint, t(8;21) (q22;q22.3), in acute myelogenous leukemia. Proc Natl Acad Sci USA 1991; 88:4882–4886.
13. Pandolfi PP. In vivo analysis of the molecular genetics of acute promyelocytic leukemia. Oncogene 2001; 20:5726–5623.
14. Kozubek S, Lukasova E, Mareckova A, et al. The topological organization of chromosomes 9 and 22 in cell nuclei has a determinative role in the induction of t(9,22) translocations and in the pathogenesis of t(9,22) leukemias. Chromosoma 1999; 108:426–435.
15. Rowley JD. Mapping of human chromosomal regions related to neoplasia: evidence from chromosomes 1 and 17. Proc Natl Acad Sci USA 1977; 74:5729–5733.
16 Sawyers CL. Rational therapeutic intervention in cancer: kinases as drug targets. Curr Opin Genet Dev 2002; 12:111–115.
17. Pearson P, Van der Luijt RB. The genetic analysis of cancer. J Intern Med 1998; 243:413–417.
18. Taylor JG, Choi EH, Foster CB, Chanock SJ. Using genetic variation to study human disease. Trends Mol Med 2001; 7:507–512.
19. Weinstein IB. Cancer. Addiction to oncogenes—the Achilles heal of cancer. Science 2002; 297:63–64.
20. Ingelman-Sundberg M, Oscarson M, Daly AK, Garte S, Nebert DW. Human cytochrome P-450 (CYP) genes: a web page for the nomenclature of alleles. Cancer Epidemiol Biomark Prev 2001; 10: 1307–1308.
21. Garte S, Gaspari L, Alexandrie AK, et al. Metabolic gene polymorphism frequencies in control populations. Cancer Epidemiol Biomark Prev2001; 10:1239–1248.
22. Bartsch H, Nair Y, Rsich A, et al. Genetic polymorphism of CYP genes, alone or in combination, as a risk modifier of tobacco-related cancers. Cancer Epidemiol Biomark Prev 2000; 9:3–28.
23. Guengerich FP, Shimada T. Activation of procarcinogens by human cytochrome P450 enzymes. Mutat Res 1998; 400:201–213.
24. Neber DW, Roe AL. Ethnic and genetic differences in metabolism genes and risk of toxicity and cancer. Sci Total Environ 2001; 274:93–102.
25. Vainio, H. Metabolic cytochrome P450 genotypes and assessment of individual susceptibility to lung cancer. Pharmacogenetics 1992; 2:259–263.
26. Sugimura H, Wakai K, Genka K, et al. Association of Ile462Val (exon 7) polymorphism of cytochrome P450 IA1 with lung cancer in the Asian population: further evidence from a case-control study in Okinawa. Cancer Epidemiol Biomark Prev 1998; 7:413–417.
27. Kiyohara C, Nakanishi Y, Inutsuka A, et al. The relationship between CYP1A1 aryl hydrocarbon hydroxylase activity and lung cancer in a Japanese population. Pharmacogenetics 1998; 8:315–323.
28. Nakachi K, Imai K, Hayashi S, Kawajiri K. Polymorphisms of the CYP1A1 and glutathione S-transferase genes associated with susceptibility to lung cancer in relation to cigarette dose in a Japanese population. Cancer Res 1993 53:2994–2999.

29. Persson I, Johansson I, Lou YC, et al. Genetic polymorphism of xenobiotic metabolizing enzymes among Chinese lung cancer patients. Int J Cancer 1999; 81:325–329.

30. Nebert DW, Roe AL, Vandale SE, Bingham E, Oakley GG. NAD(P)H:quinone oxidoreductase (NQO1) polymorphism, exposure to benzene, and predisposition to disease: a HuGE review. Genet Med 2002; 4:62–70.

31. Rothman N, Smith MT, Hayes RB, et al. Benzene poisoning, a risk factor for hematological malignancy, is associated with the NQO1 609C→T mutation and rapid fractional excretion of chlorzoxazone. Cancer Res 1997; 57:2839–2842.

32. Wiemels JL, Pagnamenta A, Taylor GM, Eden OB, Alexander FE, Greaves MF. A lack of a functional NAD(P)H:quinone oxidoreductase allele is selectively associated with pediatric leukemias that have MLL fusions. United Kingdom Childhood Cancer Study Investigators. Cancer Res 1999; 59:4095–4099.

33. Kolesar JM, Pritchard SC, Kerr KM, Nicolson MC, McLeod HL. Evaluation of *NQO1* gene expression and variant allele in human nsclc tumors and matched normal lung tissue. Int J Oncol 2002; 21: 1119–1124.

34. Anonymous. Statement of the American Society of Clinical Oncology: genetic testing for cancer susceptibility, adopted on February 20, 1996. J Clin Oncol 1996; 14:1730–1736.

35. Scheuer L, Kauff N, Robson M, et al. Outcome of preventive surgery and screening for breast and ovarian cancer in BRCA mutation carriers. J Clin Oncol 2002; 20:1260–1268.

36. McLeod HL, Krynetski EY, Relling MV, Evans WE. Genetic polymorphism of thiopurine methyltransferase and its clinical relevance for childhood acute lymphoblastic leukemia. Leukemia 2000; 14:567–572.

37. Black AJ, McLeod HL, Capell HA, et al. Thiopurine methyltransferase genotype predicts therapy-limiting severe toxicity from azathioprine. Ann Intern Med 1998; 129:716–718.

38. McLeod HL, Coulthard S, Thomas AE, et al. Analysis of thiopurine methyltransferase variant alleles in childhood acute lymphoblastic leukaemia. Br J Haematol 1999; 105:696–700.

39. Collie-Duguid ES, McLeod HL, Cassidy J. Estimation of dihydropyrimidine dehydrogenase activity: does it have a role in cancer therapy? Ann Oncol 2000; 11:255–257.

40. Marsh S, McKay JA, Curran S, Murray GI, Cassidy J, McLeod HL. Primary colorectal tumour is not an accurate predictor of thymidylate synthase in lymph node metastasis. Oncol Rep 2002; 9:231–234.

41. Collie-Duguid ES, Johnston SJ, Powrie RH, et al. Cloning and initial characterization of the human DPYD gene promoter. Biochem Biophys Res Commun 2000; 271:28–35.

42. McLeod HL, Collie-Duguid ES, Vreken P, et al. Nomenclature for human DPYD alleles. Pharmacogenetics 1998; 8:455–459.

43. Lu Z, Zhang R, Diasio RB. Dihydropyrimidine dehydrogenase activity in human peripheral blood mononuclear cells and liver: population characteristics, newly identified deficient patients, and clinical implication in 5-.uorouracil chemotherapy. Cancer Res 1993; 53:5433–5438.

44. Collie-Duguid ES, Etienne MC, Milano G, McLeod HL. Known variant DPYD alleles do not explain DPD deficiency in cancer patients. Pharmacogenetics 2000; 10:217–223.

45. Innocenti F, Ratain MJ. Update on pharmacogenetics in cancer chemotherapy. Eur J Cancer 2002; 38: 639–644.

46. Iyer L, Hall D, Das S, et al. Phenotype-genotype correlation of in vitro SN-38 (active metabolite of irinotecan) and bilirubin glucuronidation in human liver tissue with UGT1A1 promoter polymorphism. Clin Pharmacol Ther 1999; 65:576–582.

47. Schwahn B, Rozen R. Polymorphisms in the methylenetetrahydrofolate reductase gene: clinical consequences. Am J PharmacoGen 2001; 1:189–201.

48. Wang W. Marsh S. Cassidy J. McLeod HL. Pharmacogenomic dissection of resistance to thymidylate synthase inhibitors. Cancer Research 2001; 61(14):5505–5510.

49. Marsh S, McKay JA, Cassidy J, McLeod HL. Polymorphism in the thymidylate synthase promoter enhancer region in colorectal cancer. Int J Oncol 2001; 19:383–386.

50. Kaiser R, Sezer C, Papies A, et al. Patient tailored anti-emetic treatment with 5-hydroxytryptamine type 3 receptor antagonists according to cytochrome p450 genotypes. J Clin Oncol 2002; 20:2805–2811.

51. Chen ZR, Somogi AA, Bochner F. Polymorphic *O*-demethylation of codeine. Lancet 1988; 2:914–915.

52. Yue QY, Svensson JO, Alm C, et al. Codeine *O*-demethylation co-segregates wih polymorphic debrisoquin hydroxylation. Br J Clin Pharmacol 1989; 28:639–645.

53. Villalona-Calero MA, Kolesar JM. Mitomycin as a modulator of irinotecan anticancer activity. Oncology (Huntingt) 2002: 16(8 Suppl 7):21–25.

54. Biesecker BB. Goals of genetic counseling. Clin Genet 2001; 60:323–330.
55. Hemminki K. Genetic epidemiology—science and ethics on familial cancers. Acta Oncol 2001; 40: 439–444.
56. Niendorf KB, Shannon KM. The role of genetic testing and effect on patient care. Arch Dermatol 2001; 137:1515–1519.
57. Patenaude AF, Guttmacher AE, Collins FS. Genetic testing and psychology. New roles, new responsibilities. Am Psychol 2002; 57:271–282.
58. Burke W, Pinsky LE, Press NA. Categorizing genetic tests to identify their ethical, legal, and social implications. Am J Medical Genet 2001; 106:233–240.
61. Institute of Medicine (IOM). Advances in Understanding Genetic Changes in Cancer: Impact on Diagnosis and Treatment Decisions in the 1990s. Division of Health Sciences Policy, Institute of Medicine, Washington, DC: National Academy Press, 1992.
60. American College of Medical Genetics. Standards and Guidelines: Clinical Laboratory Genetics. Bethesda, MD: ACMG, 1993.
61. Meiser B, Halliday JL. What is the impact of genetic counselling in women at increased risk of developing hereditary breast cancer? A meta-analytic review. Soc Sci Med 2002; 54:1463–1470.

Index

About the Editors

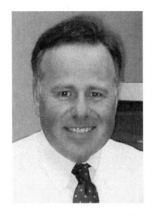

Dr. William Douglas Figg received his BS in Pharmacy from Samford University and his doctoral degree from Auburn University. He completed his internship at the University of Alabama at Birmingham and his fellowship in Drug Development at the University of North Carolina, Chapel Hill. He also received an MBA degree from a combined program at Columbia University and the London Business School. Dr. Figg joined the National Cancer Institute in 1992. The following year he became head of the Molecular Pharmacology Section and the Clinical Pharmacology Research Core. Since then his research has focused on using pharmacological principles to optimize the treatment of cancer and on identifying genes involved in the development of prostate cancer. Dr. Figg has over 240 peer reviewed publications and has given invited lectures/seminars throughout the world.

Dr. Howard McLeod received his Bachelors of Science in Pharmacy from the University of Washington in Seattle and a PharmD degree from the Philadelphia College of Pharmacy and Science. He completed research fellowship training in cancer pharmacology at St. Jude Children's Research Hospital, Memphis and the University of Glasgow, Scotland, before staying to direct the Clinical Pharmacology program at the Beatson Cancer Centre in Glasgow. He then moved to the University of Aberdeen, Scotland as Senior Lecturer in Medicine and Director of Laboratory Research for the Oncology Unit and returned to the USA in July, 2000, as an Associate Professor of Medicine at Washington University. Dr McLeod 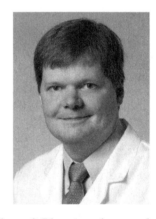 also holds appointments in the Departments of Molecular Biology & Pharmacology and Genetics at Washington University and is Director of the Siteman Cancer Center Pharmacology Core. Dr. McLeod is also the Principal Investigator for the CREATE Pharmacogenetics Research Network, a member of the NIH funded Pharmacogenetics Research Network. Dr. McLeod has published over 150 peer reviewed papers on pharmacogenomics, applied therapeutics, or clinical pharmacology and continues to work to integrate genetics principles into clinical practice to advance individualized medicine.